Normal Temperatures in Children

Age	Temperature °F	°C
3 months	99.4	37.5
6 months	99.5	37.5
1 year	99.7	37.7
3 years	99.0	37.2
5 years	98.6	37.0
7 years	98.3	36.8
9 years	98.1	36.7
11 years	98.0	36.7
13 years	97.8	36.6

Modified from Lowrey GH: *Growth and development of children*, ed 8, St Louis, 1986, Mosby.

Centigrade to Fahrenheit Temperature Conversions

°C	°F	°C	°F	°C	°F
35.0	**95.0**	**37.0**	**98.6**	**39.0**	**102.2**
35.2	95.4	37.2	99.0	39.2	102.6
35.4	95.7	37.4	99.3	39.4	102.9
35.6	96.1	37.6	99.7	39.6	103.3
35.8	96.4	37.8	100.0	39.8	103.6
36.0	**96.8**	**38.0**	**100.4**	**40.0**	**104.0**
36.2	97.2	38.2	100.8	40.2	104.4
36.4	97.5	38.4	101.1	40.4	104.7
36.6	97.9	38.6	101.5	40.6	105.1
36.8	98.2	38.8	101.8	40.8	105.4
				41.0	**105.8**

CONVERSION FORMULAS:
$$°F = (°C \times \tfrac{9}{5}) + 32 \text{ or } (°C \times 1.8) + 32$$
$$°C = (°F - 32) \times \tfrac{5}{9} \text{ or } (°F - 32) \times 0.55$$

D0763354

Normal Blood Pressure Readings for Children

GIRLS

Systolic Blood Pressure Percentile						Diastolic Blood Pressure* Percentile					
Age	5th	10th	50th	90th	95th	Age	5th	10th	50th	90th	95th
1 day	46	50	65	80	84	1 day	38	42	55	68	72
3 days	53	57	72	86	90	3 days	38	42	55	68	71
7 days	60	64	78	93	97	7 days	38	41	54	67	71
1 mo	65	69	84	98	102	1 mo	35	39	52	65	69
2 mo	68	72	87	101	106	2 mo	34	38	51	64	68
3 mo	70	74	89	104	108	3 mo	35	38	51	64	68
4 mo	71	75	90	105	109	4 mo	35	39	52	65	68
5 mo	72	76	91	106	110	5 mo	36	39	52	65	69
6 mo	72	76	91	106	110	6 mo	36	40	53	66	69
7 mo	72	76	91	106	110	7 mo	36	40	53	66	70
8 mo	72	76	91	106	110	8 mo	37	40	53	66	70
9 mo	72	76	91	106	110	9 mo	37	41	54	67	70
10 mo	72	76	91	106	110	10 mo	37	41	54	67	71
11 mo	72	76	91	105	110	11 mo	38	41	54	67	71
1 yr	72	76	91	105	110	1 yr	38	41	54	67	71
2 yr	71	76	90	105	109	2 yr	40	43	56	69	73
3 yr	72	76	91	106	110	3 yr	40	43	56	69	73
4 yr	73	78	92	107	111	4 yr	40	43	56	69	73
5 yr	75	79	94	109	113	5 yr	40	43	56	69	73
6 yr	77	81	96	111	115	6 yr	40	44	57	70	74
7 yr	78	83	97	112	116	7 yr	41	45	58	71	75
8 yr	80	84	99	114	118	8 yr	43	46	59	72	76
9 yr	81	86	100	115	119	9 yr	44	48	61	74	77
10 yr	83	87	102	117	121	10 yr	46	49	62	75	79
11 yr	86	90	105	119	123	11 yr	47	51	64	77	81
12 yr	88	92	107	122	126	12 yr	49	53	66	78	82
13 yr	90	94	109	124	128	13 yr	46	50	64	78	82
14 yr	92	96	110	125	129	14 yr	49	53	67	81	85
15 yr	93	97	111	126	130	15 yr	49	53	67	82	86
16 yr	93	97	112	127	131	16 yr	49	53	67	81	85
17 yr	93	98	112	127	131	17 yr	48	52	66	80	84
18 yr	94	98	112	127	131	18 yr	48	52	66	80	84

*K4 was used for ages less than 13; K5 was used for ages 13 and over.

Wong and Whaley's
Clinical Manual of
Pediatric Nursing

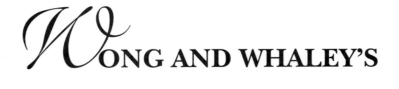

WONG AND WHALEY'S
Clinical Manual of
Pediatric Nursing

Donna L. Wong, PhD, RN, PNP, CPN, FAAN

Adjunct Associate Professor
University of Oklahoma College of Medicine—Tulsa;
Adjunct Professor
University of Oklahoma College of Nursing;
Adjunct Professor/Consultant
Oral Roberts University
Anna Vaughn School of Nursing
Tulsa, Oklahoma;
Consultant
Children's Hospital at Saint Francis
Tulsa, Oklahoma;
Texas Children's Hospital
Houston, Texas

Caryn Stoermer Hess, RN, MS

Nursing Consultant
Englewood, Colorado

With Community and Home Care Instructions *by*
Christina Algiere Kasprisin, RN, MS

Lecturer
University of Vermont College of Nursing
Burlington, Vermont

FIFTH EDITION

with 280 illustrations

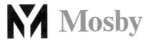 Mosby

St. Louis Baltimore Boston Carlsbad Chicago Minneapolis New York Philadelphia Portland
London Milan Sydney Tokyo Toronto

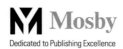
Dedicated to Publishing Excellence

Editor-in-Chief: Sally Schrefer
Senior Developmental Editor: Michele D. Hayden
Project Manager: Deborah L. Vogel
Production Editor: Ed Alderman
Designer: Bill Drone

Mosby, Inc.
A Harcourt Health Sciences Company
11830 Westline Industrial Drive
St. Louis, Missouri 63146

Printed in the United States of America

Library of Congress Cataloging-in-Publication Data

Wong, Donna L., 1948-
    Wong and Whaley's clinical manual of pediatric nursing / Donna L. Wong, Caryn
Stoermer Hess. — 5th ed.
        p.   cm.
    Includes bibliographical references and index.
    ISBN 0-323-00979-4 (alk. paper)
    1. Pediatric nursing—Handbooks, manuals, etc.   I. Title: Clinical manual of pediatric
nursing.   II. Hess, Caryn Stoermer.   III. Title.
    [DNLM: 1. Pediatric Nursing.   WY 159 W872sa 1999]
RJ245.W633   1999
610.73′62—dc21
                                                                                99-048128

99   00   01   02   03   GW/KPT   9   8   7   6   5   4   3   2   1

Reviewers/Consultants

Chantelle Bennett, BS, CCLS, CTRS
Certified Child Life Specialist
Florida Children's Hospital
Orlando, Florida

Lauren D. Blough, RN, BS, CRNI
IV Therapy Clinical Specialist/Educator
Florida Children's Hospital
Orlando, Florida

Joan Marie Carpenter, RN, MSN
Maternal-Child/Pediatric Nursing Instructor
Kauai Community College
Kauai, Hawaii

Terry Compton, RN, MS, CDE
Diabetes Nurse Coordinator
Children's Hospital
New Orleans, Louisiana

Linda S. Goodwin, RN, BSN
Saint Francis Hospital Home Care
Tulsa, Oklahoma

Mikel Gray, PhD, CUNP, CCCN, FAAN
Nurse Practitioner;
Associate Professor
Department of Urology and
School of Nursing
University of Virginia
Charlottesville, Virginia

Mary Fran Hazinski, RN, MSN, FAAN
Clinical Specialist, Division of Trauma
Departments of Surgery and Pediatrics
Vanderbilt Children's Hospital and
Vanderbilt University Medical Center
Nashville, Tennessee

Marilyn Hockenberry-Eaton, RN, CS, PhD, PNP, FAAN
Associate Professor
Department of Pediatrics
Baylor College of Medicine;
Director of Nurse Practitioners
Texas Children's Hospital
Houston, Texas

Barbara Larson, RN, MEd
Director of Education
CM Health Care Resources, Inc.
Northbrook, Illinois

Judith Ann McDonald, RN, MSN, MA
Nursing Instructor
South Suburban College
South Holland, Illinois

Chris Pasero, RN, MS
Pain Management Educator and Consultant
Rocklin, California

Denise Pflaumer, BS, CCLS
Certified Child Life Specialist
Florida Children's Hospital
Orlando, Florida

Ivy Razmus, RN, MSN
Clinical Manager
Pediatric Intensive Care Unit
Children's Hospital at Saint Francis
Tulsa, Oklahoma

Michelle Reeves, RN, MN
Endocrinology Nurse Coordinator
Children's Hospital
New Orleans, Louisiana

Judith G. Sheese, PhD
Director
Automotive Safety for Children Program
Indiana University Medical Center
Indianapolis, Indiana

Judith L. Talty, BA
Associate Program Director
Automotive Safety for Children Program
Indiana University Medical Center
Indianapolis, Indiana

David Wilson, MS, RNC
Clinical Instructor
Oral Roberts University
Anna Vaughn School of Nursing
Tulsa, Oklahoma

Preface

The fifth edition of *Wong and Whaley's Clinical Manual of Pediatric Nursing,* like its previous editions, serves a unique function in the study and practice of pediatric nursing. However, this edition benefits from the conscientious and detailed contribution of its new coauthor, Caryn Stoermer Hess. This manual is a practical guide for nurses and students engaged in the care of children and their families—a compendious collection of clinical information, resources, and data packaged for convenient use and easy access. For the practicing nurse, the book is a ready resource of material that is otherwise available only in a wide array of journal articles, texts, federal publications, professional association recommendations, and brochures. Examples of current "cutting edge" information are recommendations from the American Academy of Pediatrics, Agency for Health Care Policy and Research, American Pain Society, U.S. Department of Agriculture, and Centers for Disease Control and Prevention. For the student, it is an indispensable guide to the care of children and their families.

As an adjunct to clinical practice, the *Manual* assumes the thorough preparation and basic theoretical knowledge only a textbook can provide. Although it is not designed to accompany any particular textbook, it serves as a valuable addition to *Whaley and Wong's Nursing Care of Infants and Children* and *Whaley and Wong's Essentials of Pediatric Nursing.* The *Manual* contains more than twice as many care plans as these texts, and the outlined information and the Community and Home Care Instructions provide easy methods of self-learning for students.

The *Manual* is authoritative and up to date. Its content reflects the latest research and current clinical practice. The nursing care plans include the current NANDA nomenclature. The popular Community and Home Care Instructions reflect advances in technology, such as newer methods of measuring temperature, use of needleless connectors, and application of EMLA cream and Anesthetic Disc. Users will appreciate access to the latest information on immunizations, lead poisoning, the Food Guide Pyramid for Young Children, pain assessment and management, and laboratory values. The latest information on car seat safety design and regulations and cardiopulmonary resuscitation and choking were added by experts in these areas.

A major feature of this edition is increased focus on **community nursing care.** To highlight areas that involve a greater appreciation for broader nursing intervention, boxes called **Community Focus** have been added. Examples of this new addition include information on the early discharge of the newborn; improving immunization rates; reducing blood lead levels; collaboration between school nurses and teachers; animal safety; end-of-life care and use of "terminal sedation;" and fear of opioid addiction.

Another approach to emphasizing the importance of community nursing is the renaming of the Home Care Instructions as **Community and Home Care Instructions.** Many of the instructions can be used outside of the home setting by caregivers and health professionals in schools, daycare centers,

rehabilitation settings, etc. We anticipate that this expanded title will alert readers to a wider application of this useful information.

The *Manual* is designed to ensure that specific information can be located quickly and easily when it is needed. Color tabs printed on the cover facilitate quick access to each of the book's six units, which have black tabs coordinated with those on the cover. In addition to a detailed table of contents in the front of the book, a unit table of contents with page references is included on the front page of each unit. A list of related topics found elsewhere in the book is included in most units. Vital reference data appear inside the front and back covers, where they can be used at a moment's notice.

As in past editions, material designed for families is identified with a logo, which in this edition is a house. Permission is given to photocopy this material and provide it to caregivers to ensure that they have access to accurate, current information; to improve the quality of care; and to facilitate the nurse's teaching responsibilities.

Greater attention is given to *critical thinking* by emphasizing essential nursing observations and interventions in **Practice Alert** boxes. These call the reader's attention to considerations which, if ignored, could lead to a deteriorating or emergency situation. Key assessment data, risk factors, and danger signs are among the kinds of information in this feature. The concept of **atraumatic care**—the provision of therapeutic care in settings, by personnel, and through the use of interventions that eliminate or minimize the psychologic and physical distress experienced by children and their families in the health care system—is incorporated throughout the text and highlighted as boxed material.

Unit 1 focuses on the **assessment of the child and family.** It includes history taking; assessment of present and past physical health; and a summary of developmental achievements, both general and age-specific. New additions to this unit include a revised discussion of site of temperature measurement and vision screening guidelines and referral criteria.

Unit 2 emphasizes **health promotion** in the areas of preventive care, nutrition, immunization, safety and injury prevention, parental guidance, and play. The material on immunization of well children and car seat safety (including new illustrations) is completely revised to reflect current recommendations. A box describing combined vaccines is new. Also, a new section on the Food Guide Pyramid for Young Children has been added. Some of the material on nutrition (including sample menus for specific age groups), injury prevention, and play may be photocopied and given to families. The information on sleep and dental care has been moved to Unit 5 and is now presented as community and home care instructions.

Unit 3 outlines **basic nursing procedures** adapted for the child. This extensive collection of skills and procedures includes preparation for procedures, collecting specimens, administration of medicine, venous access devices, invasive and noninvasive oxygen monitoring, and cardiopulmonary resuscitation. An extensive new section addresses the use of restraints and the atraumatic interventions of "therapeutic hugging." Another procedure new to this edition is bladder catheterization.

Unit 4 is devoted to **health problems,** primarily those requiring hospitalization. More than 80 care plans are included. Each nursing care plan consists of assessment guidelines specific to the condition, relevant nursing diagnoses, patient/family goals, interventions, and expected patient and family outcomes. The nursing diagnoses conform to the nomenclature accepted by the North American Nursing Diagnosis Association (NANDA) and they are prioritized within the care plans.

These nursing care plans can be employed as standards of care for chart auditing and continuous quality improvement, and they can be readily individualized to meet the needs of specific patients and families. The Nursing Care Plan on pain can be used to meet the Joint Commission on Accreditation of Healthcare Agencies' new pain standards.

The health problems were selected to avoid repetition while including a large variety of disorders. Most frequently encountered disorders are included, as well as less common but more complex conditions, such as cystic fibrosis. Cross-references guide the user to generic care plans, such as The Child in Pain, or to commonly used nursing diagnoses, such as Risk for Infection. More Guidelines boxes for the busy practitioner have been added, such as instructions for a metered-dose inhaler (MDI) and peak flow meter and the new NPO guidelines for use before surgery.

Unit 5 consists of a collection of instructions for those who provide care for a child outside the clinical setting. These detailed **Community and Home Care Instructions** are designed to be copied and distributed to the parent or other care provider. The instructions are written in simple and clear language to accommodate users with a low reading level. They can be used for client teaching, for facilitating discharge planning, or for promoting continuity of care in the home or community.

Revisions include the addition of instructions for applying EMLA cream or the Anesthetic Disc, managing sleep problems, providing dental care, and newer methods of measuring temperature. The latest American Heart Association recommendations for performing cardiopulmonary resuscitation on an infant or child and for caring for a choking infant or child are included. All the instructions reflect research-based practice where possible. Where controversy exists or precise research data are lacking, the most convenient and practical suggestions are provided.

Unit 6 includes basic resource information for interpretation of **laboratory data,** including values in International Units. The extensive list of **abbreviations** and **acronyms** used in health care settings has been expanded and updated. A list of **pediatric pain resources** for families and health care professionals has been added.

Although the information in the *Manual* is carefully researched, references are included only when citations are required to appropriately credit the work. The reader is directed to the current editions of *Nursing Care of Infants and Children* and *Essentials of Pediatric Nursing* for additional references and discussion of material, especially for growth and development, interviewing, and health problems.

Every effort has been made to ensure that the information is accurate and up to date at the time of publication. However, as new research and experience broaden our practice, standards of care change accordingly. Therefore, the reader may find some differences in local and regional practices.

A number of people have contributed time and expertise to this edition. We are again grateful to Christina Algiere Kasprisin, RN, MS, for continuing to revise and expand the Community and Home Care Instructions. Numerous reviewers and consultants have provided invaluable expertise for updating the material in this manual. These outstanding experts have helped us achieve our goal of presenting data that are both current and accurate. A very special thanks is due Peggy Cook, librarian at Hillcrest Medical Center, Tulsa, Oklahoma, and Lynne Murtha, our secretary, who are wonderful friends to work with. And finally, we are so fortunate to have an outstanding Mosby team—Sally Schrefer, Shelly Hayden, Deborah Vogel, and Ed Alderman—which makes this book a reality.

As always, we thank our families for their continued love, support, and patience during the preparation of the manuscript. We are deeply indebted to our husbands, Ting and Mike, and to our children, Nina, Steven, Kyle, Brian, and Kimberly, whose presence enriches our lives immeasurably. And we will always appreciate the original writing and revisions of Lucille Whaley for the first three editions.

Donna L. Wong

Caryn Stoermer Hess

Contents

Assessment

Symbol ■ indicates material that may be photocopied and distributed to families.

Related Topics

HEALTH HISTORY

One of the most significant aspects of a health assessment is the health history. To take a thorough history, the nurse must be well versed in communication and interviewing principles. An overview of the process is presented in terms of general guidelines for communication and interviewing, with additional specific guidelines for children. Because of the frequent need for interpreters with non–English-speaking families, guidelines for using interpreters are included.

The history furnishes information about the child's physical health since birth, details the events of the present problem, and includes social and family history facts that are essential for providing comprehensive care. The objective of each assessment area is the identification of nursing diagnoses.

The summary is primarily intended for the recording of data, not the acquisition of information from the informant. There-fore it is not meant to be used as a questionnaire. The right-hand column entitled "Comments" has been added to enhance and detail sections of the history, as well as to emphasize areas of possible intervention. For a more comprehensive discussion of approaches to taking a history, see Chapter 6 in *Whaley and Wong's Nursing Care of Infants and Children* or *Whaley and Wong's Essentials of Pediatric Nursing.**

*Wong DL, Hockenberry-Eaton M, Wilson D, Winkelstein ML, Ahmann E, DiVito-Thomas PA: *Whaley and Wong's Nursing care of infants and children,* ed 6, St Louis, 1999, Mosby; and Wong DL: *Whaley and Wong's Essentials of pediatric nursing,* ed 5, St Louis, 1997, Mosby.

General Guidelines for Communication and Interviewing

Assess ability to speak and understand English.
Conduct the interview in a private, quiet area.
Begin the interview with appropriate introductions.
  Address each person by name.
Clarify the purpose of the interview.
Inform the interviewees of the confidential limits of the interview.
Demonstrate interest in the interview by sitting at eye level and close to interviewees (not across a desk), leaning slightly forward, and speaking in a calm, steady voice.
Begin with general conversation to put the interviewees at ease.
  Use comments such as, "How have things been since we talked last?" or (to the child) "What do you think is going to happen today?" to let the family express the main concern.
Include all parties in the interview.
  Direct age-appropriate questions to children (e.g., "What grade are you in school?" or "What do you like to eat?").
  Be sensitive to instances in which family members, such as adolescents, may wish to be interviewed separately.
  Recognize and respect cultural patterns of communication, e.g., avoiding direct eye contact (American Indian) or nodding for courtesy—not in actual agreement or understanding (many Asian cultures).
  Use open-ended questions or statements that begin with "What," "How," "Tell me about," or "You were saying," and reflect back key words or phrases to encourage discussion.
  Encourage continued discussion with nodding and eye contact, saying "uh-huh," "I see," or "yes."
  Use focused questions (questions that ask for a specific response, e.g., "What did you try next?") and closed questions (questions that ask for a single answer, e.g., "Did you call the doctor?") to direct the focus of the interview.
  Ensure mutual understanding by frequently clarifying and summarizing information.
  Use active listening to attend to the verbal and nonverbal aspects of the communication.
  Verbal cues to important issues include these techniques:
    Frequent reference to a topic
    Repetition of key words
    Special reference to an event or person

Nonverbal cues to important issues include the following:
    Changes in body position (e.g., looking away or leaning forward)
    Changes in pitch, rate, intonation, and volume of speech (e.g., speaking rapidly, frequent pauses, whispering, or shouting)
  Use silence to allow persons to do the following:
    Sort out thoughts and feelings
    Search for responses to questions
    Share feelings expressed by another
  Break silence constructively with statements such as, "Is there anything else you wish to say?", "I see you find it difficult to continue; how may I help?", or "I don't know what this silence means. Perhaps there is something you would like to put into words but find difficult to say."
  Convey empathy by attending to the verbal and nonverbal language of the interviewee and reflecting back the feeling of the communication (e.g., "I can see how upsetting that must have been for you.").
  Provide reassurance to acknowledge concerns and any positive efforts used to deal with problems.
  Avoid blocks to communication:
    Socializing
    Giving unrestricted and sometimes unasked-for advice
    Offering premature or inappropriate reassurance
    Giving overready encouragement
    Defending a situation or opinion
    Using stereotyped comments or cliches
    Limiting expression of emotion by asking directed, close-ended questions
    Interrupting and finishing the person's sentence
    Talking more than the interviewee
    Forming prejudged conclusions
    Deliberately changing the focus
  Watch for signs of information overload:
    Long periods of silence
    Wide eyes and fixed facial expression
    Constant fidgeting or attempting to move away
    Nervous habits (e.g., tapping, playing with hair)
    Sudden disruptions (e.g., asking to go to the bathroom)
    Looking around
    Yawning, eyes drooping
    Frequently looking at a watch or clock
    Attempting to change topic of discussion

Continued

Close the interview with an opportunity for others to bring up overlooked or sensitive concerns with a statement such as, "Have we covered everything?"

Summarize the interview, especially if problems were identified or interventions were planned.

Discuss the need for follow-up and schedule a time.

Express appreciation for each person's participation.

Specific Guidelines for Communicating with Children

Allow children time to feel comfortable.

Avoid sudden or rapid advances, broad smiles, extended eye contact, or other gestures that may be seen as threatening.

Talk to the parent if child is initially shy.

Communicate through transition objects such as dolls, puppets, or stuffed animals before questioning a young child directly.

Give older children the opportunity to talk without the parents present.

Assume a position that is at eye level with the child.

Speak in a quiet, unhurried, and confident voice.

Speak clearly, be specific, use simple words and short sentences.

State directions and suggestions *positively.*

Offer a choice only when one exists.

Be honest with children.

Allow children to express their concerns and fears.

Use a variety of communication techniques.

Creative Communication Techniques with Children

VERBAL TECHNIQUES

"I" Messages

Relate a feeling about a behavior in terms of "I."

Describe effect behavior had on the person.

Avoid use of "you."

"You" messages are judgmental and provoke defensiveness.

Example: "You" message—"You are being very uncooperative about doing your treatments."

Example: "I" message—"I am concerned about how the treatments are going because I want to see you get better."

Third-Person Technique

Involves expressing a feeling in terms of a third person ("he," "she," "they").

Is less threatening than directly asking children how they feel because it gives them an opportunity to agree or disagree without being defensive.

Example: "Sometimes when a person is sick a lot, he feels angry and sad because he cannot do what others can." Either wait silently for a response or encourage a reply with a statement such as "Did you ever feel that way?"

Approach allows children three choices: (1) to agree and, hopefully, express how they feel; (2) to disagree; or (3) to remain silent, in which case they probably have such feelings but are unable to express them at this time.

Facilitative Responding

Involves careful listening and reflecting back to patients the feelings and content of their statements.

Responses are empathic and nonjudgmental, and legitimize the person's feelings.

Formula for facilitative responses: "You feel _____ because _____ ."

Example: If child states, "I hate coming to the hospital and getting needles," a facilitative response is, "You feel unhappy because of all the things that are done to you."

Storytelling

Uses the language of children to probe into areas of their thinking while bypassing conscious inhibitions or fears.

Simplest technique is asking children to relate a story about an event, such as "being in the hospital."

Other approaches:

Show children a picture of a particular event, such as a child in a hospital with other people in the room, and ask them to describe the scene.

Cut out comic strips, remove words, and have child add statements for scenes.

Mutual Storytelling

Reveals child's thinking and attempts to change child's perceptions or fears by retelling a somewhat different story (more therapeutic approach than storytelling).

Begins by asking child to tell a story about something, followed by another story told by the nurse that is similar to child's tale but with differences that help child in problem areas.

Example: Child's story is about going to the hospital and never seeing his or her parents again. Nurse's story is also about a child (using different names but similar circumstances) in a hospital whose parents visit every day, but in the evening after work, until the child is better and goes home with them.

Bibliotherapy

Uses books in a therapeutic and supportive process.*

Provides children with an opportunity to explore an event that is similar to their own but sufficiently different to allow them to distance themselves from it and remain in control.

General guidelines for using bibliotherapy are:

Assess child's emotional and cognitive development in terms of readiness to understand the book's message.

Be familiar with the book's content (intended message or purpose) and the age for which it is written.

*See Box 1-1.

BOX 1-1

Sources of Books for Bibliotherapy

Berg PJ, Devlin MK, Gedaly-Duff V: Bibliotherapy with children experiencing loss, *Issues Compr Pediatr Nurs* 4:37-50, 1980.

Cohen L: "Here's something I want you to read," *RN* 55(10):56-59, 1992.

Cuddigan M, Hanson MB: *Growing pains: helping children deal with everyday problems through reading,* Ann Arbor, MI, 1988, Books on Demand; (800) 521-0600.

Doll B, Doll CA: *Bibliotherapy with young people: librarians and mental health professionals working together,* 1997, Libraries Unlimited, PO Box 6633, Englewood, CO 80155-6633; (800) 237-6124.

Fosson A, Husband E: Bibliotherapy for hospitalized children, *South Med J* 77(3):342-346, 1984.

Grindler MC, et al: *The right book, the right time: helping children cope,* 1997, Allyn & Bacon, 160 Gould St., Needham Heights, MA 02194; (800) 852-8024 or 781-455-1200; www.abacon.com.

Health, illness, and disability: a guide to books for children and young adults, available from Pediatric Projects Inc., PO Box 571555, Tarzana, CA 91357-1555; (800) 947-0947; fax (818) 705-3660; e-mail: medpubl@kaiwan.com.

Jaywell JF: *Using literature to help troubled teenagers cope with family issues (using literature to help troubled teenagers),* 1998, Greenwood Publishing Group, Inc., 88 Post Road West, Westport, CT 06881; (800) 225-5800 or (203) 226-3571; www.greenwood.com.

Mohr C, et al: *Books that heal: a whole language approach,* 1991, Libraries Unlimited, PO Box 6633, Englewood, CO 80155-6633; (800) 237-6124.

Pardeck JT, Pardeck JA: *Children in foster care and adoption: a guide to bibliotherapy,* 1998, Greenwood Publishing Group, 88 Post Road West, Westport, CT 06881; (800) 225-5800 or (203) 226-3571; www.greenwood.com.

Pardeck JT, Pardeck JA: *Bibliotherapy: a clinical approach for helping children (special aspects of education, vol 16),* 1993, Gordon & Breach Publishing Group, PO Box 32160, Newark, NJ 07102; (800) 545-8398; www.gbhap.com.

Pardeck JT, Pardeck JA: *Bibliotherapy: a guide to using books in clinical practice,* 1992, Edwin Mellen Press, 415 Ridge St., Lewiston, NY 14092; (716) 754-2788.

Pardeck JT, Pardeck JA: *Young people with problems: a guide to bibliotherapy,* 1986, Greenwood Publishing Group, Inc., 88 Post Road West, Westport, CT 06881; (800) 225-5800 or (203) 226-3571; www.greenwood.com.

Pearl P: *Helping children through books: a selected booklist,* 1990, Church & Synagogue Library Association, PO Box 29357, Portland, OR 97280-0357; (800) 452-2752 or (503) 244-6919; www.worldaccessnet.com.

Philpot JG: *Bibliotherapy for classroom use,* Nashville, TN, 1997, Incentive Pub.; (800) 421-2830.

Wallace NE: Special books for special children, *Child Health Care* 12(1):34-36, 1983.

Ziegler RG, et al: *Homemade books to help kids cope: an easy-to-learn technique for parents and professionals,* 1992, Magination Press, 750 First St. NE, Washington, DC 20002-4242; (800) 374-2721; www.maginationpress.com.

Web Sites for Bibliotherapy

www.amazon.com
www.ghbooks.com
www.noble.mass.edu/nobchild/biblio.htm
www.hpl.hamilton.on.ca/CHILDREN/booklist.htm

Read the book to the child if child is unable to read.
Explore the meaning of the book with the child by having child:
Retell the story
Read a special section with the nurse or parent
Draw a picture related to the story and discuss the drawing
Talk about the characters
Summarize the moral or meaning of the story

Dreams

Often reveal unconscious and repressed thoughts and feelings.
Ask child to talk about a dream or nightmare.
Explore with child what meaning the dream could have.

"What If" Questions

Encourage child to explore potential situations and to consider different problem-solving options.
Example: "What if you got sick and had to go to the hospital?" Children's responses reveal what they know already and what they are curious about and provide an opportunity for helping children learn coping skills, especially in potentially dangerous situations.

Three Wishes

Involves asking, "If you could have any three things in the world, what would they be?"

If child answers, "That all my wishes come true," ask child for specific wishes.

Rating Game

Uses some type of rating scale (numbers, sad to happy faces) to rate an event or feeling.
Example: Instead of asking youngsters how they feel, ask how their day has been "on a scale of 1 to 10, with 10 being the best."

Word Association Game

Involves stating key words and asking children to say the first word they think of when they hear each word.
Start with neutral words and then introduce more anxiety-producing words, such as "illness," "needles," "hospitals," and "operation."
Select key words that relate to some relevant event in child's life.

Sentence Completion

Involves presenting a partial statement and having child complete it.
Some sample statements are:
The thing I like best (least) about school is _____.
The best (worst) age to be is _____.
The most (least) fun thing I ever did was _____.
The thing I like most (least) about my parents is _____.
The one thing I would change about my family is _____.
If I could be anything I wanted, I would be _____.
The thing I like most (least) about myself is _____.

Pros and Cons

Involves selecting a topic, such as "being in the hospital," and having child list "five good things and five bad things" about it.
Is an exceptionally valuable technique when applied to relationships, such as things family members like and dislike about each other.

NONVERBAL TECHNIQUES

Writing

Is an alternative communication approach for older children and adults.
Specific suggestions include:
Keep a journal or diary.
Write down feelings or thoughts that are difficult to express.
Write "letters" that are never mailed (a variation is making up a "pen pal" to write to).
Keep an account of child's progress from both a physical and an emotional viewpoint.

Drawing

One of the most valuable forms of communication, it provides both nonverbal (from looking at the drawing) and verbal (from child's story of the picture) information.

Children's drawings tell a great deal about them because they are projections of their inner selves.
Spontaneous drawing involves giving child a variety of art supplies and providing the opportunity to draw.
Directed drawing involves a more specific direction, such as "draw a person" or the "three themes" approach (state three things about child and ask child to choose one and draw a picture).

Guidelines for Evaluating Drawings

Use spontaneous drawings and evaluate more than one drawing whenever possible.
Interpret drawings in light of other available information about child and family.
Interpret drawings as a whole rather than concentrating on specific details of the drawing.
Consider individual elements of the drawing that may be significant:
Sex of figure drawn first—Usually relates to child's perception of own sex role.
Size of individual figures—Expresses importance, power, or authority.
Order in which figures are drawn—Expresses priority in terms of importance.
Child's position in relation to other family members—Expresses feelings of status or alliance.
Exclusion of a member—May denote feeling of not belonging or desire to eliminate.
Accentuated parts—Usually express concern for areas of special importance (e.g., large hands may be a sign of aggression).
Absence of or rudimentary arms and hands—Suggest timidity, passivity, or intellectual immaturity; tiny, unstable feet may be an expression of insecurity, and hidden hands may mean guilt feelings.
Placement of drawing on the page and type of stroke—Free use of paper and firm, continuous strokes express security, whereas drawings restricted to a small area and lightly drawn in broken or wavering lines may be a sign of insecurity.
Erasures, shading or cross-hatching—Expresses ambivalence, concern, or anxiety with a particular area.

Magic

Uses simple magic tricks to help establish rapport with child, encourage compliance with health interventions, and provide effective distraction during painful procedures.
Although "magician" talks, no verbal response from child is required.

Play

Is universal language and "work" of children.
Tells a great deal about children because they project their inner selves through the activity.
Spontaneous play involves giving child a variety of play materials and providing the opportunity to play.
Directed play involves a more specific direction, such as providing medical equipment, a doll, or a dollhouse for focused reasons, such as exploring child's fear of injections or exploring family relationships.

Guidelines for Using an Interpreter

Explain to interpreter the reason for the interview and the type of questions that will be asked.

Clarify whether a detailed or brief answer is required and whether the translated response can be general or literal.

Introduce interpreter to family and allow some time before the actual interview so that they can become acquainted.

Give reassurance that interpreter will maintain confidentiality.

Communicate directly with family members when asking questions to reinforce interest in them and to observe nonverbal expressions, but do not ignore interpreter.

Pose questions to elicit only one answer at a time, such as "Do you have pain?" rather than "Do you have any pain, tiredness, or loss of appetite?"

Refrain from interrupting family members and interpreter while they are conversing.

Avoid commenting to interpreter about family members, since they may understand some English.

Be aware that some medical words, such as "allergy," may have no similar word in another language; avoid medical jargon whenever possible.

Respect cultural differences; it is often best to pose questions about sex, marriage, or pregnancy indirectly—ask about "child's father" rather than "mother's husband."

Allow time following the interview for interpreter to share something that he or she felt could not be said earlier; ask about interpreter's impression of nonverbal clues to communication and family members' reliability or ease in revealing information.

Arrange for family to speak with same interpreter on subsequent visits whenever possible.

Outline of a Health History

A. Identifying information
1. Name
2. Address
3. Telephone number
4. Age and birthdate
5. Birthplace
6. Race/ethnic group
7. Sex
8. Religion
9. Nationality
10. Date of interview
11. Informant

B. Chief complaint

C. Present illness
1. Onset
2. Characteristics
3. Course since onset

D. Past history
1. Pregnancy (maternal)
2. Labor and delivery
3. Perinatal period
4. Previous illnesses, operations, or injuries
5. Allergies
6. Current medications
7. Immunizations
8. Growth and development
9. Habits

E. Review of systems
1. General
2. Integument
3. Head
4. Eyes
5. Nose
6. Ears
7. Mouth
8. Throat
9. Neck
10. Chest
11. Respiratory
12. Cardiovascular
13. Gastrointestinal
14. Genitourinary
15. Gynecologic
16. Musculoskeletal
17. Neurologic
18. Endocrine
19. Lymphatic

F. Nutrition history*
1. Patterns of eating
2. Dietary intake

G. Family medical history
1. Family pedigree
2. Familial diseases and congenital anomalies
3. Family habits
4. Geographic location

H. Family personal/social history*
1. Family structure
2. Family function

I. Sexual history
1. Sexual concerns/activity of youngster
2. Sexual concerns/activity of adults if warranted

J. Patient profile (summary)
1. Health status
2. Psychologic status
3. Socioeconomic status

---

*Because of the importance of the nutrition history and family personal/social history, separate sections devoted to assessment of these two topics are on pp. 94 and 69, respectively.

Summary of a Health History

Information	Comments

Identifying Information

1. Name
2. Address
3. Telephone number
4. Age
5. Birthdate
6. Race/ethnic group
7. Sex
8. Religion/spiritual beliefs
9. Nationality
10. Date of interview
11. Informant

Additional information appropriate to older adolescent may include occupation, marital status, and temporary and permanent addresses

Under "informant" include subjective impression of reliability, general attitude, willingness to communicate, overall accuracy of data, and any special circumstances, such as use of an interpreter.

Informants should include parent and child, as well as others who may be primary caregivers, such as grandparent.

Chief Complaint (CC)

To establish the major specific reason for the individual's seeking professional health attention

Record in patient's own words; include duration of symptoms.

If informant has difficulty isolating *one* problem, ask which problem or symptom led person to seek help *now*.

In case of routine physical examination, state *CC* as reason for visit.

Present Illness (PI)

To obtain all details related to the chief complaint

1. **Onset**
   a. Date of onset
   b. Manner of onset (gradual or sudden)
   c. Precipitating and predisposing factors related to onset (emotional disturbance, physical exertion, fatigue, bodily function, pregnancy, environment, injury, infection, toxins and allergens, or therapeutic agents)
2. **Characteristics**
   a. Character (quality, quantity, consistency, or other)
   b. Location and radiation (e.g., pain)
   c. Intensity or severity
   d. Timing (continuous or intermittent, duration of each, temporal relationship to other events)
   e. Aggravating and relieving factors
   f. Associated symptoms
3. **Course since onset**
   a. Incidence
      (1) Single acute attack
      (2) Recurrent acute attacks
      (3) Daily occurrences
      (4) Periodic occurrences
      (5) Continuous chronic episode
   b. Progress (better, worse, unchanged)
   c. Effect of therapy

In its broadest sense, *illness* denotes any problem of a physical, emotional, or psychosocial nature.

Present information in chronologic order; may be referenced according to one point in time, such as *prior to admission* (PTA).

Concentrate on reason for seeking help now, especially if problem has existed for some time.

Past History (PH)

To elicit a profile of the individual's previous illnesses, injuries, or operations

1. **Pregnancy (maternal)**
   a. Number (gravida)
      (1) Dates of delivery
   b. Outcome (parity)
      (1) Gestation (full-term, premature, postmature)
      (2) Stillbirths, abortions
   c. Health during pregnancy
   d. Medications taken

Importance of perinatal history depends on child's age; the younger the child, the more important the perinatal history.

Explain relevance of obstetric history in revealing important factors relating to the child's health.

Assess parents' emotional attitudes toward the pregnancy and birth.

Summary of a Health History—cont'd

Information	Comments

2. Labor and delivery
  a. Duration of labor
  b. Type of delivery
  c. Place of delivery
  d. Medications
	Assess parent's feelings regarding delivery; investigate factors that may affect bonding, such as separation from infant.

3. Perinatal period
  a. Weight and length at birth
  b. Time of regaining birth weight
  c. Condition of health immediately after birth
  d. Apgar score
  e. Presence of problems including congenital anomalies
  f. Date of discharge from nursery
	If birth problems are reported, inquire about treatment, such as use of oxygen, phototherapy, surgery, and so on, and parents' emotional response to the event.

4. Previous illnesses, operations, or injuries
  a. Onset, symptoms, course, termination
  b. Occurrence of complications
  c. Incidence of disease in other family members or in community
  d. Emotional response to previous hospitalization
  e. Circumstances and nature of injuries
	Ask about diphtheria, scarlet fever, measles, rubella, chickenpox, mumps, tonsillitis, strep throat, pertussis, allergies, and common illnesses such as colds and earaches.
	Elicit a description of disease to verify the diagnosis.
	Be alert to areas of injury prevention.

5. Allergies
  a. Hay fever, asthma, or eczema
  b. Unusual reactions to foods, drugs, animals, plants, latex products, or household products
	Have parent describe the type of allergic reaction and its severity.

6. Current medications a. Name, dose, schedule, duration, and reason for administration	Assess parents' knowledge of correct dosage of common drugs, such as acetaminophen; note underuse or overuse.

7. Immunizations
  a. Name, number of doses, age when given
  b. Occurrence of reaction
  c. Administration of horse or other foreign serum, gamma globulin, or blood transfusion
	Parents may refer to immunizations as "baby shots."
	Whenever possible, confirm information by checking medical or school records.

 PRACTICE ALERT

Inquire about previous administration of any horse or other foreign serum, recent administration of gamma globulin or blood transfusion, and anaphylactic reactions to neomycin or chicken eggs.

Information	Comments

8. Growth and development
  a. Weight at birth, 6 months, 1 year, and present
  b. Dentition
    (1) Age of eruption/shedding
    (2) Number
    (3) Problems with teething
  c. Age of head control, sitting unsupported, walking, first words
  d. Present grade in school, scholastic achievement
  e. Interaction with peers and adults
  f. Participation in organized activities such as Scouting, sports, and so on
	Compare parents' responses with own observations of child's achievement and results from objective tests, such as Denver II or DASE. (See pp. 127 and 134.)
	
	School and social history can be more thoroughly explored under Family Assessment, p. 69.

9. Habits
  a. Behavior patterns
    (1) Nail biting
    (2) Thumb sucking
    (3) Pica
    (4) Rituals, such as "security blanket"
    (5) Unusual movements (headbanging, rocking)
    (6) Temper tantrums
	Assess parents' attitudes toward habits and any remedies used to curtail them, such as punishment for bed-wetting.
	Pica, the habitual ingestion of nonfood items, may be risk factor for lead poisoning.

Continued

Summary of a Health History—cont'd

Information	Comments
9. Habits, cont'd	
b. Activities of daily living	
(1) Hour of sleep and arising	
(2) Duration of nighttime sleep/naps	
(3) Age of toilet training	
(4) Pattern of stools and urination; occurrence of enuresis or encopresis	Record child's usual terms for defecation and urination.
(5) Type of exercise	
c. Use/abuse of drugs, alcohol, coffee (caffeine), tobacco, or alternative therapies (Comunity Focus: alternative therapies)	With adolescents, ask about quantity and frequency of chemicals used.
d. Usual disposition; response to frustration	

Review of Systems (ROS)

To elicit information concerning any potential health problem (Box 1-2)	Explain relevance of questioning to parents (similar to pregnancy section) in composing total health history of child. Make positive statements about each system (e.g., "Mother denies headaches, bumping into objects, squinting, or excessive rubbing of eyes."). Use terms parents are likely to understand, such as "bruises" for ecchymoses.

Nutrition History

To elicit information about adequacy of child's dietary intake and eating patterns (See p. 94.)

Family Medical History

To identify the presence of genetic traits or diseases that have familial tendencies; to assess family habits and exposure to a communicable disease that may affect family members	Choose terms wisely when asking about child's parentage: for example, inquire about paternal history by referring to the child's "father" rather than mother's husband; use term "partner" rather than spouse.
1. **Family pedigree** (Fig. 1-1) and guidelines for construction (boxed material)	A pedigree is a pictorial representation or diagram of a family tree to visualize patterns of disease transmission.
2. **Familial diseases** such as heart disease, hypertension, cancer, diabetes mellitus, obesity, congenital anomalies, allergy, asthma, tuberculosis, seizures, sickle cell disease, depression, mental retardation, mental illness or other emotional problems, syphilis, or rheumatic fever; indicate symptoms, treatment, and sequelae	

COMMUNITY FOCUS

Alternative Therapies

Many families are using alternative therapies such as herbal preparations when treating their children. This is of concern because, despite research currently being done on herbs, there is no standardization or FDA approval for herbs. Much of the information available on herbs is anecdotal and more research is needed.

Nurses need to recognize the growing trend of alternative therapies. Families may consult the nurse when using or considering alternative approaches for their children. However, some parents will not tell the nurse or practitioner about any alternative products or care their children are receiving. Therefore, it is important for the nurse to:

- Learn more about alternative therapies, including their indications and dosages, contraindications, and side effects.
- Include alternative therapies when taking a health history.
- Ask questions in a nonjudgmental manner.
- Document the use of alternative therapies on child's record.
- Encourage families to read labels on all products carefully.
- Have reference books on alternative therapies available.

Hadley S: Medicinal herbs for children: what nurses should know, *Small Talk* 10(5):1-14, 1998.

BOX 1-2

Review of Systems

General—Overall state of health, fatigue, recent and/or unexplained weight gain or loss (period of time for either), contributing factors (change of diet, illness, altered appetite), exercise tolerance, fevers (time of day), chills, night sweats (unrelated to climatic conditions), frequent infections, general ability to carry out activities of daily living

Integument—Pruritus, pigment or other color changes, acne, moles, discoloration, eruptions, rashes (location), tendency toward bruising, petechiae, excessive dryness, general texture, disorders or deformities of nails, hair growth or loss, hair color change (for adolescent, use of hair dyes or other potentially toxic substances such as hair straighteners)

Head—Headaches, dizziness, injury (specific details)

Eyes—Visual problems (ask about behaviors indicative of blurred vision, such as bumping into objects, clumsiness, sitting very close to the television, holding a book close to the face, writing with head near desk, squinting, rubbing the eyes, bending the head in an awkward position), cross-eye (strabismus), eye infections, edema of lids, excessive tearing, use of glasses or contact lenses, date of last optic examination

Nose—Nosebleeds (epistaxis), constant or frequent running or stuffy nose, nasal obstruction (difficulty in breathing), alteration or loss of sense of smell

Ears—Earaches, discharge, evidence of hearing loss (ask about behaviors such as need to repeat requests, loud speech, inattentive behavior), results of any previous auditory testing

Mouth—Mouth breathing, gum bleeding, toothaches, toothbrushing, use of fluoride, difficulty with teething (symptoms), last visit to dentist (especially if temporary dentition is complete), response to dentist

Throat—Sore throats, difficulty in swallowing, choking (especially when chewing food—may be from poor chewing habits), hoarseness or other voice irregularities

Neck—Pain, limitation of movement, stiffness, difficulty in holding head straight (torticollis), thyroid enlargement, enlarged nodes or other masses

Chest—Breast enlargement, discharge, masses, enlarged axillary nodes (for adolescent female, ask about breast self-examination)

Respiratory—Chronic cough, frequent colds (number per year), wheezing, shortness of breath at rest or on exertion, difficulty in breathing, sputum production, infections (pneumonia, tuberculosis), date of last chest x-ray examination, and skin reaction from tuberculin testing

Cardiovascular—Cyanosis or fatigue on exertion, history of heart murmur or rheumatic fever, anemia, date of last blood count, blood type, recent transfusion

Gastrointestinal—(Much of this in regard to appetite, food tolerance, and elimination habits is asked elsewhere) nausea, vomiting (not associated with eating, may be indicative of brain tumor or increased intracranial pressure), jaundice or yellowing skin or sclera, belching, flatulence, recent change in bowel habits (blood in stools, change in color, diarrhea, and constipation)

Genitourinary—Pain on urination, frequency, hesitancy, urgency, hematuria, nocturia, polyuria, unpleasant odor to urine, force of stream, discharge, change in size of scrotum, date of last urinalysis (for adolescent, sexually transmitted disease, type of treatment; for male adolescent, ask about testicular self-examination)

Gynecologic—Menarche, date of last menstrual period, regularity or problems with menstruation, vaginal discharge, pruritus, date and result of last Pap smear (include obstetric history as discussed under birth history when applicable); if sexually active, type of contraception

Musculoskeletal—Weakness, clumsiness, lack of coordination, unusual movements, back or joint stiffness, muscle pains or cramps, abnormal gait, deformity, fractures, serious sprains, activity level

Neurologic—Seizures, tremors, dizziness, loss of memory, general affect, fears, nightmares, speech problems, any unusual habit

Endocrine—Intolerance to weather changes, excessive thirst and urination, excessive sweating, salty taste to skin, signs of early puberty

Lymphatic—History of frequent infections, enlarged lymph nodes in any region, swelling, tenderness, red streaks

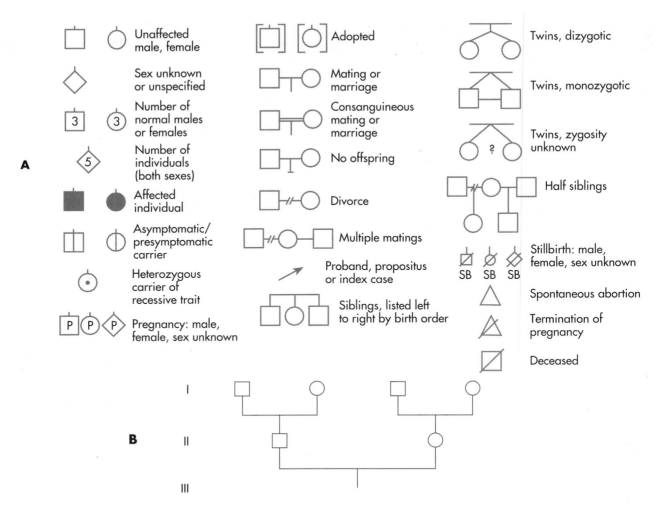

Fig. 1-1 **A,** Common pedigree symbols. **B,** Example of a standardized pedigree form. Roman numerals indicate generations: I—grandparents; II—parents; and III—offspring.

GUIDELINES

Pedigree Construction

1. Begin diagram in the middle of a large sheet of paper.
2. Represent males by a square placed to the left and females by a circle placed to the right (Fig. 1-1, *A*).
3. Represent the proband (index case, original patient) with an arrow (if the counselee or patient is different, place a *C* under that person's symbol).
4. Use a horizontal line between a square and a circle for a mating or marriage.
5. Suspend offspring vertically from the mating line and place in order of birth with oldest to the left (regardless of sex).
6. Symbolize generations by Roman numerals with the earliest generation at the top.
7. Include three generations: (1) grandparents, (2) parents, and (3) offspring; may include aunts, uncles, and first cousins of proband (Fig. 1-1, *B*).
8. Include name of each person (maiden names for married women), the person's date of birth, health problems, and date and cause of death.
9. Date the pedigree.

For a detailed description of pedigree construction, see Nelson-Anderson DL, Waters CV: *Genetic connections: a guide to documenting your individual and family health history,* Washington, MO, 1995, Sonters Pub.

Summary of a Health History—cont'd

Information	Comments

Family Medical History—cont'd

3. *Family members with congenital anomalies*
4. *Family habits,* such as smoking or chemical use
5. *Geographic location,* including birthplace, present location, and travel or contact with foreign visitors

Important for identification of endemic diseases

Family Personal/Social History

To gain an understanding of the family's structure and function (See p. 69.)

Sexual History

To elicit information concerning young person's concerns and/or activities and any pertinent data regarding adults' sexual activity that influences child

1. *Sexual concerns/activity of youngster*
2. *Sexual concerns/activity of adults if warranted*

Sexual history is an essential component of preadolescents' and adolescents' health assessments.

Degree of investigation into parents' sexual history depends on its relevance to the child's health. It may be limited to family planning concerns or it may be more detailed if overt sexual activity or abuse is suspected.

Investigate toward end of history when rapport is greatest.

Respect sensitive and complex nature of questioning.
  Give parents and youngster option of discussing sexual matters alone with nurse.
  Assure confidentiality.
  Clarify terms such as "sexually active" or "having sex"
  Refer to sexual contacts as "partners" not "girlfriends" or "boyfriends" to avoid biasing discussion of homosexual activity.

Discussion may flow easily after review of genitourinary tract, such as asking female about menstruation or male about urinary problems.

Suggestions for beginning discussion include the following:
  "Tell me about your social life."
  "Who are your closest friends?"
  "Is there one very special friend?"
  "Some teenagers have decided to have sex. What do you think about that?"

Take detailed history of all contacts if sexually transmitted disease is suspected or diagnosed.

Patient Profile (P/P)

To summarize the interviewer's overall impression of the child's and family's physical, psychologic, and socioeconomic background:

1. *Health status*
2. *Psychologic status*
3. *Socioeconomic status*

A comprehensive summary often identifies nursing diagnoses (See pp. 265-267.) based on subjective and objective findings.

PHYSICAL ASSESSMENT

Physical assessment is a continuous process that begins during the interview, primarily by using inspection or observation. During the more formal examination, the tools of percussion, palpation, and auscultation are added to enhance and refine the assessment of body systems. Like the health history, the objective of the physical assessment is to formulate nursing diagnoses and evaluate the effectiveness of therapeutic interventions.

Because of important differences in physical assessment of the child and newborn, separate guidelines and summaries for conducting the physical examination of each age group are presented.

The summary of the physical assessment of the newborn is also presented according to: the area to be assessed, usual findings, common variations/minor abnormalities, and potential signs of distress/major abnormalities. Common variations/minor abnormalities should be recorded but generally do not require further evaluation. Potential signs of distress/major abnormalities are recorded and need to be reported for further evaluation. The procedures for assessment are not presented here but in the summary of physical assessment of the child. In addition to the newborn summary, assessment of clinical gestational age is also described.

The summary of the physical assessment of the child is presented according to: the area to be assessed, the procedure for assessment, usual findings, and comments. The comments column includes findings that deviate from the normal and should be reported, special significance of certain findings, and areas for nursing intervention. This section includes detailed instructions for various assessment procedures.

For a more comprehensive discussion of performing a physical assessment, see Chapters 7 and 8 in *Whaley and Wong's Nursing Care of Infants and Children* or *Whaley and Wong's Essentials of Pediatric Nursing.**

─────────

*Wong DL, Hockenberry-Eaton M, Wilson D, Winkelstein ML, Ahmann E, DiVito-Thomas PA: *Whaley and Wong's Nursing care of infants and children,* ed 6, St Louis, 1999, Mosby; or Wong DL: *Whaley and Wong's Essentials of pediatric nursing,* ed 5, St Louis, 1997, Mosby.

General Guidelines for Physical Examination of the Newborn

Provide a comfortably warm and nonstimulating examination area.
  To prevent heat loss, undress only the body area to be examined unless the newborn is already under a heat source such as a radiant warmer.
Proceed in an orderly sequence (usually head to toe) with the following exceptions:
  Perform first all procedures that require quiet observation (position, attitude), then proceed with quiet procedures such as auscultating the lungs, heart, and abdomen.
  Perform disturbing procedures, such as testing reflexes, last.

Measure head, chest, and length at same time to compare results.
Proceed quickly to avoid stressing the infant.
  Check that equipment and supplies are working properly and are accessible.
Comfort the infant during and after the examination if upset.
  Talk softly.
  Hold infant's hands against his or her chest.
  Swaddle and hold.
  Give pacifier.

Summary of Physical Assessment of the Newborn

Usual Findings	Common Variations/ Minor Abnormalities	Potential Signs of Distress/ Major Abnormalities
General Measurements		
Head circumference—33-35 cm (13-14 inches); about 2-3 cm (1 inch) larger than chest circumference	Molding after birth may decrease head circumference	Head circumference <10th or >90th percentile
Chest circumference—30.5-33 cm (12-13 inches)	Head and chest circumference may be equal for first 1-2 days after birth	
Crown-to-rump length—31-35 cm (12.5-14 inches); approximately equal to head circumference		
Head-to-heel length—48-53 cm (19-21 inches)		
Birth weight—2700-4000 g (6-9 pounds)	Loss of 10% of birth weight in first week; regained in 10-14 days	Birth weight <10th or >90th percentile
Vital Signs		
Temperature		
Axillary—36.5°-37° C (97.7°-98.6° F)	Crying may increase body temperature slightly	Hypothermia
	Radiant warmer will falsely increase axillary temperature	Hyperthermia
Heart Rate		
Apical—120-140 beats/min	Crying will increase heart rate; sleep will decrease heart rate	Bradycardia—Resting rate below 80-100 beats/min
	During first period of reactivity (6 to 8 hours), rate can reach 180 beats/min	Tachycardia—Rate above 160-180 beats/min
		Irregular rhythm

Summary of Physical Assessment of the Newborn—cont'd

Usual Findings	Common Variations/ Minor Abnormalities	Potential Signs of Distress/ Major Abnormalities
Respirations		
30-60 breaths/min	Crying will increase respiratory rate; sleep will decrease respiratory rate During first period of reactivity (6 to 8 hours), rate can reach 80 breaths/min	Tachypnea—Rate above 60 breaths/min Apnea >15 seconds
Blood Pressure (BP)		
Oscillometric—65/41 mm Hg in arm and calf	Crying and activity will increase BP Placing cuff on thigh may agitate infant; thigh BP may be higher than arm or calf BP by 4-8 mm Hg	Oscillometric systolic pressure in calf 6-9 mm Hg less than in upper extremity (sign of coarctation of aorta)
General Appearance		
Posture—Flexion of head and extremities, which rest on chest and abdomen	*Frank breech*—Extended legs, abducted and fully rotated thighs, flattened occiput, extended neck	Limp posture, extension of extremities
Skin		
At birth, bright red, puffy, smooth Second to third day, pink, flaky, dry Vernix caseosa Lanugo Edema around eyes, face, legs, dorsa of hands, feet, and scrotum or labia *Acrocyanosis*—Cyanosis of hands and feet *Cutis marmorata*—Transient mottling when infant is exposed to stress, decreased temperature, or overstimulation	Neonatal jaundice after first 24 hours Ecchymoses or petechiae caused by birth trauma *Milia*—Distended sebaceous glands that appear as tiny white papules on cheeks, chin, and nose *Miliaria* or *sudamina*—Distended sweat (eccrine) glands that appear as minute vesicles, especially on face *Erythema toxicum*—Pink papular rash with vesicles superimposed on thorax, back, buttocks, and abdomen; may appear in 24 to 48 hours and resolve after several days *Harlequin color change*—Clearly outlined color change as infant lies on side; lower half of body becomes pink or red, and upper half is pale *Mongolian spots*—Irregular areas of deep blue pigmentation, usually in sacral and gluteal regions; seen predominantly in newborns of African, Native American, Asian, or Hispanic descent *Telangiectatic nevi ("stork bites")*— Flat, deep pink, localized areas usually seen on back of neck	Progressive jaundice, especially in first 24 hours Cracked or peeling skin Generalized cyanosis Pallor Mottling Grayness Plethora Hemorrhage, ecchymoses, or petechiae that persist *Sclerema*—Hard and stiff skin Poor skin turgor Rashes, pustules, or blisters *Café-au-lait spots*—Light brown spots *Nevus flammeus*—Port-wine marks

Summary of Physical Assessment of the Newborn—cont'd

Usual Findings	Common Variations/ Minor Abnormalities	Potential Signs of Distress/ Major Abnormalities
Head		
Anterior fontanel—Diamond shaped, 2.5-4.0 cm (1-1.75 inches) (Fig. 1-2)	Molding following vaginal delivery	Fused sutures
Posterior fontanel—Triangular, 0.5-1 cm (0.2-0.4 inch)	Third sagittal (parietal) fontanel	Bulging or depressed fontanels when quiet
Fontanels should be flat, soft, and firm	Bulging fontanel because of crying	Widened sutures and fontanels
Widest part of fontanel measured from bone to bone, not suture to suture	*Caput succedaneum*—Edema of soft scalp tissue	*Craniotabes*—Snapping sensation along lambdoidal suture that resembles indentation of Ping-Pong ball
	Cephalhematoma (uncomplicated)—Hematoma between periosteum and skull bone	

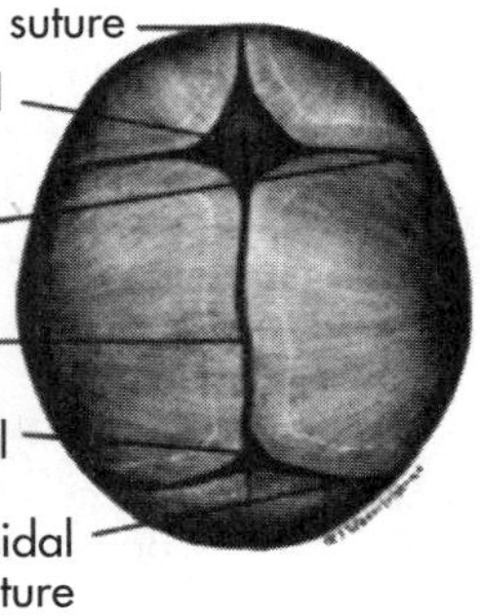

Frontal suture
Anterior fontanel
Coronal suture
Sagittal suture
Posterior fontanel
Lambdoidal suture

Fig. 1-2 Locations of sutures and fontanels.

Usual Findings	Common Variations/ Minor Abnormalities	Potential Signs of Distress/ Major Abnormalities
Eyes		
Lids usually edematous	Epicanthal folds in Oriental infants	Pink color of iris
Iris color—Slate gray, dark blue, brown	Searching nystagmus or strabismus	Purulent discharge
Absence of tears	*Subconjunctival (scleral) hemorrhages*—Ruptured capillaries, usually at limbus	Upward slant in non-Orientals
Presence of red reflex		Hypertelorism (3 cm or greater)
Corneal reflex in response to touch		Hypotelorism
Pupillary reflex in response to light		Congenital cataracts
Blink reflex in response to light or touch		Constricted or dilated fixed pupil
Rudimentary fixation on objects and ability to follow to midline		Absence of red reflex
		Absence of pupillary or corneal reflex
		Inability to follow object or bright light to midline
		Blue sclera
		Yellow sclera
Ears		
Position—Top of pinna on horizontal line with outer canthus of eye	Inability to visualize tympanic membrane because of filled aural canals	Low placement of ears
Startle reflex elicited by a loud, sudden noise	Pinna flat against head	Absence of startle reflex in response to loud, sudden noise
Pinna flexible, cartilage present	Irregular shape or size	Minor abnormalities may be signs of various syndromes, especially renal
	Pits or skin tags	
Nose		
Nasal patency	Flattened and bruised	Nonpatent canals
Nasal discharge—Thin, white mucus		Thick, bloody nasal discharge
Sneezing		Flaring of nares (alae nasi)
		Copious nasal secretions or stuffiness (may be minor)

Summary of Physical Assessment of the Newborn—cont'd

Usual Findings	Common Variations/ Minor Abnormalities	Potential Signs of Distress/ Major Abnormalities
Mouth and Throat		
Intact, high-arched palate Uvula in midline Frenulum of tongue Frenulum of upper lip Sucking reflex—Strong and coordinated Rooting reflex Gag reflex Extrusion reflex Absent or minimal salivation Vigorous cry	*Natal teeth*—Teeth present at birth; benign but may be associated with congenital defects *Epstein pearls*—Small, white epithelial cysts along midline of hard palate	Cleft lip Cleft palate Large, protruding tongue or posterior displacement of tongue Profuse salivation or drooling *Candidiasis (thrush)*—White, adherent patches on tongue, palate, and buccal surfaces Inability to pass nasogastric tube Hoarse, high-pitched, weak, absent, or other abnormal cry
Neck		
Short, thick, usually surrounded by skinfolds Tonic neck reflex	*Torticollis* (wry neck)—Head held to one side with chin pointing to opposite side	Excessive skinfolds Resistance to flexion Absence of tonic neck reflex Fractured clavicle
Chest		
Anteroposterior and lateral diameters equal Slight sternal retractions evident during inspiration Xiphoid process evident Breast enlargement	Funnel chest (pectus excavatum) Pigeon chest (pectus carinatum) Supernumerary nipples Secretion of milky substance from breasts ("witch's milk")	Depressed sternum Marked retractions of chest and intercostal spaces during respiration Asymmetric chest expansion Redness and firmness around nipples Wide-spaced nipples
Lungs		
Respirations chiefly abdominal Cough reflex absent at birth, present by 1-2 days Bilateral equal bronchial breath sounds	Rate and depth of respirations may be irregular; periodic breathing Crackles shortly after birth	Inspiratory stridor Expiratory grunt Retractions Persistent irregular breathing Periodic breathing with repeated apneic spells Seesaw respirations (paradoxical) Unequal breath sounds Persistent fine crackles Wheezing Diminished breath sounds Peristaltic sounds on one side with diminished breath sounds on same side
Heart		
Apex—Fourth to fifth intercostal space, lateral to left sternal border S_2 slightly sharper and higher in pitch than S_1	*Sinus arrhythmia*—Heart rate increases with inspiration and decreases with expiration Transient cyanosis on crying or straining	*Dextrocardia*—Heart on right side Displacement of apex, muffled Cardiomegaly Abdominal shunts Murmurs Thrills Persistent cyanosis Hyperactive precordium

Summary of Physical Assessment of the Newborn—cont'd

Usual Findings	Common Variations/ Minor Abnormalities	Potential Signs of Distress/ Major Abnormalities
Abdomen		
Cylindric in shape *Liver*—Palpable 2-3 cm below right costal margin *Spleen*—Tip palpable at end of first week of age *Kidneys*—Palpable 1-2 cm above umbilicus *Umbilical cord*—Bluish white at birth with two arteries and one vein *Femoral pulses*—Equal bilaterally	Umbilical hernia *Diastasis recti*—Midline gap between recti muscles *Wharton's jelly*—Unusually thick umbilical cord	Abdominal distention Localized bulging Distended veins Absent bowel sounds Enlarged liver and spleen Ascites Visible peristaltic waves Scaphoid or concave abdomen Green umbilical cord Presence of only one artery in cord Urine or stool leaking from cord Palpable bladder distention following scanty voiding Absent femoral pulses Cord bleeding or hematoma
Female Genitalia		
Labia and clitoris usually edematous Urethral meatus behind clitoris Vernix caseosa between labia Urination within 24 hours	*Pseudomenstruation*—Blood-tinged or mucoid discharge Hymenal tag	Enlarged clitoris with urethral meatus at tip Fused labia Absence of vaginal opening Meconium from vaginal opening No urination within 24 hours Masses in labia Ambiguous genitalia
Male Genitalia		
Urethral opening at tip of glans penis Testes palpable in each scrotum Scrotum usually large, edematous, pendulous, and covered with rugae; usually deeply pigmented in dark-skinned ethnic groups Smegma Urination within 24 hours	Urethral opening covered by prepuce Inability to retract foreskin *Epithelial pearls*—Small, firm, white lesions at tip of prepuce Erection or priapism Testes palpable in inguinal canal Scrotum small	*Hypospadias*—Urethral opening on ventral surface of penis *Epispadias*—Urethral opening on dorsal surface of penis *Chordee*—Ventral curvature of penis Testes not palpable in scrotum or inguinal canal No urination within 24 hours Inguinal hernia Hypoplastic scrotum *Hydrocele*—Fluid in scrotum Masses in scrotum Meconium from scrotum Discoloration of testes Ambiguous genitalia
Back and Rectum		
Spine intact; no openings, masses, or prominent curves Trunk incurvation reflex Anal reflex Patent anal opening Passage of meconium within 48 hours	Green liquid stools in infant under phototherapy Delayed passages of meconium in very-low-birth-weight neonates	Anal fissures or fistulas Imperforate anus Absence of anal reflex No meconium within 36 hours Pilonidal cyst or sinus Tuft of hair along spine Spina bifida (any degree)

Summary of Physical Assessment of the Newborn—cont'd

Usual Findings	Common Variations/ Minor Abnormalities	Potential Signs of Distress/ Major Abnormalities
Extremities		
Ten fingers and ten toes	Partial syndactyly between second and third toes	***Polydactyly***—Extra digits
Full range of motion	Second toe overlapping into third toe	***Syndactyly***—Fused or webbed digits
Nail beds pink, with transient cyanosis immediately after birth	Wide gap between first (hallux) and second toes	***Phocomelia***—Hands or feet attached close to trunk
Creases on anterior two thirds of sole	Deep crease on plantar surface of foot between first and second toes	***Hemimelia***—Absence of distal part of extremity
Sole usually flat	Asymmetric length of toes	Hyperflexibility of joints
Symmetry of extremities	Dorsiflexion and shortness of hallux	Persistent cyanosis of nail beds
Equal muscle tone bilaterally, especially resistance to opposing flexion		Yellowing of nail beds
Equal bilateral brachial pulses		Sole covered with creases
		Transverse palmar (simian) crease
		Fractures
		Decreased or absent ROM
		Dislocated or subluxated hip
		Limitation in hip abduction
		Unequal gluteal or leg folds (Fig. 1-3)
		Unequal knee height (Allis or Galeazzi sign)
		Audible clunk on abduction (Ortolani sign)
		Asymmetry of extremities
		Unequal muscle tone or range of motion

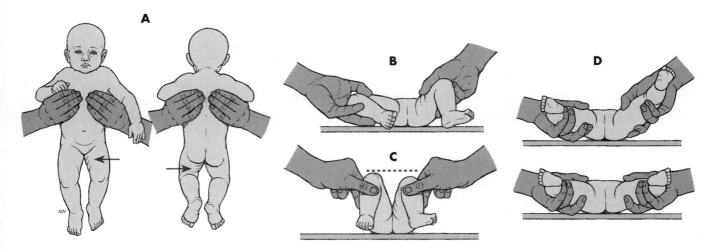

Fig. 1-3 Signs of developmental dysplasia of the hip. **A,** Asymmetry of gluteal and thigh folds. **B,** Limited hip abduction, as seen in flexion. **C,** Apparent shortening of the femur, as indicated by the level of the knees in flexion. **D,** Ortolani click, heard when affected leg is abducted in infant under 4 weeks of age.

Unit 1

Summary of Physical Assessment of the Newborn—cont'd

Usual Findings	Common Variations/ Minor Abnormalities	Potential Signs of Distress/ Major Abnormalities
Neuromuscular System		
Extremities usually maintain some degree of flexion	Quivering or momentary tremors	***Hypotonia***—Floppy, poor head control, extremities limp
Extension of an extremity followed by previous position of flexion		***Hypertonia***—Jittery, arms and hands tightly flexed, legs stiffly extended, startles easily
Head lag while sitting, but momentary ability to hold head erect		Asymmetric posturing (except tonic neck reflex)
Able to turn head from side to side when prone		***Opisthotonic posturing***—Arched back
Able to hold head in horizontal line with back when held prone		Signs of paralysis
		Tremors, twitches, and myoclonic jerks
		Marked head lag in all positions

Assessment of Reflexes

Reflexes	Expected Behavioral Responses

Localized

Eyes

Blinking or corneal reflex	Infant blinks at sudden appearance of a bright light or at approach of an object toward cornea; persists throughout life
Pupillary	Pupil constricts when a bright light shines toward it; persists throughout life
Doll's eye	As head is moved slowly to right or left, eyes lag behind and do not immediately adjust to new position of head; disappears as fixation develops; if persists, indicates neurologic damage

Nose

Sneeze	Spontaneous response of nasal passages to irritation or obstruction; persists throughout life
Glabellar	Tapping briskly on glabella (bridge of nose) causes eyes to close tightly

Mouth and Throat

Sucking	Infant begins strong sucking movements of circumoral area in response to stimulation; persists throughout infancy, even without stimulation, such as during sleep
Gag	Stimulation of posterior pharynx by food, suction, or passage of a tube causes infant to gag; persists throughout life
Rooting	Touching or stroking the cheek along side of mouth causes infant to turn head toward that side and begin to suck; should disappear at about age 3-4 months, but may persist for up to 12 months
Extrusion	When tongue is touched or depressed, infant responds by forcing it outward; disappears by age 4 months
Yawn	Spontaneous response to decreased oxygen by increasing amount of inspired air; persists throughout life
Cough	Irritation of mucous membranes of larynx or tracheobronchial tree causes coughing; persists throughout life; usually present 1 day after birth

Extremities

Grasp	Touching palms of hands or soles of feet near base of digits causes flexion of hands and toes; palmar grasp lessens after age 3 months, to be replaced by voluntary movement; plantar grasp lessens by 8 months of age
Babinski	Stroking outer sole of foot upward from heel and across ball of foot causes toes to hyperextend and hallux to dorsiflex; disappears after age 1 year
Ankle clonus	Briskly dorsiflexing foot while supporting knee in partially flexed position results in one or two oscillating movements ("beats"); eventually no beats should be felt

Mass (Body)

Moro*	Sudden jarring or change in equilibrium causes sudden extension and abduction of extremities and fanning of fingers, with index finger and thumb forming a C shape, followed by flexion and adduction of extremities; legs may weakly flex; infant may cry; disappears after age 3-4 months, usually strongest during first 2 months
Startle*	A sudden loud noise causes abduction of the arms with flexion of elbows; hands remain clenched; disappears by age 4 months
Perez	While infant is prone on a firm surface, thumb is pressed along spine from sacrum to neck; infant responds by crying, flexing extremities, and elevating pelvis and head; lordosis of the spine, as well as defecation and urination, may occur; disappears by age 4-6 months
Asymmetric tonic neck	When infant's head is turned to one side, arm and leg extend on that side, and opposite arm and leg flex; disappears by age 3-4 months, to be replaced by symmetric positioning of both sides of body
Trunk incurvation (Galant) reflex	Stroking infant's back alongside spine causes hips to move toward stimulated side; disappears by age 4 weeks
Dance or step	If infant is held so that sole of foot touches a hard surface, there is a reciprocal flexion and extension of the leg, simulating walking; disappears after age 3-4 weeks, to be replaced by deliberate movement
Crawl	When placed on abdomen, infant makes crawling movements with arms and legs; disappears at about age 6 weeks
Placing	When infant is held upright under arms and dorsal side of foot is briskly placed against hard object, such as table, leg lifts as if foot is stepping on table; age of disappearance varies

*Some authorities consider Moro and startle reflexes to be the same response.

Assessment of Gestational Age

Assessment of gestational age is an important criterion because perinatal morbidity and mortality are related to gestational age and birth weight. One of the most frequently used methods of determining gestational age is based on physical and neurologic findings. The scale in Fig. 1-4, *A,* assesses six external physical and six neuromuscular signs. Each sign has a number score and the cumulative score correlates with a maturity rating from 20 to 44 weeks (see maturity rating box on scale).

This new **Ballard Scale,** a revision of the original scale, can be used with newborns as young as 20 weeks of gestation. The tool has the same physical and neuromuscular sections but includes −1 and −2 scores that reflect signs of extremely premature infants, such as fused eyelids; imperceptible breast tissue; sticky, friable, transparent skin; no lanugo; and square-window (flexion of wrist) angle of greater than 90 degrees. The examination of infants with a gestational age of 20 weeks or less should be performed at a postnatal age of less than 12 hours. For infants with a gestational age of at least 26 weeks, the examination can be performed up to 96 hours after birth, although shortly after birth, preferably within 2 to 8 hours, is suggested. The scale overestimates gestational age by 2 to 4 days in infants less than 37 weeks' gestation, especially between 32 and 37 weeks' gestation. Neurologic maturity may require retesting once the infant has stabilized. The Ballard gestational age scale has greater validity when performed before 96 hours of age in preterm infants. It is also important to note that the infant's state and period of reactivity will affect the neuromuscular rating. An infant in the second stage of the first period of reactivity may not have an accurate neuromuscular score.

Fig. 1-4, *B,* is a classification of newborns based on maturity and intrauterine growth. The newborn's length, weight, and head circumference are plotted according to the estimated gestational age. Values that fall within 10th to 90th percentiles classify the newborn as appropriate for gestational age (AGA). Values that fall below the 10th percentile classify the newborn as small for gestational age (SGA). Values that fall above the 90th percentile classify the newborn as large for gestational age (LGA).

To facilitate the use of Fig. 1-4, *A,* the following tests and observations are described:

Test	Assessment/Description
Posture	With the infant quiet and in a supine position, observe the degree of flexion in the arms and legs. Muscle tone and degree of flexion increase with maturity. Full flexion of the arms and legs = 4.
Square window	With the thumb supporting the back of the arm below the wrist, apply gentle pressure with index and third fingers on dorsum of hand without rotating the infant's wrist. Measure the angle between the base of the thumb and forearm. Full flexion (hand lies flat on ventral surface of forearm) = 4.
Arm recoil	With the infant supine, fully flex both forearms on upper arms, hold for 5 seconds; pull down on hands to fully extend and rapidly release arms. Observe the rapidity and intensity of recoil to a state of flexion. A brisk return to full flexion = 4.
Popliteal angle	With the infant supine and the pelvis flat on a firm surface, flex lower leg on thigh and then flex thigh on abdomen. While holding knee with thumb and index finger, extend lower leg with index finger of other hand. Measure the degree of the angle behind the knee (popliteal angle). An angle less than 90° = 5.
Scarf sign	With the infant supine, support the head in the midline with one hand; use other hand to pull infant's arm across the shoulder so that infant's hand touches the opposite shoulder. Determine location of elbow in relation to midline. Elbow does not reach midline = 4.
Heel to ear	With the infant supine and the pelvis flat on a firm surface, pull the foot as far as possible up toward the ear on the same side. Measure the distance of the foot from the ear and degree of knee flexion (same as popliteal angle). Knees flexed with a popliteal angle less than 90° = 4.

Estimation of Gestational Age by Maturity Rating

NEUROMUSCULAR MATURITY

	−1	0	1	2	3	4	5
Posture							
Square Window (wrist)	> 90°	90°	60°	45°	30°	0°	
Arm Recoil		180°	140°-180°	110° 140°	90°-110°	< 90°	
Popliteal Angle	180°	160°	140°	120°	100°	90°	< 90°
Scarf Sign							
Heel to Ear							

A

PHYSICAL MATURITY

Skin	sticky friable transparent	gelatinous red, translucent	smooth pink, visible veins	superficial peeling &/or rash, few veins	cracking pale areas rare veins	parchment deep cracking no vessels	leathery cracked wrinkled
Lanugo	none	sparse	abundant	thinning	bald areas	mostly bald	
Plantar Surface	heel-toe 40-50 mm: -1 <40 mm: -2	>50 mm no crease	faint red marks	anterior transverse crease only	creases ant. 2/3	creases over entire sole	
Breast	imperceptible	barely perceptible	flat areola no bud	stippled areola 1-2 mm bud	raised areola 3-4 mm bud	full areola 5-10 mm bud	
Eye/Ear	lids fused loosely: -1 tightly: -2	lids open pinna flat stays folded	sl. curved pinna; soft; slow recoil	well-curved pinna; soft but ready recoil	formed & firm instant recoil	thick cartilage ear stiff	
Genitals (male)	scrotum flat, smooth	scrotum empty faint rugae	testes in upper canal rare rugae	testes descending few rugae	testes down good rugae	testes pendulous deep rugae	
Genitals (female)	clitoris prominent labia flat	prominent clitoris small labia minora	prominent clitoris enlarging minora	majora & minora equally prominent	majora large minora small	majora cover clitoris & minora	

MATURITY RATING

score	weeks
-10	20
-5	22
0	24
5	26
10	28
15	30
20	32
25	34
30	36
35	38
40	40
45	42
50	44

Fig. 1-4 **A,** New Ballard Scale for newborn maturity rating. Expanded scale includes extremely premature infants and has been refined to improve accuracy in more mature infants. (From Ballard JL and others: New Ballard Score, expanded to include extremely premature infants, *J Pediatr* 119(3):417-423, 1991.) (Courtesy Mead Johnson & Company, Evansville, IN 47721. Scoring section modified from Ballard JL and others: *Pediatr Res* 11:374, 1977. Figures modified from Sweet AY: Classification of the low-birth-weight infant. In Klaus MH, Fanaroff AA: *Care of the high-risk infant,* Philadelphia, 1977, WB Saunders.)

Continued

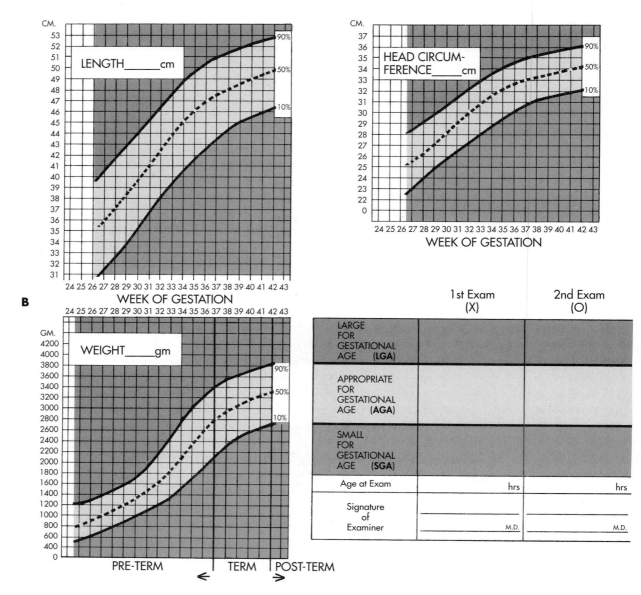

Fig. 1-4, cont'd   B, Classification of newborns based on maturity and intrauterine growth. (From Ballard JL and others: New Ballard Score, expanded to include extremely premature infants, *J Pediatr* 119(3): 417-423, 1991.) (Courtesy Mead Johnson & Company, Evansville, IN 47721. Scoring section modified from Ballard JL and others: *Pediatr Res* 11:374, 1977. Figures modified from Sweet AY: Classification of the low-birth-weight infant. In Klaus MH, Fanaroff AA: *Care of the high-risk infant,* Philadelphia, 1977, WB Saunders.)

General Guidelines for Physical Examination During Childhood

Perform examination in pleasant, nonthreatening area.
Have room well lit and decorated with neutral colors.
Have room temperature comfortably warm.
Place all strange and potentially frightening equipment out of sight.
Have some toys, dolls, stuffed animals, and games available for the child.
If possible, have rooms decorated and equipped for different age children.
Provide privacy, especially for school-age children and adolescents.
Check that equipment and supplies are working properly and are accessible to avoid disruption.
Provide time for play and becoming acquainted:
Talking to the nurse
Making eye contact
Accepting the offered equipment
Allowing physical touching
Choosing to sit on examining table rather than parent's lap
If signs of readiness are not observed, use the following techniques:
Talk to the parent while essentially "ignoring" the child; gradually focus on the child or a favorite object, such as a doll.
Make complimentary remarks about the child, such as his or her appearance, dress, or a favorite object.
Tell a funny story or perform a simple magic trick.
Have a nonthreatening "friend," such as a hand or finger puppet available to "talk" to the child for the nurse.
If the child refuses to cooperate, use the following techniques:
Assess reason for uncooperative behavior; consider that a child who is unduly afraid of a male examiner may have had a previous traumatic experience, including sexual abuse.
Try to involve child and parent in process or, if appropriate, ask parent to leave.
Avoid prolonged explanations about examining procedure.
Use a firm, direct approach regarding expected behavior.
Perform examination as quickly as possible.
Have attendant gently restrain child.
Minimize any disruptions or stimulation:
Limit number of people in room.
Use isolated room.
Use quiet, calm, confident voice.
Begin the examination in a nonthreatening manner for young children or children who are fearful (Atraumatic Care box).
Use those activities that can be presented as games, such as tests for cranial nerves (See p. 68.) or parts of developmental testing. (See p. 127.)
Use approaches such as "Simon says" to encourage child to make a face, squeeze a hand, stand on one foot, and so on.

Use the "paper doll" technique:
Lay the child supine on an examining table or floor that is covered with a large sheet of paper.
Trace outline around the child's body.
Use the body outline to demonstrate what will be examined, such as drawing a heart and listening with the stethoscope before performing the activity on the child.
If several children in the family will be examined, begin with the most cooperative child.
Involve child in the examination process:
Provide choices, such as sitting either on the table or on the parent's lap.
Allow child to handle or hold equipment.
Encourage child to use equipment on a doll, family member, or examiner.
Explain each step of the procedure in simple language.
Examine child in a comfortable and secure position:
Sitting in parent's lap
Sitting upright if in respiratory distress
Proceed to examine the body in an organized sequence (usually head to toe) with following exceptions:
Alter sequence to accommodate needs of different age children. (See p. 26.)
Examine painful areas last.
In emergency situation, examine vital functions (airway, breathing, and circulation) and injured area first.
Reassure child throughout examination, especially about bodily concerns that arise during puberty.
Discuss the findings with the family at the end of the examination.
Praise child for cooperation during examination; give reward such as an inexpensive toy or paper sticker.

ATRAUMATIC CARE

Reducing Young Children's Fears

Young children, especially preschoolers, fear intrusive procedures because of their poorly defined body boundaries. Therefore avoid invasive procedures, such as measuring rectal temperature, whenever possible. Also, avoid using the word "take" when measuring vital signs, because young children interpret words literally and may think that their temperature or other function will be taken away. Instead, say, "I want to know how warm you are."

Age-Specific Approaches to Physical Examination During Childhood

Position	Sequence	Preparation
Infant		
Before sits alone: supine or prone, preferably in parent's lap; before 4 to 6 months: can place on examining table After sits alone: sit in parent's lap whenever possible If on table, place with parent in full view	If quiet, auscultate heart, lungs, abdomen Record heart and respiratory rates Palpate and percuss same areas Proceed in usual head-to-toe direction Perform traumatic procedures last (eyes, ears, mouth [while crying]) Elicit reflexes as body part examined Elicit Moro reflex last	Completely undress if room temperature permits Leave diaper on male Gain cooperation with distraction, bright objects, rattles, talking Have older infants hold a small block in each hand; until voluntary release develops toward end of the first year, infants will be unable to grasp other objects (e.g., stethoscope, otoscope)* Smile at infant; use soft, gentle voice Pacify with bottle of sugar water or feeding Enlist parent's aid in restraining to examine ears, mouth Avoid abrupt, jerky movements
Toddler		
Sitting or standing on/by parent Prone or supine in parent's lap	Inspect body area through play: "count fingers," "tickle toes" Use minimal physical contact initially Introduce equipment slowly Auscultate, percuss, palpate whenever quiet Perform traumatic procedures last (same as for infant)	Have parent remove child's outer clothing Remove underwear as body part examined Allow child to inspect equipment; demonstrating use of equipment is usually ineffective If uncooperative, perform procedures quickly Use restraint when appropriate; request parent's assistance Talk about examination if cooperative; use short phrases Praise for cooperative behavior
Preschool Child		
Prefer standing or sitting Usually cooperative prone/supine Prefer parent's closeness	If cooperative, proceed in head-to-toe direction If uncooperative, proceed as with toddler	Request self-undressing Allow to wear underpants Offer equipment for inspection; briefly demonstrate use Make up "story" about procedure: "I'm seeing how strong your muscles are" (blood pressure) Use paper-doll technique Give choices when possible Expect cooperation; use positive statements: "Open your mouth"
School-Age Child		
Prefer sitting Cooperative in most positions Younger child prefers parent's presence Older child may prefer privacy	Proceed in head-to-toe direction May examine genitalia last in older child Respect need for privacy	Request self-undressing Allow to wear underpants Give gown to wear Explain purpose of equipment and significance of procedure, such as otoscope to see eardrum, which is necessary for hearing Teach about body functioning and care

*Farber JM: The invisible handcuffs, *Contemp Pediatr* 8(1):110, 1991.

Age-Specific Approaches to Physical Examination During Childhood—cont'd

Position	Sequence	Preparation
Adolescent		
Same as for school-age child Offer option of parent's presence	Same as for older school-age child	Allow to undress in private Give gown Expose only area to be examined Respect need for privacy Explain findings during examination: "Your muscles are firm and strong" Matter-of-factly comment about sexual development: "Your breasts are developing as they should be" Emphasize normalcy of development Examine genitalia as any other body part; may leave to end

Outline of a Physical Assessment

A. **Growth measurements**
   1. Length/height
   2. Crown-to-rump length or sitting height
   3. Weight
   4. Head circumference
   5. Chest circumference
   6. Skinfold thickness and arm circumference
B. **Physiologic measurements**
   1. Temperature
   2. Pulse
   3. Respiration
   4. Blood pressure
C. **General appearance**
D. **Skin**
E. **Accessory structures**
F. **Lymph nodes**
G. **Head**
H. **Neck**
I. **Eyes**

J. **Ears**
K. **Nose**
L. **Mouth and throat**
M. **Chest**
N. **Lungs**
O. **Heart**
P. **Abdomen**
Q. **Genitalia**
   1. Male
   2. Female
R. **Anus**
S. **Back and extremities**
T. **Neurologic assessment**
   1. Mental status
   2. Motor functioning
   3. Sensory functioning
   4. Reflexes (deep tendons)
   5. Cranial nerves

Summary of Physical Assessment of the Child

Assessment	Procedure
GROWTH MEASUREMENTS (Fig. 1-5, *A* and *B*)	Plot length, weight, and head circumference on standard percentile charts. (See pp. 113-121.) Charts for 0 to 36 months and 2 to 18 years both include children ages 24 to 36 months; record only recumbent length on 0 to 36 month chart and only stature on 2 to 18 year chart. The prepubescent charts are only appropriate for plotting values for prepubescent boys and girls, regardless of chronologic age, and not for any child showing signs of pubescence, such as breast budding, testicular enlargement, or growth of axillary or pubic hair.

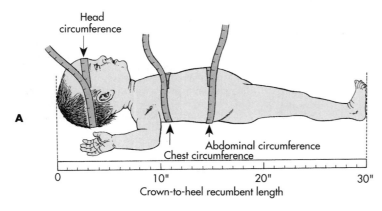

Fig. 1-5 A, Measurement of head, chest, and abdominal circumference and crown-to-heel (recumbent) length.

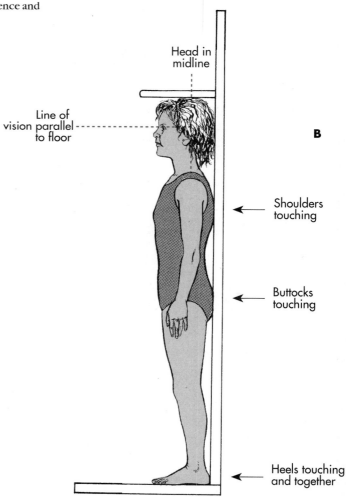

Fig. 1-5 B, Measurement of height (stature). (Redrawn from *Human growth and growth disorders: an update,* South San Francisco, 1989, Genentech.)

Usual Findings

Measurements of length, weight, and head circumference between the 25th and 75th percentiles are likely to represent normal growth (Practice Alert).

Measurements between the 10th and 25th and between the 75th and 90th percentiles may or may not be normal, depending on previous and subsequent measurements and on genetic and environmental factors.

Growth curve remains generally within same percentile, except during rapid growth periods.

 PRACTICE ALERT

The 50th percentile represents the median growth (or midpoint of all the growth measurements for each age). The 5th percentile represents the lowest 5%, and the 95th percentile represents the highest 5% of growth measurements for each age.

Comments

Questionable results may include the following:

1. Children whose height and weight are below the 5th or above the 95th percentile.
2. Children whose height and weight percentiles are widely disparate, for example, height in the 10th percentile and weight in the 90th percentile, especially with above average skinfold thickness.
3. Children who fail to show the expected gain in height and weight, especially during the rapid growth periods of infancy and adolescence.
4. Children who show a sudden increase, except during puberty, or decrease in a previously steady growth pattern.

Compare findings with growth patterns of other family members; consider genetic influence on growth determination. (See Chinese growth charts, p. 126.)

Compare children's growth trends (height and weight) with midparental height (MPH). Most children with normal birth weights and heights and normal childhood growth will achieve an adult height within ±2 inches of MPH. Special charts are available for parent-specific adjustments for evaluation of the child's height (Himes and others, 1985*).

To calculate MPH, use the following formulas:

For girls:

$$\frac{(\text{Father's height} - 13 \text{ cm or } 5 \text{ inches}) + \text{Mother's height}}{2}$$

For boys:

$$\frac{(\text{Father's height} + 13 \text{ cm or } 5 \text{ inches}) + \text{Mother's height}}{2}$$

*Himes JH and others: Parent-specific adjustments for evaluation of recumbent length and stature of children, *Pediatrics* 75(2):304-313, 1985.

Summary of Physical Assessment of the Child—cont'd

Assessment	Procedure

Length/Height	Recumbent length in children below 24 to 36 months:
	  Place supine with head in midline.
	  Grasp knees and push gently toward table to *fully* extend legs.
	  Measure from vertex (top) of head to heels of feet (toes pointing upward).
	Standing height (stature) in children over 24 to 36 months:
	  Remove socks and shoes.
	  Have child stand as tall as possible, back straight, head in midline, and eyes looking straight ahead. (See Fig. 1-5, *B*.)
	  Check for flexion of knees, slumping shoulders, raising of heels.
	  Measure from top of head to standing surface.
	  Measure to the nearest cm or ⅛ inch.

Weight	Weigh infants and young children nude on platform-type scale; protect infant by placing hand above body to prevent falling off scale. Weigh older children in underwear (and gown if privacy is a concern; no shoes) on standing-type upright scale. Check that scale is balanced before weighing. Cover scale with clean sheet of paper for each child. Measure to the nearest 10 g or ½ ounce for infants and 100 g or ¼ pound for children.
Head Circumference (HC)	Measure with paper or steel tape at greatest circumference, from top of the eyebrows and pinna of the ear to occipital prominence of skull.
Chest Circumference	Measure around chest at nipple line. Ideally, take measurements during inhalation and expiration; record the average of the two values.
Skinfold Thickness and Arm Circumference	**Measurement of Triceps Skinfold Thickness** With child's right arm flexed 90° at elbow, mark midpoint between acromion and olecranon on posterior aspect of arm. With arm hanging freely, grasp a fold of skin between thumb and forefinger 1 cm above midpoint. Gently pull fold away from underlying muscle and continue to hold until measurement is completed. Place caliper jaws over skinfold at midpoint mark; if a plastic caliper (e.g., Ross Adipometer) is used, apply pressure with thumb to align lines on caliper; follow directions for using other calipers. Estimate reading to nearest 1.0 mm, 2 to 3 seconds after applying pressure. Take measurements until duplicates agree within 1 mm. **Measurement of Midarm Circumference** Follow procedure as above, but instead of grasping a fold of skin and using calipers, wrap a paper or steel measuring tape around upper arm at midpoint. Measure to nearest 1 cm.

Usual Findings	Comments

Plot on growth chart (pp. 113-120).
Compare value with percentile for weight.
Rule of thumb guide*:
　At 1 year = 1½ × birth length
　2 to 12 years = age (years) × 2½ + 30 = length (inches)

For accurate measurements, use infant-measuring device for recumbent length and stadiometer for standing height.
Normally height is less if measured in the afternoon than in the morning. To minimize this variation, apply modest upward pressure under the jaw or the mastoid processes.

Expected Growth Rates at Various Ages*

Age	Expected Growth Rate (cm/yr)
1 to 6 months	18-22
6 to 12 months	14-18
2nd year	11
3rd year	8
4th year	7
5th to 10th years	5-6

*From *Human growth and growth disorders: an update,* South San Francisco, 1989, Genentech.

Plot on growth chart. (See pp. 113-120.)
Compare value with percentile for length.
Rule of thumb guides*:
　At 1 year = 3 × birth weight
　1 to 9 years: age (years) × 5 + 17 = weight (pounds)
　9 to 12 years: age (years) × 9 − 20 = weight (pounds)

Compare weight with appearance, for example, excessive fat, well-developed musculature, flabby, loose skin, bony prominences (for skinfold measurement, see below).
Assess nutritional status; compare with weight.

Plot on growth chart. (See pp. 114, 118, or 121.)
Compare percentile with those of height and weight.
Compare with chest circumference:
　At birth, HC exceeds chest circumference by 2 to 3 cm (1 inch).
　At 1 to 2 years, HC equals chest circumference.
　During childhood, chest circumference exceeds HC by about 5 to 7 cm (2 to 3 inches).

Usually taken in children under 36 months of age.
Taken in any child whose head size appears abnormal.

Compare with head circumference (see above).

May be measured during examination of chest.

Plot on percentile charts. (See pp. 122, 123.)
For interpretation of measurements, see Comments.

Skinfold thickness is an index of total body fat.
Arm circumference is an indirect measure of total muscle mass.
Measurements of skinfold thickness can be taken at triceps (most common site), subscapula, suprailiac, abdomen, or upper thigh with special calipers.
Percentiles for skinfold thickness and arm circumference may be used as reference data but should not be considered "standards" or "norms"; percentiles between 5th and 95th are not normal ranges.
Because of lack of standard data, these measurements should probably not be used as a routine screening measurement in well child care, but rather in follow-up and monitoring of children who are identified as having potential or actual obesity or malnutrition.

*Based on NCHS growth charts for boys, 50th percentile. (See pp. 113-116.) For explanation of percentiles, see Practice Alert, p. 29.

Summary of Physical Assessment of the Child—cont'd

Assessment	Procedure
PHYSIOLOGIC MEASUREMENTS (Vital signs)	Ideally, record when child is quiet; otherwise, record value and note activity such as crying.

Temperature*

PRACTICE ALERT

No universal agreement exists regarding the length of time mercury thermometers should be kept in place. Recommendations based on research are 7 minutes for an oral reading, 4 minutes for a rectal reading, and 5 minutes for an axillary reading. However, these times may vary widely within practice settings and may not represent clinically significant differences from temperature readings taken for shorter intervals.

If in doubt about the optimum length of insertion time, reinsert the mercury thermometer after the first reading for a short time and recheck the scale for a rise. If the value is increased, reinsert the thermometer until the next reading is the same as the previous reading.

Mercury Glass Thermometer

Heat causes mercury to expand and rise in glass tube. (See Practice Alert.)

Oral Temperature

Place under tongue in right or left posterior sublingual pocket, not in front of tongue; have child keep mouth closed without biting on thermometer.

Axillary Temperature

Place under arm with tip in center of axilla and kept close to skin, not clothing; hold child's arm firmly against side.

Rectal Temperature

Place well-lubricated tip not more than 2.5 cm (1 inch) into rectum; securely hold thermometer close to anus.

May place child in side-lying, supine, or prone position (i.e., supine with knees flexed toward abdomen); cover penis, because procedure often stimulates urination.

A small child may be placed prone across parent's lap.

Electronic Thermometer

Senses temperature with electronic component called thermistor mounted at tip of plastic and stainless steel probe, which is connected to electronic recorder; temperature measurement appears on digital display within 60 seconds.

Place probe in mouth, axilla, or rectum as with mercury thermometer.

Use predictive mode for oral/rectal temperatures; use monitor mode for axillary temperatures in most models.

*For Community and Home Care Instructions on taking temperature, see p. 586.

Usual Findings	Comments
(See inside front cover.)	Compare present value with past recordings. Note obvious differences, such as a sudden increase. Assess possible physiologic/psychologic factors influencing the recordings.

(For average body temperatures in well children under basal conditions, see inside front cover.)

Only difference in selection of mercury thermometers is that rectal type has more rounded tip as compared with oral type, which has more slender, elongated tip.

Sublingual site indicates rapid changes in core body temperature *better* than rectal site.

Several factors affect temperature of mouth, such as hot or cold beverages, smoking, open-mouth breathing, and ambient temperature.

Oxygen by mask lowers oral temperature, but clinical significance of difference is questionable.

Recommended for children who object strongly to rectal temperature but for whom an oral temperature is not feasible.

Has advantage of avoiding intrusive procedure and eliminating risk of rectal perforation and possible peritonitis.

May be affected by poor peripheral perfusion (lower value) or use of radiant warmers or presence of brown fat in cold-stressed neonates (higher value).

Taken only when no other route or device can be used (e.g., in children whose mental age or temperament prevents cooperation and understanding instructions, agitated children, and those who have had injuries or surgery that precludes using other routes).

Not recommended, because core temperature is not obtained unless thermometer is inserted to depth of at least 5 cm, which incurs risk of rectal perforation, especially in neonates less than 3 months of age, since colon curves at depth of 3 cm (Fig. 1-6); also not recommended in anyone who has had rectal surgery; or in children with diarrhea or those receiving chemotherapy that affects mucosa.

Accuracy is affected by stool in rectum (higher value).

Ideally suited to pediatric use because plastic sheath is unbreakable, and child's mouth can remain open when oral temperature is taken.

Accuracy for axillary temperature is supported by some research but not by other studies.

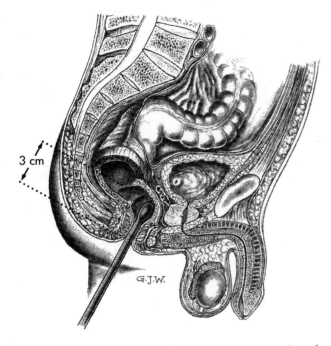

Fig. 1-6   Cross-section of rectum illustrates curve at approximately 3 cm from anus where risk of perforation from thermometer is greatest in infants under 3 months of age.

Summary of Physical Assessment of the Child—cont'd

Assessment	Procedure

Temperature (cont'd)

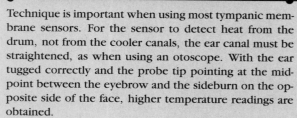

Technique is important when using most tympanic membrane sensors. For the sensor to detect heat from the drum, not from the cooler canals, the ear canal must be straightened, as when using an otoscope. With the ear tugged correctly and the probe tip pointing at the midpoint between the eyebrow and the sideburn on the opposite side of the face, higher temperature readings are obtained.

Infrared Thermometry

Infrared thermometer measures thermal radiation from axilla, ear canal opening, or tympanic membrane; temperature measurement appears on digital display in approximately 1 second.

Tympanic Membrane Sensor

Insert covered probe tip gently in ear canal, pointing toward midpoint between opposite eyebrow and sideburn (Practice Alert box).

For most accurate results, straighten ear canal so that sensor can measure heat from drum, not sides of canal; take three measurements and record highest reading.

Most models use "offsets" or internal calculations that translate ear temperature into supposedly equivalent oral or rectal temperatures.

Ear Sensor (OTOTEMP)*

Measures infrared heat energy radiating from canal opening, scans canal for highest temperature reading, and then calculates arterial temperature (correlates highly with core or internal body temperature).

Insert hemispherical probe in ear opening; ear tug is not necessary.

Axillary Sensor (OTOTEMP LighTouch Neonate)*

Measures infrared heat energy radiating from axilla.

Touch covered probe to axilla, depress and release button, remove and read.

Digital Thermometer

Consists of a probe that is connected to a microprocessor chip, which translates signals into degrees and sends temperature measurements to a digital display.

Used like oral mercury thermometer.

Chemical Dot Thermometer

Single-use disposable thermometer with specific chemical mixture in each circle that changes color to measure temperature in increments of two tenths of a degree.

Used like mercury thermometer; kept in mouth (1 minute), axilla (3 minutes), and rectum (3 minutes); color change is read 10-15 seconds after removing thermometer.

Plastic Strip Thermometer (Thermograph)

Changes color in response to sensed temperature changes.

Place strip on forehead until color change occurs; usually takes less than 15 seconds.

Some strips are used like oral mercury thermometer.

*Manufactured by Exergen Corporation, 51 Water Street, Watertown, MA 02172; (800) 422-3006, (617) 923-9900; fax, (617) 923-9911; Web site: www.exergen.com.

Usual Findings	Comments

Three types of infrared thermometers are available for aural use: tympanic, ear, and arterial heat balance via the ear canal (AHBE); often these devices are referred to as tympanic thermometers; all temperatures are a reflection of arterial temperature.

Tympanic membrane is excellent site because both eardrum and hypothalamus (temperature-regulating center) are perfused by same circulation.
Sensor is unaffected by pressure-equalizing tubes or cerumen; presence of suppurative or nonsuppurative otitis media does not significantly affect measurement.
Warm, ambient temperature may increase aural temperature.
Procedure is well accepted by infants and children.
Because of difficulty with correct placement in young infants' ears, accuracy may be affected.

Available in two sizes; smaller size of LighTouch Pedi-Q is for smaller children.
Does not calculate offsets; therefore reading is only for arterial temperature (not equivalent to other sites).

Can be used on wet skin, in incubators, or under radiant heaters, warming pads, or other heat sources.

More accurate and easier to read but somewhat more expensive than mercury or plastic strip thermometer.
Often useful when single-patient use is needed (e.g., patients in isolation).

May underestimate oral temperature and overestimate axillary temperature.
Tempa-Dot found to be accurate and reliable for children with and without fever, especially for temperature below 38° C (100.4° F).
Easier to read than mercury or plastic strip thermometer.
Safer than glass thermometers (disposable and flexible).
Read thermometer away from heat source (e.g., radiant warmer).
If unused thermometer changes color because of storage in warm area (above 35° C [95° F]), place in freezer for 1 hour and then at room temperature for 24 hours before using.

Accuracy is variable; best used for screening.
Advantages for home and community use include simple instructions and minimal cost.

Summary of Physical Assessment of the Child—cont'd

Assessment	Procedure
Pulse	Take apical pulse in children under 2 to 3 years. 　Point of maximum intensity located lateral to nipple at fourth to fifth interspace at or near midclavicular line. Take radial pulse in children over 2 to 3 years. Count pulse for 1 full minute, especially if any irregularity is present. For repeated measurement, count pulse for 15 or 30 seconds and multiply by 4 or 2, respectively.
Respiration	Observe rate of breathing for 1 full minute. In infants and young children, observe abdominal movement. In older children, observe thoracic movement.
Blood Pressure	Use an appropriately sized cuff (cuff size refers only to inner inflatable bladder, not cloth or plastic covering). **Report of the Second Task Force** (1987) recommends (Table 1-1): 　Width sufficient to cover approximately 75% of upper arm between top of shoulder and olecranon (Fig. 1-7, *A*) 　Length sufficient to completely encircle circumference of limb with or without overlapping 　Enough room at antecubital fossa to place stethoscope 　Enough room at upper edge of cuff to prevent obstruction of axilla **American Heart Association*** recommends (Table 1-2): 　Width 40% to 50% limb circumference; measured at upper arm midway between top of shoulder and olecranon 　Length sufficient to completely or nearly completely encircle circumference of limb without overlapping These suggested guidelines can be used for other measurement sites (See Fig. 1-7, *B, C,* and *D.*), although the shape of the limb (e.g., conical shape of thigh) may prevent appropriate placement of the cuff. Use same position (i.e., lying down or, preferably, sitting) and right arm for measurement. Position limb at level of heart. Rapidly inflate cuff to about 20 mm Hg above point at which radial pulse disappears. Release cuff pressure at a rate of about 2 to 3 mm Hg per second during auscultation of artery. Read mercury-gravity manometer at eye level.

TABLE 1-1　Commonly Available Blood Pressure Cuffs

Cuff Name*	Bladder Width (cm)	Bladder Length (cm)
Newborn	2.5-4.0	5.0-9.0
Infant	4.0-6.0	11.5-18.0
Child	7.5-9.0	17.0-19.0
Adult	11.5-13.0	22.0-26.0
Large arm	14.0-15.0	30.5-33.0
Thigh	18.0-19.0	36.0-38.0

From Report of the Second Task Force on Blood Pressure Control in Children—1987, *Pediatrics* 79(1):1-25, 1987.
*Cuff name does not guarantee that the cuff will be appropriate size for a person within that age range.

*Frohlich ED and others: Recommendations for human blood pressure determination by sphygmomanometers: report of a special task force appointed by the Steering Committee, American Heart Association, *Circulation* 77(2):509A, 1988.

Usual Findings

(For average pulse rates at rest, see inside front cover.)

(For average respiratory rates at rest, see inside front cover.)

(For blood pressure values at various ages using auscultation see inside front cover; and first Practice Alert on p. 39.)
These norms are based on:
    K4 diastolic pressure for children up to 12 years
    K5 diastolic pressure for adolescents 13 to 18 years
Rule of thumb guides:
    Use the following quick formula for normal *systolic BP* using auscultation:
       1 to 7 years: age in years + 90
       8 to 18 years: (2 × age in years) + 83
    Use the following quick formula for normal *diastolic BP* using auscultation:
       1 to 5 years: 56
       6 to 18 years: age in years + 52
(For blood pressure values at various ages using oscillometry, see Table 1-3.)
Normal blood pressure: systolic and diastolic pressure less than 90th percentile for age and sex
Normal high blood pressure: systolic and diastolic pressure between the 90th and 95th percentiles for age and sex

Comments

Pulse rate normally may increase with inspiration and decrease with expiration (sinus arrhythmia).
(See also Table 1-8.)
May grade pulses:
    Grade 0   Not palpable
    Grade +1 Difficult to palpate, thready, weak, easily obliterated with pressure
    Grade +2 Difficult to palpate, may be obliterated with pressure
    Grade +3 Easy to palpate, not easily obliterated with pressure (normal)
    Grade +4 Strong, bounding, not obliterated with pressure

(See also pp. 52-55.)

Blood pressure should be measured once a year in:
    Children 3 years of age through adolescence
    Children with symptoms of hypertension
    Children in emergency rooms and intensive care units
    High-risk infants
    Low-risk neonates (not universal agreement)
Task Force guidelines using limb length for selecting cuff width may produce satisfactory blood pressure readings in children with average weight for height, but inaccurate readings in children with thick arms; using limb circumference for selecting cuff width more accurately reflects direct arterial blood pressure than using length. (See second Practice Alert on p. 39.)
Using a small cuff causes a falsely elevated reading.
Use of a large cuff, or compression of brachial artery by clothing pushed up on arm, may result in lower reading; wide cuffs tend to affect blood pressure readings less than small cuffs.
    Use larger size on thigh: place cuff above knee and auscultate popliteal artery (Fig. 1-7, *C*).
    Use smaller size on forearm: place cuff above wrist and auscultate radial artery (Fig. 1-7, *B*).
    Use larger size on calf: place cuff above malleolus or at midcalf and auscultate posterior tibial or dorsal pedal artery (Fig. 1-7, *D*).
Blood pressure differences between measurement sites vary depending on the type of measurement technique; generally, pressure in upper sites is less than the pressure in lower sites (i.e., systolic pressure in thigh is higher than in upper arm using noninvasive techniques) (Table 1-4).
Compare blood pressure in upper and lower extremities at least once to detect abnormalities (e.g., coarctation of the aorta, in which the lower extremity pressure is less than the upper extremity pressure).

Summary of Physical Assessment of the Child—cont'd

Assessment	Procedure

Blood Pressure—cont'd

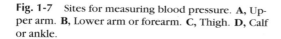

TABLE 1-2 Recommended Bladder Dimensions for Blood Pressure Cuffs

Arm Circumference at Midpoint (cm)	Cuff Name*	Bladder Width (cm)	Bladder Length (cm)
5-7.5	Newborn	3	5
7.5-13	Infant	5	8
13-20	Child	8	13
24-32	Adult	13	24
32-42	Wide adult	17	32
42-50	Thigh	20	42

From Frohlich ED and others: Recommendations for human blood pressure determination by sphygmomanometers: report of a special task force appointed by the Steering Committee, American Heart Association, *Circulation* 77(2): 509A, 1988.
*Cuff name does not guarantee that the cuff will be the appropriate size for a child within that age range.

Record systolic value as onset of a clear tapping sound (first Korotkoff sound).

Record diastolic pressure as fourth Korotkoff sound (K4, low-pitched, muffled sound) for children up to age 12 years or fifth Korotkoff sound (K5, disappearance of all sound) for children ages 13 to 18 years along with systolic pressure, limb, position, cuff size, and method (e.g., BP = 100/60 mm Hg, right arm, sitting, with child cuff by auscultation).

If using electronic monitor, follow manufacturer's instructions and above guidelines for correct cuff size.

With oscillometric device (e.g., Dinamap), all four sites in Fig. 1-7 can be used, but reserve the thigh for last since it is most uncomfortable.

Stabilize the limb during cuff deflation, because movement interferes with the device's ability to measure blood pressure accurately.

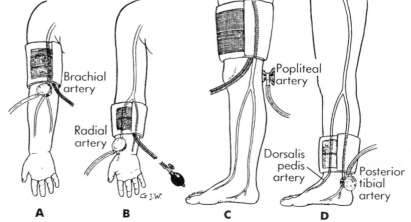

Fig. 1-7 Sites for measuring blood pressure. **A,** Upper arm. **B,** Lower arm or forearm. **C,** Thigh. **D,** Calf or ankle.

Usual Findings

TABLE 1-3 Normative Dinamap (Oscillometry) BP Values (Systolic/Diastolic, Mean in Parentheses)

Age Group	n	Mean	90th Percentile	95th Percentile
Newborn (1 to 3 days)	219	65/41(50)	75/49(59)	78/52(62)
1 month to 2 years	660	95/58(72)	106/68(83)	110/71(86)
2 to 5 years	631	101/57(74)	112/66(82)	115/68(85)

Data from Park M, Menard S: Normative oscillometric blood pressure values in the first five years in an office setting. *Am J Dis Child* 143(7):860-864, 1989.

PRACTICE ALERT

Published norms for BP, such as those on the inside front cover, are valid only if the same method of measurement (auscultation and limb length for cuff size) is used in clinical practice.

The 50th percentile represents the median BP (or midpoint of all the BP measurements for each age). The 5th percentile represents the lowest 5% of the BP and the 95th percentile represents the highest 5% of the BP for each age. The 99th percentile represents the highest 1% of the BP for each age.

PRACTICE ALERT

In choosing cuff sizes, use an appropriately sized cuff. When the correct size is not available, use an oversized cuff rather than an undersized one or use another site that more appropriately fits the cuff size. Do not choose a cuff based on the name of the cuff (e.g., an "infant" cuff may be too small for some infants).

Comments

Repeat measurements above 90th percentile later during initial visit when child is least anxious; if a high reading persists, repeat measurements at least three times during subsequent visits to detect hypertension (Table 1-5):

Significant hypertension: blood pressure persistently between 95th and 99th percentile for age and sex

Severe hypertension: blood pressure persistently at or above 99th percentile for age and sex

Consider body size when blood pressure values are in normal high range because larger children have higher blood pressures than smaller children of same age (e.g., a tall child whose BP is at 90th percentile for age is considered normal).

Refer children with consistently high blood pressure readings or significant differences in pressure between upper and lower extremities for further evaluation (e.g., in newborns a calf pressure less than 6 to 9 mm Hg compared to upper arm pressure).*

Blood pressure readings using oscillometry are generally higher than those using auscultation, but correlate better with direct radial artery blood pressure than auscultation readings.†

TABLE 1-4 Differences in Oscillometric Systolic BP Between Arm and Lower Extremity Sites in Normal Children

Age Group (years)	Systolic BP × (Mean ± SD)	
	Arm-Thigh	Arm-Calf
4-8	−7.1 ± 6.8	−9.3 ± 7.4
9-16	−2.4 ± 77	−5.0 ± 26.9

From Park M, Lee D, Johnson GA: Oscillometric blood pressures in the arm, thigh, and calf in healthy children and those with aortic coarctation, *Pediatrics* 91(4):761-765, 1993.

TABLE 1-5 Classification of Hypertension by Age Group

Age Group	Significant Hypertension (mm Hg)	Severe Hypertension (mm Hg)
Newborns (7 days)	Systolic BP ≥96	Systolic BP ≥106
(8-30 days)	Systolic BP ≥104	Systolic BP ≥110
Infants (<2 years)	Systolic BP ≥112	Systolic BP ≥118
	Diastolic BP ≥74	Diastolic BP ≥82
Children (3-5 years)	Systolic BP ≥116	Systolic BP ≥124
	Diastolic BP ≥76	Diastolic BP ≥84
Children (6-9 years)	Systolic BP ≥122	Systolic BP ≥130
	Diastolic BP ≥78	Diastolic BP ≥86
Children (10-12 years)	Systolic BP ≥126	Systolic BP ≥134
	Diastolic BP ≥82	Diastolic BP ≥90
Adolescents (13-15 years)	Systolic BP ≥136	Systolic BP ≥144
	Diastolic BP ≥86	Diastolic BP ≥92
Adolescents (16-18 years)	Systolic BP ≥142	Systolic BP ≥150
	Diastolic BP ≥92	Diastolic BP ≥98

From Report of the Second Task Force on Blood Pressure Control in Children—1987, *Pediatrics* 79(1):1-25, 1987.

*Park M, Lee D: Normative arm and calf blood pressure values in the newborn, *Pediatrics* 83(2):240-243, 1989.
†Park M, Menard S: Accuracy of blood pressure measurement by the Dinamap monitor in infants and children, *Pediatrics* 79(6):907-914, 1987.

Summary of Physical Assessment of the Child—cont'd

Assessment	Procedure
GENERAL APPEARANCE	Observe the following: 　Facies 　Posture 　Body movement 　Hygiene 　Nutrition 　Behavior 　Development 　State of awareness
SKIN	Observe skin in natural daylight or neutral artificial light. *Color*—Most reliably assessed in sclera, conjunctiva, nail beds, tongue, buccal mucosa, palms, and soles. *Texture*—Note moisture, smoothness, roughness, integrity of skin, and temperature. *Temperature*—Compare each part of body for even temperature. *Turgor*—Grasp skin on abdomen between thumb and index finger, pull taut, and release quickly. Indent skin with finger.

ACCESSORY STRUCTURES

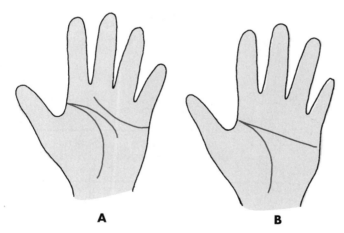

A

B

Hair—Inspect color, texture, quality, distribution, elasticity, and hygiene.

Nails—Inspect color, shape, texture, quality, distribution, elasticity, and hygiene.

Dermatoglyphics—Observe flexion creases of palm (Fig. 1-8).

Fig. 1-8 A, Example of normal flexion crease on palm. **B,** Transpalmar crease.

LYMPH NODES

(See Fig. 1-9.)

Palpate using distal portion of fingers.
Press gently but firmly in a circular motion.
Note size, mobility, temperature, tenderness, and any change in enlarged nodes.
Submaxillary—Tilt head slightly downward.
Cervical—Tilt head slightly upward.
Axillary—Have arms relaxed at side but slightly abducted.
Inguinal—Place child supine.

Usual Findings	Comments
Evaluated in terms of a comprehensive assessment; often gives clues to underlying problems such as poor hygiene and nutrition from parental neglect or poverty.	Record actual observations that lead to a conclusion such as signs of poor hygiene; give examples of present development milestones. Follow up on clues that may indicate problems, for example, investigate feeding practices of family if child appears undernourished.
	Reveals significant clues to problems such as poor hygiene, child abuse, inadequate nutrition, and serious physical disorders.

Genetically determined:
   Light-skinned—From milky white to rosy colored
   Dark-skinned—Various shades of brown, red, yellow, olive, and bluish tones
	Observe for abnormalities such as pallor, cyanosis, erythema, ecchymosis, petechiae, and jaundice (Table 1-6).
	Factors affecting color include natural skin tone, melanin production, edema, hygiene, hemoglobin levels of blood, amount of lighting, color of room, atmospheric temperature, and use of cosmetics.

Smooth, slightly dry to touch, with even temperature	Note obvious changes, such as clammy skin, oily skin, obvious lesions, and excessive dryness.
Usually same all over body, although exposed parts, such as hands, may be cooler	Note obvious differences, such as warm upper extremities and cold lower extremities.
Resumes shape immediately with no tenting, wrinkling, or prolonged depression	Good skin turgor indicates adequate hydration and possibly nutrition. Note "tenting" or poor elasticity of the pulled skin (sign of dehydration and/or malnutrition) or obvious pitting of skin upon indentation or signs of swelling (signs of edema).
Lustrous, silky, strong, elastic hair Genetic factors influence appearance; for example, a black child's hair is usually coarser, duller, and curlier.	Signs of poor nutrition include stringy, friable, dull, dry, depigmented hair. Note areas of baldness, unusual hairiness, and any evidence of infestation. During puberty, secondary hair growth indicates normal pubertal changes.
Pink, convex, smooth, and flexible, not brittle In dark-skinned child, color is darker.	Note color changes, such as blueness or yellow tint. Observe for uncut or short, ragged nails (nail biting). Report any signs of clubbing (base of the nail becomes swollen and feels springy or floating when palpated), a sign of serious respiratory or cardiac dysfunction.
Three flexion creases	If pattern differs, draw a sketch to describe it. Observe for transpalmar crease (one horizontal crease; Fig. 1-8, *B*), a characteristic of children with Down syndrome.
Generally not palpable, although small, nontender, movable nodes are normal	Note tender, enlarged, warm nodes, which usually indicate infection or inflammation *proximal* to their location.

Summary of Physical Assessment of the Child—cont'd

Assessment	Procedure

LYMPH NODES—cont'd

TABLE 1-6   Differences in Color Changes of Racial Groups

Color Change	Appearance in Light Skin	Appearance in Dark Skin
Cyanosis	Bluish tinge, especially in palpebral conjunctiva (lower eyelid), nail beds, earlobes, lips, oral membranes, soles, and palms	Ashen gray lips and tongue
Pallor	Loss of rosy glow in skin, especially face	Ashen gray appearance in black skin More yellowish-brown color in brown skin
Erythema	Redness easily seen anywhere on body	Much more difficult to assess; palpate for warmth or edema
Ecchymoses	Purplish to yellow-green areas; may be seen anywhere on skin	Very difficult to see unless in mouth or conjunctiva
Petechiae	Purplish pinpoints most easily seen on buttocks, abdomen, and inner surfaces of the arms or legs	Usually invisible except in oral mucosa, conjunctiva of eyelids, and conjunctiva covering eyeball
Jaundice	Yellow staining seen in sclera of eyes, skin, fingernails, soles, palms, and oral mucosa	Most reliably assessed in sclera, hard palate, palms, and soles

Assessment	Procedure
HEAD	Note shape and symmetry.
	Note head control (especially in infants) and head posture.
	Evaluate range of motion (ROM). Palpate skull for fontanels, nodes, or obvious swellings.
	Transilluminate skull in darkened room; firmly place rubber-collared flashlight against skull at various points. Examine scalp for hygiene, lesions, infestation, signs of trauma, loss of hair, discoloration. Percuss frontal sinuses in children over 7 years.
NECK	Inspect size.
	Trachea—Palpate for deviation; place thumb and index finger on each side and slide fingers back and forth.
	Thyroid—Palpate, noting size, shape, symmetry, tenderness, nodules; place pads of index and middle finger below cricoid cartilage; feel for isthmus (tissue connecting lobes) rising during swallowing; feel each lobe laterally and posteriorly.
	Carotid arteries—Palpate on both sides.

Usual Findings   **Comments**

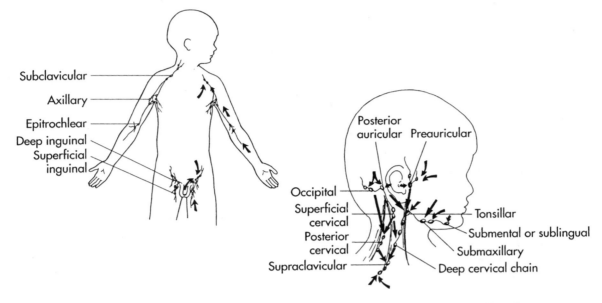

Fig. 1-9 Locations of superficial lymph nodes. Arrows indicate directional flow of lymph.

Usual Findings	Comments

Even molding of head, occipital prominence
Symmetric facial features
Head control well-established by 6 months of age
Head in midline
Moves head up, down, and from side to side
Smooth, fused except for fontanels (See p. 16.)
   Posterior fontanel closes by 2 months
   Anterior fontanel closes by 12 to 18 months
Absence of halo around rubber collar
 	
Clean, pink (more deeply pigmented in dark-skinned children)
Resonant, nontender
	Report any deviations from expected findings.
	Clues to problems include the following:
	   Uneven molding—Premature closure of sutures
	   Asymmetry—Paralysis
	   Head lag—Retarded motor/mental development
	   Head tilt—Poor vision
	   Limited ROM—Torticollis (wryneck)
	   Resistance to movement and pain—Meningeal irritation
	   Halo of light through skull—Loss of cortex (hydrocephaly)
	   Ecchymotic areas on scalp—Trauma (possibly abuse)
	   Loss of hair—Trauma (hair pulling), lack of stimulation (lying in same position)
	   Painful sinuses—Infection

During infancy, normally short with skinfolds During early childhood, lengthens In midline; rises with swallowing In midline; rises with swallowing; lobes equal but often are not palpable	Note any webbing. Note any deviation, masses, or nodules when palpating neck structures. Thyroid is often difficult to palpate. Inquire if child ever received radiation therapy to neck or upper chest area.
Equal bilaterally	Note unequal pulses and protruding neck veins.

Summary of Physical Assessment of the Child—cont'd

Assessment	Procedure
EYES	Inspect placement and alignment.
	If abnormality is suspected, measure inner canthal distance.

Palpebral slant—Draw imaginary line through two points of medial (inner) canthi (Fig. 1-10).

Epicanthal fold—Observe for excess fold from roof of nose to inner termination of eyebrow (Fig. 1-11).

Lids—Observe placement, movement, and color (Fig. 1-10).

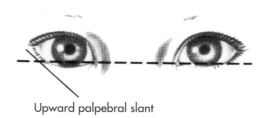

Upward palpebral slant

Fig. 1-10   Upward palpebral slant.

Palpebral conjunctiva

Pull lower lid down while child looks up.

Evert upper lid by holding lashes and pulling *down* and forward.

Observe color.

Bulbar conjunctiva—Observe color.

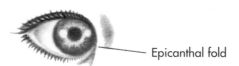

Epicanthal fold

Fig. 1-11   Epicanthal fold.

Lacrimal punctum—Observe color.

Eyelashes and **eyebrows**—Observe distribution and direction of growth.

Sclera—Observe color (Fig. 1-12).

Cornea—Check for opacities by shining light toward eye.

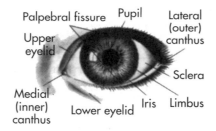

Palpebral fissure   Pupil   Lateral (outer) canthus

Upper eyelid

Sclera

Medial (inner) canthus   Lower eyelid   Iris   Limbus

Fig. 1-12   Normal structures of the eye.

Pupils (Fig. 1-12)

Compare size, shape, and movement.

Test reaction to light; shine light source toward and away from eye.

Test accommodation; have child focus on object from distance and bring object close to face.

Iris—Observe shape, color, size, and clarity (Fig. 1-12).

Lens—Inspect.

Fundus (Fig. 1-13)

Examine with ophthalmoscope set at 0; approach the child from a 15-degree angle; change to plus or minus diopters to produce clear focus.

Measure structures in relationship to disc's diameter (DD).

To facilitate locating macula, have child momentarily look *directly* at light.

Assess vision:

(For visual acuity, see pp. 134-143.)

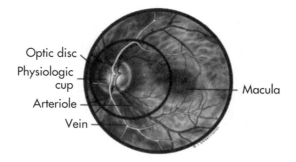

Optic disc
Physiologic cup
Arteriole
Vein

Macula

Fig. 1-13   Structures of the fundus. Interior circle represents approximate size of area seen with ophthalmoscope.

Usual Findings	Comments
Placement is symmetric. Inner canthal distance averages 3 cm (1.2 inches).	Note asymmetry, abnormal spacing (hypertelorism).
Usually palpebral fissures lie horizontally on imaginary line; in Orientals, there may be an upward slant.	Presence of upward slant and epicanthal folds in children who are not Oriental is significant finding in Down syndrome.
Often present in Oriental children.	May give false impression of strabismus.

When eye is open, falls between upper iris and pupil.
When eye is closed, sclera, cornea, and palpebral conjunctiva are completely covered.
Symmetric blink
Color is same as surrounding skin.
	Observe for deviations:
	    Ptosis (upper lid covers part of pupil or lower iris)
	    Setting sun sign (upper lid above iris)
	    Inability to completely close eye
	    Malposition of lids, **ectropion** (turning out) or **entropion** (turning in)
	    Asymmetric, excessive, or infrequent blinking
	    Signs of inflammation along lid margin or on lid

Pink and glossy Vertical yellow striations along edge near hair follicle	Note any signs of inflammation. Excessive pallor may indicate anemia.
Transparent and white color of underlying sclera	A reddened conjunctiva may indicate eyestrain, fatigue, infection, or irritation such as from excessive rubbing or exposure to environmental irritants.
Same color as lid	Excessive discharge, tearing, pain, redness, or swelling indicates dacryocystitis.
Eyelashes curl away from eye Eyebrows are above eye, do not meet in midline	Note inward growth of lashes and unusual hairiness of brows.
White Tiny black marks normal in deeply pigmented children.	Note any yellow staining, which may indicate jaundice.
Transparent	Note any opacities or ulcerations.
Round, clear, and equal Pupils constrict when light approaches, dilate when light fades. Pupils constrict as object is brought near face.	*PERRLA* is common notation for "pupils equal, round, react to light and accommodation." Note any asymmetry in size and movement.
Round, equal, clear Color varies from shades of brown, green, or blue	Note asymmetry in size, lack of clarity, coloboma (cleft at limbus [junction of iris and sclera]), absence of color (a pinkish glow is seen in albinism), or black and white speckling (Brushfield spots are commonly found in Down syndrome).
Should not be seen	Note any opacities.

Red reflex—Brilliant, uniform reflection of red; appears darker color in deeply pigmented children, lighter in infants
Optic disc—Creamy pink but lighter than surrounding fundus, round or vertically oval
Physiologic cup—Small, pale depression in center of disc
Blood vessels—Emanate from disc; veins are darker and about one fourth larger than arteries; narrow band of light, the *arteriolar light reflex*, is reflected from center of arteries, not veins; branches cross each other; may see obvious pulsations
Macula—One DD in size, darker in color than disc or surrounding fundus, located 2 DD temporal to the disc
Fovea centralis—Minute, glistening spot of reflected light in center of macula
	Visualization of red reflex virtually rules out most serious defects of cornea, lens, and aqueous and vitreous chambers.
	Observe for abnormalities:
	    Partial red or white reflex
	    Blurring of disc margins
	    Bulging of disc
	    Loss of depression
	    Dilated blood vessels
	    Tortuous vessels
	    Hemorrhages
	    Absence of pulsations
	    Notching or indenting at crossing of vessels

Summary of Physical Assessment of the Child—cont'd

Assessment	Procedure
EYES—cont'd	Use following tests for binocular vision:
	Corneal light reflex test (also called **red reflex gemini** or **Hirschberg test**)—Shine a light directly into the eyes from a distance of about 40.5 cm (16 inches).
	Cover test—Have child fixate on near (33 cm or 13 inches) or distant (50 cm or 20 inches) object; cover one eye and observe movement of the uncovered eye.
	Alternate cover test—Same as cover test, except rapidly cover one eye then the other eye several times; observe movement of covered eye when it is uncovered.
	Peripheral vision—Have child look straight ahead; move an object, such as your finger, from beyond child's field of vision into view; ask the child to signal as soon as the object is seen; estimate the angle from straight line of vision to first detection of peripheral vision.
	Color vision—Use Ishihara or Hardy-Rand-Rittler test.
EARS 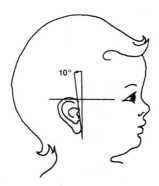 Fig. 1-14 Placement and alignment of pinna.	***Pinnae***—Inspect placement and alignment (Fig. 1-14). 1. Measure height of pinna by drawing an imaginary line from outer orbit of eye to occiput of skull. 2. Measure angle of pinna by drawing a perpendicular line from the imaginary horizontal line and aligning pinna next to this mark. Observe the usual landmarks of the pinna.
	Note presence of any abnormal openings, tags of skin, or sinuses.
	Inspect hygiene (odor, discharge, color).

A T R A U M A T I C   C A R E

Reducing Distress from Otoscopy in Young Children

Make examining the ear a game by explaining that you are looking for a "big elephant" in the ear. This kind of "fairy tale" is an absorbing distraction and usually elicits cooperation. After the ear has been examined, clarify that "looking for elephants" was only pretending and thank the child for letting you look in his or her ear.

Examine external canal and middle ear structures with otoscope (Atraumatic Care box and Practice Alert):
Child below 3 years—Position prone with ear to be examined toward ceiling; lean over child, using upper portion of body to restrain arms and trunk and examining hand to restrain the head.
Alternate position: Seat child sideways in parent's lap; have parent hug child securely around trunk and arms and top of head.
Introduce speculum between 3 and 9 o'clock position in a *downward* and *forward* slant.
Pull pinna *down* and *back* to the 6 to 9 o'clock range (Fig. 1-15, *A*).
Child over 3 years—Examine while seated with head tilted slightly away from examiner (if child needs restraining, use one of the previously mentioned positions).

Usual Findings	Comments
Binocularity is well established by 3 to 4 months of age.	Refer any child with nonbinocular vision due to malalignment (strabismus) for further evaluation.
Light falls symmetrically within each pupil.	Abnormal if light falls asymmetrically in each pupil.
Uncovered eye does not move. Neither eye moves when covered or uncovered.	Abnormal if uncovered eye moves when other eye is covered. Abnormal if covered eye moves as soon as occluder is removed.
In each quadrant, sees object at 50 degrees upward, 70 degrees downward, 60 degrees nasalward, and 90 degrees temporally.	Inability to see object until it is brought closer to straight line of vision indicates need for further evaluation.
Able to see a letter or figure within the colored dots.	Each test consists of cards on which a color field composed of spots of a certain "confusion" color is printed; against the field is a number (Ishihara) or symbol (Hardy-Rand-Rittler) similarly printed in dots but of a color likely to be confused with the field color by the person with a color vision deficit. Counsel the affected child and parents about the practical inconveniences caused by the disorder, the mode of genetic transmission, and its irreversibility.
Slightly crosses or meets this line Lies within a 10-degree angle of the vertical line	Low-set ears are commonly associated with renal anomalies or mental retardation.
Extends slightly forward from the skull Prominences and depressions symmetric	Flattened ears may indicate infrequent change of positioning from a side-lying placement; masses or swelling may make the pinna protrude. Abnormal landmarks are often signs of possible middle ear anomalies.
Adherent lobule (normal variation)	If abnormal opening is present, note any discharge.
Soft yellow cerumen	If ear needs cleaning, discuss hygiene with parent or child. If ear is free of wax, ascertain the method of cleaning, advise against the use of cotton-tipped applicators or sharp or pointed objects in the canal.
External canal—Pink (more deeply colored in dark-skinned child), outermost portion lined with minute hairs, some soft yellow cerumen	Note signs of irritation, infection, foreign bodies, and desiccated, packed wax (may interfere with hearing). If discharge is present, change speculum to examine other ear.

Tympanic membrane (Fig. 1-16)
  Translucent, light pearly pink or gray color
  Slight redness seen normally in infants and children as a result of crying
  Light reflex—Cone-shaped reflection, normally points away from face at 5 or 7 o'clock position
  Bony landmarks present
	Note the following:
	  Red, tense, bulging drum
	  Dull, transparent gray color
	  Black areas
	  Absence of light reflex or bony prominences
	  Retraction of drum with abnormal prominence of landmarks

Summary of Physical Assessment of the Child—cont'd

Assessment	Procedure

EAR—cont'd

Child over 3 years—cont'd
> Pull pinna *up* and *back* toward a 10 o'clock position (Fig. 1-15, *B*).
> Insert speculum ¼ to ½ inch; use widest speculum that diameter of canal easily accommodates.

Assess hearing. (See also pp. 143-146.)

Rinne test—Place vibrating stem and tuning fork against mastoid bone until child no longer hears sound; move prongs close to auditory meatus.

Weber test—Hold tuning fork in midline of head or forehead.

PRACTICE ALERT

Sometimes it takes an extra hand to examine a child's ear—one hand to hold the otoscope, a second hand to use the bulb (or a curette), and a third hand to straighten the canal. To gain a third hand, enlist a cooperative child's help. Have the child raise the arm opposite the affected ear up and over the head toward the opposite side. Then ask the child to grasp the upper edge of the earlobe at about the 10 or 1 o'clock position and pull the lobe gently up and back.

Fig. 1-15 Positions of eardrum. **A,** Infant. **B,** Child over 3 years of age.

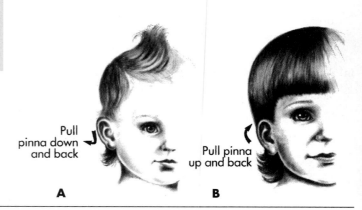

Pull pinna down and back

Pull pinna up and back

A　　　　**B**

NOSE
(Fig. 1-17)

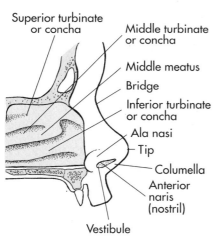

Superior turbinate or concha

Middle turbinate or concha

Middle meatus

Bridge

Inferior turbinate or concha

Ala nasi

Tip

Columella

Anterior naris (nostril)

Vestibule

Inspect size, placement, and alignment; draw imaginary vertical line from center point between eyes to notch of upper lip.

> ***Anterior vestibule***—Tilt head backward; push tip of nose up, and illuminate cavity with flashlight; to detect perforated septum, shine light into one naris and observe for admittance of light through perforation.

Fig. 1-17 External landmarks and internal structures of the nose.

MOUTH AND THROAT

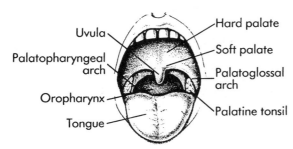

Uvula

Palatopharyngeal arch

Oropharynx

Tongue

Hard palate

Soft palate

Palatoglossal arch

Palatine tonsil

Fig. 1-18 Interior structures of the mouth.

Lips—Note color, texture, any obvious lesions.
Internal structures (Fig. 1-18)
> Ask cooperative child to open mouth wide and say "Ahh"; usually not necessary to use tongue blade (Atraumatic Care box).
> With young child, place supine with both arms extended along side of head; have parent maintain arm position to immobilize head; may be necessary to use a tongue blade, but avoid eliciting gag reflex by depressing only toward the side of the tongue; use flashlight for good illumination.

Usual Findings	Comments

Hears sound when prongs are brought close to ear

Hears sound equally in both ears

Rinne and Weber tests distinguish between bone and air conduction; both tests require cooperation and are better suited to children of school age or older.

Note abnormal results:
Rinne positive—Sound is not audible through ear.
Weber positive—Sound is heard better in *affected* ear.

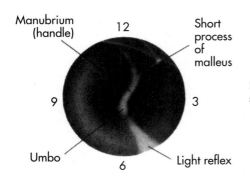

Fig. 1-16 Landmarks of tympanic membrane with "clock" superimposed.

Lies exactly vertical to imaginary line, with each side symmetric.
Both nostrils equal in size.
Bridge of nose flattened in black or Oriental children.

Mucosal lining—Redder than oral membranes, moist, but no discharge

Turbinate and meatus—Same color as mucosal lining

Septum—In midline

Note any deviation to one side, inequality in size of nostrils, or flaring of alae nasi (sign of respiratory distress).
Usually do not use a nasal spectrum to examine internal structures.
Note the following:
Abnormally pale, grayish pink, swollen, and boggy membranes
Red, swollen membranes
Any discharge
Foreign object in nose
Deviated septum
Perforated septum

More deeply pigmented than surrounding skin; smooth, moist
Mucous membranes—Bright pink, glistening, smooth, uniform, and moist
Gingiva—Firm, coral pink, and stippled; margins are "knife-edged"
Teeth—Number appropriate for age, white, good occlusion of upper/lower jaws
General rule for estimating number of teeth in children under 2 years: age (in months) minus 6 (e.g., 12 months minus 6 = 6 teeth)

Note cyanosis, pallor, lesions, or cracks, especially at corners.
Note lesions, bleeding, sensitivity, odor.

Note redness, puffiness (especially at margin), tendency to bleed.
Note loss of teeth, delayed eruption, malocclusion, obvious discoloration.
Compare dental findings with parental report of dental hygiene.

Summary of Physical Assessment of the Child—cont'd

Assessment	Procedure

MOUTH AND THROAT—cont'd

ATRAUMATIC CARE

Encouraging Opening the Mouth for Examination

Perform the examination in front of a mirror.

Let child first examine someone else's mouth, such as the parent, the nurse, or a puppet; then examine child's mouth.

Instruct child to tilt the head back slightly, breathe deeply through the mouth, and hold the breath; this action lowers the tongue to the floor of the mouth without using a tongue blade.

CHEST

(Fig. 1-19)

Inspect size, shape, symmetry, movement, and breast development.

Describe findings according to geographic and imaginary landmarks (Fig. 1-20).

Locate intercostal space (ICS), the space directly below rib, by palpating chest inferiorly from 2nd rib.

Other landmarks:

  Nipples usually at 4th ICS

  Tip of 11th rib felt laterally

  Tip of 12th rib felt posteriorly

  Tip of scapula at 8th rib or ICS

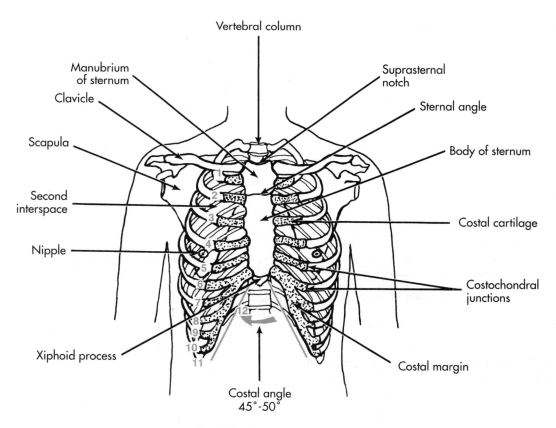

Fig. 1-19 Structures of the rib cage.

Usual Findings	Comments
Teeth—cont'd	Assess need for further dental counseling: Eating habits, such as bottle-feeding or prolonged breastfeeding during day for use as "pacifier" or at bedtime, excessive sugar Toothbrushing Sources of fluoride, need for supplementation Periodic, regular examinations by dentist
Tongue—Rough texture, freely movable, tip extends to lips, no lesions or masses under the tongue	Note smoothness, fissuring, coating on the tongue, excessive redness, swelling, or inability to move the tongue forward to lips; can interfere with speech.
Palate—Intact, slightly arched	Note presence of any clefts.
Uvula—Protrudes from back of soft palate, moves upward during gag reflex	Note if a bifid (divided in midline) uvula is present.
Palatine tonsils—Same color as surrounding mucosa, glandular rather than smooth, may be large in prepubertal children	Note exudate and enlargement that could become obstructive.
Posterior pharynx—Same color as surrounding mucosa, smooth, moist	Assess for signs of infection (erythema, edema, white lesions, or exudate).

Usual Findings	Comments
In infants, shape is almost circular; with growth, the lateral diameter increases in proportion to anteroposterior diameter. Both sides of chest symmetric Costal angle between 45 and 50 degrees Points of attachment between ribs and costal cartilage smooth ***Movement***—During inspiration chest expands, costal angle increases, and diaphragm descends; during expiration, reverse occurs. ***Nipples***—Darker pigmentation, located slightly lateral to midclavicular line between fourth and fifth ribs	Measurement of chest and palpation of axillary nodes may be done here. Note deviations: Barrel-shaped chest Asymmetry Wide or narrow costal angle Bony prominences **Pectus carinatum (pigeon breast)**—Sternum protrudes outward **Pectus excavatum (funnel chest)**—Lower portion of sternum is depressed Retractions (Fig. 1-21) Asymmetric or decreased movement
Breast development depends on age; no masses.	Compare breast development with expected stage for age. (See p. 111.) Discuss importance of monthly breast self-examination with female adolescents.

Summary of Physical Assessment of the Child—cont'd

Assessment	Procedure

CHEST—cont'd

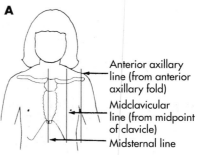

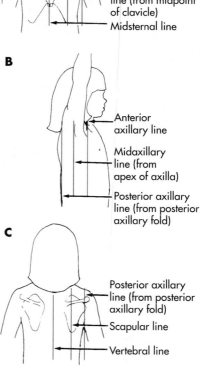

Fig. 1-20   Imaginary landmarks of the chest. **A,** Anterior. **B,** Right lateral. **C,** Posterior.

LUNGS

(Fig. 1-22)

Evaluate respiratory movements for rate, rhythm, depth, quality, and character. (See Atraumatic Care box, p. 54.)

With child sitting, place each hand flat against back or chest with thumbs in midline along lower costal margins.

Vocal fremitus—Palpate as above and have child say "99," "eee."

Percuss each side of chest in sequence from apex to base (Fig. 1-23):

For anterior lungs, child sitting or supine
For posterior lungs, child sitting

Usual Findings   **Comments**

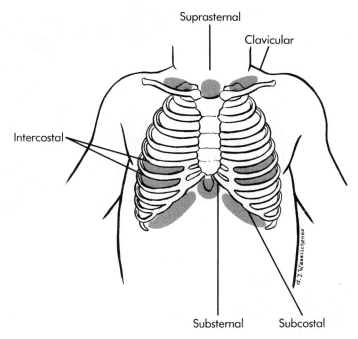

Fig. 1-21   Locations of retractions.

Usual Findings	Comments
Rate expected for age (See inside front cover.), regular, effortless, and quiet	Note abnormal rate, irregular rhythm, shallow depth, difficult breathing, or noisy, grunting respirations (Table 1-7).
Moves symmetrically with each breath; posterior base descends 5 to 6 cm (2 to 2.3 inches) during deep inspiration	
Vibrations are symmetric and most intense in thoracic area and least intense at base.	Note asymmetric vibrations or sudden absence or decrease in intensity.
	Note abnormal vibrations such as pleural friction rub or crepitation.
	Note deviation from expected sounds.

Lobes are resonant except for (Fig. 1-23):
    Dullness at fifth interspace right midclavicular line (liver)
    Dullness from second to fifth interspace over left sternal border to midclavicular line (heart)
    Tympany below left fifth interspace (stomach)	

Summary of Physical Assessment of the Child—cont'd

Assessment	Procedure
LUNGS—cont'd	Auscultate breath and voice sounds for intensity, pitch, quality, and relative duration of inspiration and expiration.

ATRAUMATIC CARE

Encouraging Deep Breaths

Ask child to "blow out" the light on an otoscope or pocket flashlight; discreetly turn off the light on the last try so that the child feels successful.

Place a cotton ball in child's palm; ask child to blow the ball into the air and have parent catch it.

Place a small tissue on the top of a pencil and ask child to blow the tissue off.

Have child blow a pinwheel, a party horn, or bubbles.

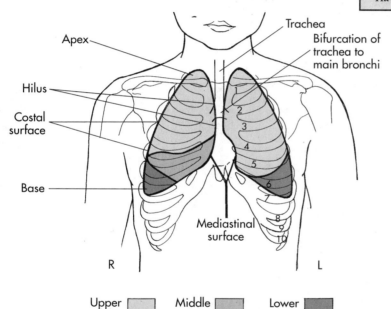

Fig. 1-22 Location of anterior lobes of lungs within thoracic cavity.

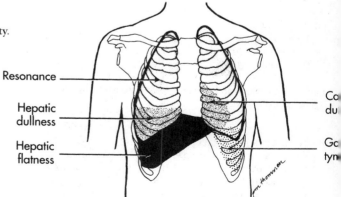

Fig. 1-23 Percussion sounds in thorax.

Usual Findings

Vesicular breath sounds—Heard over entire surface of lungs except upper intrascapular area and beneath manubrium; inspiration louder, longer, and of higher pitch than expiration.

Bronchovesicular breath sounds—Heard in upper intrascapular area and manubrium; inspiration and expiration almost equal in duration, pitch, and intensity.

Bronchial breath sounds—Heard only over trachea near suprasternal notch; expiration longer, louder, and of higher pitch than inspiration.

Voice sounds—Heard but syllables are indistinct.

Comments

Note deviations from expected breath sounds, particularly if diminished; note absence of sounds.
Note adventitious sounds.

Crackles—Discrete, noncontinuous crackling sound, heard primarily during inspiration from passage of air through fluid or moisture; if crackles clear with deep breathing, they are not pathologic.

Wheezes—Continuous musical sounds; caused by air passing through narrowed passages, regardless of cause (exudate, inflammation, foreign body, spasm, tumor).
Audible inspiratory wheeze (stridor)—Sonorous, musical wheeze heard without a stethoscope; indicates a high obstruction (e.g., epiglottitis).
Audible expiratory wheeze—Whistling, sighing wheeze heard without a stethoscope; indicates a low obstruction.
Pleural friction rub—Crackling, grating sound during inspiration and expiration; occurs from inflamed pleural surfaces; not affected by coughing.

Consolidation of lung tissue produces three types of abnormal voice sounds:
Whispered pectoriloquy—The child whispers words and the nurse hears the syllables.
Bronchophony—The child speaks words that are not distinguishable but the vocal resonance is increased in intensity and clarity.
Egophony—The child says "ee," which is heard as the nasal sound "ay" through the stethoscope.

TABLE 1-7	**Various Patterns of Respiration**
Tachypnea	Increased rate
Bradypnea	Decreased rate
Dyspnea	Distress during breathing
Apnea	Cessation of breathing
Hyperpnea	Increased depth
Hypoventilation	Decreased depth (shallow) and irregular rhythm
Hyperventilation	Increased rate and depth
Kussmaul breathing	Hyperventilation, gasping and labored respiration, usually seen in respiratory acidosis (e.g., diabetic coma)
Cheyne-Stokes respiration	Gradually increasing rate and depth with periods of apnea
Biot breathing	Periods of hyperpnea alternating with apnea (similar to Cheyne-Stokes except that the depth remains constant)
Seesaw (paradoxic) respirations	Chest falls on inspiration and rises on expiration
Agonal	Last gasping breaths before death

Summary of Physical Assessment of the Child—cont'd

Assessment	Procedure

HEART

(Fig. 1-24)

General Instructions

Begin with inspection, followed by palpation, then auscultation.

Percussion is not done because it is of limited value in defining the borders or the size of the heart.

Inspect size with child in semi-Fowler position; observe chest wall from an angle.

Palpate to determine the location of the **apical impulse (AI)**, the most lateral cardiac impulse that may correspond to the apex.

TABLE 1-8   Various Patterns of Heart Rate or Pulse

Tachycardia	Increased rate
Bradycardia	Decreased rate
Pulsus alternans	Strong beat followed by weak beat
Pulsus bigeminus	Coupled rhythm in which beat is felt in pairs because of premature beat
Pulsus paradoxus	Intensity or force of pulse decreases with inspiration
Sinus arrhythmia	Rate increases with inspiration, decreases with expiration
Water-hammer or Corrigan pulse	Especially forceful beat caused by a very wide pulse pressure (systolic blood pressure minus diastolic blood pressure)
Dicrotic pulse	Double radial pulse for every apical beat
Thready pulse	Rapid, weak pulse that seems to appear and disappear

Palpate skin for capillary filling time:
Lightly press skin on central site, such as forehead, and peripheral site, such as top of hand or foot, to produce slight blanching.
Assess time it takes for blanched area to return to original color.

Auscultate for heart sounds:
Listen with child in sitting and reclining positions.
Use both diaphragm and bell chest pieces.
Evaluate sounds for quality, intensity, rate, and rhythm (Table 1-8).

Follow sequence (Fig. 1-25):
Aortic area—Second right intercostal space close to sternum
Pulmonic area—Second left intercostal space close to sternum
Erb point—Second and third left intercostal space close to sternum
Tricuspid area—Fifth right and left intercostal space close to sternum
Mitral or apical area—Fifth intercostal space, left midclavicular line (third to fourth intercostal space and lateral to left midclavicular line in infants)

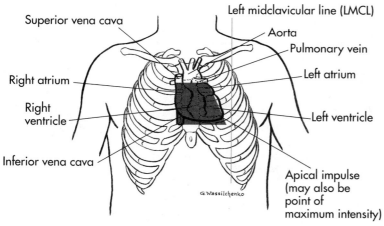

Fig. 1-24   Position of heart within thorax.

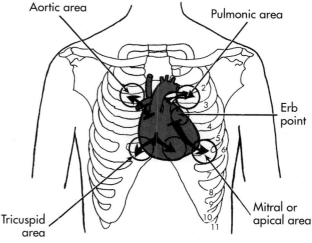

Fig. 1-25   Directions of heart sounds from anatomic valve sites.

Usual Findings	Comments
Symmetric chest wall Apical impulse sometimes apparent (in thin children)	Note obvious bulging. Infant's heart is larger in proportion to chest size and lies more centrally.
Just lateral to the left MCL and fourth ICS in children <7 years of age At the left MCL and fifth ICS in children >7 years of age	Although the AI gives a general idea of the size of the heart (with enlargement, the apex is lower and more lateral), its normal location is quite variable, making it a rather unreliable indicator of heart size; **point of maximum intensity (PMI)**, area of most intense pulsation, usually is located at same site as AI, but it can occur elsewhere. For this reason, the two terms should not be used synonymously. During palpation, may feel abnormal vibrations called **thrills** that are similar to cat's purring; they are produced by blood flowing through narrowed or abnormal opening, such as stenotic valve or septal defect.
Capillary refilling in 1 to 2 seconds	Refilling taking longer than 2 seconds is abnormal and indicates impaired skin perfusion; cool temperature prolongs capillary refill time.
S_1S_2-Clear, distinct, rate equal to radial pulse; rhythm regular and even	To distinguish S_1 from S_2, palpate for carotid pulse, which is synchronous with S_1.
Aortic area—S_2 heard louder than S_1	A normal arrhythmia is **sinus arrhythmia**, in which heart rate increases with inspiration and decreases with expiration.
Pulmonic area—Splitting of S_2 heard best (normally widens on inspiration)	Identify abnormal sounds; note presence of adventitious sounds such as pericardial friction rubs (similar to pleural friction rubs but not affected by change in respiration).
Erb point—Frequent site of innocent murmurs	Record murmurs in relation to the following:
Tricuspid area—S_1 louder sound preceding S_2	Area best heard

Mitral or apical area—S_1 heard loudest; splitting of S_1 may be audible	Timing within S_1-S_2 cycle
	   Change with position
	   Loudness and quality

Quality—Clear and distinct	
Intensity—Strong, but not pounding	
Rate—Same as radial pulse	
Rhythm—Regular and even	
Usual findings of innocent murmurs:	Grading of the intensity of heart murmurs:
Timing within S_1-S_2 cycle—Systolic, that is, they occur with or after S_1	**I**—Very faint, frequently not heard if child sits up **II**—Usually readily heard, slightly louder than grade I, audible in all positions
Quality—Usually of a low-pitched, musical, or groaning quality	**III**—Loud but not accompanied by a thrill **IV**—Loud, accompanied by a thrill
Loudness—Grade III or less in intensity and do not increase over time	**V**—Loud enough to be heard with the stethoscope barely on the chest, accompanied by a thrill
Area best heard—Usually loudest in the pulmonic area with no transmission to other areas of the heart	**VI**—Loud enough to be heard with the stethoscope not touching the chest, often heard with the human ear close to the chest, accompanied by a thrill
Change with position—Audible in the supine position but absent in the sitting position	
Other physical signs—Not associated with any physical signs of cardiac disease	

Summary of Physical Assessment of the Child—cont'd

Assessment	Procedure
ABDOMEN	**General Instructions**

Inspection is followed by auscultation, percussion, and palpation, which may distort the normal abdominal sounds.

Palpation may be uncomfortable for the child; deep palpation causes a feeling of pressure and superficial palpation causes a tickling sensation.

To minimize any discomfort and encourage cooperation, use the following:

Position child supine with legs flexed at hips and knees.

Distract child with statements such as "I am going to guess what you ate by feeling your tummy."

Have child "help" with palpation by placing own hand over examiner's palpating hand.

Have child place own hand on abdomen with fingers spread wide apart and palpate between the fingers.

Inspect contour, size, and tone.

Note condition of skin.
Note movement.

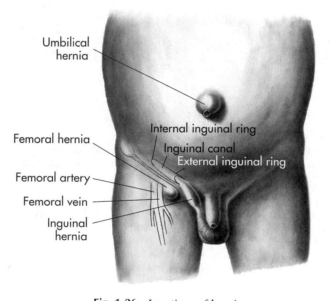

Umbilical hernia

Femoral hernia

Femoral artery

Femoral vein

Inguinal hernia

Internal inguinal ring
Inguinal canal
External inguinal ring

Fig. 1-26   Locations of hernias.

Inspect umbilicus for herniation, fistulas, hygiene, and discharge.

Observe for hernias (Fig. 1-26).

Inguinal—Slide little finger into external inguinal ring at base of scrotum; ask child to cough.

Femoral—Place finger over femoral canal (located by placing index finger over femoral pulse and middle finger against skin toward midline).

Auscultate for bowel sounds and aortic pulsations.
Percuss the abdomen.

Usual Findings	Comments

Infants and young children—cylindric and prominent in erect position, flat when supine
Adolescents—characteristic adult curves, fairly flat when erect
Circumference decreases in relation to chest size with age
Firm tone; muscular in adolescent males
	Contour, size, and tone are good indicators of nutritional status and muscular development.
	Note deviations:
	  Prominent, flabby
	  Distention
	  Concave
	  Tense, boardlike
	  Loose, wrinkled
	  Midline protrusion
	  Silvery, whitish striae
	  Distended veins

Smooth, uniformly taut In children under 7 or 8 years, rises with inspiration and synchronous with chest movement In older children, less respiratory movement In thin children, visible pulsations from descending aorta sometimes seen in epigastric region Flat to slight protrusion; no herniation or discharge	Paradoxical respirations (chest rises while abdomen falls) Visible peristaltic waves If herniation is present, palpate for abdominal contents. Discuss with parents any "home remedies" used to reduce the herniation, especially umbilical hernias; discourage use of any such remedies (e.g., belly binders, taping umbilicus flat).
None	
Bowel sounds—Short, metallic, tinkling sounds like gurgles, clicks, or growls heard every 10 to 30 seconds *Aortic pulsations*—Heard in epigastrium, slightly left of midline Tympany over stomach on left side and most of abdomen, except for dullness or flatness just below right costal margin (liver)	Bowel sounds may be stimulated by stroking abdominal wall with a fingertip. Note hyperperistalsis or absence of bowel sounds. Note percussion sounds other than those expected.

Assessment	Procedure

ABDOMEN—cont'd

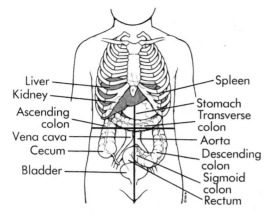

Fig. 1-27   Locations of structures in abdomen.

Liver
Kidney
Ascending colon
Vena cava
Cecum
Bladder

Spleen
Stomach
Transverse colon
Aorta
Descending colon
Sigmoid colon
Rectum

Palpate abdominal organs (Fig. 1-27):
   Place one hand flat against back and use palpating hand to "feel" organs between both hands.
   Proceed from lower quadrants *upward* to avoid missing edge of enlarged organ.
Use imaginary lines at umbilicus to divide the abdomen into quadrants (Fig. 1-27):
   Right upper quadrant (RUQ)
   Right lower quadrant (RLQ)
   Left upper quadrant (LUQ)
   Left lower quadrant (LLQ)

Palpate femoral pulses simultaneously—Place tips of two or three fingers about midway between iliac crest and pubic symphysis
Elicit abdominal reflex—Scratch skin from side to midline in each quadrant

GENITALIA
Male
(Fig.1-28)

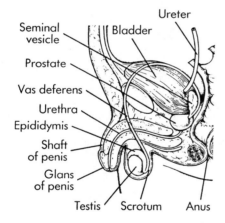

Seminal vesicle
Prostate
Vas deferens
Urethra
Epididymis
Shaft of penis
Glans of penis

Ureter
Bladder

Testis   Scrotum   Anus

Fig. 1-28   Major structures of genitalia in circumcised prepubertal male.

General Instructions

Proceed in same manner as examination of other areas; explain procedure and its significance before doing it, such as palpating for testes.
Respect privacy at all times.
Use opportunity to discuss concerns about sexual development with older child and adolescent.
Use opportunity to discuss sexual safety with young children, that this is their private area and if someone touches them in a way that is uncomfortable they should always tell their parent or some other trusted person.
If in contact with body substances, wear gloves.

Penis

Inspect size.

Glans and *shaft*—Inspect for signs of swelling, skin lesions, inflammation.
Prepuce—Inspect in uncircumcised male.

Urethral meatus—Inspect location and note any discharge.

Scrotum

Inspect size, location, skin, and hair distribution.

Testes

Palpate each scrotal sac using thumb and index finger.

Usual Findings	Comments
Liver—1 to 2 cm below right costal margin in infants and young children	Usually not palpable in older children. Considered enlarged if 3 cm below costal margin. Normally descends with inspiration; should not be considered a sign of enlargement.
Spleen—Sometimes 1 to 2 cm below left costal margin in infants and young children	Usually not palpable in older children. Considered enlarged if more than 2 cm below left costal margin; also descends with inspiration. Other structures that sometimes are palpable include kidneys, bladder, cecum, and sigmoid colon; know their location to avoid mistaking them for abnormal masses; most common palpable mass is feces. In sexually active females, consider a palpable mass in the lower abdomen a pregnant uterus.
Equal and strong bilaterally	Note absence of femoral pulse. Normally may be absent in children under 1 year of age.
Umbilicus moves toward quadrant that was stroked.	Note asymmetry or absence.
	Examination may be anxiety producing for older children, and adolescents; may be left to end of physical examination.
Generally, size is insignificant in prepubescent male. Compare growth to expected sexual development during puberty. (See p. 110.) None	Note large penis, possible sign of precocious puberty. In obese child, penis may be obscured by fat pad over pubic symphysis.
Easily retracted to expose glans and urethral meatus	In infants, prepuce is tight for up to 3 years and should not be retracted. Discuss importance of hygiene.
Centered at tip of glans No discharge	Note location on ventral or dorsal surface of penis, possible sign of ambiguous genitalia, hypospadias, or epispadias. Whenever possible, note strength and direction of urinary stream.
May appear large in infants Hangs freely from perineum behind penis One sac hangs lower than other. Loose, wrinkled skin, usually redder and coarser in adolescents Compare hair distribution to that expected for pubertal stage; typical mature male pattern forms a diamond shape from umbilicus to anus. (See p. 110.)	Note scrota that are small, close to perineum, with any degree of midline separation. Well-formed rugae indicate descent of testes.

Small ovoid bodies about 1.5 to 2 cm long
Double in size during puberty
	Prevent cremasteric reflex that retracts testes by:
	    Warming hands
	    Having child sit in tailor fashion
	    Blocking pathway of ascent by placing thumb and index finger over upper part of scrotal sac along inguinal canal
	Note failure to palpate testes after taking these precautions.
	Discuss testicular self-examination with adolescent male.

Summary of Physical Assessment of the Child—cont'd

Assessment	Procedure

GENITALIA—cont'd
Female
(Fig. 1-29)

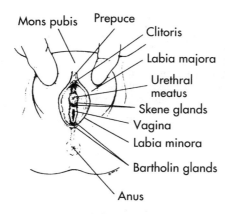

External genitalia—Inspect structures; place young child in semireclining position in parent's lap with knees bent and soles of feet in apposition.

Labia—Palpate for any masses.

Urethral meatus—Inspect for location; identified as V-shaped slit by wiping downward from clitoris to perineum.
Skene glands—Palpate or inspect.

Vaginal orifice—Internal examination usually not performed; inspect for obvious opening.

Bartholin glands—Palpate or inspect.

Fig. 1-29 External structures of genitalia in prepubertal female. Labia are spread to reveal deep structures.

ANUS

Anal area—Inspect for general firmness, condition of skin.
Anal reflex—Elicit by gently pricking or scratching perianal area.

BACK AND EXTREMITIES

Inspect curvature and symmetry of spine.
Test for scoliosis:
  Have child stand erect; observe from behind and note asymmetry of shoulders and hips.
  Have child bend forward at the waist until back is parallel to floor; observe from side and note asymmetry or prominence of rib cage.
Note mobility of spine.

Inspect each extremity joint for symmetry, size, temperature, color, tenderness, and mobility.
Test for developmental dysplasia of the hip. (See p. 19.)

Assess shape of bones:
  Measure distance between the knees when child stands with malleoli in apposition.
  Measure distance between the malleoli when the child stands with knees together.
Inspect position of feet; test if foot deformity at birth is result of fetal position or development by scratching outer, then inner, side of sole; if self-correctable, foot assumes right angle to leg.
Inspect gait:
  Have child walk in straight line.
  Estimate angle of gait by drawing imaginary line through center of foot and line of progression (Fig. 1-30).

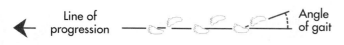

Line of progression   Angle of gait

Fig. 1-30 Measurement of angle of gait.

Usual Findings	Comments
Mons pubis—Fat pad over symphysis pubis; covered with hair in adolescence; usual hair distribution is triangular. (See p. 112.)	
Clitoris—Located at anterior end of labia minora; covered by small flap of skin (prepuce).	Note evidence of enlargement (may be small phallus).
Labia majora—Two thick folds of skin from mons to posterior commissure; inner surface pink and moist.	Note any palpable masses (may be testes), evidence of fusion, enlargement, or signs of female circumcision.
Labia minora—Two folds of skin interior to labia majora, usually invisible until puberty; prominent in newborn. Located posterior to clitoris and anterior to vagina.	Note opening from clitoris or inside vagina.
Surround meatus; no lesions	Common sites of cysts and venereal warts (condylomata acuminata).
Located posterior to urethral meatus; may be covered by crescent-shaped or circular membrane (**hymen**); discharge usually clear or whitish	Note excessive, foul-smelling, or colored discharge.
Surround vaginal opening; no lesions, secrete clear mucoid fluid	
Buttocks—Firm; gluteal folds symmetric	Note evidence of diaper rash; inquire about hygiene and type of diaper (cloth or ultra-absorbent paper; the latter can decrease diaper dermatitis).
Quick contraction of external anal sphincter; no protrusion of rectum	Note: Fissures Polyps Rectal prolapse Hemorrhoids Warts
Rounded or C-shaped in the newborn Cervical secondary curve forms about 3 months of age. Lumbar secondary curve forms about 12 to 18 months, resulting in typical double-S curve. Lordosis normal in young children, but decreases with age. Shoulders, scapula, and iliac crests symmetric	Note any abnormal curvatures and presence of masses or lesions Other signs of scoliosis include: Slight limp Crooked hem or waistline Complaint of backache
Flexible, full range of motion, no pain or stiffness	Note stiffness and pain upon movement of neck or back; requires immediate evaluation. Note any deviations.
Symmetric length Equal size Correct number of digits Nails pink (See assessment of skin, p. 40.) Temperature equal, although feet may be cooler than hands Full range of motion	Note warmth, swelling, tenderness, and immobility of joints.
Less than 5 cm (2 inches) in children over 2 years of age	Greater distance indicates **genu varum (bowleg)** (Fig. 1-31).
Less than 7.5 cm (3 inches) in children over 7 years of age	Greater distance indicates **genu valgum (knock-knee)** (Fig. 1-32). Note foot and ankle deformities (Box 1-3).
Held at right angle to leg; pointed straight ahead or turned slightly outward when standing	
Fat pads on sole give appearance of flat feet; arch develops after child is walking.	
"Toddling" or broad-based gait normal in young children; gradually assumes graceful gait with feet close together.	Note abnormal gait: Waddling Scissor Toeing-in Broad-based in older children
Feet turn outward less than 30° and inward less than 10°	

Summary of Physical Assessment of the Child—cont'd

Assessment	Procedure
BACK AND EXTREMITIES—cont'd	***Plantar reflex***—Elicit by stroking lateral sole from heel upward to little toe across to hallux. Inspect development and tone of muscles. Test strength: 　***Arms***—Have child raise arms while applying counterpressure with your hands. 　***Legs***—Have child sit with legs dangling; proceed as with arms. 　***Hands***—Have child squeeze your fingers as tightly as possible. 　***Feet***—Have child plantar flex (push soles toward floor) while applying counter-pressure to the soles.

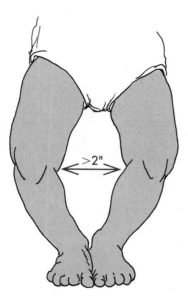

Fig. 1-31　Genu varum (bowleg).

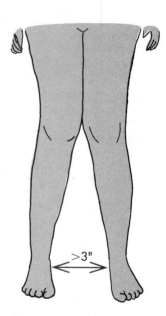

Fig. 1-32　Genu valgum (knock-knee).

NEUROLOGIC ASSESSMENT **Mental Status**	Observe behavior, mood, affect, general orientation to surroundings, level of consciousness. (See p. 459.)
Motor Functioning	Test muscle strength, tone, and development. (See p. 127.) Test cerebellar functioning: 　***Finger-to-nose test***—With the child's arm extended, have child touch nose with the index finger. 　***Heel-to-skin test***—With child standing, have child run the heel of one foot down the shin of the other leg. 　***Romberg test***—Have child stand erect with feet together and eyes closed. Have child touch tip of each finger to thumb in rapid succession. Have child pat leg with first one side, then the other side of hand in rapid sequence. Have child tap your hand with ball of foot as quickly as possible.

Usual Findings	Comments
Flexion of toes in children above 1 year	Babinski reflex seen in younger children. (See p. 21.)
Symmetric Increase in tone during muscle contraction Equal bilaterally	Note atrophy, hypertrophy, spasticity, flaccidity, rigidity, or weakness.

BOX 1-3

Types of Foot and Ankle Deformities

Pes planus (flatfoot)—Normal finding in infancy; may be result of muscular weakness in older child

Pes valgus—Eversion of entire foot but sole rests on ground

Pes varus—Inversion of entire foot but sole rests on ground

Metatarsus valgus—Eversion of forefoot while heel remains straight. Also called toeing out or duck walk

Talipes valgus—Eversion (turning outward) of foot so that only inner side of foot rests on ground

Talipes varus—Inversion (turning inward) of foot so that only outer sole of foot rests on ground

Talipes equinus—Extension or plantar flexion of foot so that only ball and toes rest on ground; commonly combined with talipes varus (most common of clubfoot deformities)

Talipes calcaneus—Dorsal flexion of foot so that only heel rests on ground

---

	Subjective impressions are based on observation throughout the examination. Objective findings can be attained through developmental testing such as Denver II.
Performs each test successfully with eyes opened and closed. During heel-to-shin and Romberg tests, stand close to child to prevent falls.	May be difficult to test in children younger than preschool age. Note any awkwardness or lack of coordination in performance.
Romberg test—Does not lean to side or fall.	Falling or leaning to one side is abnormal and is called the *Romberg sign.*

Summary of Physical Assessment of the Child—cont'd

Assessment	Procedure
NEUROLOGIC ASSESSMENT—cont'd **Sensory Functioning**	Test vision and hearing. (See pp. 134-146.)
	Sensory intactness—Touch skin lightly with a pin and have child point to stimulated area while keeping eyes closed.
	Sensory discrimination: Touch skin with pin and cotton; have child describe it as sharp or dull. Touch skin with cold and warm object (such as metal and rubber heads of reflex hammer); have child differentiate between temperatures. Using two pins, touch skin simultaneously with both or only one pin; have child discriminate when one or two pins are used.
Reflexes (Deep Tendon)	*Biceps*—Hold the child's arm by placing the partially flexed elbow in your hand with the thumb over the antecubital space; strike your thumbnail with the hammer. *Triceps*—Bend the arm at the elbow and rest the palm in your hand; strike the triceps tendon. *Alternate procedure*—If the child is supine, rest arm over chest and strike the triceps tendon.
	Brachioradialis—Rest the forearm on the lap or abdomen, with the arm flexed at the elbow and palm down; strike the radius about 1 inch (depending on child's size) above the wrist. *Knee jerk or patellar reflex*—Sit child on the edge of the examining table or on parent's lap with the lower legs flexed at the knee and dangling freely; tap the patellar tendon just below the knee cap. *Achilles*—Use the same position as for the knee jerk; support the foot lightly in your hand and strike the Achilles tendon. *Ankle clonus*—See p. 21. *Kernig sign*—Flex child's leg at hip and knee while supine; note pain or resistance. *Brudzinski sign*—With child supine, flex the head; note pain and involuntary flexion of hip and knees.
Cranial Nerves	(See Assessment of Cranial Nerves, p. 68.)

Usual Findings	Comments
Localizes pinprick	Use sterile pin or other sharp object (e.g., toothpick), being careful not to puncture skin.
	Compare sensation in symmetric areas at both distal and proximal points.
Able to distinguish types of sensation and temperature	Note difficulty in performing test, especially in older child.
Minimal distance for discrimination on finger is about 2 to 3 mm.	
Biceps—Partial flexion of forearm	Use distraction techniques to prevent child from inhibiting reflex activity:
	For upper extremity reflexes, ask child to clench teeth or to squeeze thigh with the hand on the side not being tested.
Triceps—Partial extension of forearm	For lower extremity reflexes, have child lock fingers and pull one hand against the other or grip hands together.

Usual grading of reflexes:

Grade 0	0 Absent
Grade 1	+ Diminished
Grade 2	++ Normal, average
Grade 3	+++ Brisker than normal
Grade 4	++++ Hyperactive (clonus)

Note asymmetric, absent, diminished, or hyperactive reflexes.

Brachioradialis—Flexion of the forearm and supination (turning upward) of the palm

Patellar—Partial extension of lower leg

Achilles—Plantar flexion of foot (foot pointing downward)

Ankle clonus—Absence of beats
Kernig—Absence of pain or resistance

These special reflexes are elicited when meningeal irritation is suspected.

Brudzinski—Absence of pain or associated movements

Signs of pain, resistance, or associated movements require immediate referral.

Testing of cranial nerves may be done as part of the neurologic examination or integrated into assessment of each system, such as cranial nerves II, III, IV, and VI with the eye.

Cranial nerves can usually be tested in children of preschool age and older.

Note inability to perform any of the items correctly.

Assessment of Cranial Nerves

Cranial Nerve	Distribution/Function	Test
I—Olfactory (S)*	Olfactory mucosa of nasal cavity	With eyes closed, have child identify odors such as coffee, alcohol, or other smells from a swab; test each nostril separately.
II—Optic (S)	Rods and cones of retina, optic nerve	Check for perception of light, visual acuity, peripheral vision, color vision, and normal optic disc.
III—Oculomotor (M)*	Extraocular muscles (EOM) of eye: **Superior rectus (SR)**—Moves eyeball up and in **Inferior rectus (IR)**—Moves eyeball down and in **Medial rectus (MR)**—Moves eyeball nasally **Inferior oblique (IO)**—Moves eyeball up and out	Have child follow an object (toy) or light in the six cardinal positions of gaze (Fig. 1-33).
	Pupil constriction and accommodation	Perform PERRLA. (See pp. 44-45.)
	Eyelid closing	Check for proper placement of lid. (See pp. 44-45.)
IV—Trochlear (M)	**Superior oblique muscle (SO)**—Moves eye down and out	Have child look down and in (Fig. 1-33).
V—Trigeminal (M, S)	Muscles of mastication	Have child bite down hard and open jaw; test symmetry and strength.
	Sensory: face, scalp, nasal and buccal mucosa	With child's eyes closed, see if child can detect light touch in the mandibular and maxillary regions. Test corneal and blink reflex by touching cornea lightly (approach child from the side so that child does not blink before cornea is touched).
VI—Abducens (M)	**Lateral rectus (LR) muscle**—Moves eye temporally	Have child look toward temporal side (Fig. 1-33).
VII—Facial (M, S)	Muscles for facial expression	Have child smile, make funny face, or show teeth to see symmetry of expression.
	Anterior two thirds of tongue (sensory)	Have child identify a sweet or salty solution; place each taste on anterior section and sides of protruding tongue; if child retracts tongue, solution will dissolve toward posterior part of tongue.
	Nasal cavity and lacrimal gland, sublingual and submandibular salivary glands	Not tested
VIII—Auditory, Acoustic, or Vestibulocochlear (S)	Internal ear Hearing, balance	Test hearing; note any loss of equilibrium or presence of vertigo (dizziness).

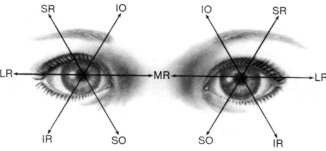

Fig. 1-33 Testing cardinal positions of gaze.

*S—sensory; M—motor.

Assessment of Cranial Nerves—cont'd

Cranial Nerve	Distribution/Function	Test
IX—Glossopharyngeal (M, S)	Pharynx, tongue	Stimulate the posterior pharynx with a tongue blade; the child should gag.
	Posterior one third of tongue (sensory)	Test sense of sour or bitter taste on posterior segment of tongue.
X—Vagus (M, S)	Muscles of larynx, pharynx, some organs of gastrointestinal system, sensory fibers of root of tongue, heart, lung, and some organs of gastrointestinal system	Note hoarseness of the voice, gag reflex, and ability to swallow.
		Check that uvula is in midline; when stimulated with a tongue blade, should deviate upward and to the stimulated side.
XI—Accessory (M)	Sternocleidomastoid and trapezius muscles of shoulder	Have child shrug shoulders while applying mild pressure; with the hands placed on shoulders, have child turn head against opposing pressure on either side; note symmetry and strength.
XII—Hypoglossal (M)	Muscles of tongue	Have child move tongue in all directions; have child protrude tongue as far as possible; note any midline deviation.
		Test strength by placing tongue blade on one side of tongue and having child move it away.

FAMILY ASSESSMENT

Family assessment involves the collection of data about:
   Family structure—The composition of the family (who lives in the home) and those social, cultural, religious, and economic characteristics that influence the child's and family's overall psychobiologic health
   Family function—How the family behaves toward one another, the roles family members assume, and the quality of their relationships

In its broadest sense, "family" refers to all those individuals who are significant to the nuclear unit, including relatives, friends, and other social groups, such as the school and church. The more common method of eliciting information on family structure and function is by interviewing family members. However, several family assessment tools can be used to collect and graphically record data about family composition, environment, and relationships. These tools include screening questionnaires and diagrams.

Theoretic Framework

Family systems theory—The family is viewed as part of an open social system in that the family continually interacts with itself and the environment.
Key features include the following:
   Ability of the family system to adapt
   Change in any member causes a reciprocal change in other members ("ripple" effect)

No family member is identified as the "problem"; the problem lies in the type of interactions engaged in by the family. Change can occur at any point in the family system.

Indications for Comprehensive Family Assessment

Children receiving comprehensive well-child care
Children experiencing major stressful life events, such as chronic illness, disability, parental divorce, foster care, or death of a family member
Children requiring extensive home care

Children with developmental delays
Children with repeated injuries and those with suspected child abuse
Children with behavioral or physical problems that suggest family dysfunction as the etiology

Family Assessment Interview

GENERAL GUIDELINES FOR FAMILY INTERVIEW

Schedule the interview with the family at a time that is most convenient for all parties; include as many family members as possible; clearly state the purpose of the interview.

Begin the interview by asking each person's name and relationship to others in the family.

Restate the purpose and the objective of the interview.

Keep the initial conversation general to put members at ease and to learn the "big picture" of the family.

Identify major concerns and reflect these back to the family to be certain that all parties perceive the same message.

Terminate the interview with a summary of what was discussed and a plan for additional sessions if needed.

STRUCTURAL ASSESSMENT AREAS

Family Composition

Immediate members of the household (names, ages, and relationships)

Significant extended family members

Previous marriages, separations, deaths of spouses, or divorces

Home and Community Environment

Type of dwelling/number of rooms/occupants

Sleeping arrangements

Number of floors, accessibility of stairs, elevators

Adequacy of utilities

Safety features (fire escape, smoke detector, guardrails on windows, use of car restraint) and firearms

Environmental hazards (e.g., chipped paint, poor sanitation, pollution, heavy street traffic)

Availability and location of health facilities, schools, play areas

Relationship with neighbors

Recent crises or changes in home

Child's reaction/adjustment to recent stresses

Occupation and Education of Family Members

Types of employment

Work schedules

Work satisfaction

Exposure to environmental/industrial hazards

Sources of income and adequacy

Effect of illness on financial status

Highest degree or grade level attained

Cultural and Religious Traditions

Religious beliefs and practices

Cultural/ethnic beliefs and practices

Language spoken in home

Assessment questions include:

Does the family identify with a particular religious/ethnic group? Are both parents from that group?

How is religious/ethnic background part of family life?

What special religious/cultural traditions are practiced in the home (e.g., food choices and preparation)?

Where were family members born, and how long have they lived in this country?

What language does the family speak most frequently?

Do they speak/understand English?

What do they believe causes health or illness?

What religious/ethnic beliefs influence the family's perception of illness and its treatment?

What methods are used to prevent/treat illness?

How does the family know when a health problem needs medical attention?

Who is the person the family contacts when a member is ill?

Does the family rely on cultural/religious healers or remedies? If so, ask them to describe the type of healer or remedy.

Who does the family go to for support (clergy, medical healer, relatives)?

Does the family experience discrimination because of their race, beliefs, or practices? Ask them to describe.

FUNCTIONAL ASSESSMENT AREAS

Family Interactions and Roles

Interactions refers to ways family members relate to each other

Chief concern is amount of intimacy and closeness among the members, especially spouses

Roles refers to behaviors of people as they assume a different status or position

Observations include:

Family members' responses to each other (cordial, hostile, cool, loving, patient, short-tempered)

Obvious roles of leadership vs submission

Support and attention shown to various members

Assessment questions include:

What activities do the family members perform together?

Whom do family members talk to when something is bothering them?

What are members' household chores?

Who usually oversees what is happening with the children, such as at school or concerning their health?

How easy or difficult is it for the family to change or to accept new responsibilities for household tasks?

Power, Decision-Making, and Problem Solving

Power refers to an individual member's control over others in family; manifested through family decision-making and problem solving

Chief concern is clarity of boundaries of power between parents and children

One method of assessment involves offering a hypothetical conflict or problem, such as a child failing school, and asking family members how they would handle the situation

Assessment questions include:

Who usually makes the decisions in the family?

If one parent makes a decision, can the child appeal to the other parent to change it?

What input do children have in making decisions or discussing rules?

Who makes and enforces the rules?

What happens when a rule is broken?

Communication

Concerned with clarity and directness of communication patterns

Observations include:

Who speaks to whom

If one person speaks for or interrupts another

If members appear disinterested when certain individuals speak

If there is agreement between verbal and nonverbal messages

Further assessment, such as periodically asking family members if they understood what was just said and to repeat the message

Assessment questions include:

How often do family members wait until others are through talking before "having their say"?

Do parents or older siblings tend to lecture and preach?

Do parents tend to "talk down" to the children?

Expression of Feelings and Individuality

Concerned with personal space and freedom to grow within limits and structure needed for guidance

Family Assessment Questionnaires
General Guidelines for Administration

Be familiar with the questionnaire, especially training requirements, complexity of questions, and expected length of time for completion.

Explain to the family why the questionnaire is being administered and how the information will be used.

Observing patterns of communication offers clues to how freely feelings are expressed

Assessment questions include:

Is it OK for family members to get angry or sad?

Who gets angry most of the time? What does this person do?

If someone is upset, how do other family members try to comfort this person?

Who comforts specific family members?

When someone wants to do something, such as try out for a new sport or get a job, what is the family's response (offer assistance, discouragement, or no advice)?

Discuss the results with the family.

Use the responses to help the family clarify and define what they perceive as any concerns or needs.

Restate the needs to be certain that all parties perceive the same message.

*Family APGAR**

Brief screening questionnaire designed to reflect a family member's satisfaction with the functional state of the family and to record members of household (Fig. 1-34).

Acronym APGAR is for Adaptation, Partnership, Growth, Affection, and Resolve (commitment) (Box 1-4).

Can be used with nuclear families as well as families with alternative lifestyles.

Requires about 5 minutes to complete.

Training is not required to administer the Family APGAR.

Scoring: Choices are scored as follows: "Almost always," 2; "Some of the time," 1; "Hardly ever," 0. Scores for the five statements are totaled. Scores of 7 to 10 suggest a highly functional family; 4 to 6, a moderately dysfunctional family; 0 to 3, a severely dysfunctional family.

A low score in any single item could signal family dysfunction. The Family APGAR is not recommended for use with individuals from enmeshed (overly close) or "psychosomatic" families. Persons with health problems, such as asthma, atopic dermatitis, or irritable bowel syndrome, may report falsely high scores.†

---

*Smilkstein G: The Family APGAR: a proposal for a family function test and its use by physicians, *J Fam Pract* 6(6):1231-1239, 1978.

†Smilkstein G: Family APGAR analyzed, *Fam Med* 25(5):293-294, 1993 (letter to the editor).

*Feetham Family Functioning Survey**†

Provides information about family members' *perceptions* of relationships that contribute to or are affected by family functioning.

Consists of questions relating to (1) relationships between the family and individuals, (2) relationships between the family and subsystems, such as housework and division of labor,

---

*Roberts C, Feetham S: Assessing family functioning across three areas of relationship, *Nurs Res* 31(4):231-235, 1982. The survey is available for a fee from Nursing Systems and Research, Children's Hospital National Medical Center, 111 Michigan Ave., NW, Washington, DC 20010; (202) 939-4980.

†Feetham S, Perkins M, Carroll R: Exploratory analysis: a technique for analysis of dyadic data in research of families. In Feetham S and others: *Nursing in families: theory/research/education/practice*, Newport, CA, 1993, Sage Publications.

and (3) relationships between the family and broader social units; 27 questions specifically address family functioning in terms of household tasks; child care; sexual and marital relationships; interactions with family, children, and friends; community involvement; and sources of emotional support.

Developed as a research instrument; for clinical use, the items should not be scored to determine a family's functional state but to identify areas that may be of concern.

Questions on family functioning are rated on three 7-point scales of "How much is there now?" "How much should there be?" and "How important is this to me?" (Box 1-5); discrepancy between the first two ratings, together with degree of importance, contributes to clinical assessment of the family members' perceptions of those family functions included in the survey and to the identification of areas that may be of concern to the family.

Family APGAR questionnaire

PART I

The following questions have been designed to help us better understand you and your family. You should feel free to ask questions about any item in the questionnaire.

The space for comments should be used when you wish to give additional information or if you wish to discuss the way the question is applied to your family. Please try to answer all questions.

Family is defined as the individual(s) with whom you usually live. If you live alone, your "family" consists of persons with whom you now have the strongest emotional ties.*

For each question, check only one box

	Almost always	Some of the time	Hardly ever
I am satisfied that I can turn to my family for help when something is troubling me. Comments:	☐	☐	☐
I am satisfied with the way my family talks over things with me and shares problems with me. Comments:	☐	☐	☐
I am satisfied that my family accepts and supports my wishes to take on new activities or directions. Comments:	☐	☐	☐
I am satisfied with the way my family expresses affection and responds to my emotions, such as anger, sorrow, and love. Comments:	☐	☐	☐
I am satisfied with the way my family and I share time together. Comments:	☐	☐	☐

*According to which member of the family is being interviewed the interviewer may substitute for the word 'family' either spouse, significant other, parents, or children.

Fig. 1-34 Family APGAR questionnaire. (Modified from Smilkstein G, Ashworth C, Montano D: Validity and reliability of the family APGAR as a test of family function, *J Fam Pract* 15(2):303-311, 1982.)

Family APGAR questionnaire

PART II

Who lives in your home?* List by relationship (e.g., spouse, significant other,†child, or friend).

Please check below the column that best describes how you now get along with each member of the family listed.

Relationship	Age	Sex	Well	Fairly	Poorly
_____	__	__	☐	☐	☐
_____	__	__	☐	☐	☐
_____	__	__	☐	☐	☐
_____	__	__	☐	☐	☐
_____	__	__	☐	☐	☐
_____	__	__	☐	☐	☐

If you don't live with your own family, please list below the individuals to whom you turn for help most frequently. List by relationship, (e.g., family member, friend, associate at work, or neighbor).

Please check below the column that best describes how you now get along with each person listed.

Relationship	Age	Sex	Well	Fairly	Poorly
_____	__	__	☐	☐	☐
_____	__	__	☐	☐	☐
_____	__	__	☐	☐	☐
_____	__	__	☐	☐	☐
_____	__	__	☐	☐	☐
_____	__	__	☐	☐	☐

*If you have established your own family, consider home to be the place where you live with your spouse, children, or significant other; otherwise, consider home as your place of origin, e.g., the place where your parents or those who raise you live.
†"Significant other" is the partner you live with in a physically and emotionally nurturing relationship, but to whom you are not married.

Fig. 1-34, cont'd

BOX 1-4

Family APGAR

Definition	Functions Measured by the Family APGAR	Relevant Open-Ended Questions*
Adaptation is the use of intrafamilial and extrafamilial resources for problem solving when family equilibrium is stressed during a crisis.	How resources are shared, or the degree to which a member is satisfied with the assistance received when family resources are needed	How have family members aided each other in time of need? In what way have family members received help or assistance from friends and community agencies?
Partnership is the sharing of decision-making and nurturing responsibilities by family members.	How decisions are shared, or the member's satisfaction with mutuality in family communication and problem solving	How do family members communicate with each other about such matters as vacations, finances, medical care, large purchases, and personal problems?
Growth is the physical and emotional maturation and self-fulfillment that is achieved by family members through mutual support and guidance.	How nurturing is shared, or the member's satisfaction with the freedom available within the family to change roles and attain physical and emotional growth or maturation	How have family members changed during the past years? How has this change been accepted by family members? In what ways have family members aided each other in growing or developing independent lifestyles? How have family members reacted to your desires for change?
Affection is the caring or loving relationship that exists among family members.	How emotional experiences are shared, or the member's satisfaction with the intimacy and emotional interaction that exists in the family	How have members of your family responded to emotional expressions such as affection, love, sorrow, or anger?
Resolve is the commitment to devote time to other members of the family for physical and emotional nurturing. It also usually involves a decision to share wealth and space.	How time (and space and money) is shared, or the member's satisfaction with the time commitment that has been made to the family by its members	How do members of your family share time, space, and money?

Modified from Smilkstein G: The Family APGAR: a proposal for a family function test and its use by physicians, *J Fam Pract* 6(6):1231-1239, 1978.

*Suggested questions to be used with Family APGAR form.

BOX 1-5

Sample Questions from the Feetham Family Functioning Survey

1. The amount of talk with your *friends* regarding your concerns and problems.
   (15) a. How much is there now?

   LITTLE   MUCH
   1   2   3   4   5   6   7

   (16) b. How much should there be?

   LITTLE   MUCH
   1   2   3   4   5   6   7

   (17) c. How important is this to me?

   LITTLE   MUCH
   1   2   3   4   5   6   7

2. The amount of talk with your *relatives* (do not include your spouse) regarding your concerns and problems.
   (18) a. How much is there now?

   LITTLE   MUCH
   1   2   3   4   5   6   7

   (19) b. How much should there be?

   LITTLE   MUCH
   1   2   3   4   5   6   7

   (20) c. How important is this to me?

   LITTLE   MUCH
   1   2   3   4   5   6   7

Reproduced with the permission of Suzanne L Feetham, PhD, RN, FAAN. Developed from research funded by Division of Nursing, HRA, HHS, NU00632, Wayne State University, Detroit, MI, 1977-1980.

Feetham Family Functioning Survey—cont'd

Requires less than 10 minutes to complete; can be used with single-parent and two-parent families.

Training is not required to administer the survey provided the user has general knowledge of administering measurement instruments; instructions for administration for research and clinical use purposes are included with the survey forms.

Coping-Health Inventory for Parents (CHIP)†*

Assesses parents' perceptions of behaviors they are currently using to manage family life with seriously ill or chronically ill child.

Self-report checklist of 45 coping behaviors defined as personal or collective (with other individuals, programs) efforts to manage the hardships associated with health problems in the family (Box 1-6).

Records how helpful each behavior was on a scale of 0 to 3: "extremely helpful," 3; "moderately helpful," 2; "minimally helpful," 1; and "not helpful," 0.

For behavior not used, parent records why by checking either "I do not cope this way because" (1) "chose not to" or (2) "not possible."

---

*CHIP is available for a fee from Family Stress Coping and Health Project, 1300 Linden Drive, University of Wisconsin-Madison, Madison, WI 53706; (608) 262-5712.

†McCubbin H, Thompson A: *Family assessment inventories for research and practice,* ed 2, Madison, WI, 1991, The University of Wisconsin-Madison.

BOX 1-6

Coping-Health Inventory for Parents

Sample coping behaviors from Coping-Health Inventory for Parents (CHIP):

1. Trying to maintain family stability
2. Engaging in relationships and friendships which help me to feel important and appreciated
3. Trusting my spouse (or former spouse) to help support me and my child(ren)
4. Sleeping
5. Talking with the medical staff (nurses, social worker, etc.) when we visit the medical center
6. Believing that my child(ren) will get better
7. Working, outside employment
8. Showing that I am strong
9. Purchasing gifts for myself and/or other family members
10. Talking with other individuals/parents in my same situation

From McCubbin H, Thompson A: *Family assessment inventories for research and practice,* ed 2, Madison, WI, 1991, The University of Wisconsin-Madison.

Home Screening Questionnaire (HSQ)†*

Assesses child's home environment

Includes two separate forms for children ages birth to 3 years and 3 to 6 years (Fig. 1-35, *A* and *B*)

Completed by parent in any setting

Requires about 15 to 20 minutes for completion

Scoring is based on credits for different answers; for each age group there is a minimal score for determining suspect or nonsuspect results

Training is suggested but not required to administer the HSQ

---

*The forms and manual are available for a fee from Denver Developmental Materials, Inc., PO Box 371075, Denver, CO 80237-5075; call (303) 355-4729 or (800) 419-4729.

†Frankenburg W, Coons C: Home Screening Questionnaire: its validity in assessing home environment, *J Pediatr* 108(4):624-626, 1986.

SAMPLE

Child's Name _____ Birthdate _____ Age _____

Parent's Name _____ Phone No. _____

Address _____ Date _____

HOME SCREENING QUESTIONNAIRE
Ages 0-3 Years

Please answer **all** of the following questions about how your child's time is spent and some of the activities of your family. On some questions, you may want to check more than one blank.

A

FOR OFFICE USE ONLY	

_____   1. How often do you and your child see relatives?
    _____ never
    _____ at least once a year
    _____ at least 6 times a year
    _____ at least once a month
    _____ at least once a week

_____   2. Do you subscribe to any magazines?
    YES   NO   If yes, what kind?
    _____ home and family magazines
    _____ news magazines
    _____ children's magazines
    _____ other

_____   3. About how many hours each day does your child spend in a playpen, jumpchair, infant swing or infant seat?
    _____ none
    _____ up to 1 hour
    _____ 1 to 3 hours
    _____ more than 3 hours

_____   4. Does your child have a toy box or other special place where he/she keeps his/her toys?   YES   NO

_____   5. How many children's books does your child have of his/her *own?*
    _ _ 0: too young
    _____ 1 or 2
    _____ 5-9
    _____ 10 or more

_____   6. How many books do you own?
    _____ 0-9
    _____ 10-20
    _____ more than 20

    Where do you keep them?
    _____ in boxes

    _____ on a bookcase
    _____ other — explain _____
    _____

_____   7. How often does someone take your child into a grocery store?
    _____ hardly ever; prefer to go alone
    _____ at least once a month
    _____ at least twice a month
    _____ at least once a week

_____   8. How many different babysitters or day care centers have you used in the past 3 months? _____

_____   9. Do you have any pets?   YES   NO (include dog, cat, fish, birds, etc.)

_____ 10. About how many times in the past week did you have to spank or slap your child to get him/her to mind? _____

_____ 11. Did you start talking to your child when he/she was
    _____ 0-3 months
    _____ 3-9 months
    _____ 9-15 months
    _____ when he/she was old enough to understand?

_____ 12. Most of the time do you feel that your child
    _____ is usually smiling and pleasant
    _____ prefers to be by himself/herself
    _____ responds readily to affection
    _____ gets angry when he/she doesn't get his/her way
    _____ is often cranky

_____ 13. Do you talk to your child as you are doing the housework?
    YES   NO   TOO YOUNG

Fig. 1-35   Sample Home Screening Questionnaires. **A,** Ages 0 to 3 years.

SAMPLE

Child's Name _____ Birthdate _____ Age _____

Parent's Name _____ Phone No. _____

Address _____ Date _____

HOME SCREENING QUESTIONNAIRE
Ages 3-6 Years

Please answer **all** of the following questions about how your child's time is spent and some of the activities of your family. On some questions, you may want to check more than one blank.

FOR OFFICE USE ONLY	

1. a) Do you get any magazines in the mail?
    YES   NO
    b) If yes, what kind?
    ____ home and family magazines
    ____ news magazines
    ____ children's magazines
    ____ other

2. Does your child have a toy box or other special place where he/she keeps his/her toys?   YES   NO

3. How many children's books does your family own?
    ____ 0 to 2
    ____ 3 to 9
    ____ 10 or more

4. How many books do you have besides children's books?
    ____ 0 to 9
    ____ 10 to 20
    ____ more than 20

5. How often does someone take your child into a grocery store?
    ____ hardly ever; I prefer to go alone
    ____ at least once a month
    ____ at least twice a month
    ____ at least once a week

6. About how many times in the past week did you have to spank your child? _____

7. Do you have a TV?   YES   NO
    About how many hours is the TV on each day? _____

8. How often does someone get a chance to read stories to your child?
    ____ hardly ever
    ____ at least once a week
    ____ at least 3 times a week
    ____ at least 5 times a week

9. Do you ever sing to your child when he/she is nearby?   YES   NO

10. Does your child put away his/her toys by himself/herself *most of the time?*
    YES   NO

11. Is your child allowed to walk or ride his tricycle by himself/herself to the house of a friend or relative?   YES   NO

12. What do you do with your child's art work?
    ____ let him/her keep it
    ____ put it away
    ____ hang it somewhere in the house
    ____ throw it away shortly after looking at it

13. In the space below write what you might say if your child said, "Look at that big truck".

14. What do you usually do when a friend is visiting you in your home and your child has nothing to do?
    ____ suggest something for him/her to do
    ____ offer him/her a toy
    ____ give him/her a cookie or something to eat
    ____ put him/her to bed for a nap
    ____ play with him/her

B

Fig. 1-35, cont'd   **B,** Ages 3 to 6 years. (Reprinted with permission of William K. Frankenburg, M.D. Copyright 1981, 1988, WK Frankenburg.)

Home Observation and Measurement of the Environment (HOME)†*

Assesses child's home environment and interactions with family members

Includes three separate forms for children ages birth to 3 years, 3 to 6 years, and 6 to 10 (Fig. 1-36); forms are also available for children with moderate to severe disabilities in each of the three age groups and for each of the following conditions: visual, auditory, orthopedic, and cognitive impairments

Requires semi-structured interview and direct observation of child and parent in the home

---

*An administration manual is available for a fee from Lorraine Culson (501) 565-7627.

†Caldwell B, Bradley R: *Home observation and measurement of the environment,* rev ed, Little Rock, AR, 1984, University of Arkansas.

Requires approximately 1 hour to administer

All items are scored in binary (plus or minus) fashion; scoring is based on total number of plus (+) answers and compared to percentile scores for ages birth to 6 years (percentile scores are not available for children ages 6 to 10 years or for children with disabilities)

Some items require direct observation

"No" responses indicate possible areas for intervention and counseling

Training is not required to administer the HOME; with careful study and knowledge of child development and family dynamics, the manual serves as an instructional guide, although establishing reliability with a person trained in the use of the HOME is recommended

May not identify strengths or risks in single-parent families or those in low-income groups

Family Resource Questionnaires†*

Several scales are available to measure the adequacy of different resources in households with children, parents' needs for different types of help and assistance, and the helpfulness of sources of support to families with young children.

---

*An excellent source of family resource scales and family functioning scales by Dunst, Trivette, and Deal may be purchased for a fee from Brookline Books, Inc., PO Box 1047, Cambridge, MA 02238-1047; call (617) 868-0360 or (800) 666-2665.

†Dunst C, Trivette C, Deal A: *Enabling and empowering families: principles and guidelines for practice,* Cambridge, MA, 1988, Brookline Books.

Family Assessment Diagrams
General Guidelines for Administration

Be familiar with the diagram, especially directions for its use.

Explain to the family why the diagram is being administered and how the information will be used.

Discuss the diagram with the family.

Use the diagram to help the family clarify and define what they perceive as a concern or need.

Restate the needs to be certain that all parties perceive the same message.

Infant/Toddler HOME Inventory

Bettye M. Caldwell and Robert H. Bradley

Family Name _____ Visitor _____ Date _____

Address _____ Phone _____

Child's Name _____ Birthdate _____ Age _____ Sex _____

Parent Present _____ If other than parent, relationship to child _____

Family Composition _____
(persons living in household, including sex and age of children)

Family
Ethnicity _____ Language Spoken _____ Maternal Education _____ Paternal Education _____

Is Mother Employed? _____ Type of work when employed _____ Is Father Employed? _____ Type of work when employed _____

Current child care arrangements _____

Summarize past year's arrangement _____

Other persons present during visit _____

Comments: _____

SUMMARY

	Subscale	Score Fourth	Lowest Half	Middle Fourth	Upper
I.	RESPONSIVITY		0 - 6	7 - 9	10 - 11
II.	ACCEPTANCE		0 - 4	5 - 6	7 - 8
III.	ORGANIZATION		0 - 3	4 - 5	6
IV.	LEARNING MATERIALS		0 - 4	5 - 7	8 - 9
V.	INVOLVEMENT		0 - 2	3 - 4	5 - 6
VI.	VARIETY		0 - 1	2 - 3	4 - 5
	TOTAL SCORE		0 - 25	26 - 36	37 - 45

A

Fig. 1-36 Home Inventory Questionnaires. **A,** For families of infants and toddlers.

Continued

Infant/Toddler HOME

Place a plus (+) or minus (-) in the box alongside each item if the behavior is observed during the visit or if the parent reports that the conditions or events are characteristic of the home environment. Count the number of +s and enter the subtotal and the total on the front side of the Record Sheet.

I. RESPONSIVITY		24. Child has a special place for toys and treasures.
1. Parent spontaneously vocalizes to child at least twice.		25. Child's play environment is safe.
2. Parent responds verbally to child's vocalizations or verbalizations.		**IV. LEARNING MATERIALS**
3. Parent tells child name of object or person during visit.		26. Muscle activity toys or equipment.
4. Parent's speech is distinct, clear and audible.		27. Push or pull toy.
5. Parent initiates verbal interchanges with Visitor.		28. Stroller or walker, kiddie car, scooter, or tricycle.
6. Parent converses freely and easily.		29. Parent provides toys for child to play with during visit.
7. Parent permits child to engage in "messy" play.		30. Cuddly toy or role-playing toys.
8. Parent spontaneously praises child at least twice.		31. Learning facilitators—mobile, table and chair, high chair, play pen.
9. Parent's voice conveys positive feelings toward child.		32. Simple eye-hand coordination toys.
10. Parent caresses or kisses child at least once.		33. Complex eye-hand coordination toys.
11. Parent responds positively to praise of child offered by Visitor.		34. Toys for literature and music.
II. ACCEPTANCE		**V. INVOLVEMENT**
12. Parent does not shout at child.		35. Parent keeps child in visual range, looks at often.
13. Parent does not express overt annoyance with or hostility to child.		36. Parent talks to child while doing household work.
14. Parent neither slaps nor spanks child during visit.		37. Parent consciously encourages developmental advance.
15. No more than 1 instance of physical punishment during past week.		38. Parent invests maturing toys with value via personal attention.
16. Parent does not scold or criticize child during visit.		39. Parent structures child's play periods.
17. Parent does not interfere with or restrict child 3 times during visit.		40. Parent provides toys that challenge child to develop new skills.
18. At least 10 books are present and visible.		**VI. VARIETY**
19. Family has a pet.		41. Father provides some care daily.
III. ORGANIZATION		42. Parent reads stories to child at least 3 times weekly.
20. Child care, if used, is provided by one of three regular substitutes.		43. Child eats at least one meal a day with mother and father.
21. Child is taken to grocery store at least once a week.		44. Family visits relatives or receives visits once a month or so.
22. Child gets out of house at least 4 times a week.		45. Child has 3 or more books of his/her own.

23. Child is taken regularly to doctor's office or clinic.		**I**	**II**	**III**	**IV**	**V**	**VI**	**TOTAL**
	TOTALS							

Fig. 1-36, A, cont'd

HOME Inventory for Families of Preschoolers (Three to Six)

Bettye M. Caldwell and Robert H. Bradley

Family Name _____ Date _____ Visitor _____

Child's Name _____ Birthdate _____ Age _____ Sex _____

Caregiver for visit _____ Relationship to child _____

Family Composition _____
(persons living in household, including sex and age of children)

Family
Ethnicity _____   Language
Spoken _____   Maternal
Education _____   Paternal
Education _____

Is Mother
Employed? _____   Type of work
when employed _____   Is Father
Employed? _____   Type of work
when employed _____

Address _____ Phone _____

Current child care arrangements _____

Summarize past year's arrangement _____

Caregiver for visit _____   Other persons
present _____

B

SUMMARY

Subscale	Score	Percentile Range		
		Lowest Fourth	Middle Half	Upper Fourth
I. LEARNING STIMULATION		0 - 2	3 - 9	10 - 11
II. LANGUAGE STIMULATION		0 - 4	5 - 6	7
III. PHYSICAL ENVIRONMENT		0 - 3	4 - 6	7
IV. WARMTH AND AFFECTION		0 - 3	4 - 5	6 - 7
V. ACADEMIC STIMULATION		0 - 2	3 - 4	5
VI. MODELING		0 - 1	2 - 3	4 - 5
VII. VARIETY IN EXPERIENCE		0 - 4	5 - 7	8 - 9
VIII. ACCEPTANCE		0 - 2	3	4
TOTAL SCORE		0 - 29	30 - 45	46 - 55

For rapid profiling of a family, place an X in the box that corresponds to the raw score.

Fig. 1-36, cont'd   B, For families of preschoolers.

Continued

HOME Inventory (Preschool)

Place a plus (+) or minus (-) in the box alongside each item if the behavior is observed during the visit or if the parent reports that the conditions or events are characteristic of the home environment. Count the number of +s and enter the subtotals and the total on the front side of the Record Sheet.

I. LEARNING STIMULATION

1. Child has toys which teach color, size, shape.	
2. Child has three or more puzzles.	
3. Child has record player and at least five children's records.	
4. Child has toys permitting free expression.	
5. Child has toys or games requiring refined movements.	
6. Child has toys or games which help teach numbers.	
7. Child has at least 10 children's books.	
8. At least 10 books are visible in the apartment.	
9. Family buys and reads a daily newspaper.	
10. Family subscribes to at least one magazine.	
11. Child is encouraged to learn shapes.	
Subtotal	

II. LANGUAGE STIMULATION

12. Child has toys that help teach the names of animals.	
13. Child is encouraged to learn the alphabet.	
14. Parent teaches child simple verbal manners (please, thank you).	
15. Mother uses correct grammar and pronunciation.	
16. Parent encourages child to talk and takes time to listen.	
17. Parent's voice conveys positive feeling to child.	
18. Child is permitted choice in breakfast or lunch menu.	
Subtotal	

III. PHYSICAL ENVIRONMENT

19. Building appears safe.	
20. Outside play environment appears safe.	
21. Interior of apartment not dark or perceptually monotonous.	
22. Neighborhood is esthetically pleasing.	

23. House has 100 square feet of living space per person.	
24. Rooms are not overcrowded with furniture.	
25. House is reasonably clean and minimally cluttered.	
Subtotal	

IV. WARMTH AND ACCEPTANCE

26. Parent holds child close 10-15 minutes per day.	
27. Parent converses with child at least twice during visit.	
28. Parent answers child's questions or requests verbally.	
29. Parent usually responds verbally to child's speech.	
30. Parent praises child's qualities twice during visit.	
31. Parent caresses, kisses, or cuddles child during visit.	
32. Parent helps child demonstrate some achievement during visit.	
Subtotal	

V. ACADEMIC STIMULATION

33. Child is encouraged to learn colors.	
34. Child is encouraged to learn patterned speech (songs, etc.).	
35. Child is encouraged to learn spatial relationships.	
36. Child is encouraged to learn numbers.	
37. Child is encouraged to learn to read a few words.	
Subtotal	

VI. MODELING

38. Some delay of food gratification is expected.	
39. TV is used judiciously.	
40. Parent introduces visitor to child.	
41. Child can express negative feelings without reprisal.	
42. Child can hit parent without harsh reprisal.	
Subtotal	

Fig. 1-36, B, cont'd

VII.	VARIETY IN EXPERIENCE	
43.	Child has real or toy musical instrument.	
44.	Child is taken on outing by family member at least every other week.	
45.	Child has been on trip more than 50 miles during last year.	
46.	Child has been taken to a museum during past year.	
47.	Parent encourages child to put away toys without help.	
48.	Parent uses complex sentence structure and vocabulary.	
49.	Child's art work is displayed some place in the house.	
50.	Child eats at least one meal per day with mother and father.	
51.	Parent lets child choose some foods or brands at grocery store.	
	Subtotal	

VIII.	ACCEPTANCE	
52.	Parent does not scold or derogate child more than once.	
53.	Parent does not use physical restraint during visit.	
54.	Parent neither slaps nor spanks child during visit.	
55.	No more than one instance of physical punishment during past week.	
	Subtotal	

COMMENTS _____

_____

_____

_____

_____

Fig. 1-36, B, cont'd

HOME Inventory for Families of Elementary Children

Bettye M. Caldwell and Robert H. Bradley

Family Name _____ Date of Visit _____

Observed Child's Name _____ Birthdate _____ Age _____ Sex _____

Caregiver for visit _____ Relationship to child _____

Family Composition _____
(persons living in household, including sex and age of children)

| Family Ethnicity _____ | Maternal Education _____ | Paternal Education _____ | Home Visitor _____ |

Is Mother Employed? _____   Type of work when employed _____   Is Father Employed? _____   Type of work when employed _____

Address _____ How long? _____ Phone _____

Current child care arrangements _____

Summarize past year's arrangement _____

Persons in home at time of visit _____

C

Summary

		Score
I.	EMOTIONAL AND VERBAL RESPONSIVITY	
II.	ENCOURAGEMENT OF MATURITY	
III.	EMOTIONAL CLIMATE	
IV.	GROWTH FOSTERING MATERIALS AND EXPERIENCES	
V.	PROVISION FOR ACTIVE STIMULATION	
VI.	FAMILY PARTICIPATION IN DEVELOPMENTALLY STIMULATING EXPERIENCES	
VII.	PATERNAL INVOLVEMENT	
VIII.	ASPECTS OF THE PHYSICAL ENVIRONMENT	

COMMENTS _____

_____

_____

_____

_____

Fig. 1-36, cont'd   C, For families of elementary children. Home Inventory Questionnaires are available from the Center for Research on Teaching and Learning, College of Education, University of Arkansas at Little Rock, 2801 S. University Ave., Little Rock, AR 72204; (501) 569-3422. (From Caldwell B, Bradley R: *Manual of home observation for measurement of the environment,* rev ed, Little Rock, AR, 1984, University of Arkansas.)

HOME Inventory (Elementary)

Place a plus (+) or minus (-) in the box alongside each item if the behavior is observed during the visit or if the parent reports that the conditions or events are characteristic of the home environment. Count the number of +s and enter the subtotals and the total on the front side of the Record Sheet.

I. EMOTIONAL AND VERBAL RESPONSITIVITY

1. Family has fairly regular and predictable daily schedule for child (meals, daycare, bedtime, TV, homework, etc.).

2. Parent sometimes yields to child's fears or rituals (allows nightlight, accompanies child to new experiences, etc.).

3. Child has been praised at least twice during past week for doing something.

4. Child is encouraged to read on his or her own.

5. *Parent encourages child to contribute to the conversation during visit.

6. *Parent shows some positive emotional responses to praise of child by visitor.

7. *Parent responds to child's questions during interview.

8. *Parent uses complete sentence structure and some long words in conversing.

9. *When speaking of or to child, parent's voice conveys positive feelings.

10. *Parent initiates verbal interchanges with visitor, asks questions, makes spontaneous comments.

Subtotal

II. ENCOURAGEMENT OF MATURITY

11. Family requires child to carry out certain selfcare routines, e.g., makes bed, cleans room, cleans up after spills, bathes self. (A YES requires 3 out of 4).

12. Family requires child to keep living and play area reasonably clean and straight.

13. Child puts his outdoor clothing, dirty clothes, night clothes in special place.

14. Parents set limits for child and generally enforce them (curfew, homework before TV, or other regulations that fit family pattern).

15. Parent introduces interviewer to child.

16. *Parent is consistent in establishing or applying family rules.

17. *Parent does not violate rules of common courtesy.

Subtotal

III. EMOTIONAL CLIMATE

18. Parent has not lost temper with child more than once during previous week.

19. Mother reports no more than one instance of physical punishment occurred during past month.

20. Child can express negative feelings toward parents without harsh reprisals.

21. Parent has not cried or been visbly upset in child's presence more than once during past week.

22. Child has a special place in which to keep his possessions.

23. *Parent talks to child during visit (beyond correction and introduction).

24. *Parent uses some term of endearment or some dimunitive for child's name when talking about child at least twice during visit.

25. *Parent does not express overannoyance with or hostility toward child (complains, describes child as "bad," says he won't mind, etc.)

Subtotal

IV. GROWTH FOSTERING MATERIALS AND EXPERIENCES

26. Child has free access to record player or radio.

27. Child has free access to musical instrument (piano, drum, ukelele, or guitar, etc.).

28. Child has free access to at least 10 appropriate books.

29. Parents buys and reads a newspaper daily

30. Child has free access to desk or other suitable place for reading or studying.

31. Family has a dictionary and encourages child to use it.

32. Child has visited a friend by him/herself in the past week.

33. *House has at least two pictures or other type of artwork on the walls.

Subtotal

V. PROVISION FOR ACTIVE STIMULATION

34. Family has a television, and it is used judiciously, not left on continuously. (No TV requires an automatic NO – any scheduling scores YES).

35. Family encourages child to develop or sustain hobbies.

36. Child is regularly included in family's recreational hobby.

37. Family provides lessons to organizational membership to support child's talents (especially Y membership, gymnastic lessons, art center, etc.).

Subtotal

Fig. 1-36, C, cont'd

Continued

V.	PROVISION FOR ACTIVE STIMULATION (cont'd)	
38.	Child has ready access to at least two pieces of playground equipment in the immediate vacinity.	
39.	Child has access to a library card, and family arranges for child to go to library once a month.	
40.	Family member has taken child or arranged for child to go to a scientific, historical or art museum within the past year.	
41.	Family member has taken child or arranged for child to take a trip on a plane, train, or bus within the last year.	
	Subtotal	

VI.	FAMILY PARTICIPATION IN DEVELOPMENTALLY STIMULATING EXPERIENCES	
42.	Family visits or receives visits from relatives or friends at least once every other week.	
43.	Child has accompanied parent on a family business venture 3-4 times within the past year (e.g., to garage, clothing shop, appliance repair shop, etc.).	
44.	Family member has taken child or arranged for child to attend some type of live musical or theatre performance.	
45.	Family member has taken child or arranged for child to go on a trip of more than 50 miles from his home (50-mile radial distance, not total distance).	
46.	Parents discuss television programs with child.	
47.	Parent helps child to achieve motor skills—ride a two-wheel bicycle, roller skate, ice skate, play ball, etc.	
	Subtotal	

VII.	PATERNAL INVOLVEMENT	
48.	Father (or father substitute) regularly engages in outdoor recreation with child.	
49.	Child sees and spends some time with father or father figure, 4 days a week.	
50.	Child eats at least one meal per day, on most days, with mother and father (or mother and father figures). (One parent families rate an automatic NO.)	
51.	Child has remained with this primary family group for ALL his life aside from 2-3 week vacations, illnesses of mother, visits of grandmother, etc. (A YES requires no changes in mother's, father's, grandmother's or grandfather's presence since birth).	
	Subtotal	

VIII.	ASPECTS OF THE PHYSICAL ENVIRONMENT	
52.	Child's room has a picture or wall decoration appealing to children.	
53.	*The interior of the apartment is not dark or perceptually monotonous.	
54.	*In terms of available floor space, the rooms are not overcrowded with furniture.	
55.	*All visible rooms of the house are reasonably clean and minimally cluttered.	
56.	*There is at least 100 square feet of living space per person in the house.	
57.	*House is not overly noisy—television, shouts of children, radio, etc.	
58.	*Building has no potentially dangerous structural or health defects (e.g., plaster coming down from ceiling, stairway with boards missing, rodents, etc.)	
59.	* Child's outside play environment appears safe and free of hazards. (No outside play area requires an automatic NO).	
	Subtotal	

Fig. 1-36, C, cont'd

Genogram (Family Tree, Family Diagram)

Modified pedigree (See p. 12.) that records composition of family members, usually from three generations

Uses symbols (Fig. 1-37) to represent attachment or intensity of relationship; if symbols other than these are used, add to the genogram a key to explain their meaning

Nuclear family or family members living in household may be designated by drawing a broken line around them.

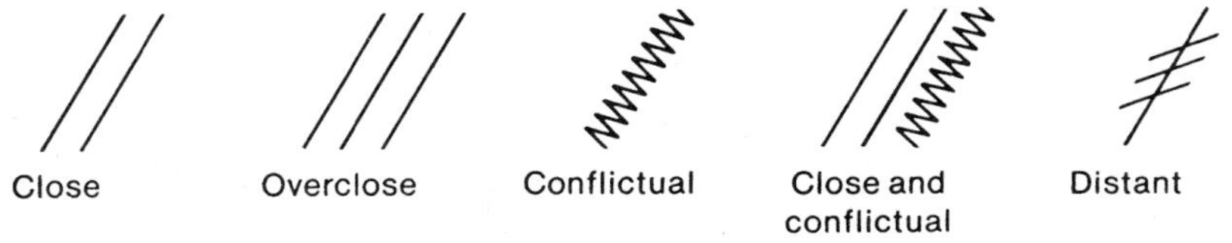

Close   Overclose   Conflictual   Close and conflictual   Distant

Fig. 1-37 Symbols of attachment or intensity of relationship. If symbols other than these are used, add a key that explains their meaning to the genogram.

Sociogram

Use of drawing to identify significant persons in individual's life

Instructions: "Draw a circle to represent you. Around the circle draw circles to represent the most significant persons in your life and label each. Draw the circles in proximity to your circle to represent closeness. For example, the most significant person is the circle closest to you."

Family Circle*

Purpose is same as sociogram but directions differ slightly: "Draw a circle to represent your family. Draw in smaller circles to represent you and the most significant persons in your life. People can be inside or outside the family circle. Draw the circles large or small depending on their significance or influence to you."

In either drawing, family members can label relationships as supportive with a plus sign or negative with a minus sign.

Drawings in both the sociogram and the family circle can be used with children as young as 5 years of age.

Questions for discussion of either drawing include these:

How would you change the circles to improve relationships?

How do you think you could accomplish these changes?

If one person in the circle were to change, how do you think that would affect others?

---

*Thrower S, Bruce W, Walton R: The Family Circle Method for integrating family systems concepts in family medicine, *J Fam Pract* 15(3): 451-457, 1982.

*Ecomap**

Visual presentation of family's support system outside the home

Begins with genogram of immediate family inside one circle and uses other, smaller circles to represent each member's relationships with other significant people, agencies, or institutions (Fig. 1-38)

Size of circles is not important.

Symbols of attachment (See Fig. 1-37.) are used to signify the type of relationship.

Arrows may be drawn along connecting lines to denote flow of energy or resources.

*Hartman A: *Finding families: an ecological approach to family assessment in adoption*, Beverly Hills, CA, 1979, Sage Publications.

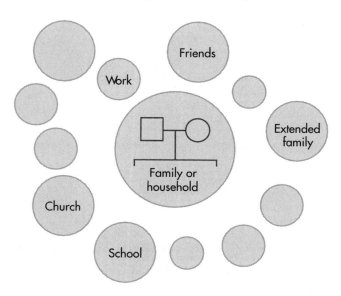

Fig. 1-38 Ecomap. Genogram is completed for immediate family members, and circles are labeled as appropriate. (Modified from Hartman A: *Finding families: an ecological approach to family assessment in adoption*, Beverly Hills, CA, 1979, Sage Publications.)

Role Rating Scale

Provides a numeric rating of the individual's investment in three or more key areas of life, (e.g., parental rating of investment in roles as individual, parent, spouse)

For children, may ask siblings to rate investment in roles as individual, student, son or daughter, or athlete (select roles as appropriate to child)

Instructions for spouses: "In the box, circle if you are the husband or wife. Imagine that your life as an individual, parent, and spouse makes up 100 points. In the appropriate space, write in how many of the 100 points you devote to each part of your life. In the opposite space write in how many points you think your spouse devotes to each part of his/her life" (Fig. 1-39).

SPOUSES' ROLE RATING SCALE		
	Husband	Wife
Individual		
Parent		
Spouse		

Fig. 1-39 Spouses' role rating scale.

ASSESSMENT OF TEMPERAMENT

Temperament is the *behavioral style* or the *how* rather than the what or why of behavior. Nine temperament variables have been identified.*

1. **Activity level**—The activity level of the child.
   Scored in terms of movement during bathing, eating, playing, dressing, handling, reaching, crawling, walking, and sleep-wake cycles.
   High activity refers to high motor activity, such as preference for running or inability to sit still.
   Low activity refers to low motor activity, such as preference for reading or other quiet games and ability to sit still for prolonged periods.
2. **Rhythmicity**—The predictability and/or unpredictability of the child's functions.
   Scored in terms of sleep-wake cycles, hunger, feeding pattern, and elimination schedule.
   High rhythmicity refers to a child with regular bodily habits.
   Low rhythmicity refers to a child with irregular bodily habits.
3. **Approach-withdrawal**—The initial response of the child to a new stimulus.
   Scored in terms of response to new food, toy, person, or experience, such as first day at school.
   Approach refers to predominantly positive response, such as smiling, verbalizations, and reaching for the stimulus.
   Withdrawal refers to predominantly negative response, such as fussing, crying, and moving away from or refusing the stimulus.
4. **Adaptability**—The child's ability to adapt or adjust the routine to fit a new situation.
   Scored in terms of ease of adjusting to new or altered situation (similar to approach-withdrawal), but is concerned with more than the nature of the initial response.
   High adaptability refers to the ability to settle in easily.
   Low adaptability refers to the inability to adjust easily.
5. **Intensity**—The energy level of response, irrespective of its quality or direction.
   Scored in terms of reactions to sensory stimuli, environmental objects, and social contacts.
   High intensity refers to behavioral reactions such as loud crying or laughing in response to a stimulus, such as receiving a new toy.
   Low intensity refers to behavioral reactions such as whimpering or failing to react to a stimulus.
6. **Threshold**—How much stimulus is required before the child reacts to a given situation.

---

*Chess S, Thomas A: Dynamics of individuality: individual behavioral development. In Levine MD and others, editors: *Developmental-behavioral pediatrics*, ed 2, Philadelphia, 1992, WB Saunders.

Scored in terms of level of sensory stimuli needed before child responds.
   Low threshold indicates high intensity to slight stimulus such as waking up to soft sounds.
   High threshold indicates low intensity to moderate to strong stimulus such as lack of discomfort with a wet diaper.
7. **Mood**—The amount of happy, joyful behavior in contrast to unhappy, crying, whining behavior.
   Scored in terms of response to sensory stimuli, environmental objects, and social contacts.
   Positive mood refers to child who is generally pleasant and cooperative.
   Negative mood refers to child who is generally fussy and complaining.
8. **Attention-persistence**—The length of time that a given activity is pursued by the child and the continuation of an activity in spite of obstacles.
   Scored in terms of the child's ability to pursue an activity, such as read a book, or try to master a skill without giving up.
   Long attention–high persistence refers to a child who can pay attention for prolonged periods and continues working on a project or playing despite obstacles, such as a parent telling him to stop or someone interrupting his activity.
   Short attention–low persistence refers to a child who has difficulty paying attention and gives up easily.
9. **Distractibility**—The effectiveness of outside stimuli in diverting the child's behavior or attention.
   Low distractibility refers to the child who is not easily distracted.
   High distractibility refers to the child who is easily distracted.

The three most common patterns of child temperament, which describe most but not all children, are described in Table 1-9.

Approximately one third of children do not fall into the above categories but are characterized by a variety of combinations of temperament variables.

Samples of questionnaires that can be used to assess children's temperament are presented on pp. 90-93. The questionnaires focus on the nine temperament variables through questions that relate to activities appropriate to each age group, such as sleep, feeding, play, diapering, dressing, and response to new experiences. Low scores refer to low activity, high rhythmicity, approachability, adaptability, mild intensity, high threshold, positive mood, high attention-persistence, and low distractibility. High scores reflect the opposite temperament variables. The purpose of the questionnaires is to acquaint parents with their child's type of temperament and to guide them regarding appropriate childrearing techniques.

TABLE 1-9	Three Common Patterns of Child Temperament					
	Temperament Variables					
Pattern (% of Children)	**Activity**	**Rhythmicity**	**Approach/Withdrawal**	**Adaptability**	**Intensity**	**Mood**
Easy (40%)	Moderate	High	Approach	High	Low	Positive
Difficult (10%)	High	Low	Withdrawal	Low	High	Negative
Slow to warm up (15%)	Low	Moderate	Withdrawal	Low	Low	Negative

SAMPLE*

INFANT TEMPERAMENT QUESTIONNAIRE (ITQ)
(FOR 4- TO 8-MONTH-OLD INFANTS)

Child's Name _____ Sex _____

Date of Birth _____ Present Age _____
Month   Day   Year

Rater's Name _____ Relationship to Child _____

Date of Rating _____
Month   Day   Year

The purpose of this questionnaire is to determine the general pattern of your infant's reactions to his/her environment.

The questionnaire consists of several pages of statements about your infant. Please circle the number indicating the frequency with which you think the statement is true for your infant. Although some of the statements seem to be similar, they are not the same and should be rated independently. If any item cannot be answered or does not apply to your infant, just draw a line through it. If your infant has changed with respect to any of the areas covered, use the response that best describes the recently established pattern. There are no good and bad or right and wrong answers, only descriptions of what your infant does. When you have completed the questionnaire, which will take about 25-30 minutes, you may make any additional comments at the end.

USING THE FOLLOWING SCALE, PLEASE CIRCLE THE NUMBER THAT INDICATES HOW OFTEN THE INFANT'S RECENT AND CURRENT BEHAVIOR HAS BEEN LIKE THAT DESCRIBED BY EACH ITEM.

	Almost never 1	Rarely 2	Variable usually does not 3	Variable usually does 4	Frequently 5	Almost always 6
1. The infant eats about the same amount of solid food (within 1 oz.) from day to day.	almost never	1	2	3	4	5	6	almost always
2. The infant is fussy on waking up and going to sleep (frowns, cries).	almost never	1	2	3	4	5	6	almost always
3. The infant plays with a toy for under a minute and then looks for another toy or activity.	almost never	1	2	3	4	5	6	almost always
4. The infant sits still while watching TV or other nearby activity.	almost never	1	2	3	4	5	6	almost always
5. The infant accepts right away any change in place or position of feeding or person giving it.	almost never	1	2	3	4	5	6	almost always
6. The infant accepts nail cutting without protest.	almost never	1	2	3	4	5	6	almost always
7. The infant's hunger cry can be stopped for over a minute by picking up, pacifier, putting on bib, etc.	almost never	1	2	3	4	5	6	almost always
8. The infant plays continuously for more than 10 min. at a time with a favorite toy.	almost never	1	2	3	4	5	6	almost always
9. The infant accepts his/her bath any time of the day without resisting it.	almost never	1	2	3	4	5	6	almost always
10. The infant takes feedings quietly with mild expression of likes and dislikes.	almost never	1	2	3	4	5	6	almost always
11. The infant indicates discomfort (fusses or squirms) when diaper is soiled with bowel movement.	almost never	1	2	3	4	5	6	almost always
12. The infant lies quietly in the bath.	almost never	1	2	3	4	5	6	almost always
13. The infant wants and takes milk feedings at about the same times (within one hour) from day to day.	almost never	1	2	3	4	5	6	almost always
14. The infant is shy (turns away or clings to mother) on meeting another child for the first time.	almost never	1	2	3	4	5	6	almost always

From Carey W, McDevitt S: Revision of the Infant Temperament Questionnaire, *Pediatrics* 61:735-739, 1978.

A copy of the complete questionnaire can be obtained by sending a check for $10.00 to Dr. William B. Carey, Division of General Pediatrics, Children's Hospital of Philadelphia, 34th St. and Civic Center Blvd., Philadelphia, PA 19104, USA; or call (215) 590-4167.

*The first page of the scale is reprinted by permission of the authors.

SAMPLE*

TODDLER TEMPERAMENT QUESTIONNAIRE (TTQ)
(FOR 1-TO 3-YEAR-OLD CHILDREN)

DATA SHEET

Child's Name _____ Sex _____

Date of Birth _____ Present Age _____
              Month   Day   Year

Rater's Name _____ Relationship to Child _____

Date of Rating _____
               Month   Day   Year

RATING INFORMATION

1. Please base your rating on the child's *recent* and *current* behavior (the last *four to six* weeks).
2. Consider only *your own* impressions and observations of the child.
3. Rate each question *independently*. Do not purposely attempt to present a consistent picture of the child.
4. Use *extreme ratings* where appropriate. Avoid rating only near the middle of the scale.
5. Rate each item *quickly*. If you cannot decide, skip the item and come back to it later.
6. *Rate every item*. Circle the number of any item that you are unable to answer due to lack of information or any item that does not apply to your child.

USING THE SCALE SHOWN BELOW, PLEASE MARK AN ''X'' IN THE SPACE THAT TELLS HOW OFTEN THE CHILD'S RECENT AND CURRENT BEHAVIOR HAS BEEN LIKE THE BEHAVIOR DESCRIBED BY EACH ITEM.

	Almost never 1	Rarely 2	Variable usually does not 3	Variable usually does 4	Frequently 5	Almost always 6
1. The child gets sleepy at about the same time each evening (within ½ hour).	almost never	1	2	3	4	5	6	almost always
2. The child fidgets during quiet activities (story telling, looking at pictures).	almost never	1	2	3	4	5	6	almost always
3. The child takes feedings quietly with mild expression of likes and dislikes.	almost never	1	2	3	4	5	6	almost always
4. The child is pleasant (smiles, laughs) when first arriving in unfamiliar places.	almost never	1	2	3	4	5	6	almost always
5. A child's initial reaction to seeing the doctor is acceptance.	almost never	1	2	3	4	5	6	almost always
6. The child pays attention to game with parent for only a minute or so.	almost never	1	2	3	4	5	6	almost always
7. The child's bowel movements come at different times from day to day (over one hour difference).	almost never	1	2	3	4	5	6	almost always
8. The child is fussy on waking up (frowns, complains, cries).	almost never	1	2	3	4	5	6	almost always
9. The child's initial reaction to a new babysitter is rejection (crying, clinging to mother, etc.)	almost never	1	2	3	4	5	6	almost always
10. The child reacts to a disliked food even if it is mixed with a preferred one.	almost never	1	2	3	4	5	6	almost always
11. The child accepts delays (for several minutes) for desired objects or activities (snacks, treats, gifts).	almost never	1	2	3	4	5	6	almost always
12. The child moves little (stays still) when being dressed.	almost never	1	2	3	4	5	6	almost always
13. The child continues an activity in spite of noises in the same room.	almost never	1	2	3	4	5	6	almost always
14. The child shows strong reactions (cries, stamps feet) to failure.	almost never	1	2	3	4	5	6	almost always

From Fullard W, McDevitt S, Carey W: Assessing temperament in one- to three-year-old children, *J Pediatr Psychol* 9(2):205-217, 1984.

*The first page of the scale is reprinted by permission of the authors.

Unit 1

SAMPLE*

BEHAVIORAL STYLE QUESTIONNAIRE (BSQ)
(FOR 3- TO 7-YEAR-OLD CHILDREN)

DATA SHEET

Child's Name _____ Sex _____

Date of Birth _____ Present Age _____

Month   Day   Year

Rater's Name _____ Relationship to Child _____

Date of Rating _____

Month   Day   Year

RATING INFORMATION

1. Please base your rating on the child's *recent* and *current* behavior (the last *four to six* weeks).
2. Consider only *your own* impressions and observations of the child.
3. Rate each question *independently*. Do not purposely attempt to present a consistent picture of the child.

4. Use *extreme ratings* where appropriate. Avoid rating only near the middle of the scale.
5. Rate each item *quickly*. If you cannot decide, skip the item and come back to it later.
6. *Rate every item.* Circle the number of any item that you are unable to answer due to lack of information or any item that does not apply to your child.

USING THE SCALE SHOWN BELOW, PLEASE MARK AN "X" IN THE SPACE THAT TELLS HOW OFTEN THE CHILD'S RECENT AND CURRENT BEHAVIOR HAS BEEN LIKE THE BEHAVIOR DESCRIBED BY EACH ITEM.

	Almost never 1	Rarely 2	Variable usually does not 3	Variable usually does 4	Frequently 5	Almost always 6	
1. The child is moody for more than a few minutes when corrected or disciplined.	almost never	1	2	3	4	5	6	almost always
2. The child seems not to hear when involved in a favorite activity.	almost never	1	2	3	4	5	6	almost always
3. The child can be coaxed out of a forbidden activity.	almost never	1	2	3	4	5	6	almost always
4. The child runs ahead when walking with the parent.	almost never	1	2	3	4	5	6	almost always
5. The child laughs or smiles when playing.	almost never	1	2	3	4	5	6	almost always
6. The child moves slowly when working on a project or activity.	almost never	1	2	3	4	5	6	almost always
7. The child responds intensely to disapproval.	almost never	1	2	3	4	5	6	almost always
8. The child needs a period of adjustment to get used to changes in school or at home.	almost never	1	2	3	4	5	6	almost always
9. The child enjoys games that involve running or jumping.	almost never	1	2	3	4	5	6	almost always
10. The child is slow to adjust to changes in household rules.	almost never	1	2	3	4	5	6	almost always
11. The child has bowel movements at about the same time each day.	almost never	1	2	3	4	5	6	almost always
12. The child is willing to try new things.	almost never	1	2	3	4	5	6	almost always
13. The child sits calmly while watching TV or listening to music.	almost never	1	2	3	4	5	6	almost always
14. The child leaves or wants to leave the table during meals.	almost never	1	2	3	4	5	6	almost always

From McDevitt S, Carey W: The measurement of temperament in 3-7 year old children, *J Child Psychol Psychiatry* 19(3):245-253, 1978.

*The first partial page of the scale is reprinted by permission of the authors.

SAMPLE*

MIDDLE CHILDHOOD TEMPERAMENT QUESTIONNAIRE
(FOR 8- TO 12-YEAR-OLD CHILDREN)

DATA SHEET

Child's Name _____ Sex _____

Date of Birth _____ **Present Age** _____
                  Month   Day   Year

Rater's Name _____ **Relationship to Child** _____

Date of Rating _____
                  Month   Day   Year

INSTRUCTIONS TO PARENT

1. There are no *right* or *wrong* or good or bad answers, only descriptions of your child.
2. Please base your rating on the child's *recent* and *current* behavior (the last *four to six* weeks).
3. Rate each question *separately*. Do not purposely try to present a consistent picture of your child.
4. Use *extreme ratings* where appropriate. Try to avoid rating only near the middle of each scale.
5. Rate each item *quickly*. If you cannot decide, skip the item and come back to it later.
6. *Rate every item*. Please circle any item you are unable to answer due to lack of information or any item that does not apply to your child.
7. Consider only *your own* impressions and observations of the child.

USING THE SCALE SHOWN BELOW, PLEASE MARK AN "X" IN THE SPACE THAT TELLS HOW OFTEN THE CHILD'S RECENT AND CURRENT BEHAVIOR HAS BEEN LIKE THE BEHAVIOR DESCRIBED BY EACH ITEM.

	Almost never 1	Rarely 2	Variable usually does not 3	Variable usually does 4	Frequently 5	Almost always 6
1. Runs to get where he/she wants to go.	almost never	1	2	3	4	5	6	almost always
2. Avoids (stays away from, doesn't talk to) a new sitter on first meeting.	almost never	1	2	3	4	5	6	almost always
3. Easily excited by praise (laughs, claps, yells, etc.).	almost never	1	2	3	4	5	6	almost always
4. Frowns or complains when asked by the parent to do a chore.	almost never	1	2	3	4	5	6	almost always
5. Notices (looks toward) minor changes in lighting (changes in shadows, turning on lights, etc.).	almost never	1	2	3	4	5	6	almost always
6. Loses interest in a new toy or game the same day she/he gets it.	almost never	1	2	3	4	5	6	almost always
7. Has difficulty (asks for advice, takes a long time, etc.) making decisions.	almost never	1	2	3	4	5	6	almost always
8. Uncomfortable with wet or dirty clothes, wants to change right away.	almost never	1	2	3	4	5	6	almost always
9. Shows strong reactions (yells, shouts, etc.) when pleasantly surprised.	almost never	1	2	3	4	5	6	almost always
10. Responses to parent's instructions are predictable.	almost never	1	2	3	4	5	6	almost always
11. Remains pleasant (smiles, etc.) even when tired.	almost never	1	2	3	4	5	6	almost always
12. Looks up right away from play when telephone or doorbell rings.	almost never	1	2	3	4	5	6	almost always
13. Moves right into a new place (store, theater, playground).	almost never	1	2	3	4	5	6	almost always
14. Adjusts within a day or two to changes in routine (different bed time, new chores, etc.).	almost never	1	2	3	4	5	6	almost always

From Hegvik R, McDevitt S, Carey W. The Middle Childhood Temperament Questionnaire, *J Develop Behavior Pediatr* 3:197-200, 1982.
*The first page of the scale is reprinted by permission of the authors.

NUTRITIONAL ASSESSMENT

A nutritional assessment is an essential part of a complete health appraisal. Its purpose is to evaluate the child's nutritional status—the state of balance between nutrient intake and nutrient expenditure or need. A thorough nutritional assessment includes information about dietary intake, clinical assessment of nutritional status, and biochemical status.

Information about dietary intake usually begins with a dietary history (see below) and may be coupled with a more detailed account of actual food intake. Two methods of recording food intake are a food diary and food frequency record. The *food diary* is a record of every food and liquid consumed for a certain number of days, usually 2 weekdays and 1 weekend day (p. 95). A *food frequency record* provides information about the number of times in a day or week items from the Food Guide Pyramid (p. 180) are consumed.

Clinical assessment of nutritional status provides information regarding signs of adequate nutrition and deficient or excess nutrition. The overview on pp. 97-99 also identifies specific nutrients that may be responsible for abnormal clinical findings. In addition, measurement of height, weight, head circumference, skinfold thickness, and arm circumference are assessed. Techniques for measurement are on pp. 28-31 and expected norms are on pp. 113-126.

A number of biochemical tests are available for studying nutritional status. Common laboratory procedures for nutritional status include measurement of hemoglobin, hematocrit, transferrin, albumin, creatinine, and nitrogen. (See Common Laboratory Tests in Unit 6.)

Dietary History

What are the family's usual mealtimes?
Do family members eat together or at separate times?
Who does the family grocery shopping and meal preparation?
How much money is spent to buy food each week?
How are most foods prepared—baked, broiled, boiled, microwaved, stir-fried, deep-fried, other?
How often does the family or your child eat out?
    What kinds of restaurants do you go to?
    What kinds of food does your child typically eat at restaurants?
Does your child eat breakfast regularly?
Where does your child eat lunch?
What are your child's favorite foods, beverages, and snacks?
    What are the average amounts eaten per day?
    What foods are artificially sweetened?
    What are your child's snacking habits?
    When are sweet foods usually eaten?
    What are your child's toothbrushing habits?

What special cultural practices are followed?
    What ethnic foods are eaten?
What foods and beverages does your child dislike?
How would you describe your child's usual appetite (hearty eater, picky eater)?
What are your child's feeding habits (breast, bottle, cup, spoon, eats by self, needs assistance, any special devices)?
Does your child take vitamins or other supplements; do they contain iron or fluoride?
Are there any known or suspected food allergies; is your child on a special diet?
Has your child lost or gained weight recently?
Are there any feeding problems (excessive fussiness, spitting up, colic, difficulty sucking or swallowing); any dental problems or appliances, such as braces, that affect eating?
What types of exercise does your child do regularly?
Is there a family history of cancer, diabetes, heart disease, high blood pressure, or obesity?

Additional Questions for Infant Feeding

What was your infant's birth weight; when did it double, triple?
Was your infant premature?
Are you breast-feeding or have you breast-fed your infant? For how long?
If you use a formula, what is the brand?
    How long has your infant been taking it?
    How many ounces does your infant drink a day?
Are you giving your infant cow's milk (whole, low-fat, skim)? When did you start?
    How many ounces does your infant drink a day?
Do you give your infant extra fluids (water, juice)?
If your infant takes a bottle to bed at nap or nighttime, what is in the bottle?

At what age did you start feeding cereal, vegetables, meat or other protein sources, fruit/juice, finger food, and table food?
Do you make your own baby food or use commercial foods, such as infant cereal?
Does your infant take a vitamin/mineral supplement? If so, what type?
Has your infant shown an allergic reaction to any food(s)? If so, list the foods and describe the reaction.
Does your infant spit up frequently, have unusually loose stools, or have hard, dry stools? If so, how often?
How often do you feed your infant?
How would you describe your infant's appetite?

Food Diary

Meals and Snacks		Description of Food Items			With Whom Eaten?	Any Related Factors? (Associated Activity, Place, Persons, Money, Feelings, Hunger, etc.)
TOTAL FOOD INTAKE						**COMMENTS**
Time	Place	Food	Amount	Type of Preparation		

From Williams S: *Handbook of material and infant nutrition*, Berkeley, CA, 1976, SRW Productions, Inc.

Food Frequency Record*

Food group	Number of servings (day, week)	Serving size (in cup, tablespoon, or ounce portions)	Food group	Number of servings (day, week)	Serving size (in cup, tablespoon, or ounce portions)
BREADS/CEREALS/RICE/PASTA			**MILK/CHEESE/YOGURT**		
Bread, tortilla			Milk		
Cooked pasta, rice, hot cereal			Cheese		
Dry cereal (not pre-sweetened)			Yogurt		
Crackers			Pudding		
Muffins			Ice cream		
Other			Other		
VEGETABLES			**OTHER PROTEIN FOODS**		
Yellow or orange			Meat		
Green/leafy			Fish		
Other			Poultry		
			Egg		
			Peanut butter		
			Legumes (dried beans, peas)		
			Nuts		
			Other		
FRUITS/JUICE			**FATS/OILS/SWEETS**		
Citrus (orange, grapefruit, tangerine)			Butter, oil, margarine, mayonnaise, salad dressing		
Non-citrus			Soda, punch		
Other			Cake/cookie, etc.		
			Candy		
			Presweetened cereal		

*For comparison of actual intake with recommended intake, see Food Guide Pyramid, p. 180.

Clinical Assessment of Nutritional Status

Evidence of Adequate Nutrition	Evidence of Deficient or Excess Nutrition	Deficiency/Excess*
GENERAL GROWTH		
Within 5th and 95th percentiles for height, weight, and head circumference	Below 5th or above 95th percentiles for growth	Protein, calories, fats, and other essential nutrients, especially vitamin A, pyridoxine, niacin, calcium, iodine, manganese, zinc
Steady gain with expected growth spurts during infancy and adolescence	Absence of or delayed growth spurts; poor weight gain	
Sexual development appropriate for age	Delayed sexual development	Excess vitamin A, D
SKIN		
Smooth, slightly dry to touch	Hardening and scaling	Vitamin A
Elastic and firm	Seborrheic dermatitis	Excess niacin
Absence of lesions	Dry, rough, pectechiae	Riboflavin
Color appropriate to genetic background	Delayed wound healing	Vitamin C
	Scaly dermatitis on exposed surfaces	Riboflavin, vitamin C, zinc
	Wrinkled, flabby	Niacin
	Crusted lesions around orifices, especially nares	Protein and calories
		Zinc
	Pruritus	Excess vitamin A, riboflavin, niacin
	Poor turgor	Water, sodium
	Edema	Protein, thiamin
		Excess sodium
	Yellow tinge (jaundice)	Vitamin B$_{12}$
		Excess vitamin A, niacin
	Depigmentation	Protein, calories
	Pallor (anemia)	Pyridoxine, folic acid, vitamin B$_{12}$, C, E (in premature infants), iron
		Excess vitamin C, zinc
	Paresthesia	Excess riboflavin
HAIR		
Lustrous, silky, strong, elastic	Stringy, friable, dull, dry, thin	Protein, calories
	Alopecia	Protein, calories, zinc
	Depigmentation	Protein, calories, copper
	Raised areas around hair follicles	Vitamin C
HEAD		
Even molding, occipital prominence, symmetric facial features	Softening of cranial bones, prominence of frontal bones, skull flat and depressed toward middle	Vitamin D
Fused sutures after 18 months	Delayed fusion of sutures	Vitamin D
	Hard tender lumps in occiput	Excess vitamin A
	Headache	Excess thiamin
NECK		
Thyroid not visible, palpable in midline	Thyroid enlarged; may be grossly visible	Iodine
EYES		
Clear, bright	Hardening and scaling of cornea and conjunctiva	Vitamin A
Good night vision	Night blindness	
Conjunctiva—Pink, glossy	Burning, itching, photophobia, cataracts, corneal vascularization	Riboflavin

*Nutrients listed are deficient unless specified as excess.

Continued

Clinical Assessment of Nutritional Status—cont'd

Evidence of Adequate Nutrition	Evidence of Deficient or Excess Nutrition	Deficiency/Excess*
EARS		
Tympanic membrane—Pliable	Calcified (hearing loss)	Excess vitamin D
NOSE		
Smooth, intact nasal angle	Irritation and cracks at nasal angle	Riboflavin Excess vitamin A
MOUTH		
Lips—Smooth, moist, darker color than skin	Fissures and inflammation at corners	Riboflavin Excess vitamin A
Gums—Firm, coral pink, stippled	Spongy, friable, swollen, bluish red or black, bleed easily	Vitamin C
Mucous membranes—Bright pink, smooth, moist	Stomatitis	Niacin
Tongue—Rough texture, no lesions, taste sensation	Glossitis Diminished taste sensation	Niacin, riboflavin, folic acid Zinc
Teeth—Uniform white, smooth, intact	Brown mottling, pits, fissures Defective enamel Caries	Excess fluoride Vitamins A, C, D, calcium, phosphorus Excess carbohydrates
CHEST		
In infants, shape is almost circular	Depressed lower portion of rib cage	Vitamin D
In children, lateral diameter increases in proportion to anteroposterior diameter	Sharp protrusion of sternum	
Smooth costochondral junctions	Enlarged costochondral junctions	Vitamin C, D
Breast development—Normal for age	Delayed development	(See General Growth p. 97, especially zinc.)
CARDIOVASCULAR SYSTEM		
Pulse and blood pressure (BP) within normal limits	Palpitations Rapid pulse	Thiamin Potassium Excess thiamin
	Arrhythmias	Magnesium, potassium Excess niacin, potassium
	Increased BP Decreased BP	Excess sodium Thiamin; excess niacin
ABDOMEN		
In young children, cylindric and prominent	Distended, flabby, poor musculature Prominent, large	Protein, calories Excess calories
In older children, flat	Potbelly, constipation	Vitamin D
Normal bowel habits	Diarrhea	Niacin Excess vitamin C
	Constipation	Excess calcium, potassium

*Nutrients listed are deficient unless specified as excess.

Clinical Assessment of Nutritional Status—cont'd

Evidence of Adequate Nutrition	Evidence of Deficient or Excess Nutrition	Deficiency/Excess*
MUSCULOSKELETAL SYSTEM		
Muscles—Firm, well-developed, equal strength bilaterally	Flabby, weak, generalized wasting	Protein, calories
	Weakness, pain, cramps	Thiamin, sodium, chloride, potassium, phosphorus, magnesium
		Excess thiamin
	Muscle twitching, tremors	Magnesium
	Muscular paralysis	Excess potassium
Spine—Cervical and lumbar curves (double S curve)	Kyphosis, lordosis, scoliosis	Vitamin D
Extremities—Symmetric; legs straight with minimum bowing	Bowing of extremities, knock-knees	Vitamin D, calcium, phosphorus
	Epiphyseal enlargement	Vitamin A, D
	Bleeding into joints and muscles, joint swelling, pain	Vitamin C
Joints—Flexible, full range of motion, no pain or stiffness	Thickening of cortex of long bones with pain and fragility; hard, tender lumps in extremities	Excess vitamin A
	Osteoporosis of long bones	Calcium; excess vitamin D
NEUROLOGIC SYSTEM		
Behavior—Alert, responsive, emotionally stable	Listless, irritable, lethargic, apathetic (sometimes apprehensive, anxious, drowsy, mentally slow, confused)	Thiamin, niacin, pyridoxine, vitamin C, potassium, magnesium, iron, protein, calories
	Masklike facial expression, blurred speech, involuntary laughing	Excess vitamin A, D, thiamin, folic acid, calcium
		Excess manganese
Absence of tetany and convulsions	Convulsions	Thiamin, pyridoxine, vitamin D, calcium, magnesium
		Excess phosphorus (in relation to calcium)
Intact peripheral nervous system	Peripheral nervous system toxicity (unsteady gait, numb feet and hands, fine motor clumsiness)	Excess pyridoxine
Intact reflexes	Diminished or absent tendon reflexes	Thiamin, vitamin E

*Nutrients listed are deficient unless specified as excess.

Recommended Dietary Allowances[a]
(Designed for the maintenance of good nutrition of practically all healthy people in the United States)

Category	Age (Years) or Condition	Weight[b] (kg)	Weight[b] (lb)	Height[b] (cm)	Height[b] (in)	Protein (g)	Fat-Soluble Vitamins Vitamin A (µg RE)[c]	Vitamin D (µg)[d]	Vitamin E (mg α-TE)[e]	Vita-min K (µg)
Infants	0.0-0.5	6	13	60	24	13	375	7.5	3	5
	0.5-1.0	9	20	71	28	14	375	10	4	10
Children	1-3	13	29	90	35	16	400	10	6	15
	4-6	20	44	112	44	24	500	10	7	20
	7-10	28	62	132	52	28	700	10	7	30
Males	11-14	45	99	157	62	45	1,000	10	10	45
	15-18	66	145	176	69	59	1,000	10	10	65
	19-24	72	160	177	70	58	1,000	10	10	70
	25-50	79	174	176	70	63	1,000	5	10	80
	51+	77	170	173	68	63	1,000	5	10	80
Females	11-14	46	101	157	62	46	800	10	8	45
	15-18	55	120	163	64	44	800	10	8	55
	19-24	58	128	164	65	46	800	10	8	60
	25-50	63	138	163	64	50	800	5	8	65
	51+	65	143	160	63	50	800	5	8	65
Pregnant						60	800	10	10	65
Lactating	1st 6 months					65	1,300	10	12	65
	2nd 6 months					62	1,200	10	11	65

From Food and Nutrition Board, National Academy of Sciences-National Research Council, Washington, D.C., 1989.

[a]The allowances, expressed as average daily intakes over time, are intended to provide for individual variations among most normal persons as they live in the United States under usual environmental stresses. Diets should be based on a variety of common foods in order to provide other nutrients for which human requirements have been less well defined.

[b]Weights and heights of Reference Adults are actual medians for the U.S. population of the designated age, as reported by NHANES II. The median weights and heights of those under 19 years of age were taken from Hamill and others (1979). The use of these figures does not imply that the height-to-weight ratios are ideal.

[c]Retinol equivalents. 1 Retinol equivalent = 1 µg retinol or 6 µg β-carotene.

[d]As cholecalciferol. 10 µg cholecalciferol = 400 IU vitamin D.

[e]α-Tocopherol equivalents. 1 mg d-α-tocopherol = 1 α-TE.

[f]1 NE (niacin equivalent) is equal to 1 mg of niacin or 60 mg of dietary tryptophan.

Water-Soluble Vitamins							Minerals						
Vita-min C (mg)	Thi-amin (mg)	Ribo-flavin (mg)	Niacin (mg NE)^f	Vita-min B$_6$ (mg)	Folate (µg)	Vita-min B$_{12}$ (µg)	Cal-cium (mg)	Phos-phorus (mg)	Mag-nesium (mg)	Iron (mg)	Zinc (mg)	Iodine (µg)	Sele-nium (µg)
30	0.3	0.4	5	0.3	25	0.3	400	300	40	6	5	40	10
35	0.4	0.5	6	0.6	35	0.5	600	500	60	10	5	50	15
40	0.7	0.8	9	1.0	50	0.7	800	800	80	10	10	70	20
45	0.9	1.1	12	1.1	75	1.0	800	800	120	10	10	90	20
45	1.0	1.2	13	1.4	100	1.4	800	800	170	10	10	120	30
50	1.3	1.5	17	1.7	150	2.0	1,200	1,200	270	12	15	150	40
60	1.5	1.8	20	2.0	200	2.0	1,200	1,200	400	12	15	150	50
60	1.5	1.7	19	2.0	200	2.0	1,200	1,200	350	10	15	150	70
60	1.5	1.7	19	2.0	200	2.0	800	800	350	10	15	150	70
60	1.2	1.4	15	2.0	200	2.0	800	800	350	10	15	150	70
50	1.1	1.3	15	1.4	150	2.0	1,200	1,200	280	15	12	150	45
60	1.1	1.3	15	1.5	180	2.0	1,200	1,200	300	15	12	150	50
60	1.1	1.3	15	1.6	180	2.0	1,200	1,200	280	15	12	150	55
60	1.1	1.3	15	1.6	180	2.0	800	800	280	15	12	150	55
60	1.0	1.2	13	1.6	180	2.0	800	800	280	10	12	150	55
70	1.5	1.6	17	2.2	400	2.2	1,200	1,200	320	30	15	175	65
95	1.6	1.8	20	2.1	280	2.6	1,200	1,200	355	15	19	200	75
90	1.6	1.7	20	2.1	260	2.6	1,200	1,200	340	15	16	200	75

COMMUNITY FOCUS

Dietary Reference Intakes*

For many years, Recommended Dietary Allowances (RDAs) have been the standard for nutritional adequacy in the United States. The Food and Nutrition Board of the National Academy of Sciences is in the process of changing the system used for nutritional recommendations. Dietary Reference Intakes (DRIs) will be the new standard for planning and assessing diets for healthy people. DRIs will include the RDA as well as three new values: Estimated Average Requirement (EAR), Adequate Intake (AI), and Tolerable Upper Intake Level (UL). DRIs will be published according to nutrient groups as soon as the research and review process is completed.

*Updates on the DRI process are available on the The National Academy of Sciences Web site, www2.nas.edu/fnb; or by calling the National Academy Press at (800) 624-6242.

Estimated Safe and Adequate Daily Dietary Intakes of Selected Vitamins and Minerals[a]

Category	Age (Years)	Vitamins	
		Biotin (µg)	Pantothenic Acid (mg)
Infants	0-0.5	10	2
	0.5-1	15	3
Children and adolescents	1-3	20	3
	4-6	25	3-4
	7-10	30	4-5
	11+	30-100	4-7
Adults		30-100	4-7

Category	Age (Years)	Trace Elements[b]				
		Copper (mg)	Manganese (mg)	Fluoride (mg)	Chromium (µg)	Molybdenum (µg)
Infants	0-0.5	0.4-0.6	0.3-0.6	0.1-0.5	10-40	15-30
	0.5-1	0.6-0.7	0.6-1.0	0.2-1.0	20-60	20-40
Children and adolescents	1-3	0.7-1.0	1.0-1.5	0.5-1.5	20-80	25-50
	4-6	1.0-1.5	1.5-2.0	1.0-2.5	30-120	30-75
	7-10	1.0-2.0	2.0-3.0	1.5-2.5	50-200	50-150
	11+	1.5-2.5	2.0-5.0	1.5-2.5	50-200	75-250
Adults		1.5-3.0	2.0-5.0	1.5-4.0	50-200	75-250

From Food and Nutrition Board, National Academy of Sciences-National Research Council, Washington, DC, 1989.

[a]Because there is less information on which to base allowances, these figures are not given in the main table of RDA and are provided here in the form of ranges of recommended intakes.

[b]Since the toxic levels for many trace elements may be only several times usual intakes, the upper levels for the trace elements given in this table should not be habitually exceeded.

Estimated Sodium, Chloride, and Potassium Minimum Requirements of Healthy Persons[a]

Age	Weight (kg)[a]	Sodium (mg)[a,b]	Chloride (mg)[a,b]	Potassium (mg)[c]
Months				
0-5	4.5	120	180	500
6-11	8.9	200	300	700
Years				
1	11.0	225	350	1,000
2-5	16.0	300	500	1,400
6-9	25.0	400	600	1,600
10-18	50.0	500	750	2,000
>18[d]	70.0	500	750	2,000

From Food and Nutrition Board, National Academy of Sciences-National Research Council, Washington, DC, 1989.

[a]No allowance has been included for large, prolonged losses from the skin through sweat.

[b]There is no evidence that higher intakes confer any health benefit.

[c]Desirable intakes of potassium may considerably exceed these values (~3,500 mg for adults).

[d]No allowance included for growth. Values for those below 18 years assume a growth rate at the 50th percentile reported by the National Center for Health Statistics and averaged for males and females.

Median Heights and Weights and Recommended Energy Intake

Category	Age (Year) or Condition	Weight (kg)	Weight (lb)	Height (cm)	Height (in)	REE[a] (kcal/day)	Average Energy Allowance (kcal)[b] Multiples of REE	Average Energy Allowance (kcal)[b] Per kg	Average Energy Allowance (kcal)[b] Per Day[c]
Infants	0.0-0.5	6	13	60	24	320		108	650
	0.5-1.0	9	20	71	28	500		98	850
Children	1-3	13	29	90	35	740		102	1,300
	4-6	20	44	112	44	950		90	1,800
	7-10	28	62	132	52	1,130		70	2,000
Males	11-14	45	99	157	62	1,440	1.70	55	2,500
	15-18	66	145	176	69	1,760	1.67	45	3,000
	19-24	72	160	177	70	1,780	1.67	40	2,900
	25-50	79	174	176	70	1,800	1.60	37	2,900
	51+	77	170	173	68	1,530	1.50	30	2,300
Females	11-14	46	101	157	62	1,310	1.67	47	2,200
	15-18	55	120	163	64	1,370	1.60	40	2,200
	19-24	58	128	164	65	1,350	1.60	38	2,200
	25-50	63	138	163	64	1,380	1.55	36	2,200
	51+	65	143	160	63	1,280	1.50	30	1,900
Pregnant	1st trimester								+0
	2nd trimester								+300
	3rd trimester								+300
Lactating	1st 6 months								+500
	2nd 6 months								+500

From Recommended Dietary Allowances, Food and Nutrition Board, National Academy of Sciences-National Research Council, Washington, DC, 1989. The data in this table have been assembled from the observed median heights and weights of children together with desirable weights for adults for the mean heights of men (70 inches) and women (64 inches) between the ages of 18 and 34 years as surveyed in the United States population (HEW/NCHS data). The energy allowances for the young adults are for men and women doing light work. The allowances for the two older age groups represent mean energy needs over these age spans, allowing for a 2% decrease in basal (resting) metabolic rate per decade and a reduction in activity of 200 kcal/day for men and women between 51 and 75 years, 500 kcal for men over 75 years and 400 kcal for women over 75. The customary range of daily energy output is shown for adults and is based on a variation in energy needs of ±400 kcal at any one age, emphasizing the wide range of energy intakes appropriate for any group of people. Energy allowances for children through age 18 are based on medium energy intakes of children these ages followed in longitudinal growth studies.

[a]Resting energy expenditure.
[b]In the range of light to moderate activity, the coefficient of variation is ±20%.
[c]Figure is rounded.

Ranges of Daily Caloric Requirements at Different Weights Under Normal Conditions

*Holliday-Segar Method**

Body Weight (kg)	Caloric Expenditure/Day
Up to 10	100 kcal/kg†
11-20	1,000 kcal + 50 kcal/kg for each kg above 10 kg
Above 20	1,500 kcal + 20 kcal/kg for each kg above 20 kg

From Johnson KB: *The Harriet Lane Handbook: a manual for pediatric house officers,* St Louis, 1993, Mosby.
*Not suitable for neonates less than 2 weeks old or for conditions associated with abnormal losses.
†For each 100 kilocalories metabolized, 100 cc H_2O is required.

Standard Basal Caloric Output

| Weight (kg) | Output (kcal/24 hr) | | |
	Male	Male and Female	Female
3		140	
5		270	
7		400	
9		500	
11		600	
13		650	
15		710	
17		780	
19		830	
21		880	
25	1,020		960
29	1,120		1,040
33	1,210		1,120
37	1,300		1,190
41	1,350		1,260
45	1,410		1,320
49	1,470		1,380
53	1,530		1,440
57	1,590		1,500
61	1,640		1,560

Increments or decrements:
1. Add or subtract 12% of above for each degree Celsius (8% for each degree Fahrenheit) above or below rectal temperature of 37.8° C (100° F).
2. Add 0% to 30% increments for activity.
3. Water requirements for normal maintenance therapy are 115 ml for every 100 kcal metabolized.

From Behrman RE and others: *Nelson textbook of pediatrics,* ed 14, Philadelphia, 1992, WB Saunders.

Ranges of Daily Water Requirements at Different Ages Under Normal Conditions

Age	Average Body Weight (kg)	Total Water Requirements Per 24 Hours (ml)	Water Requirements Per kg Per 24 Hours (ml)
3 days	3.0	250-300	80-100
10 days	3.2	400-500	125-150
3 months	5.4	750-850	140-160
6 months	7.3	950-1100	130-155
9 months	8.6	1100-1250	125-145
1 year	9.5	1150-1300	120-135
2 years	11.8	1350-1500	115-125
4 years	16.2	1600-1800	100-110
6 years	20.0	1800-2000	90-100
10 years	28.7	2000-2500	70-85
14 years	45.0	2000-2700	50-60
18 years	54.0	2200-2700	40-50

From Behrman RE, Vaughan VC, editors: *Nelson textbook of pediatrics,* ed 3, Philadelphia, 1987, WB Saunders.

SLEEP ASSESSMENT

A sleep history is usually taken during the general health history. However, when sleep problems are identified, a more detailed history of sleep and awake patterns is needed for planning appropriate intervention. (See p. 106.) The following information includes a summary of a comprehensive sleep history, a chart for parents to record the child's sleep/awake habits, and a chart of typical sleep requirements in infancy and childhood.

Assessment of Sleep Problems in Children*
General History of Chief Complaint

Ask parents/child to describe sleep problems; record in their words.

Inquire about onset, duration, character, frequency, and consistency of sleep problems:

———

*Not all of these areas need to be assessed with every family. For example, if night wakings are not a problem, this section of the interview can be eliminated.

Circumstances surrounding onset (e.g., birth of sibling, start of toilet training, death of significant other, move from crib to bed)

Circumstances that aggravate problem (e.g., overtiredness, family conflict, or disrupted routine [visitors])

Remedies used to correct problem and results of interventions

24-Hour Sleep History

Time and regularity of meals*
  Family members present
  Activities afterward, especially evening meal

Time of night and day sleep periods
  Hours of sleep and waking
  Hours of being put to bed and taken out of bed
  How bedtime is decided (when child looks tired or at a time decided by parent; do both parents agree on bedtime?)

Pre-bedtime or nap rituals (bath, bottle or breast-feeding, snack, television, active or quiet playing, story)
  Mood before nap or bedtime (wide awake, sleepy, happy, cranky)
  Which parent(s) participates in nap or bedtime rituals?

Nap and bedtime rituals
  Where is child allowed to fall asleep? (own bed or crib, couch, parent's bed, someone's lap, other)
  Is child helped to fall asleep? (rocked; walked; patted; given pacifier or bottle; placed in room with light; television, radio, or tape recorder on; other)
  Are patterns consistent each time or do they vary?
  Does child awake if sleep aids are changed or taken away? (placed in own bed, television turned off, other)

———

*A convenient point to start the 24-hour history is the evening meal.
Adapted from Ferber R: Assessment procedures for diagnosis of sleep disorders in children. In Noshpitz J, editor: *Sleep disorders for the clinician,* London, 1987, Butterworths, pp. 185-193.

Does child verbally insist that parents stay in room?
Child's behaviors if refuses to go to sleep or stay in room
If child complains of fears, how convincing are the fears?

Sleep environment
  Number of bedrooms
  Location of bedrooms, especially in relation to parent(s)' room
  Sensory features (light on, door open or closed, noise level, temperature)

Night wakings
  Time, frequency, and duration
  Child's behavior (call out, cry, come out of room, appear frightened, confused, or upset)
  Parental responses (let child cry, go in immediately, take to own bed, feed, pick up, rock, give pacifier, talk, scold, threaten, other)
  Conditions that reestablish sleep
    Do they always work?
    How long do the interventions take to work?
    Which parents intervene?
    Do both parents use same or different approach?

Daytime sleepiness
  Occurrence of falling asleep at inappropriate times (circumstances, suddenness and irresistibility of onset, length of sleep, mood on awakening)
  Signs of fatigue (yawning or lying down, as well as overactivity, impulsivity, distractibility, irritability, temper tantrums)

Past Sleep History

Sleep patterns since infancy, especially ages when started to sleep through the night, stopped daytime naps, began later bedtime

Response to changes in sleep arrangements (crib to bed, different room or house, other)

Sleep behaviors (restlessness, snoring, sleepwalking, nightmares, partial wakings [young child may wake confused, crying, and thrashing, but does not respond to parent; falls asleep without intervention if not excessively disturbed])

Parental perception of child's sleep habits (good or poor sleeper, light or deep sleeper, needs little sleep)

Family history of sleep problems (sibling behavior imitated by child; some sleep disorders [e.g., narcolepsy and enuresis] tend to recur in families)

2-Week Sleep Record

PATIENT'S NAME _____ PARENT'S NAME _____

PATIENT'S DATE OF BIRTH _____ ADDRESS _____

DATE OF SLEEP RECORD: FROM __ TO __ TELEPHONE NUMBER _____

INSTRUCTIONS:

Leave blank the periods your child is awake.	Mark your child's bedtimes with downward-pointing arrows. ↓
Fill in the times your child is asleep with shaded boxes.	Mark the times your child gets up in the morning and after naps with arrows pointing upwards. ↑

Day	Midnight	_____ AM _____					Noon	_____ PM _____					Midnight
		2:00	4:00	6:00	8:00	10:00		2:00	4:00	6:00	8:00	10:00	

SPECIAL OBSERVATIONS AND NOTES: _____

_____

_____

_____

_____

_____

Modified from Ferber R: *Solve your child's sleep problems,* New York, 1985, Simon & Schuster.

This section may be photocopied and distributed to families.

From Wong DL, Hess CS: *Wong and Whaley's Clinical manual of pediatric nursing,* ed 5. Copyright © 2000, Mosby, St Louis.

Typical Sleep Requirements in Infancy and Childhood

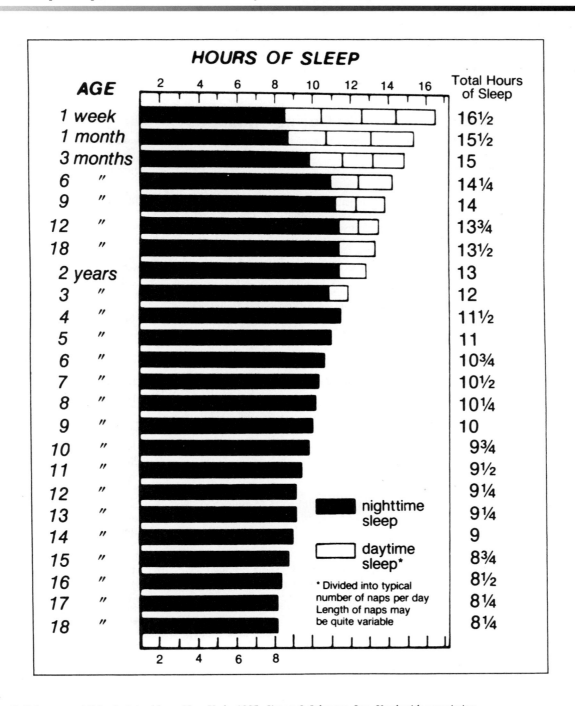

From Ferber R: *Solve your child's sleep problems*, New York, 1985, Simon & Schuster, Inc. Used with permission.
This section may be photocopied and distributed to families.
From Wong DL, Hess CS: *Wong and Whaley's Clinical manual of pediatric nursing*, ed 5. Copyright © 2000, Mosby, St Louis.

GROWTH MEASUREMENTS

This section primarily includes reference data for evaluating and recording a child's growth. It begins with a comparison of the general trends in physical growth throughout childhood and a chart illustrating the sequence of tooth eruption and shedding (Fig. 1-40). Included next is summary of pubertal sexual development (Figs. 1-41 through 1-45). The remainder of the section consists of tables and charts of height, weight, head circumference, triceps skinfold measurements, and mid-arm circumference for girls and boys at different ages (Figs. 1-46 through 1-56).

General Trends in Physical Growth During Childhood

Age	Weight*	Height*
INFANTS		
Birth to 6 months	Weekly gain: 140-200 g (5-7 ounces) Birth weight doubles by end of first 6 months†	Monthly gain: 2.5 cm (1 inch)
6 to 12 months	Weekly gain: 85-140 g (3-5 ounces) Birth weight triples by end of first year† (Practice Alert)	Monthly gain: 1.25 cm (0.5 inch) Birth length increases by approximately 50% by end of first year
TODDLERS	Birth weight quadruples by age 2½ years Yearly gain: 2-3 kg (4.4-6.6 pounds)	Height at 2 years is approximately 50% of eventual adult height Gain during second year: about 12 cm (4.8 inches) Gain during third year: about 6-8 cm (2.4-3.2 inches)
PRESCHOOLERS	Yearly gain: 2-3 kg (4.4-6.6 pounds)	Birth length doubles by 4 years of age Yearly gain: 6-8 cm (2.4-3.2 inches)
SCHOOL-AGE CHILDREN	Yearly gain: 2-3 kg (4.4-6.6 pounds)	Yearly gain after age 6 years: 5.0 cm (2 inches) Birth length triples by about 13 years of age
PUBERTAL GROWTH SPURT		
Females—Between 10 and 14 years	Weight gain: 7-25 kg (15-55 pounds) Mean: 17.5 kg (38.1 pounds)	Height gain: 5-25 cm (2-10 inches); approximately 95% of mature height achieved by onset of menarche or skeletal age of 13 years Mean: 20.5 cm (8.2 inches)
Males—Between 12 and 16 years	Weight gain: 7-30 kg (15-65 pounds) Mean: 23.7 kg (52.1 pounds)	Height gain: 10-30 cm (4-12 inches); approximately 95% of mature height achieved by skeletal age of 15 years Mean: 27.5 cm (11 inches)

*Yearly height and weight gains for each age group represent averaged estimates from a variety of sources.
†A study (Jung E, Czaijka-Narins DM: Birth weight doubling and tripling times: an updated look at the effects of birth weight, sex, race, and type of feeding, *Am J Clin Nutr* 42:182-189, 1985) has shown the mean doubling time for birth weight to be 4.7 months and mean tripling time to be 14.7 months. (See Practice Alert, p. 109.)

PRACTICE ALERT

Breast-Feeding and Infant Weight Gain

Mothers with breast-fed infants who fail to gain weight according to the standard growth curves may be told that their milk, although nutritionally good for the baby from an immunologic standpoint, lacks fat for adequate growth. There is evidence, however, which indicates that the standard growth charts may not reflect normal growth patterns of infants who are breast-fed. Infants who are breast-fed grow more rapidly during the first 2 months of life, but growth is slower from 3 to 12 months when compared with the current NCHS growth reference data charts. In the second year of life, breast-fed infants gain weight faster than is reflected by reference charts, and by 24 months their average weight approximates current growth charts. Breast-fed infants are leaner than formula-fed infants, but growth in head circumference is greater in the breast-fed group. Even with the introduction of solid foods, breast-fed infants demonstrate self-

regulation in regard to energy intake. The conclusions from the studies are that infants who are breast-fed during the first year of life are at risk for being labeled as "growth deficient" when compared with current NCHS growth charts (Dewey and others, 1995). Efforts are currently being made to collect data for growth reference charts that will reflect a wider range of ethnic backgrounds, feeding methods, and parental stature.

Nurses can share these findings with parents to allay fears of an inadequate milk supply, which can discourage mothers from continuing to breast-feed. Also, an evaluation of growth, especially if weight falls below the 5th percentile, must be viewed carefully to avoid the diagnosis of failure to thrive in infants with no other evidence of inadequate nutrition.

Data from Dewey KG and others: Growth of breast-fed infants deviates from current reference data: a pooled analysis of U.S., Canadian, and European data sets, *Pediatrics* 96(3):495-503, 1995.

Sequence of Tooth Eruption and Shedding

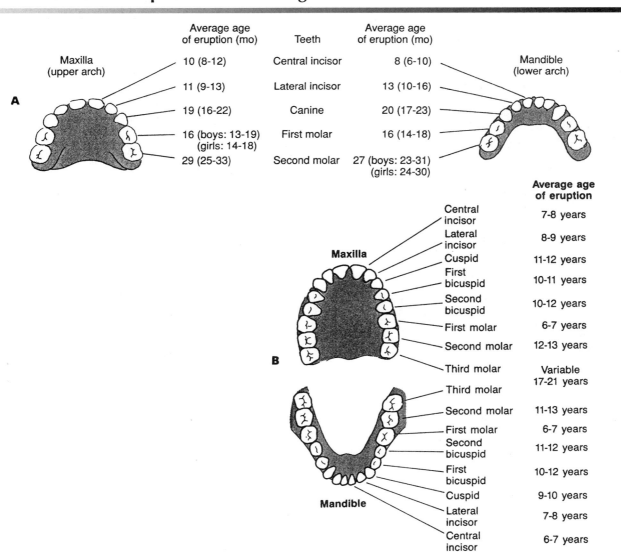

Fig. 1-40 **A,** Sequence of eruption of primary teeth. Range represents ± standard deviation or 67% of subjects studied. **B,** Sequence of eruption of secondary teeth. (Data from McDonald RE, Avery DR: *Dentistry for the child and adolescent,* ed 6, St Louis, 1994, Mosby.)

Sexual Development in Adolescent Males

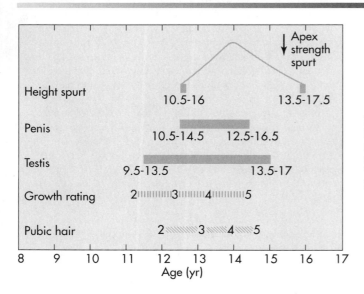

Fig. 1-41 Approximate timing of the developmental changes in boys. Numbers across from growth rating and pubic hair indicate stages of development. Range of ages during which some of the changes occur is indicated by inclusive numbers. (From Marshall WA, Tanner JM: Variations in the pattern of pubertal changes in boys, *Arch Dis Child* 45(239):13-23, 1970.)

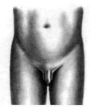

Stage 1 (prepubertal)

No pubic hair; essentially the same as during childhood; no distinction between hair on pubis and over the abdomen

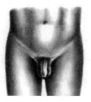

Stage 2 (pubertal)

Initial enlargement of scrotum and testes; reddening and textural changes of scrotal skin; sparse growth of long, straight, downy, and slightly pigmented hair at base of penis

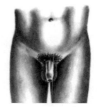

Stage 3

Initial enlargement of penis, mainly in length; testes and scrotum further enlarged; hair darker, coarser, and curly and spread sparsely over entire pubis

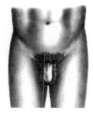

Stage 4

Increased size of penis with growth in diameter and development of glans; glans larger and broader; scrotum darker; pubic hair more abundant with curling but restricted to pubic area

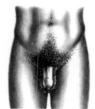

Stage 5

Testes, scrotum, and penis adult in size and shape; hair adult in quantity and type with spread to inner surface of thighs

Fig. 1-42 Developmental stages of secondary sex characteristics and genital development in boys. Average age span is 12 to 16 years. (Modified from Marshall WA, Tanner JM: Variations in the pattern of pubertal changes in boys, *Arch Dis Child* 45(239):13-23, 1970; and Daniel WA, Paulshock BZ: *Patient Care,* May 13, 1979, pp. 122-124.)

Sexual Development in Adolescent Females

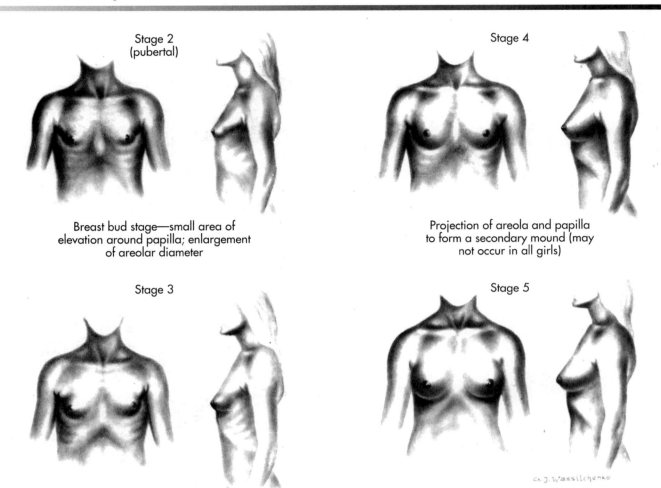

Stage 2
(pubertal)

Breast bud stage—small area of
elevation around papilla; enlargement
of areolar diameter

Stage 3

Further enlargement of breast and areola
with no separation of their contours

Stage 4

Projection of areola and papilla
to form a secondary mound (may
not occur in all girls)

Stage 5

Mature configuration; projection of papilla
only caused by recession of areola
into general contour

Fig. 1-43 Development of the breast in girls. Average age span is 11 to 13 years. Stage 1 (prepubertal—elevation of papilla only) is not shown. (Modified from Marshall WA, Tanner JM: Variations in pattern of pubertal changes in girls, *Arch Dis Child* 44(235):291-303, 1969; and Daniel WA, Paulshock BZ: *Patient Care,* May 13, 1979, pp. 122-124.)

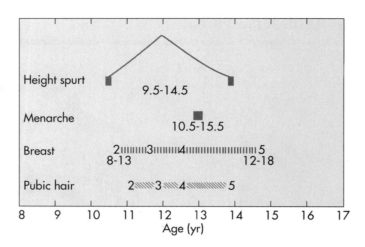

Fig. 1-44 Approximate timing of developmental changes in girls. Numbers across from breast and pubic hair indicate stages of development. Range of ages during which some of the changes occur is indicated by inclusive numbers. (From Marshall WA, Tanner JM: Variations in the pattern of pubertal changes in girls, *Arch Dis Child*, 44(235):291-303, 1969.)

Stage 1
(prepubertal)

No pubic hair; essentially the same as during childhood; no distinction between hair on pubis and over the abdomen

Stage 2

Sparse growth of long, straight, downy, and slightly pigmented hair extending along labia; between stages 2 and 3 begins to appear on pubis

Stage 3

Hair darker, coarser, and curly and spread sparsely over entire pubis in the typical female triangle

Stage 4

Pubic hair denser, curled, and adult in distribution but less abundant and restricted to the pubic area

Stage 5

Hair adult in quantity, type, and pattern with spread to inner aspect of thighs

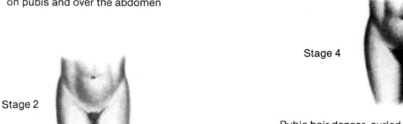

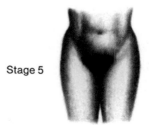

Fig. 1-45 Growth of pubic hair in girls. Average age span for stages 2 through 5 is 11 to 14 years. (Adapted from Marshall WA, Tanner JM: Variations in the pattern of pubertal changes in girls, *Arch Dis Child* 44(235): 291-303, 1969; and Daniel WA, Paulshock BZ: *Patient Care,* May 13, 1979, pp. 122-124.)

Boys: Birth to Age 36 Months—Physical Growth (Length, Weight), NCHS Percentiles

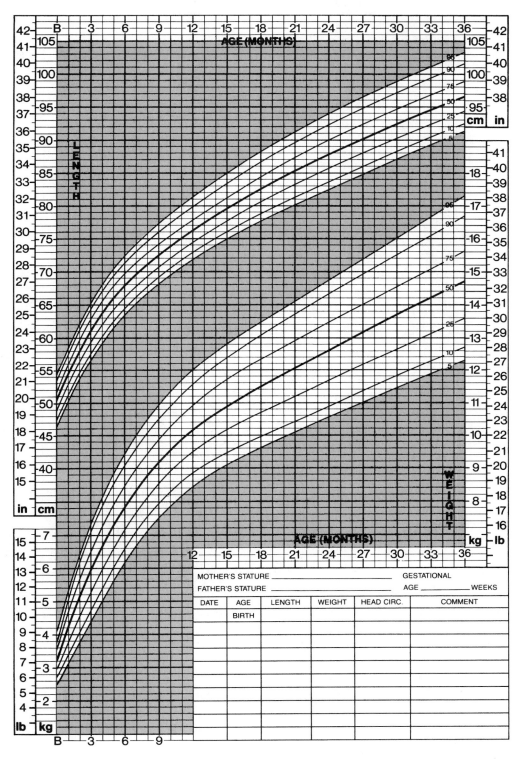

Fig. 1-46 Modified from Hamill PV and others: Physical growth: National Center for Health Statistics percentiles, *Am J Clin Nutr* 32(3):607-629, 1979. Data from the Fels Longitudinal Study, Wright State University School of Medicine, Yellow Springs, OH. Provided as a service of Ross Products Division, Abbott Laboratories, 1982.

Boys: Birth to Age 36 Months—Physical Growth (Head Circumference, Length, Weight), *NCHS Percentiles*

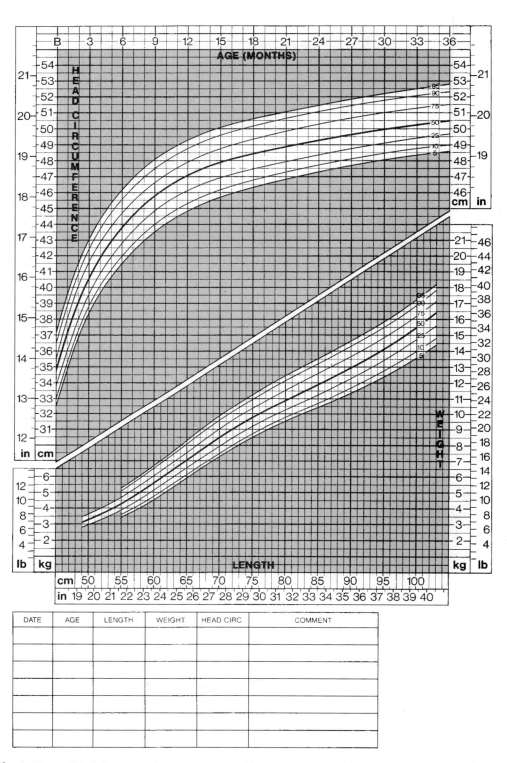

DATE	AGE	LENGTH	WEIGHT	HEAD CIRC	COMMENT

Fig. 1-47   Modified from Hamill PV and others: Physical growth: National Center for Health Statistics percentiles, *Am J Clin Nutr* 32(3):607-629, 1979. Data from the Fels Longitudinal Study, Wright State University School of Medicine, Yellow Springs, OH. Provided as a service of Ross Products Division, Abbott Laboratories, 1982.

Boys: Ages 2 to 18 Years—Physical Growth (Stature, Weight), NCHS Percentiles

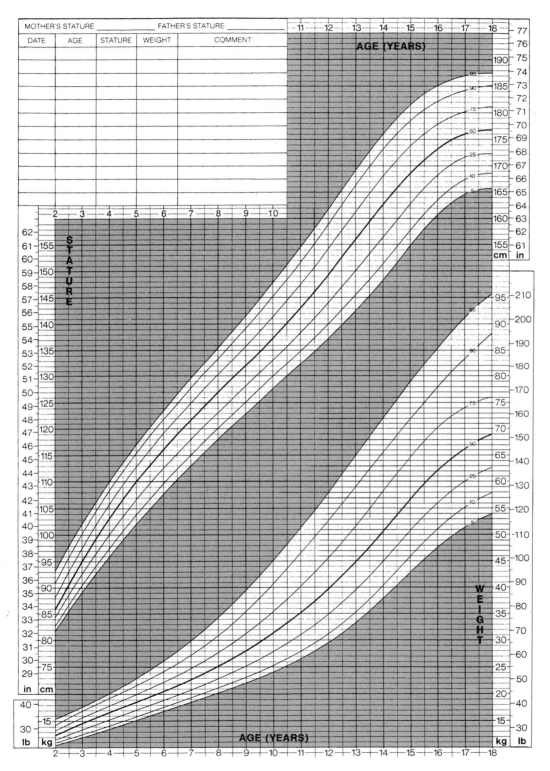

Fig. 1-48 Modified from Hamill PV and others: Physical growth: National Center for Health Statistics percentiles, *Am J Clin Nutr* 32(3):607-629, 1979. Data from the National Center for Health Statistics (NCHS), Hyattsville, MD. Provided as a service of Ross Products Division, Abbott Laboratories, 1982.

Boys: Prepubescent—Physical Growth (Stature, Weight), NCHS Percentiles

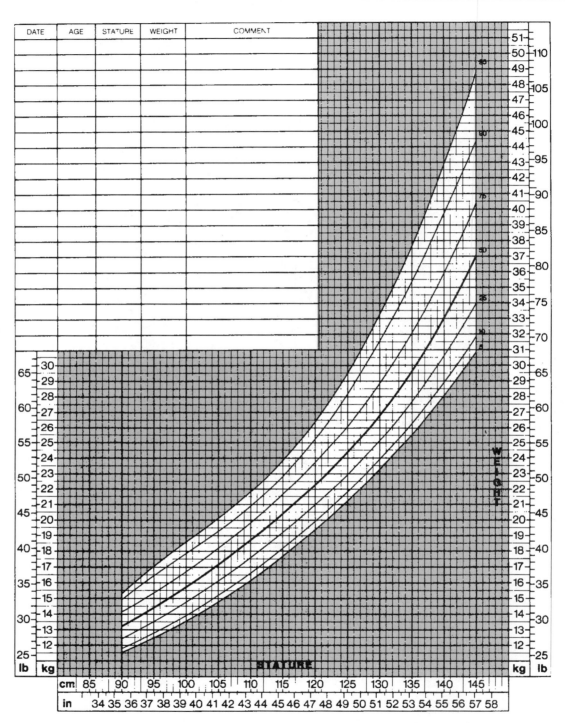

Fig. 1-49   Modified from Hamill PV and others: Physical growth: National Center for Health Statistics percentiles, *Am J Clin Nutr* 32(3):607-629, 1979. Data from the National Center for Health Statistics (NCHS), Hyattsville, MD. Provided as a service of Ross Products Division, Abbott Laboratories, 1982.

Girls: Birth to Age 36 Months—Physical Growth (Length, Weight), NCHS Percentiles

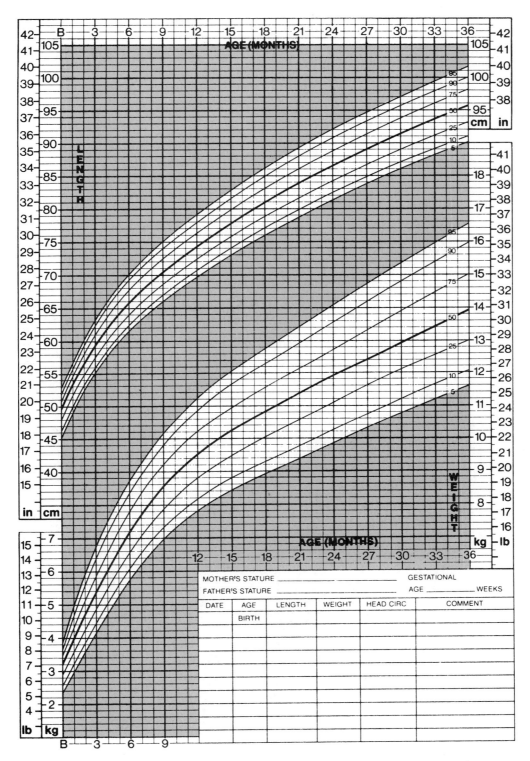

Fig. 1-50 Modified from Hamill PV and others: Physical growth: National Center for Health Statistics percentiles, *Am J Clin Nutr* 32(3):607-629, 1979. Data from the Fels Longitudinal Study, Wright State University School of Medicine, Yellow Springs, OH. Provided as a service of Ross Products Division, Abbott Laboratories, 1982.

Girls: Birth to Age 36 Months—Physical Growth (Head Circumference, Length, Weight), NCHS Percentiles

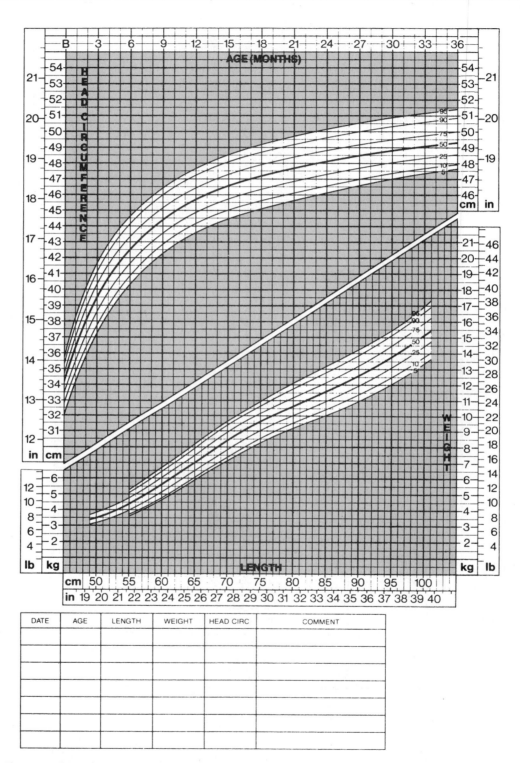

DATE	AGE	LENGTH	WEIGHT	HEAD CIRC	COMMENT

Fig. 1-51 Modified from Hamill PV and others: Physical growth: National Center for Health Statistics percentiles, *Am J Clin Nutr* 32(3):607-629, 1979. Data from the Fels Longitudinal Study, Wright State University School of Medicine, Yellow Springs, OH. Provided as a service of Ross Products Division, Abbott Laboratories, 1982.

Girls: Ages 2 to 18 Years—Physical Growth (Stature, Weight), NCHS Percentiles

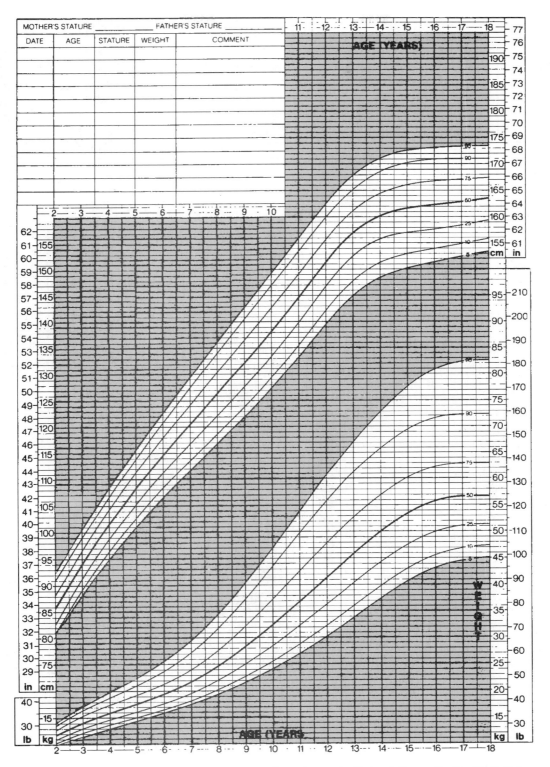

Fig. 1-52 Modified from Hamill PV and others: Physical growth: National Center for Health Statistics percentiles, *Am J Clin Nutr* 32(3):607-629, 1979. Data from the National Center for Health Statistics (NCHS), Hyattsville, MD. Provided as a service of Ross Products Division, Abbott Laboratories, 1982.

Girls: Prepubescent—Physical Growth (Stature, Weight), NCHS Percentiles

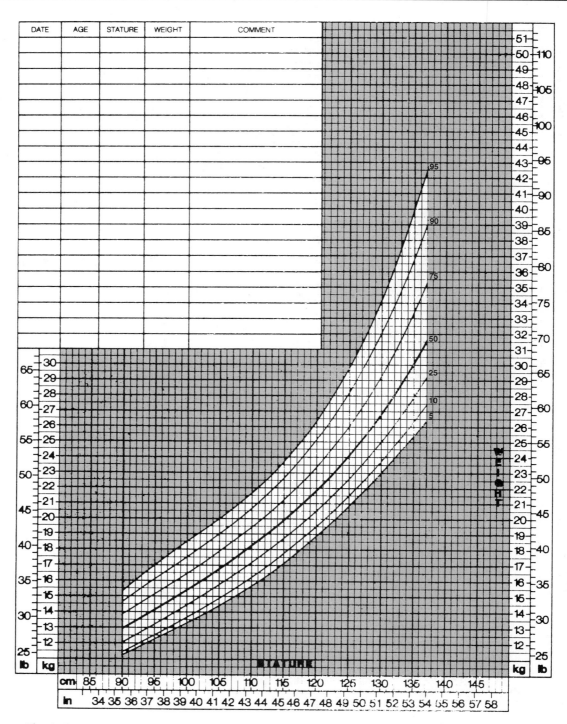

Fig. 1-53 Modified from Hamill PV and others: Physical growth: National Center for Health Statistics percentiles, *Am J Clin Nutr* 32(3):607-629, 1979. Data from the National Center for Health Statistics (NCHS), Hyattsville, MD. Provided as a service of Ross Products Division, Abbott Laboratories, 1982.

Head Circumference Charts

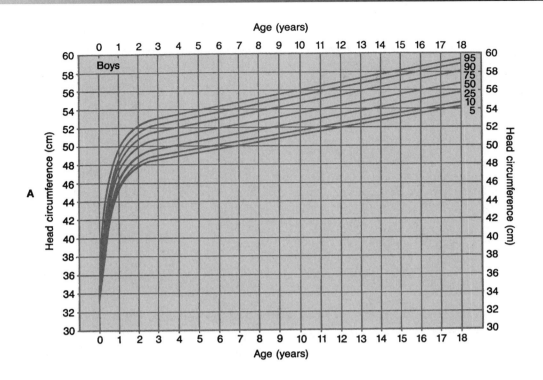

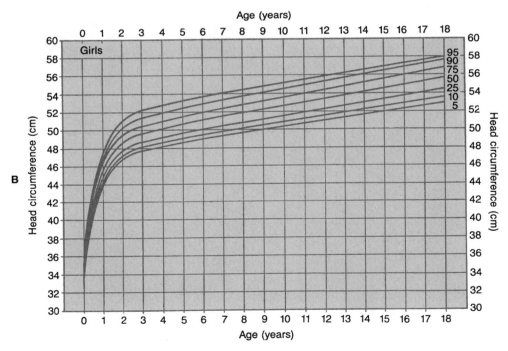

Fig. 1-54 Selected percentiles for smoothed head circumference values of children from birth to 18 years. **A,** Boys. **B,** Girls. (From Roche AF and others: Head circumference reference data: birth to 18 years, *Pediatrics* 79(5):706-712, 1987.)

Triceps Skinfold Thickness

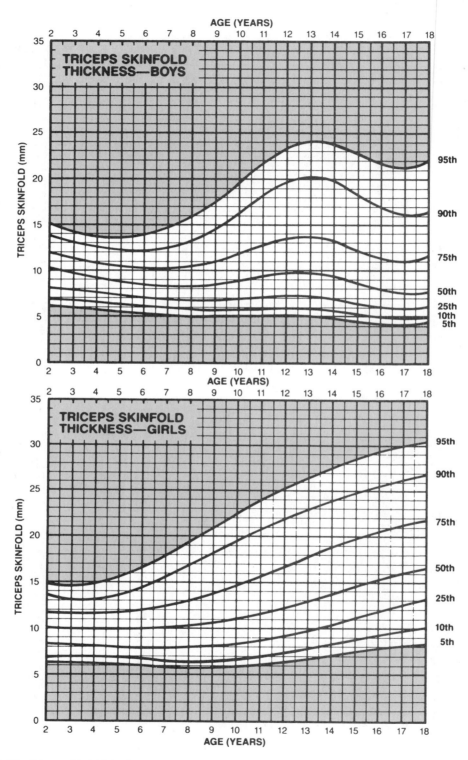

Fig. 1-55 Triceps skinfold thickness. (Modified from Johnson CL and others: Basic data on anthropometric measurements and angular measurements of the hip and knee joints for selected age groups, 1-74 years of age, United States, 1972-1975. Vital and Health Statistics Series 11, No. 219. DHHS Publication No. [PHS] 81-1669, 1981. Provided as a service of Ross Laboratories, Copyright 1983, Columbus, OH, 43216. May be copied for individual patient use.)

Midarm Circumference

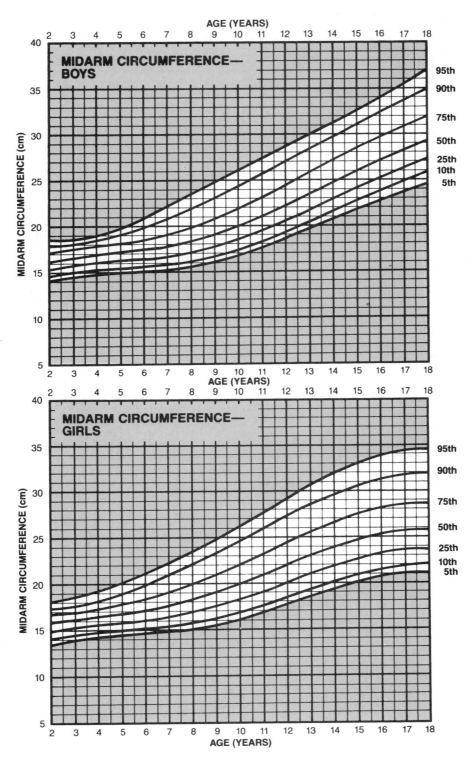

Fig. 1-56　Midarm circumference. (Modified from Johnson CL and others: Basic data on anthropometric measurements and angular measurements of the hip and knee joints for selected age groups, 1-74 years of age, United States, 1972-1975. Vital and Health Statistics Series 11, No. 219. DHHS Publication No. [PHS] 81-1669, 1981. Provided as a service of Ross Laboratories, Copyright 1983, Columbus, OH, 43216. May be copied for individual patient use.)

Height and Weight Measurements for Boys in the United States

Age*	Height by Percentiles‡						Weight by Percentiles					
	5		50		95		5		50		95	
	cm	inches	cm	inches	cm	inches	kg	lb	kg	lb	kg	lb
Birth	46.4	18¼	50.5	20	54.4	21½	2.54	5½	3.27	7¼	4.15	9¼
3 months	56.7	22¼	61.1	24	65.4	25¾	4.43	9¾	5.98	13¼	7.37	16¼
6 months	63.4	25	67.8	26¾	72.3	28½	6.20	13¾	7.85	17¼	9.46	20¾
9 months	68.0	26¾	72.3	28½	77.1	30¼	7.52	16½	9.18	20¼	10.93	24
1	71.7	28¼	76.1	30	81.2	32	8.43	18½	10.15	22½	11.99	26½
1½	77.5	30½	82.4	32½	88.1	34¾	9.59	21¼	11.47	25¼	13.44	29½
2†	82.5	32½	86.8	34¼	94.4	37¼	10.49	23¼	12.34	27¼	15.50	34¼
2½†	85.4	33½	90.4	35½	97.8	38½	11.27	24¾	13.52	29¾	16.61	36½
3	89.0	35	94.9	37¼	102.0	40¼	12.05	26½	14.62	32¼	17.77	39¼
3½	92.5	36½	99.1	39	106.1	41¾	12.84	28¼	15.68	34½	18.98	41¾
4	95.8	37¾	102.9	40½	109.9	43¼	13.64	30	16.69	36¾	20.27	44¾
4½	98.9	39	106.6	42	113.5	44¾	14.45	31¾	17.69	39	21.63	47¾
5	102.0	40¼	109.9	43¼	117.0	46	15.27	33¾	18.67	41¼	23.09	51
6	107.7	42½	116.1	45¾	123.5	48½	16.93	37¼	20.69	45½	26.34	58
7	113.0	44½	121.7	48	129.7	51	18.64	41	22.85	50¼	30.12	66½
8	118.1	46½	127.0	50	135.7	53½	20.40	45	25.30	55¾	34.51	76
9	122.9	48½	132.2	52	141.8	55¾	22.25	49	28.13	62	39.58	87¼
10	127.7	50¼	137.5	54¼	148.1	58¼	24.33	53¾	31.44	69¼	45.27	99¾
11	132.6	52¼	143.3	56½	154.9	61	26.80	59	35.30	77¾	51.47	113½
12	137.6	54¼	149.7	59	162.3	64	29.85	65¾	39.78	87¾	58.09	128
13	142.9	56¼	156.5	61½	169.8	66¾	33.64	74¼	44.95	99	65.02	143¼
14	148.8	58½	163.1	64¼	176.7	69½	38.22	84¼	50.77	112	72.13	159
15	155.2	61	169.0	66½	181.9	71½	43.11	95	56.71	125	79.12	174½
16	161.1	63½	173.5	68¼	185.4	73	47.74	105¼	62.10	137	85.62	188¾
17	164.9	65	176.2	69¼	187.3	73¾	51.50	113½	66.31	146¼	91.31	201¼
18	165.7	65¼	176.8	69½	187.6	73¾	53.97	119	68.88	151¾	95.76	211

Adapted from National Center for Health Statistics, Health Resources Administration, Department of Health, Education and Welfare, Hyattsville, MD. Values correspond with NCHS percentile curves. (See Figs. 1-46 to 1-49.) Conversion of metric data to approximate inches and pounds by Ross Laboratories.

*Years unless otherwise indicated.

†Height data include some recumbent length measurements, which make values slightly higher than if all measurements had been of stature (standing height).

‡For an explanation of percentiles, see Practice Alert, p. 29.

Height and Weight Measurements for Girls in the United States

Age*	Height by Percentiles‡						Weight by Percentiles					
	5		50		95		5		50		95	
	cm	inches	cm	inches	cm	inches	kg	lb	kg	lb	kg	lb
Birth	45.4	17¾	49.9	19¾	52.9	20¾	2.36	5¼	3.23	7	3.81	8½
3 months	55.4	21¾	59.5	23½	63.4	25	4.18	9¼	5.4	12	6.74	14¾
6 months	61.8	24¼	65.9	26	70.2	27¾	5.79	12¾	7.21	16	8.73	19¼
9 months	66.1	26	70.4	27¾	75.0	29½	7.0	15½	8.56	18¾	10.17	22½
1	69.8	27½	74.3	29¼	79.1	31¼	7.84	17¼	9.53	21	11.24	24¾
1½	76.0	30	80.9	31¾	86.1	34	8.92	19¾	10.82	23¾	12.76	28¼
2†	81.6	32¼	86.8	34¼	93.6	36¾	9.95	22	11.8	26	14.15	31¼
2½†	84.6	33¼	90.0	35½	96.6	38	10.8	23¾	13.03	28¾	15.76	34¾
3	88.3	34¾	94.1	37	100.6	39½	11.61	25½	14.1	31	17.22	38
3½	91.7	36	97.9	38½	104.5	41¼	12.37	27¼	15.07	33¼	18.59	41
4	95.0	37½	101.6	40	108.3	42¾	13.11	29	15.96	35¼	19.91	44
4½	98.1	38½	105.0	41¼	112.0	44	13.83	30½	16.81	37	21.24	46¾
5	101.1	39¾	108.4	42¾	115.6	45½	14.55	32	17.66	39	22.62	49¾
6	106.6	42	114.6	45	122.7	48¼	16.05	35½	19.52	43	25.75	56¾
7	111.8	44	120.6	47½	129.5	51	17.71	39	21.84	48¼	29.68	65½
8	116.9	46	126.4	49¾	136.2	53½	19.62	43¼	24.84	54¾	34.71	76½
9	122.1	48	132.2	52	142.9	56¼	21.82	48	28.46	62¾	40.64	89½
10	127.5	50¼	138.3	54½	149.5	58¾	24.36	53¾	32.55	71¾	47.17	104
11	133.5	52½	144.8	57	156.2	61½	27.24	60	36.95	81½	54.0	119
12	139.8	55	151.5	59¾	162.7	64	30.52	67¼	41.53	91½	60.81	134
13	145.2	57¼	157.1	61¾	168.1	66¼	34.14	75¼	46.1	101¾	67.3	148¼
14	148.7	58½	160.4	63¼	171.3	67½	37.76	83¼	50.28	110¾	73.08	161
15	150.5	59¼	161.8	63¾	172.8	68	40.99	90¼	53.68	118¼	77.78	171½
16	151.6	59¾	162.4	64	173.3	68¼	43.41	95¾	55.89	123¼	80.99	178½
17	152.7	60	163.1	64¼	173.5	68¼	44.74	98¾	56.69	125	82.46	181¾
18	153.6	60½	163.7	64½	173.6	68¼	45.26	99¾	56.62	124¾	82.47	181¾

Adapted from National Center for Health Statistics, Health Resources Administration, Department of Health, Education and Welfare, Hyattsville, MD. Values correspond with NCHS percentile curves. (See Figs. 1-50 to 1-53.) Conversion of metric data to approximate inches and pounds by Ross Laboratories.

*Years unless otherwise indicated.

†Height data include some recumbent length measurements, which make values slightly higher than if all measurements had been of stature (standing height).

‡For an explanation of percentiles, see Practice Alert, p. 29.

Growth Standards of Healthy Chinese Children

Age	Weight (kg)		Height (cm)		Head Circumference (cm)	
	Boys	Girls	Boys	Girls	Boys	Girls
Birth	3.27	3.17	50.6	50.0	34.3	33.7
1 month	4.97	4.64	56.5	55.5	38.1	37.3
2 months	5.95	5.49	59.6	58.4	39.7	38.7
3 months	6.73	6.23	62.3	60.9	41.0	40.0
4 months	7.32	6.69	64.4	52.9	42.0	41.0
5 months	7.70	7.19	65.9	64.5	42.9	41.9
6 months	8.22	7.62	68.1	66.7	43.9	42.8
8 months	8.71	8.14	70.6	69.0	44.9	43.7
10 months	9.14	8.57	72.9	71.4	45.7	44.5
12 months	9.56	9.04	75.6	74.1	46.3	45.2
15 months	10.15	9.54	78.3	76.9	46.8	45.6
18 months	10.67	10.08	80.7	79.4	47.3	46.2
21 months	11.18	10.56	83.0	81.7	47.8	46.7
24 months	11.95	11.37	86.5	85.3	48.2	47.1
2.5 years	12.84	12.28	90.4	89.3	48.8	47.7
3 years	13.63	13.16	93.8	92.8	49.1	48.1
3.5 years	14.45	14.00	97.2	96.3	49.4	48.5
4 years	15.26	14.89	100.8	100.1	49.7	48.9
4.5 years	16.07	15.63	103.9	103.1	50.0	49.1
5 years	16.88	16.46	107.2	106.5	50.2	49.4
5.5 years	17.65	17.18	110.1	109.2	50.5	49.6
6 years	19.25	18.67	114.7	113.9	50.8	50.0
7 years	21.01	20.35	120.6	119.3	51.1	50.2
8 years	23.08	22.43	125.3	124.6	51.4	50.6
9 years	25.33	24.57	130.6	129.5	51.7	50.9
10 years	27.15	27.05	134.4	134.8	51.9	51.3
11 years	30.13	30.51	139.2	140.6	52.3	51.7
12 years	33.05	34.74	144.2	146.6	52.7	52.3
13 years	36.90	38.52	149.8	150.7	53.0	52.8

Data from Beijing Children's Hospital, 1987, Beijing, China.

ASSESSMENT OF DEVELOPMENT
Denver II*

The Denver II is a major revision and a restandardization of the Denver Developmental Screening Test (DDST) and the Revised

---

*To ensure that the Denver II is administered and interpreted in the prescribed manner, it is recommended that those intending to administer the Denver II receive the appropriate training, which can be obtained with the forms and instructional manual from Denver Developmental Materials, PO Box 371075, Denver, CO 80237-5075, USA; (303) 355-4729, (800) 419-4729.

Denver Developmental Screening Test (DDST-R). It differs from the earlier screening tests in items included as well as in the form, the interpretation, and the referral (Fig. 1-57, *A* and *B*). Like the other tests, it assesses gross motor, language, fine motor, adaptive, and personal-social development in children from 1 month to 6 years.

Item Differences

The previous total of 105 items has been increased to 125, including an increase from 21 DDST to 39 Denver II language items.

Previous items that were difficult to administer and/or interpret have either been modified or eliminated. Many items that were previously tested by parental report now require observation by the examiner.

Each item was evaluated to determine if significant differences existed on the basis of sex, ethnic group, maternal educa-

tion, and place of residence. Items for which clinically significant differences existed were replaced or, if retained, are discussed in the Technical Manual. When evaluating children delayed on one of these items, the examiner can look up norms for the subpopulations to determine if the delay may be due to sociocultural differences.

Test Form Differences

The age scale is similar to the American Academy of Pediatrics suggested periodicity schedule for health maintenance visits. This facilitates use of the Denver II at these times.

In children born prematurely, the age is adjusted only until the child is 2 years old.

The items on the test form are arranged in the same format as the DDST-R.

The norms for the distribution bars were updated with the new standardization data but retained the 25th, 50th, 75th, and 90th percentile divisions. (See Practice Alert, p. 29).

The test form contains a place to rate the child's behavioral characteristics (compliance, interest in surroundings, fearfulness, and attention span).

Interpretation and Referral

Explain to the parents that the Denver II is not an intelligence test but a systematic appraisal of the child's present development. Stress that the child is not expected to perform each item.

To determine relative areas of advancement and areas of delay, sufficient items should be administered to establish the basal and ceiling levels in each sector.

By scoring appropriate items as "pass," "fail," "refusal," or "no opportunity," and relating such scores to the age of the child, each item can be interpreted as described in Box 1-7.

To identify cautions, all items intersected by the age line are administered.

To screen solely for developmental delays, only the items located totally to the *left* of the child's age line are administered.

Criteria for referral are based on the availability of resources in the community.

Unit 1

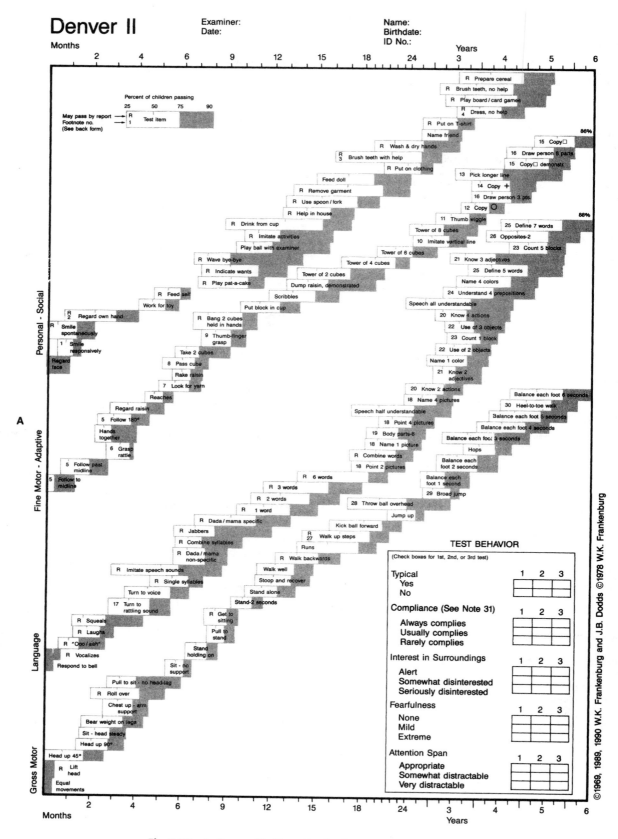

Fig. 1-57   A, Denver II. (From Frankenburg WK, Dodds JB, 1990.)

DIRECTIONS FOR ADMINISTRATION

1. Try to get child to smile by smiling, talking or waving. Do not touch him/her.
2. Child must stare at hand several seconds.
3. Parent may help guide toothbrush and put toothpaste on brush.
4. Child does not have to be able to tie shoes or button/zip in the back.
5. Move yarn slowly in an arc from one side to the other, about 8" above child's face.
6. Pass if child grasps rattle when it is touched to the backs or tips of fingers.
7. Pass if child tries to see where yarn went. Yarn should be dropped quickly from sight from tester's hand without arm movement.
8. Child must transfer cube from hand to hand without help of body, mouth, or table.
9. Pass if child picks up raisin with any part of thumb and finger.
10. Line can vary only 30 degrees or less from tester's line. /
11. Make a fist with thumb pointing upward and wiggle only the thumb. Pass if child imitates and does not move any fingers other than the thumb.

               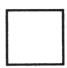

12. Pass any enclosed form. Fail continuous round motions.
13. Which line is longer? (Not bigger.) Turn paper upside down and repeat. (pass 3 of 3 or 5 of 6)
14. Pass any lines crossing near midpoint.
15. Have child copy first. If failed, demonstrate.

When giving items 12, 14, and 15, do not name the forms. Do not demonstrate 12 and 14.

16. When scoring, each pair (2 arms, 2 legs, etc.) counts as one part.
17. Place one cube in cup and shake gently near child's ear, but out of sight. Repeat for other ear.

B 18. Point to picture and have child name it. (No credit is given for sounds only.)
   If less than 4 pictures are named correctly, have child point to picture as each is named by tester.

     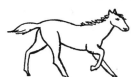   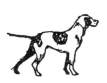   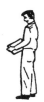

19. Using doll, tell child: Show me the nose, eyes, ears, mouth, hands, feet, tummy, hair. Pass 6 of 8.
20. Using pictures, ask child: Which one flies?... says meow?... talks?... barks?... gallops? Pass 2 of 5, 4 of 5.
21. Ask child: What do you do when you are cold?... tired?... hungry? Pass 2 of 3, 3 of 3.
22. Ask child: What do you do with a cup? What is a chair used for? What is a pencil used for? Action words must be included in answers.
23. Pass if child correctly places <u>and</u> says how many blocks are on paper. (1, 5).
24. Tell child: Put block **on** table; **under** table; **in front of** me, **behind** me. Pass 4 of 4. (Do not help child by pointing, moving head or eyes.)
25. Ask child: What is a ball?... lake?... desk?... house?... banana?... curtain?... fence?... ceiling? Pass if defined in terms of use, shape, what it is made of, or general category (such as banana is fruit, not just yellow). Pass 5 of 8, 7 of 8.
26. Ask child: If a horse is big, a mouse is __? If fire is hot, ice is __? If the sun shines during the day, the moon shines during the __? Pass 2 of 3.
27. Child may use wall or rail only, not person. May not crawl.
28. Child must throw ball overhand 3 feet to within arm's reach of tester.
29. Child must perform standing broad jump over width of test sheet (8 1/2 inches).
30. Tell child to walk forward, ⚬⚬⚬⚬➔ heel within 1 inch of toe. Tester may demonstrate. Child must walk 4 consecutive steps.
31. In the second year, half of normal children are non-compliant.

OBSERVATIONS:

Fig. 1-57, cont'd   **B,** Directions for administration of numbered items on Denver II. (From Frankenburg WK, Dodds JB, 1990.)

Revised Denver Prescreening Developmental Questionnaire*

The Revised Prescreening Developmental Questionnaire (R-PDQ) is a revision of the original PDQ. Advantages of the R-PDQ include the addition and arrangement of items to be more age-appropriate, simplified parent scoring, and easier comparison with Denver Developmental Screening Test (DDST) norms for professionals. The R-PDQ is a parent-answered prescreen consisting of 105 questions from the DDST, although only a subset of questions are asked for each age group. The form may need to be read to less educated caregivers.

Preparation and scoring of the R-PDQ include the following:

1. Calculate the child's age as detailed in the Denver II manual and choose the appropriate form* for the child: orange (0 to 9 months), purple (9 to 24 months), gold (2 to 4 years), or white (4 to 6 years). (See sample of 0 to 9 month form, Fig. 1-58.)
2. Give the appropriate form to the child's caregiver and have person note relationship to the child. Have the caregiver answer questions until: (1) 3 NOs are circled (they do not have to be consecutive); or (2) all of the questions on both sides of the form have been answered.
3. Check form to see that all appropriate questions have been answered.

---

*Forms and complete instructions are available from Denver Developmental Materials, Inc. PO Box 371075, Denver, CO 80237-5075, USA; (303) 355-4729, (800) 419-4729.

†Suggested Denver Developmental Activities are available from Denver Developmental Materials, Inc.

4. Review YES and NO responses. Ensure that the child's caregiver understood each question and scored the items correctly. Give particular attention to the scoring of questions that require verbal responses by the child and that require the child to draw.
5. Identify "delays" (items passed by 90% of children at a younger age than the child being screened). Ages at which 90% of children in the DDST sample passed the items are indicated in parentheses in the "For Office Use" column. These ages are shown in months and weeks up to 24 months, and in years and months after 24 months. Highlight "delays" by circling the 90% age in parentheses to the right of the item that the child was not able to perform.
6. Children who have no "delays" are considered to be developing normally.
7. If a child has one "delay," give the caregiver age-appropriate developmental activities to pursue with the child† and schedule the child for rescreening with the R-PDQ 1 month later. If, on rescreening a month later, the child has one or more "delays," schedule second-stage screening with the Denver II as soon as possible.
8. If a child has two or more "delays" on the first-stage screening with the R-PDQ, schedule a second-stage screening with the Denver II as soon as possible. If, on second-stage screening with the Denver II, a child receives other than normal results, schedule the child for a diagnostic evaluation.

BOX 1-7

Denver II Scoring

Interpretation of Denver II Scores

Advanced: Passed an item completely to the *right* of the age line (passed by less than 25% of children at an age older than the child)

OK: Passed, failed, or refused an item intersected by the age line between the 25th and 75th percentiles

Caution: Failed or refused items intersected by the age line on or between the 75th and 90th percentiles

Delay: Failed an item completely to the *left* of the age line; refusals to the left of the age line may also be considered delays, since the reason for the refusal may be inability to perform the task

Interpretation of Test

Normal: No delays and a maximum of one caution
Suspect: One or more delays and/or two or more cautions
Untestable: Refusals on one or more items completely to the left of the age line or on more than one item intersected by the age line in the 75th to 90th percentile area

Recommendations for Referral for Suspect and Untestable Tests

Rescreen in 1 to 2 weeks to rule out temporary factors.
If rescreen is suspect or untestable, use clinical judgment based on the following: number of cautions and delays; which items are cautions and delays; rate of past development; clinical examination and history; and availability of referral resources.

Unit 1

0-9 MONTHS (R-PDQ)

REVISED DENVER PRESCREENING DEVELOPMENTAL QUESTIONNAIRE

Child's Name _____

Person Completing R-PDQ: _____

Relation to Child: _____

For Office Use

Today's Date: _____ yr _____ mo _____ day

Child's Birthdate: _____ yr _____ mo _____ day

Subtract to get Child's Exact Age: _____ yr _____ mo _____ day

R-PDQ Age: (_____ yr _____ mo _____ completed wks)

CONTINUE ANSWERING UNTIL **3 "NOs"** ARE CIRCLED | For Office Use

1. Equal Movements
When your baby is lying on his/her back, can (s)he move each of his/her arms as easily as the other and each of the legs as easily as the other? Answer **No** if your child makes jerky or uncoordinated movements with one or both of his/her arms or legs.
Yes   No   (0)   FMA

2. Stomach Lifts Head
When your baby is on his/her stomach on a flat surface, can (s)he lift his/her head off the surface?
Yes   No   (0-3)   GM

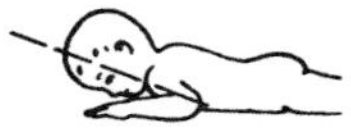

3. Regards Face
When your baby is lying on his/her back, can (s)he look at you and watch your face?
Yes   No   (1)   PS

4. Follows To Midline
When your child is on his/her back, can (s)he follow your movement by turning his/her head from one side to facing directly forward?
Yes   No   (1-1)   FMA

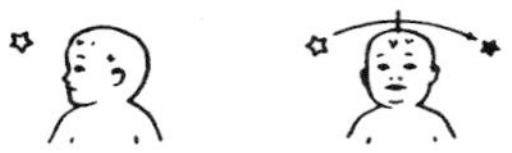

5. Responds To Bell
Does your child respond with eye movements, change in breathing or other change in activity to a bell or rattle sounded outside his/her line of vision?
Yes   No   (1-2)   L

6. Vocalizes Not Crying
Does your child make sounds other than crying, such as gurgling, cooing, or babbling?
Yes   No   (1-3)   L

7. Smiles Responsively
When you smile and talk to your baby, does (s)he smile back at you?
Yes   No   (1-3)   PS

8. Follows Past Midline
When your child is on his/her back, does (s)he follow your movement by turning his/her head from one side *almost all the way to the other side?*
Yes   No   (2-2)   FMA

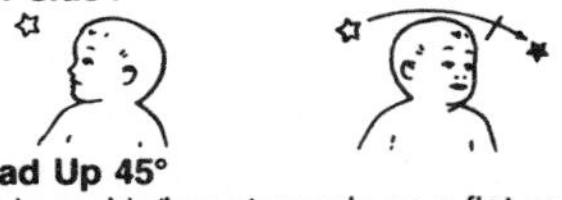

9. Stomach, Head Up 45°
When your baby is on his/her stomach on a flat surface, can (s)he lift his/her head 45°?
Yes   No   (2-2)   GM

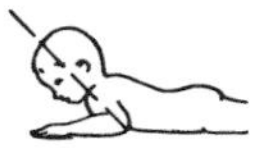

10. Stomach, Head Up 90°
When your baby is on his/her stomach on a flat surface, can (s)he lift his/her head 90°?
Yes   No   (3)   GM

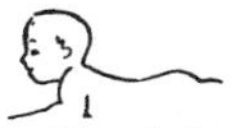

11. Laughs
Does your baby laugh out loud without being tickled or touched?
Yes   No   (3-1)   L

12. Hands Together
Does your baby play with his/her hands by touching them together?
Yes   No   (3-3)   FMA

13. Follows 180°
When your child is on his/her back, does (s)he follow your movement from one side *all the way* to the other side?
Yes   No   (4)   FMA

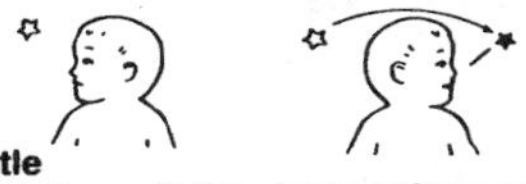

14. Grasps Rattle
It is important that you follow instructions carefully. Do **not** place the pencil in the palm of your child's hand. When you touch the pencil to the back or tips of your baby's fingers, does your baby grasp the pencil for a few seconds?
Yes   No   (4)   FMA

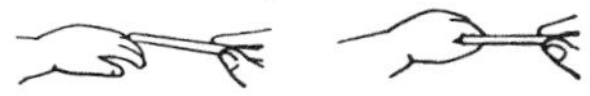

TRY THIS   NOT THIS

(Please turn page)

©Wm. K. Frankenburg, M.D., 1975, 1986

Fig. 1-58   Revised Denver Prescreening Developmental Questionnaire. (The first page is reprinted with permission of William K. Frankenburg, MD. Copyright 1975, 1986, WK Frankenburg, MD.)

ASSESSMENT OF LANGUAGE AND SPEECH
Major Developmental Characteristics of Language and Speech

Age (Years)	Normal Language Development	Normal Speech Development	Intelligibility
1	Says two or three words with meaning	Omits most final and some initial consonants	Usually no more than 25% intelligible to unfamiliar listener
	Imitates sounds of animals	Substitutes consonants "m," "w," "p," "b," "k," "g," "n," "t," "d," and "h" for more difficult sounds	Height of unintelligible jargon at age 18 months
2	Uses two- or three-word phrases Has vocabulary of about 300 words Uses "I," "me," "you"	Uses above consonants with vowels, but inconsistently and with much substitution Omission of final consonants Articulation lags behind vocabulary	At age 2 years, 50% intelligible in context
3	Says four- or five-word sentences Has vocabulary of about 900 words Uses "who," "what," and "where" in asking questions Uses plurals, pronouns, and prepositions	Masters "b," "t," "d," "k," and "g"; sounds "r" and "l" may still be unclear, omits or substitutes "w" Repetitions and hesitations common	At age 3 years, 75% intelligible
4-5	Has vocabulary of 1500 to 2100 words Able to use most grammatic forms correctly, such as past tense of verb with "yesterday" Uses complete sentences with nouns, verbs, prepositions, adjectives, adverbs, and conjunctions	Masters "f" and "v"; may still distort "r," "l," "s," "z," "sh," "ch," "y," and "th" Little or no omission of initial or final consonants	Speech is 100% intelligible, although some sounds are still imperfect
5-6	Has vocabulary of 3000 words Comprehends "if," "because," and "why"	Masters "r," "l," and "th"; may still distort "s," "z," "sh," "ch," and "j" (usually mastered by age 7½ to 8 years)	

Assessment of Communication Impairment

Key questions for language disorders:

1. How old was your child when he/she spoke his/her first words?
2. How old was your child when he/she began to put words into sentences?
3. Does your child have difficulty in learning new vocabulary words?
4. Does your child omit words from sentences (i.e., do his/her sentences sound telegraphic?) or use short or incomplete sentences?
5. Does your child have trouble with grammar, such as using the verbs *is, am, are, was,* and *were?*
6. Can your child follow two or three directions given at once?
7. Do you have to repeat directions or questions?
8. Does your child respond appropriately to questions?
9. Does your child ask questions beginning with *who, what, where,* and *why?*
10. Does it seem that your child has made little or no progress in speech and language in the last 6 to 12 months?

Key questions for speech impairment:

1. Does your child ever stammer or repeat sounds or words?
2. Does your child seem anxious or frustrated when trying to express an idea?
3. Have you noticed certain behaviors, such as blinking, jerking the head, or attempting to rephrase thoughts with different words when your child stammers?
4. What do you do when any of these occurs?
5. Does your child omit sounds from words?
6. Does it seem like your child uses *t, d, k,* or *g* in place of most other consonants when speaking?
7. Does your child omit sounds from words or replace the correct consonant with another one (such as *rabbit* with *wabbit*)?
8. Do you have any difficulty in understanding your child's speech?
9. Has anyone else ever remarked about having difficulty in understanding your child?
10. Has there been any recent change in the sound of your child's voice?

Clues for Detecting Communication Impairment

LANGUAGE DISABILITY

Assigning meaning to words
First words not uttered before second birthday
Vocabulary size reduced for age, or fails to show steady increase
Difficulty in describing characteristics of objects, although may be able to name them
Infrequent use of modifier words (adjectives or adverbs)
Excessive use of jargon past age 18 months

Organizing words into sentences
First sentences not uttered before third birthday
Short and incomplete sentences
Tendency to omit words (articles, prepositions)
Misuse of the *be, do,* and *can* verb forms
Difficulty understanding and producing questions
Plateaus at an early developmental level; uses easy speech patterns

Altering word forms
Omission of endings for plurals and tenses
Inappropriate use of plurals and tense endings
Inaccurate use of possessive words

SPEECH IMPAIRMENT

Dysfluency (stuttering)
Noticeable repetition of sounds, words, or phrases after age 4 years
Obvious frustration when attempting to communicate
Demonstration of struggling behavior while talking (head jerks, blinks, retrials, or circumlocution)
Embarrassment about own speech

Articulation deficiency
Intelligibility of conversational speech absent by age 3 years
Omission of consonants at beginning of words by age 3 years and at end of words by age 4 years
Persisting articulation faults after age 7 years
Omission of a sound where one should occur
Distortion of a sound
Substitution of an incorrect sound for a correct one

Voice disorders
Deviations in pitch (too high or too low, especially for age and sex); monotone
Deviations in loudness
Deviations in quality (hypernasality or hyponasality)

Guidelines for Referral Regarding Communication Impairment

Age	Assessment Findings
2 years	Failure to speak any meaningful words spontaneously Consistent use of gestures rather than vocalizations Difficulty in following verbal directions Failure to respond consistently to sound
3 years	Speech is largely unintelligible Failure to use sentences of three or more words Frequent omission of initial consonants Use of vowels rather than consonants
5 years	Stutters or has any other type of dysfluency Sentence structure noticeably impaired Substitutes easily produced sounds for more difficult ones Omits word endings (plurals, tenses of verbs, and so on)
School age	Poor voice quality (monotonous, loud, or barely audible) Vocal pitch inappropriate for age and sex Any distortions, omissions, or substitutions of sounds after age 7 years Connected speech characterized by use of unusual confusions or reversals
General	Any child with signs that suggest a hearing impairment Any child who is embarrassed or disturbed by own speech Parents who are excessively concerned or who pressure the child to speak at a level above that appropriate for age

Denver Articulation Screening Examination

The Denver Articulation Screening Examination (DASE) (Fig. 1-59) is designed to reliably discriminate between significant developmental delays and normal variations in the acquisition of speech sounds in children from 2½ to 6 years of age. It uses the *imitative* method for assessing speech sounds. A complete instructional manual is available.*

General guidelines include the following:

1. Tell the child to repeat a word, such as *car*. Give child several examples to ensure understanding. Beginning with the first word, *table*, have the child repeat all 22 words after you. Score the child's pronunciation of the *underlined* sounds or blends in each word. (There are 30 articulated sound elements for testing.)

2. If the child is shy or hard to test, use the simple line drawings to illustrate each word.

*Available from Denver Developmental Materials, Inc, PO Box 371075, Denver, CO 80237-5075; USA; (303) 355-4729, (800) 419-4729.

3. To determine test results, match the raw score line (number of correct sounds) with the column denoting child's age. A child is considered to be the closest *previous* age group shown on the percentile rank chart. The child's percentile rank is at the point where the line and column meet. Percentiles above the heavy line are *abnormal* and those below are *normal*.

4. Rate the child's spontaneous speech in terms of intelligibility:
   a. Easy to understand
   b. Understandable half the time
   c. Not understandable
   d. Can't evaluate (if the child does not speak in sentences or phrases during the interview)

5. Rate the child's total test results as follows:
   a. **Normal**—Normal on DASE *and* intelligibility
   b. **Abnormal**—Abnormal on DASE *and/or* intelligibility

6. Rescreen children with abnormal results within 2 weeks.

ASSESSMENT OF VISION
Major Developmental Characteristics of Vision

Age (weeks)	Development
Birth	Visual acuity 20/100-20/400* Pupillary and corneal (blink) reflexes present Able to fixate on moving object in range of 45 degrees when held 20-25 cm (8-10 inches) away Cannot integrate head and eye movements well (doll's eye reflex—eyes lag behind if head is rotated to one side)
4	Can follow in range of 90 degrees Can watch parent intently as he or she speaks to infant Tear glands begin to function Visual acuity is hyperoptic because of less spheric eyeball than in adult
6-12	Has peripheral vision to 180 degrees Binocular vision begins at age 6 weeks, is well established by age 4 months Convergence on near objects begins by age 6 weeks, is well developed by age 3 months Doll's eye reflex disappears
12-20	Recognizes feeding bottle Able to fixate on a 1.25 cm (½ inch) block Looks at hand while sitting or lying on back Able to accommodate to near objects
20-28	Adjusts posture to see an object Able to rescue a dropped toy Develops color preference for yellow and red Able to discriminate between simple geometric forms Prefers more complex visual stimuli Develops hand-eye coordination
28-44	Can fixate on very small objects Depth perception begins to develop Lack of binocular vision indicates strabismus
44-52	Visual acuity 20/40-20/60 Visual loss may develop if strabismus is present Can follow rapidly moving objects

*Measurement of visual acuity varies according to testing procedures.

DENVER ARTICULATION SCREENING EXAM
for children 2½ to 6 years of age

Instructions: Have child repeat each word after
you. Circle the underlined sounds that he pro-
nounces correctly. Total correct sounds is the
Raw Score. Use charts on reverse side to score
results.

Name:

Hosp. No.:

Address:_____

_____

Date: _____ Child's age: _____ Examiner: _____ Raw score: ____

Percentile:_____ Intelligibility:_____ Result: _____

1. table	6. zipper	11. sock	16. wagon	21. leaf
2. shirt	7. grapes	12. vacuum	17. gum	22. carrot
3. door	8. flag	13. yarn	18. house	
4. trunk	9. thumb	14. mother	19. pencil	
5. jumping	10. toothbrush	15. twinkle	20. fish	

Intelligibility: (circle one)
    1. Easy to understand
    2. Understandable ½ the time

    3. Not understandable
    4. Can't evaluate

Comments:

A

Date: _____ Child's age: _____ Examiner: _____ Raw score:____

Percentile:_____ Intelligibility:_____ Result: _____

1. table	6. zipper	11. sock	16. wagon	21. leaf
2. shirt	7. grapes	12. vacuum	17. gum	22. carrot
3. door	8. flag	13. yarn	18. house	
4. trunk	9. thumb	14. mother	19. pencil	
5. jumping	10. toothbrush	15. twinkle	20. fish	

Intelligibility: (circle one)
    1. Easy to understand
    2. Understandable ½ the time

    3. Not understandable
    4. Can't evaluate

Comments:

Date: _____ Child's age: _____ Examiner: _____ Raw score____

Percentile:_____ Intelligibility:_____ Result: _____

1. table	6. zipper	11. sock	16. wagon	21. leaf
2. shirt	7. grapes	12. vacuum	17. gum	22. carrot
3. door	8. flag	13. yarn	18. house	
4. trunk	9. thumb	14. mother	19. pencil	
5. jumping	10. toothbrush	15. twinkle	20. fish	

Intelligibility: (circle one)
    1. Easy to understand
    2. Understandable ½ the time

    3. Not understandable
    4. Can't evaluate

Fig. 1-59 **A,** Denver Articulation Screening Examination for children 2½ to 6 years of age. (From Frankenburg WK, University of Colorado Medical Center, 1971.)
Continued

Unit 1

To score DASE words: Note raw score for child's performance. Match raw score line (extreme left of chart) with column representing child's age (to the closest previous age group). Where raw score line and age column meet number in that square denotes percentile rank of child's performance when compared to other children that age. Percentiles above heavy line are ABNORMAL percentiles, below heavy line are NORMAL.

PERCENTILE RANK

Raw Score	2.5 yr.	3.0	3.5	4.0	4.5	5.0	5.5	6 years
2	1							
3	2							
4	5							
5	9							
6	16							
7	23							
8	31	2						
9	37	4	1					
10	42	6	2					
11	48	7	4					
12	54	9	6	1	1			
13	58	12	9	2	3	1	1	
14	62	17	11	5	4	2	2	
15	68	23	15	9	5	3	2	
16	75	31	19	12	5	4	3	
17	79	38	25	15	6	6	4	
18	83	46	31	19	8	7	4	
19	86	51	38	24	10	9	5	1
20	89	58	45	30	12	11	7	3
21	92	65	52	36	15	15	9	4
22	94	72	58	43	18	19	12	5
23	96	77	63	50	22	24	15	7
24	97	82	70	58	29	29	20	15
25	99	87	78	66	36	34	26	17
26	99	91	84	75	46	43	34	24
27		94	89	82	57	54	44	34
28		96	94	88	70	68	59	47
29		98	98	94	84	84	77	68
30		100	100	100	100	100	100	100

To score intelligibility:

	NORMAL	ABNORMAL
2½ years	Understandable ½ the time, or, "easy"	Not understandable
3 years and older	Easy to understand	Understandable ½ time Not understandable

Test result: 1. NORMAL on DASE and Intelligibility = NORMAL

2. ABNORMAL on DASE and/or Intelligibility = ABNORMAL

*If abnormal on initial screening, rescreen within 2 weeks.
If abnormal again, child should be referred for complete speech evaluation.

Fig. 1-59, cont'd B, Percentile rank. (From Frankenburg WK, University of Colorado Medical Center, 1971.)

Clues for Detecting Visual Impairment

REFRACTIVE ERRORS

Myopia

Nearsightedness—Ability to see objects clearly at close range but not at a distance

Pathophysiology—Results from eyeball that is too long, causing image to fall in front of retina

Clinical manifestations:
Rubs eyes excessively
Tilts head or thrusts head forward
Has difficulty in reading or other close work
Holds books close to eyes
Writes or colors with head close to table
Clumsy; walks into objects
Blinks more than usual or is irritable when doing close work
Is unable to see objects clearly
Does poorly in school, especially in subjects that require demonstration, such as arithmetic
Dizziness
Headache
Nausea following close work

Treatment—Corrected with biconcave lenses that focus image on retina

Hyperopia

Farsightedness—Ability to see objects at a distance but not at close range

Pathophysiology—Results from eyeball that is too short, causing image to focus beyond retina

Clinical manifestations:
Because of accommodative ability, child can usually see objects at all ranges
Most children normally hyperopic until about 7 years of age

Treatment—If correction is required, use convex lenses to focus rays on retina

Astigmatism

Unequal curvatures in refractive apparatus

Pathophysiology—Results from unequal curvatures in cornea or lens that cause light rays to bend in different directions

Clinical manifestations:
Depends on severity of refractive error in each eye
May have clinical manifestations of myopia

Treatment—Corrected with special lenses that compensate for refractive errors

Anisometropia

Different refractive strengths in each eye

Pathophysiology—May develop amblyopia because weaker eye is used less

Clinical manifestations:
Depends on severity of refractive error in each eye
May have clinical manifestations of myopia

Treatment—Treated with corrective lenses, preferably contact lenses, to improve vision in each eye so they work as a unit

AMBLYOPIA

Lazy eye—Reduced visual acuity in one eye

Pathophysiology:
Results when one eye does not receive sufficient stimulation (e.g., from refractive errors, cataract, or strabismus)

Each retina receives different images, resulting in diplopia (double vision)
Brain accommodates by suppressing less intense image
Visual cortex eventually does not respond to visual stimulation, with loss of vision in that eye

Clinical manifestations—Poor vision in affected eye

Treatment—Preventable if treatment of primary visual defect, such as anisometropia or strabismus, begins before 6 years of age

STRABISMUS

"Squint" or cross-eye—Malalignment of eyes
  Esotropia—Inward deviation of eye
  Exotropia—Outward deviation of eye

Pathophysiology:
May result from muscle imbalance or paralysis, poor vision, or as congenital defect
Since visual axes are not parallel, brain receives two images and amblyopia can result

Clinical manifestations:
Squints eyelids together or frowns
Has difficulty focusing from one distance to another
Inaccurate judgment in picking up objects
Unable to see print or moving objects clearly
Closes one eye to see
Tilts head to one side
If combined with refractive errors, may see any of the manifestations listed for refractive errors
Diplopia
Photophobia
Dizziness
Headache
Cross-eye

Treatment:
Treatment depends on cause of strabismus
May involve occlusion therapy (patching stronger eye) or surgery to increase visual stimulation to weaker eye
Early diagnosis is essential to prevent vision loss

CATARACTS

Opacity of crystalline lens

Pathophysiology—Prevents light rays from entering eye and being refracted on retina

Clinical manifestations:
Gradually less able to see objects clearly
May lose peripheral vision
Nystagmus (with complete blindness)
Gray opacities of lens
Strabismus
Absence of red reflex

Treatment:
Requires surgery to remove cloudy lens and replace lens (intraocular lens implant, removable contact lens, prescription glasses)
Must be treated early to prevent blindness from amblyopia

GLAUCOMA

Increased intraocular pressure

Pathophysiology:
Congenital type results from defective development of some component related to flow of aqueous humor
Increased pressure on optic nerve causes eventual atrophy and blindness

Continued

Clues for Detecting Visual Impairment—cont'd

GLAUCOMA—cont'd

Clinical Manifestations:
  Mostly seen in acquired types; loses peripheral vision
  May bump into objects not directly in front
  Sees halos around objects
  May complain of mild pain or discomfort (severe pain, nausea, vomiting, if sudden rise in pressure)
  Redness
  Excessive tearing (epiphora)
  Photophobia
  Spasmodic winking (blepharospasm)
  Corneal haziness
  Enlargement of eyeball (buphthalmos)
Treatment:
  Requires surgical treatment (goniotomy) to open outflow tracts
  May require more than one procedure

Special Tests of Visual Acuity and Estimated Visual Acuity at Different Ages

Test	Description	Birth	4 Months	1 Year	Age of 20/20 Vision
Optokinetic Nystagmus	A striped drum is rotated or a striped tape is moved in front of infant's eyes. Presence of nystagmus indicates vision. Acuity is assessed by using progressively smaller stripes.	20/400	20/200	20/60	20 to 30 months
Forced-Choice Preferential Looking*	Either a homogeneous field or a striped field is presented to infant; an observer monitors the direction of the eyes during presentation of pattern. Acuity is assessed by using progressively smaller striped fields.	20/400	20/200	20/50	18 to 24 months
Visually Evoked Potentials	Eyes are stimulated with bright light or pattern, and electrical activity to visual cortex is recorded through scalp electrodes. Acuity is assessed by using progressively smaller patterns.	20/100 to 20/200	20/80	20/40	6 to 12 months

Data from Hoyt C, Nickel B, Billson F: Ophthalmological examination of the infant: development aspects, *Surv Ophthalmol* 26:177-189, 1982.
*One type of preferential looking test is the *Teller Acuity Card Test,* in which a set of rectangular cards containing different black-and-white patterns or grading is presented to the child as an observer looks through a central peephole in the card. The observer, who is hidden from view, observes the variety of visual cues, such as fixation, eye movements, head movements, or pointing. The finest grading the child is judged to be able to see is taken as the acuity estimate. The test is appropriate for children from birth to 24 to 36 months of age (Teller D and others: Assessment of visual acuity in infants and children: the acuity card procedure, *Dev Med Child Neurol* 28:779-789, 1986).

Letter or Symbol Vision Acuity Tests

Test	Description	Comments*
Snellen Letter†	Uses letters of the English alphabet for testing at 20 feet	For most children above the second grade who are familiar with reading the alphabet
Snellen E†	Uses the capital letter E pointing in four directions; children "read" the chart by showing the direction of the letter E or using a large duplicate E to match the chart E at 20 feet	For illiterate or non–English-speaking people, preschool children, and grade 1 Preschool children often have difficulty with direction despite adequate vision
Home Eye Test for Preschoolers‡	Uses a large letter E for demonstration and an E chart for testing at 10 feet	For use by parents on children ages 3 to 6 years
Blackbird Preschool Vision Screening System§	Uses a modified E to resemble a flying bird; children identify which way the bird is flying Uses flash cards, storytelling, and disposable cardboard eyeglass occluders	For children as young as 3 years Avoids the problem with image reversal and eye-hand coordination that can occur with the letter E
Blackbird Storybook Home Eye Test§	Similar to above	For use by parents for children as young as 2½ years
HOTV or Matching Symbol†	Uses the four letters H, O, T, and V on a chart for testing at 10 or 20 feet Child names the letters on the chart or matches them to a demonstration card	For children as young as 3 years Avoids the problem with image reversal and eye-hand coordination that can occur with the letter E
Faye Symbol Chart§	Use pictures of a house, apple, and umbrella on a chart for testing at 10 feet	For children as young as 27 to 30 months
Denver Eye Screening Test (DEST)‖	Uses single cards for the letter E, one for demonstration and one for testing at 15 feet Also uses Allen Picture Cards (a tree, birthday cake, horse and rider, telephone, car, house, and teddy bear) for testing at 15 feet	For children 2½ years and older May be reliably used with cooperative children from the age of 24 months
Dot Test†	Uses a series of different-sized dots; child points to one of the nine dots randomly positioned on a disk	For children as young as 24 months

*Ages for testing are based on published reports. Proper instruction of young children is essential for successful screening.
†Available from Good-Lite Co., 1540 Hannah Ave., Forest Park, IL 60130, USA; (708) 366-3860.
‡Available from the National Society to Prevent Blindness, 500 E. Remington Rd., Schaumburg, IL 60173, USA; (800) 331-2020; e-mail: info@preventblindness.org; Web site: www.preventblindness.org.
§Available from Blackbird Vision Screening System, PO Box 277424, Sacramento, CA 95827, USA; (916) 363-6884.
‖Available from Denver Developmental Materials, Inc., PO Box 371075, Denver, CO 80237-5075, USA; (303) 355-4729, (800) 419-4729.

Vision Screening Guidelines and Referral Criteria

Function	Recommended Tests	Referral Criteria	Comments
Ages 3-5 Years			

Distance visual acuity	Snellen letters
	Snellen numbers
	Tumbling E
	HOTV
	Picture tests
	  Allen figures
	  LH test
		1. <4 of 6 correct on 20-ft line with either eye tested at 10 ft monocularly (e.g., <10/20 or 20/40)
		or
		2. Two-line difference between eyes, even within the passing range (i.e., 10/12.5 and 10/20 or 20/25 and 20/40)
			1. Tests are listed in decreasing order of cognitive difficulty; the highest test that the child is capable of performing should be used; in general, the tumbling E or the HOTV test should be used for ages 3-5 years and Snellen letters or numbers for ages 6 years and older
			2. Testing distance of 10 ft is recommended for all visual acuity tests
			3. A line of figures is preferred over single figures
			4. The nontested eye should be covered by an occluder held by the examiner or by an adhesive occluder patch applied to eye; the examiner must ensure that it is not possible to peek with the nontested eye

Ocular alignment	Unilateral cover test
	  at 10 ft or 3 m
	or
	Random-dot-E stereo
	  test at 40 cm (630
	  seconds of arc)
		Any eye movement
		
		<4 of 6 correct	

Ages 6 Years and Older			

Distance visual acuity	Snellen letters
	Snellen numbers
	Tumbling E
	HOTV
	Picture tests
	  Allen figures
	  LH test
		1. <4 of 6 correct on 15-ft line with either eye tested at 10 ft monocularly (i.e., <10/15 or 20/30)
		or
		2. Two-line difference between eyes, even within the passing range (i.e., 10/10 and 10/15 or 20/20 and 20/30)
			Same as above

Ocular alignment	Same as above		

From American Academy of Pediatrics: Eye examination and vision screening in infants, children, and young adults, *Pediatrics* 98(1):156, 1996.

Denver Eye Screening Test

The Denver Eye Screening Test (DEST) (Fig. 1-60) tests visual acuity in children 3 years or older by using a single card for the letter E (20/30) from a distance of 15 feet. A complete instructional manual is available.

General guidelines include the following:

1. Mark a distance of 15 feet for testing.
2. Use the large E (20/100) to explain and to demonstrate the testing procedure to the child. (See procedure for Snellen E, below).
3. Use the small E for actual testing. Test each eye separately using the occluder.
4. Consider the results *abnormal* if the child fails to correctly identify the direction of the small E over three trials.
5. Test children from 2½ to 2¹¹⁄₁₂ years of age or those untestable with the letter E using the picture (Allen) cards. (Cooperative children as young as 2 years can also be tested.)
6. Show each card to the child at close range to make certain he or she can identify it.

7. Present the pictures at a distance of 15 feet for actual testing. Test each eye separately if possible.
8. Consider the results *abnormal* if the child fails to correctly name three of the seven cards in three to five trials.
9. Screen children from 6 to 30 months by testing for the following:
   a. Fixation (ability to follow a moving light source or spinning toy)
   b. Squinting (observation of the child's eyes or report by parent)
   c. Strabismus (report by parent and performance on cover and pupillary light reflex tests; see pp. 44-45)
10. Consider the results *abnormal* if failure to fixate, presence of a squint, and/or failing two of the three procedures for strabismus.
11. Retest all children with abnormal findings. Refer those with a repeat failure.

Snellen Screening

PREPARATION

1. Hang the Snellen chart (Fig. 1-61) on a light-colored wall so that the 20- to 30-foot lines are at eye level when children 6 to 12 years old are tested in the standing position.
2. Secure the chart to the wall with double-stick tape on the back side of all four corners. If the chart must be reversed for use of the letter or E chart, secure it at the top and bottom with tacks. Make sure that the chart does not swing when in place.
3. The illumination intensity on the chart should be 10 to 30 footcandles, without any glare from windows or light fixtures. The illumination should be checked with a light meter.
4. Mark an exact 20-foot distance from the chart. Mark the floor with a piece of tape or "footprints" positioned so that the heels touch the 20-foot line.

PROCEDURE

1. Place the child at the 20-foot mark, with the heel edging the line if child is standing or with the back of the chair placed at the marker if the child is seated.
2. If the E chart is used, accustom the child to identifying which direction the "legs of the E" are pointing. Use a demonstration E card for this purpose.
3. Teach the child to use the occluder to cover one eye. Instruct child to keep both eyes open during the test. Provide a clean cover card for each child and discard after use.
4. If the child wears glasses, test only with glasses on.
5. Test both eyes together, then right eye, then left eye.
6. Begin with the 40- or 30-foot line and proceed with test to include the 20-foot line.

7. With a child suspected to have low vision, begin with the 200-foot line and proceed until the child can no longer correctly read three out of four or four out of six symbols on a line.
8. Use covers on the Snellen chart to expose only one symbol or one line at a time. When screening kindergarten or older children, expose one line but a pointer may be used to point to one symbol at a time.

RECORDING AND REFERRAL

1. Record the last line the child read correctly (three out of four or four out of six symbols).
2. Record visual acuity as a fraction. The numerator represents the distance from the chart, and the denominator represents the last line read correctly. For example, 20/30 means that the child read the 30-foot line at a 20-foot distance.
3. Observe the child's eyes during testing and record any evidence of squinting, head tilting, thrusting the head forward, excessive blinking, tearing, or redness.
4. Only make referrals after a second screening has been made on children who are potential candidates for referral.
5. The following children should be referred for a complete eye examination:
   a. Three-year-old children with vision in either eye of 20/50 or less (inability to correctly identify one more than half the symbols on the 40-foot line) *or* a two-line difference in visual acuity between the eyes in the passing range; for example, 20/20 in one eye and 20/40 in the other
   b. All other ages and grades with vision in either eye of 20/40 or less (inability to correctly identify one more than half the symbols on the 30-foot line)
   c. All children who consistently show any of the signs of possible visual disturbances, regardless of visual acuity

Modified from recommendations of the National Society to Prevent Blindness: *Guide to testing distance visual acuity,* Schaumburg, IL, 1988, The Society.

Unit 1

DENVER EYE SCREENING TEST

Name:
Hospital No.:
Ward:
Address:

Vision Tests	1ST SCREENING: DATE: Right Eye Normal	Right Eye Abnormal	Right Eye Untestable	Left Eye Normal	Left Eye Abnormal	Left Eye Untestable	RESCREENING: DATE: Right Eye Normal	Right Eye Abnormal	Right Eye Untestable	Left Eye Normal	Left Eye Abnormal	Left Eye Untestable
1. "E" (3 years and above—3 to 5 trials)	3P	3F	U	3P	3F	U	3P	3F	U	3P	3F	U
2. Picture card (2 1/2 – 2 11/12 yrs.—3 to 5 trials)	3P	3F	U	3P	3F	U	3P	3F	U	3P	3F	U
3. Fixation (6 months – 2 5/12 years)	P	F	U	P	F	U	P	F	U	P	F	U
4. Squinting		yes			yes			yes			yes	

Tests for Non-Straight Eyes	Normal	Abnormal	Untestable	Normal	Abnormal	Untestable
1. Do your child's eyes turn in or out, or are they ever not straight?	NO	YES	U	NO	YES	U
2. Cover Test	P	F	U	P	F	U
3. Pupillary Light Reflex	P	F	U	P	F	U

Total Test Rating (Both Eyes)	1st Screening	Rescreening
Normal (passed vision test plus no squint, plus passed 2/3 tests for non-straight eyes)	Normal	Normal
Abnormal (abnormal on any vision test, squinting or 2 of 3 procedures for non-straight eyes)	Abnormal	Abnormal
Untestable (untestable on any vision test or untestable on 2/3 tests for non-straight eyes)	Untestable	Untestable
Future Rescreening Appointment for Total Test Rating (Abnormal or Untestable)	Date:	Date:

Fig. 1-60 Denver Eye Screening Test. (From Frankenburg WK, Dodds JB, University of Colorado Medical Center, 1969.)

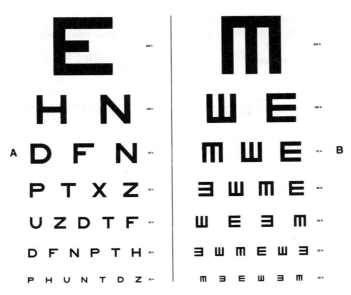

Fig. 1-61 Snellen chart. **A,** Letter (alphabet) chart. **B,** Symbol E chart. (From National Society to Prevent Blindness, Inc., Schaumburg, IL.)

ASSESSMENT OF HEARING
Major Developmental Characteristics of Hearing

Age (Months)	Development
Birth	Responds to loud noise with startle reflex Responds to sound of human voice more readily than to any other sound Becomes quiet with low-pitched sounds, such as lullaby, metronome, or heartbeat
2-3	Turns head to side when sound is made at level of ear
3-4	Locates sound by turning head to side and looking in same direction
4-6	Can localize sounds made below ear, which is followed by localization of sound made above ear; will turn head to side and then look up or down Begins to imitate sounds
6-8	Locates sounds by turning head in a curving arc Responds to own name
8-10	Localizes sounds by turning head diagonally and directly toward sound
10-12	Knows several words and their meanings, such as *no* and the names of family members Learns to control and adjust own response to sound, such as listening for sound to occur again
18	Begins to discriminate between harshly dissimilar sounds, such as the sounds of a doorbell and a train
24	Refines gross discriminative skills
36	Begins to distinguish more subtle differences in speech sounds, such as between *e* and *er*
48	Begins to distinguish between similar sounds such as *f* and *th* or between *f* and *s* Listening becomes considerably refined Able to be tested with an audiometer

Assessment of Child for Hearing Impairment

Family History

Genetic disorders associated with hearing impairment
Family members, especially siblings, with hearing disorders

Prenatal History

Miscarriages
Illnesses during pregnancy (rubella, syphilis, diabetes)
Drugs taken
Exposure to childhood diseases
Eclampsia

Delivery

Duration of labor, type of delivery
Fetal distress
Presentation (especially breech)
Drugs used
Blood incompatibility

Birth History

Birth weight <1500 g
Hyperbilirubinemia at level exceeding indications for exchange transfusion
Severe asphyxia
Prematurity
Congenital perinatal viral infection (cytomegalovirus, rubella, herpes, syphilis, toxoplasmosis)
Congenital anomalies involving head and neck

Past Health History

Immunizations
Serious illness (e.g., bacterial meningitis)
Seizures

High unexplained fevers
Ototoxic drugs
Hyperbilirubinemia (if preterm)
No history (adopted child)
Colds, ear infections, allergies
Treatment of ear problems
Visual difficulties
Exposure to excessive noise (such as monitor alarms, gunshot)

Hearing

Parental concerns regarding hearing loss (what cues, at what age)
Response to name calling, loud noises, sounds of different frequencies (crinkling paper, whisper, bell, rattle)
Results of previous audiometric testing

Speech Development

Age of babbling, first meaningful words, phrases
Intelligibility of speech
Present vocabulary

Motor Development

Age of sitting, standing, walking
Level of independence in self-care, feeding, toileting, grooming

Adaptive Behavior

Play activities
Socialization with other children
Behaviors: temper tantrums, stubbornness, self-vexation, vibratory stimulus
Educational achievement
Recent behavioral and/or personality changes

Clues for Detecting Hearing Impairment

Orientation Response

Lack of startle or blink reflex to a loud sound
Persistence of Moro reflex beyond 4 months of age (associated with mental retardation)
Failure to be awakened by loud environmental noises during early infancy
Failure to localize a source of sound by 6 months of age
General indifference to sound
Lack of response to the spoken word; failure to follow verbal directions
Response to loud noises as opposed to the voice

Vocalizations and Sound Production

Monotone quality, unintelligible speech, lessened laughter
Normal quality in central auditory loss
Lessened experimental sound play and squealing
Normal use of jargon during early infancy in central auditory loss, with persistent use later on
Absence of babble or inflections in voice by age 7 months
Failure to develop intelligible speech by age 24 months
Vocal play, head banging, or foot stamping for vibratory sensation

Yelling or screeching to express pleasure, annoyance, or need
Asking to have statements repeated or answering them incorrectly

Visual Attention

Augmented visual alertness and attentiveness
Responding more to facial expression than verbal explanation
Being alert to gestures and movement
Use of gestures rather than verbalization to express desires, especially after age 15 months
Marked imitativeness in play

Social Rapport and Adaptations

Less interest and involvement in vocal nursery games
Intense preoccupation with things rather than persons
Avoidance of social interactions; often puzzled and unhappy in such situations
Inquiring, sometimes confused facial expression
Suspicious alertness, sometimes interpreted as paranoia, alternating with cooperation
Marked reactivity to praise, attention, and physical affection

Clues for Detecting Hearing Impairment—cont'd

Shows less interest than peers in casual conversation

Is often inattentive unless the environment is quiet and the speaker is close to the child

Is more responsive to movement than to sound

Intently observes the speaker's face, responding more to facial expression than verbalization

Often asks to have statements repeated

May not follow directions exactly

Emotional Behavior

Use of tantrums to call attention to self or needs

Frequently stubborn because of lack of comprehension

Irritable at not making self understood

Shy, timid, and withdrawn

Often appears "dreamy," "in a world of his/her own," or markedly inattentive

Selected Hearing and Tympanic Membrane Compliance Tests*

Description	Comments
Clinical Hearing Tests	
In newborns, elicit the startle reflex and observe other neonatal responses to loud noises, such as facial grimaces, blinking, gross motor movement, quiet if crying or crying if quiet, opening the eyes, or ceasing sucking activity.	An objective sign of alerting to sound may be an increase in heart rate or respiratory rate.
During infancy, note child's reaction to a noise. Stand approximately 18 inches away from infant, to the side and out of child's peripheral field of vision. With the room silent and infant sitting in parent's lap, distracted by some object, make a voice sound such as "ps" or "phth" (high-pitched) or "oo" (low-pitched), ring a bell, shake a rattle, or rustle tissue paper.	Absence of alerting behaviors suggests hearing loss. Eliciting the startle reflex is used only in infants from birth to 4 months. Test is usually inadequate for children beyond infancy because of their tendency to ignore sounds or to be distracted. Compare response of localizing sound to expected age response.
Crib-O-Gram	
Neonatal screening tool that analyzes hearing responses by comparing the infant's motor activity before, during, and after a sound is introduced.	Both administration of the test and its scoring are totally automated. The test is repeated several times to increase reliability.
A motion-sensitive transducer is placed beneath the mattress, and a microprocessor "reads" the infant's movements.	A consistent change in activity that coincides with the test sound is scored as a pass. Neonates who are premature or ill may not respond to sound despite adequate hearing.
Tympanometry	
Measures tympanic membrane compliance (or mobility) and estimates middle ear air pressure. A soft rubber cuff is pressed over the external canal to produce an airtight seal; an automatic reading of air pressure registers on the machine.	Detects middle ear disease and abnormalities but does not indicate the degree of hearing loss or the interpretation of sound. Difficult to perform in young children because of inability to maintain an adequate seal or excessive movement by the child.
Conduction Tests	
Rinne test—Stem of tuning fork is placed against the mastoid bone until the sound ceases to be audible. Tuning fork is then moved so that the prongs are held near, but not touching, the auditory meatus. Child should again hear the sound **(Rinne positive).** If sound is not again audible **(Rinne negative),** some abnormality is interfering with the conduction of air through the external and middle chambers.	Requires the cooperation and ability of the child to signal when the sound is no longer audible and when it is again heard. Not useful for most children before preschool age.
Weber test—Stem of tuning fork is held in the midline of the head. Child should hear the sound equally in both ears **(Weber positive).** With air conductive loss, child will hear the sound better in the affected ear **(Weber negative).**	Often not suitable for young children because of their difficulty in discriminating between "better, more, or less."

Continued

Selected Hearing and Tympanic Membrane Compliance Tests*—cont'd

Description	Comments

Audiometry

Electrical audiometer measures the threshold of hearing for pure-tone frequencies and loudness.

A sound is transmitted to the child's ear and reduced until child indicates the sound is no longer heard; this procedure is repeated for several sounds covering the range found in conversation.

In an air conduction audiogram, the sounds are transmitted through earphones.

In a bone conduction audiogram, the sounds are passed through a plaque placed over the mastoid bone.

Provides valuable information regarding the severity of the hearing loss, the sound cycles involved, and the possible location of the defect. Requires specialized training of personnel, expensive equipment, and cooperation from the child in terms of confirming the perception of sound. For children ages 24 months to approximately 5 years, play audiometry can be used; it is based on behavior modification and involves reinforcement for correct response.

Evoked Otoacoustic Emissions (EOAEs)

Special OAE analyzer delivers a rapid series of clicks to the ear through a probe fitted with a tympanometry tip that is inserted closely in the external auditory canal.

The presence of OAEs, defined as sound energy emitted by the cochlea that is believed to be generated by movement of the outer hairs of the organ of Corti, is usually associated with normal or near-normal cochlear sensitivity; their absence indicates a hearing loss of at least 20-25 dB, provided there is no conductive dysfunction.†

Preferred method of screening neonates for sensorineural hearing loss (ototoxicity and noise-induced hearing loss).

Requires specialized equipment.

Minimal training is required.

Infants must be in a quiet sleep for testing.

Results do not indicate severity of cochlear damage; should be followed by BAER (see below).

Brainstem-Auditory Evoked Response (BAER)

Electrode wires attached to the infant's or child's scalp transmit electrical or brain wave potentials generated within the auditory system to a computer for analysis.

Following repetitive acoustic stimulation, the waveforms from a normal sleeping or quiet infant consist of several peaks and valleys that reflect activations of neural structures of the brain.

Requires expensive equipment and specialized training of personnel.

---

*Any child who is suspected of a hearing loss because of poor performance using screening tests is referred for special audiometric or BAER testing.

†Abdo MH, Feghali JG, Stapells DR: Transient evoked otoacoustic emissions: clinical applications and technical considerations, *Int J Pediatr Otorhinolaryngol* 25:61-71, 1993.

SUMMARY OF GROWTH AND DEVELOPMENT

This summary of growth and development offers a broad overview of the significant physical, psychosocial, and mental achievements during childhood. It begins with a comparison of cognitive and personality development throughout the life span according to different theorists. Following are summaries of the specific developmental milestones associated with each major age group of children.

Personality, Moral, and Cognitive Development

Stage/Age	Radius of Significant Relationships (Sullivan)	Psychosexual Stages (Freud)	Psychosocial Stages (Erikson)	Cognitive Stages (Piaget)	Moral Judgment Stages (Kohlberg)
I Infancy (Birth-1 year)	Maternal person (unipolar-bipolar)	Oral sensory	Trust vs mistrust	Sensorimotor (birth to 18 months)	
II Toddlerhood (1-3 years)	Parental persons (tripolar)	Anal-urethral	Autonomy vs shame and doubt	Preoperational thought, preconceptual phase (transductive reasoning, for example, specific to specific) (2 to 4 years)	Preconventional (premoral) level Punishment and obedience orientation
III Early Childhood (3-6 years)	Basic family	Phallic-locomotion	Initiative vs guilt	Preoperational thought, intuitive phase (transductive reasoning) (4 to 7 years)	Preconventional (premoral) level Naive instrumental orientation
IV Middle Childhood (6-12 years)	Neighborhood, school	Latency	Industry vs inferiority	Concrete operations (inductive reasoning and beginning logic)	Conventional level Good-boy, nice-girl orientation Law-and-order orientation
V Adolescence (13-18 years)	Peer groups and out-groups Models of leadership Partners in friendship, sex, competition, cooperation	Genitality	Identity and repudiation vs identity confusion	Formal operations (deductive and abstract reasoning)	Postconventional or principled level Social-contract orientation Universal ethical principle orientation (no longer included in revised theory)
VI Early Adulthood	Divided labor and shared household		Intimacy and solidarity vs isolation		
VII Young and Middle Adulthood	Mankind "My kind"		Generativity vs self-absorption		
VIII Later Adulthood			Ego integrity vs despair		

Growth and Development During Infancy

Age (Months)	Physical	Gross Motor	Fine Motor
1	Weight gain of 150 to 210 g (5 to 7 ounces) weekly for first 6 months Height gain of 2.5 cm (1 inch) monthly for first 6 months Head circumference increases by 1.5 cm (½ inch) monthly for first 6 months Primitive reflexes present and strong Doll's eye reflex and dance reflex fading Obligatory nose breathing (most infants)	Assumes flexed position with pelvis high but knees not under abdomen when prone (at birth, knees flexed under abdomen)* Can turn head from side to side when prone; lifts head momentarily from bed* Has marked head lag, especially when pulled from lying to sitting position Holds head momentarily parallel and in midline when suspended in prone position Assumes asymmetric tonic neck reflex position when supine When held in standing position, body limp at knees and hips In sitting position back is uniformly rounded, absence of head control	Hands predominantly closed Grasp reflex strong Hand clenches on contact with rattle
2	Posterior fontanel closed Crawling reflex disappears	Assumes less flexed position when prone—hips flat, legs extended, arms flexed, head to side* Less head lag when pulled to sitting position Can maintain head in same plane as rest of body when held in ventral suspension When prone, can lift head almost 45 degrees off table When held in sitting position, head is held up but bobs forward Assumes asymmetric tonic neck reflex position intermittently	Hands frequently open Grasp reflex fading
3	Primitive reflexes fading	Able to hold head more erect when sitting, but still bobs forward Has only slight head lag when pulled to sitting position Assumes symmetric body positioning Able to raise head and shoulders from prone position to a 45- to 90-degree angle from table; bears weight on forearms When held in standing position, able to bear slight fraction of weight on legs Regards own hand	Actively holds rattle but will not reach for it* Grasp reflex absent Hands kept loosely open Clutches own hand; pulls at blankets and clothes
4	Drooling begins Moro, tonic neck, and rooting reflexes have disappeared*	Has almost no head lag when pulled to sitting position* Balances head well in sitting position* Back less rounded, curved only in lumbar area Able to sit erect if propped up Able to raise head and chest off surface to angle of 90 degrees Assumes predominant symmetric position Rolls from back to side*	Inspects and plays with hands; pulls clothing or blanket over face in play* Tries to reach objects with hand but overshoots Grasps object with both hands Plays with rattle placed in hand, shakes it, but cannot pick it up if dropped Can carry objects to mouth

*Milestones that represent essential integrative aspects of development that lay the foundation for the achievement of more advanced skills

Sensory	Vocalization	Socialization/Cognition
Able to fixate on moving object in range of 45 degrees when held at a distance of 20 to 25 cm (8 to 10 inches) Visual acuity approaches 20/100† Follows light to midline Quiets when hears a voice	Cries to express displeasure Makes small, throaty sounds Makes comfort sounds during feeding	Is in sensorimotor phase—stage I, use of reflexes (birth to 1 month), and stage II, primary circular reactions (1 to 4 months) Watches parent's face intently as she or he talks to infant
Binocular fixation and convergence to near objects beginning When supine, follows dangling toy from side to point beyond midline Visually searches to locate sounds Turns head to side when sound is made at level of ear	Vocalizes, distinct from crying* Crying becomes differentiated Coos Vocalizes to familiar voice	Demonstrates social smile in response to various stimuli*
Follows object to periphery (180 degrees)* Locates sound by turning head to side and looking in same direction* Begins to have ability to coordinate stimuli from various sense organs	Squeals to show pleasure* Coos, babbles, chuckles Vocalizes when smiling "Talks" a great deal when spoken to Less crying during periods of wakefulness	Displays considerable interest in surroundings Ceases crying when parent enters room Can recognize familiar faces and objects, such as feeding bottle Shows awareness of strange situations
Able to accommodate to near objects Binocular vision fairly well established Can focus on a 1.25 cm (½-inch) block Beginning eye-hand coordination	Makes consonant sounds *n, k, g, p, b* Laughs aloud* Vocalization changes according to mood	Is in stage III, secondary circular reactions Demands attention by fussing; becomes bored if left alone Enjoys social interaction with people Anticipates feeding when sees bottle or mother if breast-feeding Shows excitement with whole body, squeals, breathes heavily Shows interest in strange stimuli Begins to show memory

†Degree of visual acuity varies according to vision measurement procedure used

Continued

Growth and Development During Infancy—cont'd

Age (Months)	Physical	Gross Motor	Fine Motor
5	Beginning signs of tooth eruption Birth weight doubles	No head lag when pulled to sitting position When sitting, able to hold head erect and steady Able to sit for longer periods when back is well supported Back straight When prone, assumes symmetric positioning with arms extended Can turn over from abdomen to back* When supine, puts feet to mouth	Able to grasp objects voluntarily* Uses palmar grasp, bidextrous approach Plays with toes Takes objects directly to mouth Holds one cube while regarding a second one
6	Growth rate may begin to decline Weight gain of 90 to 150 g (3 to 5 ounces) weekly for next 6 months Height gain of 1.25 cm (½ inch) monthly for next 6 months Teething may begin with eruption of two lower central incisors* Chewing and biting occur*	When prone, can lift chest and upper abdomen off table, bearing weight on hands When about to be pulled to a sitting position, lifts head Sits in high chair with back straight Rolls from back to abdomen When held in standing position, bears almost all of weight Hand regard absent	Resecures a dropped object Drops one cube when another is given Grasps and manipulates small objects Holds bottle Grasps feet and pulls to mouth
7	Eruption of lower central incisors	When supine, spontaneously lifts head off table Sits, leaning forward on both hands* When prone, bears weight on one hand Sits erect momentarily Bears full weight on feet When held in standing position, bounces actively	Transfers objects from one hand to the other* Has unidextrous approach and grasp Holds two cubes more than momentarily Bangs cube on table Rakes at a small object
8	Begins to show regular patterns in bladder and bowel elimination Parachute reflex appears	Sits steadily unsupported* Readily bears weight on legs when supported; may stand holding onto furniture Adjusts posture to reach an object	Has beginning pincer grasp using index, fourth, and fifth fingers against lower part of thumb Releases objects at will Rings bell purposely Retains two cubes while regarding third cube Secures an object by pulling on a string Reaches persistently for toys out of reach
9	Eruption of upper central incisor may begin	Creeps on hands and knees Sits steadily on floor for prolonged time (10 minutes) Recovers balance when leans forward but cannot do so when leaning sideways Pulls self to standing position and stands holding onto furniture*	Uses thumb and index finger in crude pincer grasp* Preference for use of dominant hand now evident Grasps third cube Compares two cubes by bringing them together

*Milestones that represent essential integrative aspects of development that lay the foundation for the achievement of more advanced skills

Sensory	Vocalization	Socialization/Cognition
Visually pursues a dropped object Is able to sustain visual inspection of an object Can localize sounds made below the ear	Squeals Makes vowel cooing sounds interspersed with consonant sounds (e.g., *ab-goo*)	Smiles at mirror image Pats bottle or breast with both hands More enthusiastically playful, but may have rapid mood swings Is able to discriminate strangers from family Vocalizes displeasure when object is taken away Discovers parts of body
Adjusts posture to see an object Prefers more complex visual stimuli Can localize sounds made above the ear Will turn head to the side, then look up or down	Begins to imitate sounds* Babbling resembles one-syllable utterances—*ma, mu, da, di, bi** Vocalizes to toys, mirror image Takes pleasure in hearing own sounds (self-reinforcement)	Recognizes parents; begins to fear strangers Holds arms out to be picked up Has definite likes and dislikes Begins to imitate (cough, protrusion of tongue) Excites on hearing footsteps Laughs when head is hidden in a towel Briefly searches for a dropped object (object permanence beginning)* Frequent mood swings—from crying to laughing with little or no provocation
Can fixate on very small objects* Responds to own name Localizes sound by turning head in an arc Beginning awareness of depth and space Has taste preferences	Produces vowel sounds and chained syllables—*baba, dada, kaka** Vocalizes four distinct vowel sounds "Talks" when others are talking	Increasing fear of strangers; shows signs of fretfulness when parent disappears* Imitates simple acts and noises Tries to attract attention by coughing or snorting Plays peekaboo Demonstrates dislike of food by keeping lips closed Exhibits oral aggressiveness in biting and mouthing Demonstrates expectation in response to repetition of stimuli
	Makes consonant sounds *t, d,* and *w* Listens selectively to familiar words Utterances signal emphasis and emotion Combines syllables, such as *dada,* but does not ascribe meaning to them	Increasing anxiety over loss of parent, particularly mother, and fear of strangers Responds to word *no* Dislikes dressing, diaper change
Localizes sounds by turning head diagonally and directly toward sound Depth perception increasing	Responds to simple verbal commands Comprehends "no-no"	Parent (usually mother) is increasingly important for own sake Shows increasing interest in pleasing parent Begins to show fears of going to bed and being left alone Puts arms in front of face to avoid having it washed

Continued

Growth and Development During Infancy—cont'd

Age (Months)	Physical	Gross Motor	Fine Motor
10	Labyrinth-righting reflex is strongest—when infant is in prone or supine position, is able to raise head	Can change from prone to sitting position Stands while holding onto furniture, sits by falling down Recovers balance easily while sitting While standing, lifts one foot to take a step	Crude release of an object beginning Grasps bell by handle
11	Eruption of lower lateral incisors may begin	When sitting, pivots to reach toward back to pick up an object Cruises or walks holding onto furniture or with both hands held*	Explores objects more thoroughly (e.g., clapper inside bell) Has neat pincer grasp Drops object deliberately for it to be picked up Puts one object after another into a container (sequential play) Able to manipulate an object to remove it from tight-fitting enclosure
12	Birth weight tripled* Birth length increased by 50%* Head and chest circumference equal (head circumference 46.5 cm [18½ inches]) Has total of six to eight deciduous teeth Anterior fontanel almost closed Landau reflex fading Babinski reflex disappears Lumbar curve develops; lordosis evident during walking	Walks with one hand held* Cruises well May attempt to stand alone momentarily; may attempt first step alone* Can sit down from standing position without help	Releases cube in cup Attempts to build two-block tower but fails Tries to insert a pellet into a narrow-necked bottle but fails Can turn pages in a book, many at a time

*Milestones that represent essential integrative aspects of development that lay the foundation for the achievement of more advanced skills

Sensory	Vocalization	Socialization/Cognition
	Says "dada," "mama" with meaning Comprehends "bye-bye" May say one word (e.g., *hi, bye, no*)	Inhibits behavior to verbal command of "no-no" or own name Imitates facial expressions; waves bye-bye Extends toy to another person but will not release it Develops object permanence* Repeats actions that attract attention and cause laughter Pulls clothes of another to attract attention Plays interactive games such as pat-a-cake Reacts to adult anger; cries when scolded Demonstrates independence in dressing, feeding, locomotive skills, and testing of parents Looks at and follows pictures in a book
	Imitates definite speech sounds	Experiences joy and satisfaction when a task is mastered Reacts to restrictions with frustration Rolls ball to another on request Anticipates body gestures when a familiar nursery rhyme or story is being told (e.g., holds toes and feet in response to "This little piggy went to market") Plays games such as up-down, "so big," or peekaboo Shakes head for "no"
Discriminates simple geometric forms (e.g., circle) Amblyopia may develop with lack of binocularity Can follow rapidly moving object Controls and adjusts response to sound; listens for sound to recur	Says three to five words besides "dada," "mama"* Comprehends meaning of several words (comprehension always precedes verbalization) Recognizes objects by name Imitates animal sounds Understands simple verbal commands (e.g., "Give it to me," "Show me your eyes")	Shows emotions such as jealousy, affection (may give hug or kiss on request), anger, fear Enjoys familiar surroundings and explores away from parent Is fearful in strange situation; clings to parent May develop habit of "security blanket" or favorite toy Has increasing determination to practice locomotor skills Searches for an object even if it has not been hidden, but searches only where object was last seen*

Growth and Development During Toddler Years

Age (Months)	Physical	Gross Motor	Fine Motor
15	Steady growth in height and weight Head circumference 48 cm (19 inches) Weight 11 kg (24 pounds) Height 78.7 cm (31 inches)	Walks without help (usually since age 13 months) Creeps up stairs Kneels without support Cannot walk around corners or stop suddenly without losing balance Assumes standing position without support Cannot throw ball without falling	Constantly casting objects to floor Builds tower of two cubes Holds two cubes in one hand Releases a pellet into a narrow-necked bottle Scribbles spontaneously Uses cup with lid well but rotates spoon
18	Physiologic anorexia from decreased growth needs Anterior fontanel closed Physiologically able to control sphincters	Runs clumsily, falls often Walks up stairs with one hand held Pulls and pushes toys Jumps in place with both feet Seats self on chair Throws ball overhand without falling	Builds tower of three or four cubes Release, prehension, and reach well developed Turns pages in a book two or three at a time In drawing, makes stroke imitatively Manages spoon without rotation
24	Head circumference 49 to 50 cm (19.5 to 20 inches) Chest circumference exceeds head circumference Lateral diameter of chest exceeds anteroposterior diameter Usual weight gain of 1.8 to 2.7 kg (4 to 6 pounds) Usual gain in height of 10 to 12.5 cm (4 to 5 inches) Adult height approximately double height at 2 years May have achieved readiness for beginning daytime control of bowel and bladder Primary dentition of 16 teeth	Goes up and down stairs alone with two feet on each step Runs fairly well, with wide stance Picks up object without falling Kicks ball forward without overbalancing	Builds tower of six or seven cubes Aligns two or more cubes like a train Turns pages of book one at a time In drawing, imitates vertical and circular strokes Turns doorknob, unscrews lid
30	Birth weight quadrupled Primary dentition (20 teeth) completed May have daytime bowel and bladder control	Jumps with both feet Jumps from chair or step Stands on one foot momentarily Takes a few steps on tiptoe	Builds tower of eight cubes Adds chimney to train of cubes Good hand-finger coordination; holds crayon with fingers rather than fist Moves fingers independently In drawing, imitates vertical and horizontal strokes, makes two or more strokes for cross

Sensory	Vocalization	Socialization/Cognition
Able to identify geometric forms; places round object into appropriate hole Binocular vision well developed Displays an intense and prolonged interest in pictures	Uses expressive jargon Says four to six words, including names "Asks" for objects by pointing Understands simple commands May use head-shaking gesture to denote "no" Uses "no" even while agreeing to the request	Tolerates some separation from parent Less likely to fear strangers Beginning to imitate parents, such as cleaning house (sweeping, dusting), folding clothes, mowing lawn May discard bottle Kisses and hugs parents, may kiss pictures in a book Expressive of emotions, has temper tantrums
	Says 10 or more words Points to a common object, such as shoe or ball, and to two or three body parts	Great imitator ("domestic mimicry") Takes off gloves, socks, and shoes and unzips Temper tantrums may be more evident Beginning awareness of ownership ("my toy") May develop dependency on transitional objects, such as "security blanket"
Accommodation well developed In geometric discrimination, able to insert square block into oblong space	Has vocabulary of approximately 300 words Uses two- to three-word phrases Uses pronouns *I, me, you* Understands directional commands Gives first name; refers to self by name Verbalizes need for toileting, food, or drink Talks incessantly	Stage of parallel play Has sustained attention span Temper tantrums decreasing Pulls people to show them something Increased independence from mother Dresses self in simple clothing
	Gives first and last name Refers to self by appropriate pronoun Uses plurals Names one color	Separates more easily from mother In play, helps put things away, can carry breakable objects, pushes with good steering Begins to notice sex differences; knows own sex May attend to toilet needs without help except for wiping

Growth and Development During Preschool Years

Age (Years)	Physical	Gross Motor	Fine Motor	Language
3	Usual weight gain of 1.8 to 2.7 kg (4 to 6 pounds) Average weight of 14.6 kg (32 pounds) Usual gain in height of 7.5 cm (3 inches) Average height of 95 cm (37.25 inches) May have achieved nighttime control of bowel and bladder	Rides tricycle Jumps off bottom step Stands on one foot for a few seconds Goes up stairs using alternate feet, may still come down using both feet on step Broad jumps May try to dance, but balance may not be adequate	Builds tower of nine or ten cubes Builds bridge with three cubes Adeptly places small pellets in narrow-necked bottle In drawing, copies a circle, imitates a cross, names what has been drawn, cannot draw stick figure but may make circle with facial features	Has vocabulary of about 900 words Uses primarily "telegraphic" speech Uses complete sentences of three or four words Talks incessantly regardless of whether anyone is paying attention Repeats sentence of six syllables Asks many questions Begins to sing songs
4	Pulse and respiration rates decrease slightly Growth rate is similar to that of previous year Average weight of 16.7 kg (36.75 pounds) Average height of 103 cm (40.5 inches) Length at birth is doubled Maximum potential for development of amblyopia	Skips and hops on one foot Catches ball reliably Throws ball overhand Walks downstairs using alternate footing	Uses scissors successfully to cut out picture following outline Can lace shoes but may not be able to tie bow In drawing, copies a square, traces a cross and diamond, adds three parts to stick figure	Has vocabulary of 1500 words or more Uses sentences of four or five words Questioning is at peak Tells exaggerated stories Knows simple songs May be mildly profane if associates with older children Obeys four prepositional phrases, such as *under, on top of, beside, in back of,* or *in front of* Names one or more colors Comprehends analogies, such as, "If ice is cold, fire is _____"
5	Pulse and respiration rates decrease slightly Average weight of 18.7 kg (41.25 pounds) Average height of 110 cm (43.25 inches) Eruption of permanent dentition may begin Handedness is established (about 90% are right-handed)	Skips and hops on alternate feet Throws and catches ball well Jumps rope Skates with good balance Walks backward with heel to toe Jumps from height of 12 inches and lands on toes Balances on alternate feet with eyes closed	Ties shoelaces Uses scissors, simple tools, or pencil very well In drawing, copies a diamond and triangle; adds seven to nine parts to stick figure; prints a few letters, numbers, or words, such as first name	Has vocabulary of about 2100 words Uses sentences of six to eight words, with all parts of speech Names coins (e.g., nickel, dime) Names four or more colors Describes drawing or picture with much comment and enumeration Knows names of days of week, months, and other time-associated words Knows composition of articles, such as, "A shoe is made of _____" Can follow three commands in succession

Socialization	Cognition	Family Relationships
Dresses self almost completely if helped with back buttons and told which shoe is right or left Has increased attention span Feeds self completely Can prepare simple meals, such as cold cereal and milk Can help set table; can dry dishes without breaking any May have fears, especially of dark and of going to bed Knows own sex and sex of others Play is parallel and associative; begins to learn simple games but often follows own rules; begins to share	Is in preconceptual phase Is egocentric in thought and behavior Has beginning understanding of time; uses many time-oriented expressions; talks about past and future as much as about present; pretends to tell time Has improved concept of space as demonstrated in understanding of prepositions and ability to follow directional command Has beginning ability to view concepts from another perspective	Attempts to please parents and conform to their expectations Is less jealous of younger sibling; may be opportune time for birth of additional sibling Is aware of family relationships and sex-role functions Boys tend to identify more with father or other male figure Has increased ability to separate easily and comfortably from parents for short periods

Very independent
Tends to be selfish and impatient
Aggressive physically as well as verbally
Takes pride in accomplishments
Has mood swings
Shows off dramatically, enjoys entertaining others
Tells family tales to others with no restraint
Still has many fears
Play is associative:
  Imaginary playmates are common
  Uses dramatic, imaginative, and imitative devices
  Sexual exploration and curiosity demonstrated through play, such as being "doctor" or "nurse"
	Is in phase of intuitive thought
	Causality is still related to proximity of events
	Understands time better, especially in terms of sequence of daily events
	Unable to conserve matter
	Judges everything according to one dimension, such as height, width, or order
	Immediate perceptual clues dominate judgment
	Is beginning to develop less egocentrism and more social awareness
	May count correctly but has poor mathematic concept of numbers
	Obeys because parents have set limits, not because of understanding of right and wrong
		Rebels if parents expect too much, such as impeccable table manners
		Takes aggression and frustration out on parents or siblings
		"Do's" and "don'ts" become important
		May have rivalry with older or younger siblings; may resent older sibling's privileges and younger sibling's invasion of privacy and possessions
		May "run away" from home
		Identifies strongly with parent of opposite sex
		Is able to run simple errands outside the home

Less rebellious and quarrelsome than at age 4 years More settled and eager to get down to business Not as open and accessible in thoughts and behavior as in earlier years Independent but trustworthy; not foolhardy; more responsible Has fewer fears; relies on outer authority to control world Eager to do things right and to please; tries to "live by the rules" Has better manners Cares for self totally except for teeth, occasionally needing supervision in dress or hygiene Not ready for concentrated close work or small print because of slight farsightedness and still unrefined eye-hand coordination Play is associative; tries to follow rules but may cheat to avoid losing	Begins to question what parents think by comparing them with age-mates and other adults May notice prejudice and bias in outside world Is more able to view another's perspective, but tolerates differences rather than understanding them May begin to show understanding of conservation of numbers through counting objects regardless of arrangement Uses time-oriented words with increased understanding Very curious about factual information regarding world	Gets along well with parents May seek out parent more often than at age 4 years for reassurance and security, especially when entering school Begins to question parents' thinking and principles Strongly identifies with parent of same sex, especially boys with their fathers Enjoys activities such as sports, cooking, shopping with parent of same sex

Growth and Development During School-Age Years

Age (Years)	Physical and Motor	Mental	Adaptive	Personal-Social
6	Growth and weight gain continues slowly Weight: 16 to 23.6 kg (35½ to 58 pounds); height: 106.6 to 123.5 cm (42 to 48 inches) Central mandibular incisors erupt Loses first tooth Gradual increase in dexterity Activity age; constant activity Often returns to finger feeding More aware of hand as a tool Likes to draw, print, and color Vision reaches maturity	Develops concept of numbers Counts 13 pennies Knows whether it is morning or afternoon Defines common objects such as fork and chair in terms of their use Obeys triple commands in succession Knows right and left hands Says which is pretty and which is ugly of a series of drawings of faces Describes the objects in a picture rather than simply enumerating them Attends first grade	At table, uses knife to spread butter or jam on bread At play, cuts, folds, and pastes paper toys, sews crudely if needle is threaded Takes bath without supervision; performs bedtime activities alone Reads from memory; enjoys oral spelling game Likes table games, checkers, simple card games Giggles a lot Sometimes steals money or attractive items Has difficulty owning up to misdeeds Tries out own abilities	Can share and cooperate better Has great need for children of own age Will cheat to win Often engages in rough play Often jealous of younger brother or sister Does what adults are seen doing May have occasional temper tantrums Is a boaster Is more independent, probably influence of school Has own way of doing things Increases socialization
7	Begins to grow at least 5 cm (2 inches) a year Weight: 17.7 to 30 kg (39 to 66½ pounds); height: 111.8 to 129.7 cm (44 to 51 inches) Maxillary central incisors and lateral mandibular incisors erupt More cautious in approaches to new performances Repeats performances to master them Jaw begins to expand to accommodate permanent teeth	Notices that certain parts are missing from pictures Can copy a diamond Repeats three numbers backward Develops concept of time; reads ordinary clock or watch correctly to nearest quarter hour; uses clock for practical purposes Attends the second grade More mechanical in reading; often does not stop at the end of a sentence, skips words such as *it, the,* and *he*	Uses table knife for cutting meat; may need help with tough or difficult pieces Brushes and combs hair acceptably without help May steal Likes to help and have a choice Is less resistant and stubborn	Is becoming a real member of the family group Takes part in group play Boys prefer playing with boys; girls prefer playing with girls Spends a lot of time alone; does not require a lot of companionship
8-9	Continues to grow at least 5 cm (2 inches) a year Weight: 19.6 to 39.6 kg (43 to 87 pounds); height: 117 to 141.8 cm (46 to 56 inches) Lateral incisors (maxillary) and mandibular cuspids erupt	Gives similarities and differences between two things from memory Counts backward from 20 to 1; understands concept of reversibility Repeats days of the week and months in order; knows the date	Makes use of common tools such as hammer, saw, or screwdriver Uses household and sewing utensils Helps with routine household tasks such as dusting, sweeping	Is easy to get along with at home Likes the reward system Dramatizes Is more sociable Is better behaved Is interested in boy-girl relationships but will not admit it

Growth and Development During School-Age Years—cont'd

Age (Years)	Physical and Motor	Mental	Adaptive	Personal-Social
8-9 (cont'd)	Movement fluid, often graceful and poised Always on the go; jumps, chases, skips Increased smoothness and speed in fine motor control; uses cursive writing Dresses self completely Likely to overdo; hard to quiet down after recess More limber; bones grow faster than ligaments	Describes common objects in detail, not merely their use Makes change out of a quarter Attends third and fourth grades Reads more; may plan to wake up early just to read Reads classic books but also enjoys comics More aware of time; can be relied on to get to school on time Can grasp concepts of parts and whole (fractions) Understands concepts of space, cause and effect, nesting (puzzles), conservation (permanence of mass and volume) Classifies objects by more than one quality; has collections Produces simple paintings or drawings	Assumes responsibility for share of household chores Looks after all of own needs at table Buys useful articles; exercises some choice in making purchases Runs useful errands Likes pictorial magazines Likes school; wants to answer all the questions Is afraid of failing a grade; is ashamed of bad grades Is more critical of self Takes music and sport lessons	Goes about home and community freely, alone, or with friends Likes to compete and play games Shows preference in friends and groups Plays mostly with groups of own sex but is beginning to mix Develops modesty Compares self with others Enjoys Scouts, group sports
10-12	*Boys:* Slow growth in height and rapid weight gain; may become obese in this period Weight: 24.3 to 58 kg (54 to 128 pounds); height: 127.5 to 162.3 cm (50 to 64 inches) Posture is more similar to an adult's; will overcome lordosis *Girls:* Pubescent changes may begin to appear; body lines soften and round out Remainder of teeth will erupt and tend toward full development (except wisdom teeth)	Writes brief stories Attends fifth to seventh grades Writes occasional short letters to friends or relatives on own initiative Uses telephone for practical purposes Responds to magazine, radio, or other advertising Reads for practical information or own enjoyment—stories or library books of adventure or romance, or animal stories	Makes useful articles or does easy repair work Cooks or sews in small way Raises pets Washes and dries own hair Is responsible for a thorough job of cleaning hair, but may need reminding to do so Is sometimes left alone at home for an hour or so Is successful in looking after own needs or those of other children left in his or her care	Loves friends; talks about them constantly Chooses friends more selectively; may have a "best friend" Enjoys conversation Develops beginning interest in opposite sex Is more diplomatic Likes family; family really has meaning Likes mother and wants to please her in many ways Demonstrates affection Likes father, who is adored and idolized Respects parents

Growth and Development During Adolescence

Early Adolescence (11-14 years)	Middle Adolescence (14-17 years)	Late Adolescence (17-20 years)
Growth		
Rapidly accelerating growth Reaches peak velocity Secondary sex characteristics appear	Growth decelerating in girls Stature reaches 95% of adult height Secondary sex characteristics well advanced	Physically mature Structure and reproductive growth almost complete
Cognition		
Explores newfound ability for limited abstract thought Clumsy groping for new values and energies Comparison of "normality" with peers of same sex	Developing capacity for abstract thinking Enjoys intellectual powers, often in idealistic terms Concern with philosophic, political, and social problems	Established abstract thought Can perceive and act on long-range operations Able to view problems comprehensively Intellectual and functional identity established
Identity		
Preoccupied with rapid body changes Trying out of various roles Measurement of attractiveness by acceptance or rejection of peers Conformity to group norms	Modifies body image Very self-centered; increased narcissism Tendency toward inner experience and self-discovery Has a rich fantasy life Idealistic Able to perceive future implications of current behavior and decisions; variable application	Body image and gender role definition nearly secured Mature sexual identity Phase of consolidation of identity Stability of self-esteem Comfortable with physical growth Social roles defined and articulated
Relationships with Parents		
Defining independence-dependence boundaries Strong desire to remain dependent on parents while trying to detach No major conflicts over parental control	Major conflicts over independence and control Low point in parent-child relationship Greatest push for emancipation; disengagement Final and irreversible emotional detachment from parents; mourning	Emotional and physical separation from parents completed Independence from family with less conflict Emancipation nearly secured
Relationships with Peers		
Seeks peer affiliations to counter instability generated by rapid change Upsurge of close idealized friendships with members of the same sex Struggle for mastery takes place within peer group	Strong need for identity to affirm self-image Behavioral standards set by peer group Acceptance by peers extremely important—fear of rejection Exploration of ability to attract the opposite sex	Peer group recedes in importance in favor of individual friendship Testing of male-female relationships against possibility of permanent alliance Relationships characterized by giving and sharing
Sexuality		
Self-exploration and evaluation Limited dating, usually group Limited intimacy	Multiple plural relationships Decisive turn toward heterosexuality (if is homosexual, knows by this time) Exploration of "self appeal" Feeling of "being in love" Tentative establishment of relationships	Forms stable relationships and attachment to another Growing capacity for mutuality and reciprocity Dating as a male-female pair Intimacy involves commitment rather than exploration and romanticism

Growth and Development During Adolescence—cont'd

Early Adolescence (11-14 years)	Middle Adolescence (14-17 years)	Late Adolescence (17-20 years)
Psychologic Health		
Wide mood swings Intense daydreaming Anger outwardly expressed with moodiness, temper outbursts, and verbal insults and name-calling	Tendency toward inner experiences; more introspective Tendency to withdraw when upset or feelings are hurt Vascillation of emotions in time and range Feelings of inadequacy common; difficulty in asking for help	More constancy of emotion Anger more apt to be concealed

Health Promotion

Symbol ■ indicates material that may be photocopied and distributed to families.

Related Topics

RECOMMENDATIONS FOR CHILD PREVENTIVE CARE

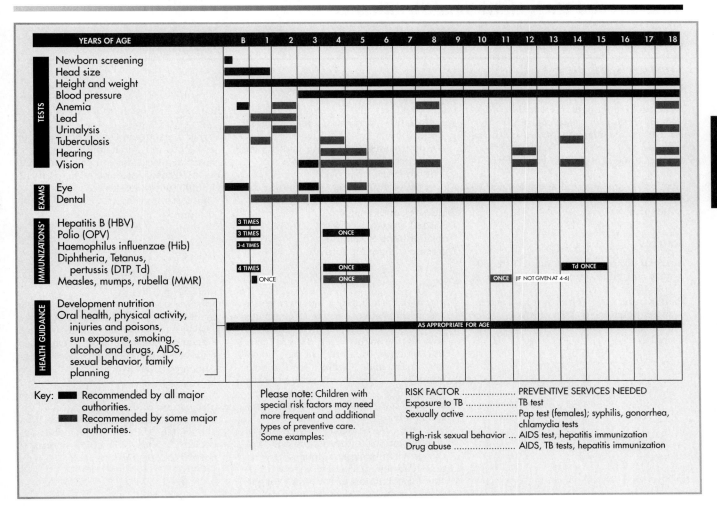

| YEARS OF AGE | B | 1 | 2 | 3 | 4 | 5 | 6 | 7 | 8 | 9 | 10 | 11 | 12 | 13 | 14 | 15 | 16 | 17 | 18 |

TESTS
- Newborn screening
- Head size
- Height and weight
- Blood pressure
- Anemia
- Lead
- Urinalysis
- Tuberculosis
- Hearing
- Vision

EXAMS
- Eye
- Dental

IMMUNIZATIONS*
- Hepatitis B (HBV) — 3 TIMES
- Polio (OPV) — 3 TIMES, ONCE
- Haemophilus influenzae (Hib) — 3-4 TIMES
- Diphtheria, Tetanus, pertussis (DTP, Td) — 4 TIMES, ONCE, Td ONCE
- Measles, mumps, rubella (MMR) — ONCE, ONCE, ONCE (IF NOT GIVEN AT 4-6)

HEALTH GUIDANCE
- Development nutrition
- Oral health, physical activity, injuries and poisons, sun exposure, smoking, alcohol and drugs, AIDS, sexual behavior, family planning — AS APPROPRIATE FOR AGE

Key:
- ▬ Recommended by all major authorities.
- ▬ Recommended by some major authorities.

Please note: Children with special risk factors may need more frequent and additional types of preventive care. Some examples:

RISK FACTOR	PREVENTIVE SERVICES NEEDED
Exposure to TB	TB test
Sexually active	Pap test (females); syphilis, gonorrhea, chlamydia tests
High-risk sexual behavior	AIDS test, hepatitis immunization
Drug abuse	AIDS, TB tests, hepatitis immunization

Unit 2

NUTRITION
Vitamins and Their Nutritional Significance

Physiologic Functions/Sources	Results of Deficiency or Excess	Nursing Considerations

VITAMIN A (RETINOL)*

Functions

Necessary component in formation of pigment rhodopsin (visual purple)

Formation and maintenance of epithelial tissue

Normal bone growth and tooth development

Needed for growth and spermatogenesis

Involved in thyroxine formation

Antioxidant

Sources

Natural form—Liver, kidney, fish oils, milk and non-skim milk products, egg yolk

Provitamin A (carotene)—Carrots, sweet potatoes, squash, apricots, spinach, collards, broccoli, cabbage, artichokes

Deficiency

Night blindness

Keratinization (hardening and scaling) of epithelium

    Xerophthalmia (hardening and scaling of cornea and conjunctiva)

    Phrynoderma (toad skin)

    Drying of respiratory, gastrointestinal, and genitourinary tracts

Defective tooth enamel

Retarded growth

Impaired bone formation

Decreased thyroxine formation

Excess

Early signs—Irritability, anorexia, pruritus, fissures at corners of nose and lips

Later signs—Hepatomegaly, jaundice, retarded growth, poor weight gain, thickening of the cortex of long bones with pain and fragility, hard tender lumps in extremities and occiput of the skull

Can cause birth defects if excessive maternal intake

NOTE: Overdose results from ingestion of large quantities of the vitamin only, not the provitamin; large amounts of carotene (carotenemia) cause yellow or orange discoloration of the skin (not the sclera, urine, or feces as in jaundice) but none of the above symptoms

Nursing Considerations (Vitamin A)

Encourage foods rich in vitamin A, such as whole cow's milk

As milk consumption decreases, encourage foods rich in vitamin A

Ensure adequate intake in preterm infants

Advise parents of safe use of supplements in child with measles

Emphasize correct use of vitamin supplements and potential hazards of excess

Investigate child's dietary habits to calculate approximate intake; if excessive, remove supplemental source (e.g., daily feeding of liver)

Advise parents of the benign nature of carotenemia; treatment is avoidance of excess pigmented fruits or vegetables, especially carrots; skin color returns to normal in 2 to 6 weeks

VITAMIN B₁ (THIAMIN)†

Functions

Coenzyme (with phosphorus) in carbohydrate metabolism

Needed for healthy nervous system

Sources

Pork, beef, liver, legumes, nuts, whole or enriched grains and cereals, green vegetables, fruits, milk, brown rice

Deficiency

Gastrointestinal—Anorexia, constipation, indigestion

Neurologic—Apathy, fatigue, emotional instability, polyneuritis, tenderness of calf muscles, partial anesthesia, muscle weakness, paresthesia, hyperesthesia, decreased or absent tendon reflexes, convulsions, and coma (in infants)

Cardiovascular—Palpitations, cardiac failure, peripheral vasodilation, edema

Excess

Headache

Irritability

Insomnia

Rapid pulse

Weakness

Vitamin B complex

Encourage foods rich in B vitamins

Stress proper cooking and storage techniques to preserve potency, such as minimum cooking of vegetables in small amount of liquid, storage of milk in opaque container

Advise against fad diets that severely restrict groups of food, such as vegetarianism (vegans or macrobiotics)

Explore need for vitamin supplements when dieting, when using goat milk exclusively for infant feeding (deficient in folic acid), or when the breast-feeding mother is a strict vegetarian (vitamin B₁₂)

Emphasize correct use of vitamin supplements and potential hazards of excess

*Fat soluble.

†Water soluble.

Vitamins and Their Nutritional Significance—cont'd

Physiologic Functions/Sources	Results of Deficiency or Excess	Nursing Considerations

VITAMIN B₂ (RIBOFLAVIN)†

Functions

Coenzyme (with phosphorus) in carbohydrate, protein, and fat metabolism

Maintains healthy skin, especially around mouth, nose, and eyes

Sources

Milk and its products, eggs, organ meat (liver, kidney, and heart), enriched cereals, some green leafy vegetables,‡ legumes

Deficiency

Ariboflavinosis

Lips—Cheilosis (fissures at corners of lips), perlèche (inflammation at corners of lips)

Tongue—Glossitis

Nose—Irritation and cracks at nasal angle

Eyes—Burning, itching, tearing, photophobia, corneal vascularization, cataracts

Skin—Seborrheic dermatitis, delayed wound healing and tissue repair

Excess

Paresthesia, pruritus

Same as vitamin B complex

NIACIN (NICOTINIC ACID, NICOTINAMIDE)†

Functions

Coenzyme (with riboflavin) in protein and fat metabolism

Needed for healthy nervous system and skin and for normal digestion

May lower cholesterol

Sources

Meat, poultry, fish, peanuts, beans, peas, whole or enriched grains (except corn and rice)

Milk and its products are sources of tryptophan (60 mg of tryptophan = 1 mg of niacin)

Deficiency

Pellagra

Oral-Stomatitis, glossitis

Cutaneous—Scaly dermatitis on exposed areas

Gastrointestinal—Anorexia, weight loss, diarrhea, fatigue

Neurologic—Apathy, anxiety, confusion, depression, dementia

Death

Excess

Release of histamine, a vasodilator (flushing, decreased blood pressure, increased cerebral blood flow; aggravates asthma)

Dermatologic problems (pruritus, rash, hyperkeratosis, acanthosis nigricans)

Increased gastric acidity (aggravates peptic ulcer disease)

Hepatotoxicity

Increased serum uric acid levels

Elevated plasma glucose levels

Certain cardiac arrhythmias

Same as vitamin B complex

If used as hypolipidemic agent, stress safe dosage to prevent child's accidental ingestion

VITAMIN B₆ (PYRIDOXINE)†

Functions

Coenzyme in protein and fat metabolism

Needed for formation of antibodies and hemoglobin

Needed for utilization of copper and iron

Aids in conversion of tryptophan to niacin

Sources

Meats, especially liver and kidney, cereal grains (wheat and corn), yeast, soybeans, peanuts, tuna, chicken, salmon

Deficiency

Scaly dermatitis, weight loss, anemia, retarded growth, irritability, convulsions, peripheral neuritis

Excess

Peripheral nervous system toxicity (unsteady gait, numb feet and hands, clumsiness of hands, sometimes perioral numbness)

May cause peptic ulcer disease or seizures

Same as vitamin B complex

Stress proper cooking and storing techniques to preserve potency

Cook food covered in small amount of water

Do not soak food in water

Store in light-resistant container

†Water soluble.

‡Green leafy vegetables include spinach, broccoli, kale, turnip greens, mustard greens, collards, dandelion greens, and beet greens.

Continued

Unit 2

Vitamins and Their Nutritional Significance—cont'd

Physiologic Functions/Sources	Results of Deficiency or Excess	Nursing Considerations

FOLIC ACID (FOLACIN; REDUCED FORM IS CALLED FOLINIC ACID OR CITROVORUM FACTOR)†

Functions	**Deficiency**	
Coenzyme for single-carbon transfer (purines, thymine, hemoglobin)	Macrocytic anemia, bone marrow depression, glossitis, intestinal malabsorption	Same as vitamin B complex
Necessary for formation of red blood cells		Stress proper cooking and storing techniques to preserve potency
May prevent neural tube defects (i.e., myelomeningocele)		Cook food covered in small amount of water
	Excess	Do not soak food in water
Sources	Rare because megadoses not available over the counter	Store in light-resistant container
Green leafy vegetables,‡ cabbage, asparagus, liver, kidneys, nuts, eggs, whole grain cereals, legumes, bananas	May cause insomnia and irritability	Women of childbearing age should supplement to prevent neural tube defects

VITAMIN B₁₂ (COBALAMIN)†

Functions	**Deficiency**	
Coenzyme in protein synthesis; indirect effect on formation of red blood cells (particularly on formation of nucleic acids and folic acid metabolism)	Pernicious anemia (one form of deficiency from absence of intrinsic factor in gastric secretions)	Same as vitamin B complex
Needed for normal functioning of nervous tissue	General signs of severe anemia	
	Lemon-yellow tinge to skin	
	Spinal cord degeneration	
	Delayed brain growth	
Sources	**Excess**	
Meat, liver, kidney, fish, shellfish, poultry, milk, eggs, cheese, nutritional yeast, sea vegetables	Excess is rare	

BIOTIN

Functions	**Deficiency**	
Coenzyme in carbohydrate, protein, and fat metabolism	Deficiency is uncommon because synthesized by bacterial flora	Same as vitamin B complex
Interrelated with functions of other B vitamins		
	Excess	
Sources	Unknown	
Liver, kidney, egg yolk, tomatoes, legumes, nuts		

PANTOTHENIC ACID†

Functions	**Deficiency**	
Coenzyme in carbohydrate, protein, and fat metabolism	Deficiency is uncommon because of its multiple food sources and synthesis by bacterial flora	Same as vitamin B complex
Synthesis of amino acids, fatty acids, and steroids		
	Excess	
Sources	Minimum toxicity (occasional diarrhea and water retention)	
Liver, kidney, heart, salmon, eggs, vegetables, legumes, whole grains		

†Water soluble.
‡Green leafy vegetables include spinach, broccoli, kale, turnip greens, mustard greens, collards, dandelion greens, and beet greens.

Vitamins and Their Nutritional Significance—cont'd

Physiologic Functions/Sources	Results of Deficiency or Excess	Nursing Considerations

VITAMIN C (ASCORBIC ACID)†

Functions

Essential for collagen formation
Increases absorption of iron for hemoglobin formation
Enhances conversion of folic acid to folinic acid
Affects cholesterol synthesis and conversion of proline to hydroxyproline
Probably a coenzyme in metabolism of tyrosine and phenylalanine
May play role in hydroxylation of adrenal steroids
May have stimulating effect on phagocytic activity of leukocytes and formation of antibodies
Antioxidant agent (spares other vitamins from oxidation)

Sources

Citrus fruits, strawberries, tomatoes, potatoes, cabbage, broccoli, cauliflower, spinach, papaya, mango, cantaloupe, watermelon, enriched fruit juice

Deficiency

Scurvy
Skin—Dry, rough, petechiae, perifollicular hyperkeratotic papules (raised areas around hair follicles)
Musculoskeletal—Bleeding muscles and joints, pseudoparalysis from pain, swelling of joints, costochondral beading (scorbutic rosary)
Gums—Spongy, friable, swollen, bleed easily, bluish red or black, teeth loosen and fall out
General disposition—Irritable, anorexic, apprehensive, in pain, refuses to move, assumes semi-froglike position when supine (scorbutic pose)
Signs of anemia
Decreased wound healing
Increased susceptibility to infection

Excess

Diarrhea
Increased excretion of uric acid and acidification of urine (may cause urate precipitation and formation of oxalate stones)
Hemolysis
Impaired leukocytosis activity
Damage to beta cells of pancreas and decreased insulin production
Reproductive failure
"Rebound scurvy" from withdrawal of large amounts

Encourage foods rich in vitamin C
Investigate infant's diet for sources of vitamin, especially when cow's milk is principal source of nutrition
Stress proper cooking and storing techniques to preserve potency
　Wash vegetables quickly; do not soak in water
　Cook vegetables in covered pot with minimum water and for short time; avoid copper or cast iron cookware
　Do not add baking soda to cooking water
　Use fresh fruits and vegetables as soon as possible; store in refrigerator
　Store juice in airtight, opaque container
　Wrap cut fruit or eat soon after exposing to air
In caring for child with scurvy:
　Position for comfort and rest
　Handle very gently and minimally
　Administer analgesics as needed
　Prevent infection
　Provide good oral care
　Provide soft, bland diet
　Emphasize rapid recovery when vitamin is replaced
Emphasize correct use of vitamin supplement and potential hazards of excess
Identify groups at risk for vitamin C supplements (e.g., those with thalassemia, or those on anticoagulant or aminoglycoside antibiotic therapy)

VITAMIN D₂ (ERGOCALCIFEROL) AND D₃ (CHOLECALCIFEROL)*

Functions

Absorption of calcium and phosphorus and decreased renal excretion of phosphorus

Sources

Direct sunlight
Cod liver oil, herring, mackerel, salmon, tuna, sardines
Enriched food sources—Milk, milk products, enriched cereals, margarine, breads, many breakfast drinks

Deficiency

Rickets
Head—Craniotabes (softening of cranial bones, prominence of frontal bones), deformed shape (skull flat and depressed toward middle), delayed closure of fontanels
Chest—Rachitic rosary (enlargement of costochondral junction of ribs), Harrison groove (horizontal depression in lower portion of rib cage), pigeon chest (sharp protrusion of sternum)
Spine—Kyphosis, scoliosis, lordosis
Abdomen—Potbelly, constipation
Extremities—Bowing of arms and legs, knock-knee, saber shins, instability of hip joints, pelvic deformity, enlargement of epiphyses at ends of long bones
Teeth—Delayed calcification, especially of permanent teeth
Rachitic tetany—Seizures

Encourage foods rich in vitamin D, especially fortified cow's milk
In breast-fed infants, encourage use of vitamin D supplements if maternal diet inadequate or if infant exposed to minimal sunlight
In caring for child with rickets:
　Maintain good body alignment
　Reposition frequently to prevent decubiti and respiratory infection
　Handle very gently and minimally
Prevent infection
Institute seizure precautions
Have 10% calcium gluconate available in case of tetany
Observe for possibility of overdose from supplements
If prescribed, supervise proper use of orthopedic splints and braces

*Fat soluble.
†Water soluble.

Continued

Unit 2

Vitamins and Their Nutritional Significance—cont'd

Physiologic Functions/Sources	Results of Deficiency or Excess	Nursing Considerations

VITAMIN D₂ (ERGOCALCIFEROL) AND D₃ (CHOLECALCIFEROL)—cont'd

Excess

Acute—Vomiting, dehydration, fever, abdominal cramps, bone pain, convulsions, coma

Chronic—Lassitude, mental slowness, anorexia, failure to thrive, thirst, urinary urgency, polyuria, vomiting, diarrhea, abdominal cramps, bone pain, pathologic fractures

Calcification of soft tissue—Kidneys, lungs, adrenal glands, vessels (hypertension), heart, gastric lining, tympanic membrane (deafness)

Osteoporosis of long bones

Elevated serum levels of calcium and phosphorus

Same as vitamin A; may include low-calcium diet during initial therapy

VITAMIN E (TOCOPHEROL)*

Functions

Production of red blood cells and protection from hemolysis

Muscle and liver integrity

Coenzyme factor in tissue respiration

Minimizes oxidation of polyunsaturated fatty acids and vitamins A and C in intestinal tract and tissues

Possible role in treatment and prevention of bronchopulmonary dysplasia and retinopathy of prematurity is under investigation

Deficiency

Hemolytic anemia from hemolysis caused by shortened life of red blood cells, especially in premature infants; and focal necrosis of tissues

Causes infertility in rats, but not in humans (does *not* increase human male virility or potency)

Excess

Little is known; less toxic than other fat-soluble vitamins

Initiate early feeding in premature infants; may need supplementation

Sources

Vegetable oils, wheat germ oil, milk, egg yolk, muscle meats, fish, whole grains, nuts, legumes, spinach, broccoli

VITAMIN K*

Functions

Catalyst for production of prothrombin and blood-clotting factors II, VII, IX, and X by the liver

Deficiency

Hemorrhage

Excess

Hemolytic anemia in individuals who are deficient in glucose-6-phosphate dehydrogenase

Administer prophylactically to all newborns

Other indications include intestinal disease, lack of bile, prolonged antibiotic therapy; may be used in management of blood-clotting time when anticoagulants such as warfarin (Coumadin) and dicumarol (bishydroxycoumarin), which are vitamin K antagonists, are used

Sources

Pork, liver, green leafy vegetables,‡ cabbage, tomatoes, egg yolk, cheese

*Fat soluble.

‡Green leafy vegetables include spinach, broccoli, kale, turnip greens, mustard greens, collards, dandelion greens, and beet greens.

Minerals and Their Nutritional Significance

Physiologic Functions/Sources	Results of Deficiency or Excess	Nursing Considerations
CALCIUM*		
Functions	**Deficiency**	
Bone and tooth development and maintenance (in combination with phosphorus)	Rickets	Encourage foods rich in calcium, especially dairy products
	Tetany	
	Impaired growth, especially of bones and teeth	Caution that oxalates in leafy vegetables (spinach), oxalates in chocolates, and a high phosphorus intake (especially from carbonated beverages) can decrease calcium absorption
Muscle contractions, especially the heart		
Blood clotting		
Absorption of vitamin B$_{12}$	**Excess**	
Enzyme activation		
Nerve conduction	Drowsiness, extreme lethargy	Discourage use of whole cow's milk in newborns because the phosphorus-to-calcium ratio favors excretion of calcium
Integrity of intracellular cement substances and various membranes	Impaired absorption of other minerals (iron, zinc, manganese)	
	Calcium deposits in tissues (renal failure)	Advise against fad diets, especially those that restrict dairy products
Sources		Emphasize correct use of calcium-supplements, especially the possible interaction between megadoses of calcium and resulting deficiency states of other minerals
Dairy products, egg yolk, sardines, canned salmon with bones, green leafy vegetables‡ (except spinach), soybeans, dried beans, peas		
CHLORIDE*		
Functions	**Deficiency**	
Acid-base and fluid balance	Acid-base disturbances (hypochloremic alkalosis, dehydration); occurs mostly in combination with sodium loss	Deficiency and excess are unusual; most diets supply adequate chloride (usually in combination with sodium)
Enzyme activation in saliva		
Component of hydrochloric acid in stomach		Disease states such as excessive vomiting can necessitate chloride replacement
	Excess	
Sources	Acid-base disturbance	
Salt, meat, eggs, dairy products, many prepared and preserved foods		
CHROMIUM†		
Functions	**Deficiency**	
Involved in glucose metabolism and energy production	Possible abnormal glucose metabolism	No specific recommendations are needed
	Excess	
Sources	Unknown	
Meat, cheese, whole-grain breads and cereals, legumes, peanuts, brewer's yeast, vegetable oils		
COPPER†		
Functions	**Deficiency**	
Production of hemoglobin	Anemia, leukopenia, neutropenia	Deficiency from inadequate food sources is less likely than from excess intake of other minerals, especially zinc and possibly iron; therefore emphasize the correct use of any vitamin supplement
Essential component of several enzyme systems		
	Excess	
Sources	Severe vomiting and diarrhea	Caution against cooking acid foods in unlined copper pots, which can lead to chronic and toxic accumulation of copper
Organ meats, oysters, nuts, seeds, legumes, corn oil margarine	Hemolytic anemia	

*Macrominerals—required intake >100 mg/day.

†Microminerals or trace elements—required intake <100 mg/day.

‡Green leafy vegetables include spinach, broccoli, kale, turnip greens, mustard greens, collards, dandelion greens, and beet greens.

Continued

Minerals and Their Nutritional Significance—cont'd

Physiologic Functions/Sources	Results of Deficiency or Excess	Nursing Considerations
FLUORINE†		
Functions	**Deficiency**	
Formation of caries-resistant teeth Strong bone development	Increased susceptibility to tooth decay	In areas with optimally fluoridated water, encourage sufficient intake to supply recommended amount of fluoride
	Excess	In areas of unfluoridated water or when ready-to-use formula, bottled water, or breast milk is used, stress the importance of fluoride supplements
Sources	Fluorosis (mottling and/or pitting of enamel) Severe bone deformities	
Fluoridated water and foods or beverages prepared with fluoridated water; fish, tea, commercially prepared chicken for infants		In areas with excess fluoride in the water, consider the use of bottled water in drinking and cooking to reduce the fluoride intake to safe levels Fluorine has the narrowest range of safe and adequate intake; therefore stress the importance of storing supplements in a safe area
IODINE†		
Functions	**Deficiency**	
Production of thyroid hormone Normal reproduction	Goiter (enlarged thyroid from decreased thyroxine formation)	Encourage use of iodized salt for individuals living far from the sea If iodine preparations are in the home, stress the importance of safe storage
Sources	**Excess**	
Seafood, kelp, iodized salt, sea salt, enriched bread, milk (from dairy processing)	Unknown from food sources; may occur from ingestion of iodine preparations, such as saturated solutions of potassium iodide (SSKI)	
IRON†		
Functions	**Deficiency**	
Formation of hemoglobin and myoglobin Essential part of several enzymes and proteins	Anemia (See p. 444.)	Encourage foods rich in iron Discourage excessive milk consumption, especially more than 1 L per day (milk is a very poor source of iron) If iron supplements are prescribed, teach parents factors that affect absorption (Box 2-1)

BOX 2-1

Factors That Affect Iron Absorption

Increase

Acidity (low pH)—Administer iron between meals (gastric hydrochloric acid)
Ascorbic acid (vitamin C)—Administer iron with juice, fruit, or multivitamin preparation
Vitamin A
Calcium
Tissue need
Meat, fish, poultry
Cooking in cast iron pots

Decrease

Alkalinity (high pH)—Avoid antacid preparations
Phosphates—Milk is unfavorable vehicle for iron administration
Phytates—Found in cereals
Oxalates—Found in many fruits and vegetables (plums, currants, green beans, spinach, sweet potatoes, tomatoes)
Tannins—Found in tea, coffee
Tissue saturation
Malabsorptive disorders
Disturbances that cause diarrhea or steatorrhea
Infection

---

†Microminerals or trace elements—required intake < 100 mg/day.

Minerals and Their Nutritional Significance—cont'd

Physiologic Functions/Sources	Results of Deficiency or Excess	Nursing Considerations
IRON—cont'd		
Sources	**Excess**	
Liver, especially pork, followed by calf, beef, and chicken; kidney, red meat, poultry, shellfish, whole grains, iron-enriched infant formula and cereal, enriched cereals and bread, legumes, nuts, seeds, green leafy vegetables‡ (except spinach), dried fruits, potatoes, molasses, tofu, prune juice	Hemosiderosis (excess iron storage in various tissues of the body, especially the spleen, liver, lymph glands, heart, and pancreas) Hemochromatosis (excess iron storage with cellular damage)	Stress the importance of storing iron supplements in a safe area
MAGNESIUM*		
Functions	**Deficiency**	
Bone and tooth formation Production of proteins Nerve conduction to muscles Activation of enzymes needed for carbohydrate and protein metabolism	Tremors, spasm Irregular heartbeat Muscular weakness Lower extremity cramps Convulsions, delirium	Deficiency and excess are unusual, except in disease states such as prolonged vomiting or diarrhea or kidney dysfunction, where replacement may be needed
Sources	**Excess**	
Whole grains, nuts, soybeans, meat, green leafy vegetables‡ (uncooked), tea, cocoa, raisins	Nervous system disturbances due to imbalance in calcium-to-magnesium ratio	
MANGANESE†		
Functions	**Deficiency**	
Activation of enzymes involved in reproduction, growth, and fat metabolism Normal bone structure Nervous system functioning	Unknown	No specific recommendations are needed
	Excess	
	Unknown	
Sources		
Nuts, whole grains, legumes, green vegetables, fruit		
MOLYBDENUM†		
Functions	**Deficiency**	
Essential component of several oxidative enzymes	Very rare; diagnosed in patients on complete total parenteral alimentation	No specific recommendations are needed
Sources	**Excess**	
Legumes, whole grains, organ meats, some dark green vegetables	Produces secondary copper deficiency (growth failure, anemia, and disturbed bone development)	

*Macrominerals—required intake >100 mg/day.
†Microminerals or trace elements—required intake <100 mg/day.
‡Green leafy vegetables include spinach, broccoli, kale, turnip greens, mustard greens, collards, dandelion greens, and beet greens.

Continued

Unit 2

Minerals and Their Nutritional Significance—cont'd

Physiologic Functions/Sources	Results of Deficiency or Excess	Nursing Considerations
PHOSPHORUS*		
Functions	**Deficiency**	
Bone and tooth development (in combination with calcium)	Weakness, anorexia, malaise, bone pain	Dietary deficiency is uncommon, although prolonged use of antacids can produce deficiency, in which case supplementation is recommended
Involved in numerous chemical reactions, including protein, carbohydrate, and fat metabolism		
Acid-base balance		
Sources	**Excess**	
Dairy products, eggs, meat, poultry, legumes, carbonated beverages	Produces secondary calcium deficiency from disturbed calcium-to-phosphorus ratio	To preserve calcium-to-phosphorus ratio in newborns, discourage use of whole cow's milk
POTASSIUM*		
Functions	**Deficiency**	
Acid-base and fluid balance (major extracellular fluid areas)	Cardiac arrhythmias	Dietary deficiency and excess are unlikely, although disease states such as prolonged nausea and vomiting or the use of diuretics can result in hypokalemia; in such instances, encourage replacement with supplements of rich food sources, such as bananas
Nerve conduction	Muscular weakness	
Muscular contraction, especially the heart	Lethargy	
Release of energy	Kidney and respiratory failure	
	Heart failure	
Sources	**Excess**	
Bananas, citrus fruit, dried fruits, meat, fish, bran, legumes, peanut butter, potatoes, coffee, tea, cocoa	Cardiac arrhythmias	
	Respiratory failure	
	Mental confusion	
	Numbness of extremities	
SELENIUM†		
Functions	**Deficiency**	
Antioxidant, especially protective of vitamin E	Keshan disease (cardiomyopathy in children; found in China)	Deficiency and excess are uncommon in North America, although selenium deficiency can occur in patients on prolonged total parenteral alimentation; in these instances, supplementation is required
Protects against toxicity of heavy metals		
Associated with fat metabolism	**Excess**	
Sources	Eye, nose, and throat irritation	
Seafood, organ meats, egg yolk, whole grains, chicken, meat, tomatoes, cabbage, garlic, mushrooms, milk	Increased dental caries	
	Liver and kidney degeneration	
SODIUM*		
Functions	**Deficiency**	
Acid-base and fluid balance (major extracellular fluid cation)	Dehydration	Deficiency intake is very rare, although losses secondary to nausea, vomiting, excessive sweating, and use of diuretics can occur and require replacement
Cell permeability; absorption of glucose	Hypotension	
Muscle contraction	Convulsions	
	Muscle cramps	Encourage parents to limit excessive use of salt in preparing foods and to limit commercial foods with high sodium content, such as smoked meats
Sources	**Excess**	
Table salt, seafood, meat, poultry, numerous prepared foods	Edema	
	Hypertension	
	Intracranial hemorrhage	

*Macrominerals—required intake >100 mg/day.
†Microminerals or trace elements—required intake <100 mg/day.

Minerals and Their Nutritional Significance—cont'd

Physiologic Functions/Sources	Results of Deficiency or Excess	Nursing Considerations
SULFUR*		
Functions	**Deficiency**	
Essential component of cell protein, especially of hair and skin	Unknown	No specific recommendations are needed
Enzyme activation	**Excess**	
Associated with energy metabolism		
Detoxification of certain chemical reactions	Unknown	
Sources		
Dairy products, eggs, meat, fish, nuts, legumes		
ZINC†		
Functions	**Deficiency**	
Component of about 100 enzymes	Loss of appetite	Encourage food sources rich in zinc, especially protein
Synthesis of nucleic acids and protein in immune system and coagulation	Diminished taste sensation	Caution that fiber, phytates, oxalates, tannins (in tea or coffee), iron, and calcium adversely affect zinc absorption
Release of vitamin A from liver	Delayed healing	Recognize groups at risk for zinc deficiency, such as vegetarians and Mexican-Americans, whose diets may have restricted or low meat content and high fiber and phytate content; and patients with malabsorption syndromes
Improved wound healing with vitamin C	***Skin lesions***—Erythematous, crusted lesions around body orifices	
	Alopecia	
Sources	Diarrhea	
Seafood (especially oysters), meat, poultry, eggs, wheat, legumes	Growth failure	
	Retarded sexual maturity	Emphasize correct use of zinc supplements and the possible interaction with other minerals
	Excess	
	Vomiting and diarrhea	
	Malaise, dizziness	
	Anemia, gastric bleeding	
	Impaired absorption of calcium and copper	

*Macrominerals—required intake >100 mg/day.
†Microminerals or trace elements—required intake <100 mg/day.

Unit 2

Normal and Special Infant Formulas*

Formula (Manufacturer)	Protein Source	Carbohydrate Source	Fat Source	Indications for Use	Comments (Nutritional Considerations)
Human and Cow's Milk Formulas					
Human breast milk	Mature human milk; whey/casein ratio—60:40	Lactose	Mature human milk	For all full-term infants except those with galactosemia; may be used with low-birth-weight infants	Recommended sole form of feeding for first 5 to 6 months; nutritionally complete except for fluoride
Evaporated cow's milk formulas	Milk protein; whey/casein ratio—18:82	Lactose, sucrose	Butterfat	For full-term infants with no special nutritional requirements; use of undiluted cow's milk after 12 months	Supplement with iron and vitamin C; A and D if not fortified; fluoride if fluoridated water is not used for formula preparation
Commercial Infant Formulas					
Enfamil (Mead Johnson)	Nonfat cow's milk, demineralized whey; whey/casein ratio—60:40	Lactose	Palm olein, soy, coconut, HOSun† oils	For full-term and premature infants with no special nutritional requirements	Available fortified with iron, 12 mg/L Also available in 24 cal/oz
Improved Similac (Ross)	Nonfat cow's milk; whey/casein ratio—48:52	Lactose	Soy, coconut oils, and high-oleic safflower oil	For full-term and premature infants with no special nutritional requirements	Available fortified with iron, 1.8 mg/100 cal, nucleotides, 72 mg/L Also available in 24 cal/oz with iron
Baby formula (Gerber)	Nonfat cow's milk; whey/casein ratio—18:82	Lactose	Palm olein, soy, coconut, HOSun oils	For full-term and premature infants with no special nutritional requirements	Available fortified with iron, 12 mg/L
Good Start H.A. (Carnation)	Hydrolyzed whey	Lactose, maltodextrin	Palm olein, soy, safflower, coconut oils	For full-term infants	Manufacturer's claim regarding hypoallergenicity has been withdrawn
Good Nature (Carnation)	Nonfat cow's milk	Corn syrup solids	Palm, corn, oleic oils	For feeding older infants	Contains more protein and calcium than "starter" formulas
Similac Natural Care Human Milk Fortifier (Ross)	Nonfat cow's milk; whey protein concentrate	Hydrolyzed corn starch, lactose	MCT,‡ coconut, soy oils	For low-birth-weight infants; fed mixed with or alternately with human milk; improves vitamin/mineral content of human milk	Protein, 2.7 g/100 cal osmolality—300 mOsm/kg water, 24 cal/oz
Similac NeoCare with Iron (Ross)	Nonfat cow's milk, whey/casein ratio—50:50	Corn syrup and lactose	MCT oils	Preterm infants, 22 cal/oz	Protein, 2.6 g/100 cal Phosphorus, 62 mg/100 cal Calcium, 105 mg/100 cal

*All formulas provide 20 kcal/oz except as noted in product information from the formula manufacturers. For the most current information, consult product labels or package enclosures.
†HOSun, high-oleic sunflower.
‡MCT, medium-chain triglycerides.
§L-Amino acids include L-cystine, L-tyrosine, and L-tryptophan, which are reduced in hydrolyzed, charcoal-treated casein.
‖Ross Laboratories and Mead Johnson manufacture several specialty formulas for metabolic disorders for infants.

Normal and Special Infant Formulas*—cont'd

Formula (Manufacturer)	Protein Source	Carbohydrate Source	Fat Source	Indications for Use	Comments (Nutritional Considerations)
Commercial Infant Formulas—cont'd					
Enfamil Human Milk Fortifier (Mead Johnson)	Whey protein concentrate, casein	Corn syrup solids	Trace	For low-birth-weight infants; fed mixed with human milk; increases protein, calories, calcium, phosphorus, and other nutrients	Used only as human milk fortifier, not as separate formula; one packet of powder supplies 3.5 kcal/ml and less than 0.1 g/dl fat
For Milk Protein–Sensitive Infants ("Milk Allergy"), Lactose Intolerance					
Prosobee (Mead Johnson)	Soy protein isolate	Corn syrup solids	Palm, soy, coconut, HOSun oils	With milk protein allergy, lactose intolerance, lactase deficiency, galactosemia	Hypoallergenic, zero band antigen; lactose- and sucrose-free
Isomil (Ross)	Soy protein isolate	Corn syrup, sucrose	Soy, coconut oils	With milk protein allergy, lactose intolerance, lactase deficiency, galactosemia	Hypoallergenic; lactose-free
Isomil SF (Ross)	Soy protein isolate	Hydrolyzed corn starch	Soy, coconut oils	For use during diarrhea	Lessens amount and duration of watery stools; contains fiber
Lactofree (Mead Johnson)	Milk protein isolate	Corn syrup solids	Palm olein, soy, HOSun oils	With lactose intolerance, lactase deficiency, galactosemia	Lactose-free
Soyalac (Loma Linda)	Soybean solids	Sucrose, corn syrup	Soy oil	With milk protein allergy, lactose intolerance, lactase deficiency, galactosemia	Lactose-free
I-Soyalac (Loma Linda)	Soy protein isolate	Sucrose, tapioca dextrin	Soy oil	With milk protein allergy, lactose intolerance, lactase deficiency, galactosemia	Lactose- and corn-free
For Infants with Malabsorption Syndromes, Milk Allergy (Hydrolysate Formulas)					
RCF (Ross Carbohydrate Free) (Ross)	Soy protein isolate		Soy, coconut oils	With carbohydrate intolerance	Carbohydrate is added according to amount infant will tolerate
Portagen (Mead Johnson)	Sodium caseinate	Corn syrup solids, sucrose, lactose	MCT (coconut source), corn oil	For impaired fat absorption secondary to pancreatic insufficiency, bile acid deficiency, intestinal resection, lymphatic anomalies	Nutritionally complete

Continued

Normal and Special Infant Formulas*—cont'd

Formula (Manufacturer)	Protein Source	Carbohydrate Source	Fat Source	Indications for Use	Comments (Nutritional Considerations)
For Infants with Malabsorption Syndromes, Milk Allergy (Hydrolysate Formulas)—cont'd					
Nutramigen (Mead Johnson)	Casein hydrolysate, L-amino acids§	Corn syrup solids, modified corn starch	Corn, soy oils	For infants and children sensitive to food proteins; use in galactosemic patients	Nutritionally complete; hypoallergenic formula; lactose- and sucrose-free
Pregestimil (Mead Johnson)	Casein hydrolysate, L-amino acids	Corn syrup solids, modified tapioca starch	MCT, soy, HOSun oils	Disaccharidase deficiencies, malabsorption syndromes, cystic fibrosis, intestinal resection	Nutritionally complete; easily digestible protein, carbohydrate, and fat; lactose- and sucrose-free
Alimentum (Ross)	Casein hydrolysate, L-amino acids	Sucrose, modified tapioca starch	MCT, oleic, soy oils	For infants and children sensitive to food proteins or with cystic fibrosis	Nutritionally complete; hypoallergenic formula; lactose-free
Specialty Formulas					
Lonalac (Mead Johnson)	Casein	Lactose	Coconut	For children with congestive heart failure, who require reduced sodium intake	For long-term management, additional sodium must be given; supplement with vitamins C and D and iron; Na = 1 mEq/L
Similac PM 60/40 (Ross)	Whey protein concentrate, sodium caseinate (60:40 ratio)	Lactose	Coconut, corn oils	For newborns predisposed to hypocalcemia and infants with impaired renal, digestive, and cardiovascular functions	Low calcium, potassium, and phosphorus; relatively low solute load; Na = 7 mEq/L; available in powder only
Diet Modifiers					
Polycose (Ross)		Glucose polymers (corn syrup solids)		Used to increase calorie intake, as in failure-to-thrive infants	Carbohydrate only; a powdered or liquid calorie supplement; powder, 23 kcal/tbsp
Moducal (Mead Johnson)		Hydrolyzed corn starch		Used to increase carbohydrate intake	Carbohydrate only; a powdered calorie supplement: 30 kcal/tbsp
Casec (Mead Johnson)	Calcium caseinate			Used to increase protein intake	Protein only; negligible fat and no carbohydrate
MCT Oil (Mead Johnson)			90% MCT (coconut source)	Supplement in fat malabsorption conditions	Fat only; 8.3 kcal/g; 115 kcal/tbsp

*All formulas provide 20 kcal/oz except as noted in product information from the formula manufacturers. For the most current information, consult product labels or package enclosures.
†HOSun, high-oleic sunflower.
‡MCT, medium-chain triglycerides.
§L-Amino acids include L-cystine, L-tyrosine, and L-tryptophan, which are reduced in hydrolyzed, charcoal-treated casein.
‖Ross Laboratories and Mead Johnson manufacture several specialty formulas for metabolic disorders for infants.

Normal and Special Infant Formulas*—cont'd

Formula (Manufacturer)	Protein Source	Carbohydrate Source	Fat Source	Indications for Use	Comments (Nutritional Considerations)
For Infants with Phenylketonuria‖					
Lofenalac (Mead Johnson)	Casein hydrolysate, L-amino acids	Corn syrup solids, modified tapioca starch	Corn oil	For infants and children	111 mg phenylalanine per quart of formula (20 cal/oz); must be supplemented with other foods to provide minimal phenylalanine
Phenyl-free (Mead Johnson)	L-Amino acids	Sucrose, corn syrup solids, modified tapioca starch	Corn, coconut oils	For children over 1 year of age	Phenylalanine-free; permits increased supplementation with normal foods
Phenex-1 (Ross)	L-Amino acids	Hydrolyzed corn starch	Soy, coconut, palm oils	For infants	Phenylalanine-free; fortified with L-tyrosine, L-glutamine, L-carnitine, and taurine; contains vitamins, minerals, and trace elements
Phenex-2 (Ross)	L-Amino acids	Hydrolyzed corn starch	Soy, coconut, palm oils	For children and adults	Phenylalanine-free; fortified with L-tyrosine, L-glutamine, L-carnitine, and taurine; contains vitamins, minerals, and trace elements
Pro-Phree (Ross)	None	Hydrolyzed corn starch	Soy, coconut, palm oils	For infants and toddlers requiring reduced protein intake	Must be supplemented with protein; has vitamins, minerals, and trace elements

Unit 2

Guidelines for Feeding During the First Year

Birth to 6 Months (Breast- or Bottle-Feeding)

Breast-Feeding

Most desirable complete diet for first half of year.*

Requires supplements of fluoride (0.25 mg)—regardless of the fluoride content of the local water supply—after 6 months of age; may require iron by 4 to 6 months of age.

Requires supplements of vitamin D (400 units) if mother's diet is inadequate.

Formula

Iron-fortified commercial formula is a complete food for the first half of the year.*

Requires fluoride supplements (0.25 mg) after 6 months of age when the concentration of fluoride in the drinking water is below 0.3 parts per million (ppm).

Evaporated milk formula requires supplements of vitamin C, iron, and fluoride (in accordance with the fluoride content of the local water supply) after 6 months of age.

6 to 12 Months (Solid Foods)

May begin to add solids by 5 to 6 months of age.

First foods are strained, pureed, or finely mashed.

Finger foods such as teething crackers, raw fruit, or vegetables can be introduced by 6 to 7 months.

Chopped table food or commercially prepared junior foods can be started by 9 to 12 months.

With the exception of cereal, the order of introducing foods is variable; a recommended sequence is weekly introduction of other foods, beginning with fruit, then vegetables, and then meat.

As the quantity of solids increases, the amount of formula should be limited to approximately 900 ml (30 oz) daily, and fruit juice to less than 360 ml (12 oz) daily.

Method of Introduction

Introduce solids when infant is hungry.

Begin spoon feeding by pushing food to back of tongue because of infant's natural tendency to thrust tongue forward.

---

*Breast-feeding or commercial formula feeding is recommended up to 12 months of age. After 1 year, whole cow's milk can be given.

This section may be photocopied and distributed to families.

From Wong DL, Hess CS: *Wong and Whaley's Clinical manual of pediatric nursing,* ed 5. Copyright © 2000, Mosby, St Louis.

Use small spoon with straight handle; begin with 1 or 2 teaspoons of food; gradually increase to 2 to 3 tablespoons per feeding.

Introduce one food at a time, usually at intervals of 4 to 7 days, to identify food allergies.

As the amount of solid food increases, decrease the quantity of milk to prevent overfeeding.

Never introduce foods by mixing them with the formula in the bottle.

Cereal

Introduce commercially prepared iron-fortified infant cereals and administer daily until 18 months of age.

Rice cereal is usually introduced first because of its low allergenic potential.

Can discontinue supplemental iron once cereal is given.

Fruits and Vegetables

Applesauce, bananas, and pears are usually well tolerated.

Avoid fruits and vegetables marketed in cans that are not specifically designed for infants because of variable and sometimes high lead content and addition of salt, sugar, and/or preservatives.

Offer fruit juice only from a cup, not a bottle, to reduce the development of "nursing caries."

Meat, Fish, and Poultry

Avoid fatty meats.

Prepare meats by baking, broiling, steaming, or poaching.

Include organ meats such as liver, which has a high iron, vitamin A, and vitamin B complex content.

If soup is given, be sure all ingredients are familiar to child's diet.

Avoid commercial meat/vegetable combinations because protein is low.

Eggs and Cheese

Serve egg yolk hard boiled and mashed, soft cooked, or poached.

Introduce egg white in small quantities (1 tsp) toward end of first year to detect an allergy.

Use cheese as a substitute for meat and as a finger food.

Developmental Milestones Associated with Feeding

Age (Months)	Development
Birth	Has sucking, rooting, and swallowing reflexes Feels hunger and indicates desire for food by crying; expresses satiety by falling asleep
1	Has strong extrusion reflex
3-4	Extrusion reflex is fading Begins to develop hand-eye coordination
4-5	Can approximate lips to the rim of a cup
5-6	Can use fingers to feed self a cracker
6-7	Chews and bites May hold own bottle, but may not drink from it (prefers for it to be held)
7-9	Refuses food by keeping lips closed; has taste preferences Holds a spoon and plays with it during feeding May drink from a straw Drinks from a cup with assistance
9-12	Picks up small morsels of food (finger foods) and feeds self Holds own bottle and drinks from it Drinks from a household cup without assistance but spills some Uses a spoon with much spilling
12-18	Drools less Drinks well from a household cup, but may drop it when finished Holds cup with both hands Begins to use a spoon but turns it before reaching mouth
24	Can use a straw Chews food with mouth closed and shifts food in mouth Distinguishes between finger and spoon foods Holds small glass in one hand; replaces glass without dropping Uses spoon correctly but with some spilling
36	Spills small amount from spoon Begins to use fork; holds it in fist Uses adult pattern of chewing, which involves rotary action of jaw
48	Rarely spills when using spoon Serves self finger foods Eats with fork held with fingers
54	Uses fork in preference to spoon
72	Spreads with knife
84	Cuts tender food with knife

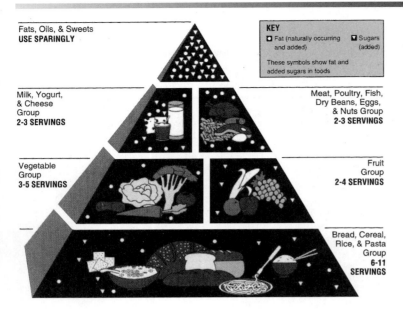

Fats, Oils, & Sweets
USE SPARINGLY

KEY
☐ Fat (naturally occurring
and added)
▼ Sugars
(added)

These symbols show fat and
added sugars in foods

Milk, Yogurt,
& Cheese
Group
2-3 SERVINGS

Meat, Poultry, Fish,
Dry Beans, Eggs,
& Nuts Group
2-3 SERVINGS

Vegetable
Group
3-5 SERVINGS

Fruit
Group
2-4 SERVINGS

Bread, Cereal,
Rice, & Pasta
Group
**6-11
SERVINGS**

Fig. 2-1 Food Guide Pyramid: a guide to daily food choices. (Courtesy U.S. Department of Agriculture, 1992.)

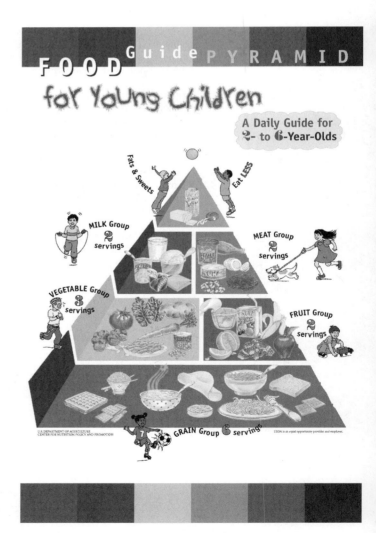

Fig. 2-2 Food Guide Pyramid for Young Children. (Courtesy U.S. Department of Agriculture Center for Nutrition Policy and Promotion, 1999.)

Unit 2

BOX 2-2

Food Guide Pyramid: Sample Serving Sizes

Bread, Cereal, Rice, and Pasta Group

1 slice of bread
1 ounce of ready-to-eat cereal
½ cup of cooked cereal, rice, or pasta

Vegetable Group

1 cup of raw leafy vegetables
½ cup of other vegetables, cooked or chopped raw
¾ cup of vegetable juice

Fruit Group

1 medium apple, banana, or orange
½ cup of chopped, cooked, or canned fruit
¾ cup of fruit juice

Milk, Yogurt, and Cheese Group

1 cup of milk or yogurt
1½ ounces of natural cheese
2 ounces of processed cheese

Meat, Poultry, Fish, Dry Beans, Eggs, and Nuts Group

2-3 ounces of cooked lean meat, poultry, or fish
½ cup of cooked dry beans, 1 egg, or 2 tablespoons of peanut butter count as 1 ounce of lean meat

COMMUNITY FOCUS

Healthy Food Choices

Current research indicates that new lower-fat recipes in school lunch programs are well-accepted by children.* However, children who were informed about healthier food choices did not consistently select healthier items.† Some schools offer fast food from various restaurants. More information on fast food can be obtained at the Web site **www.olen.com/food/** or by ordering *Fast Food Facts* by the Minnesota Attorney General's office through e-mail: **consumer.ag@state.mn.us.**

*Borja ME, Bordi PL, Lambert CU: New lower-fat dessert recipes for the school lunch program are well accepted by children, *J Am Diet Assoc* 96(9):908-910, 1996.

†Colizza DF, Colvin SP: Food choices of healthy school-age children, *J Sch Nurs* 11(4):17-20, 1995.

Sample Menus for Children and Adolescents Based on Food Guide Pyramid

YOUNG CHILD (AGE 4-6)*

Breakfast	1 oz dry, unsweetened cereal
	¼ cup orange juice
	4 oz low-fat milk
	1 slice toast
Snack	½ banana
Lunch	2 tbsp peanut butter
	2 tsp all-fruit preserves
	1 slice whole wheat bread
	½ cup peas
	4 oz low-fat milk
Snack	2 graham crackers
	4 oz low-fat milk
	½ cup carrots, raw
Dinner	1 chicken leg, roasted without skin
	½ cup macaroni and cheese
	½ cup green beans, cooked
	1 whole wheat roll
	4 oz low-fat milk
Snack	½ cup canned peaches

Total Servings

Grain group	6
Vegetable group	3
Fruit group	2
Milk group	2
Meat group	2

SCHOOL-AGE CHILD*

Breakfast	2 four-inch waffles
	2 tbsp syrup
	½ cup orange juice
Lunch	4 oz lean hamburger and bun
	½ cup raw carrot sticks
	¾ cup apple juice
Snack	1 cup frozen yogurt *or*
	1 cup unsweetened cereal with low-fat milk
Dinner	1 cup spaghetti with tomato sauce
	1 piece garlic bread
	Green salad with romaine lettuce and dressing
	½ cup broccoli
	1 banana
	1 cup low-fat milk
Snack	2 cups plain popcorn
	½ cup grape juice

Total Servings

Grain group	6-7
Vegetable group	3
Fruit group	3-4
Milk group	2
Meat group	2

ADOLESCENT*

Breakfast	8 oz of 1% milk†
	½ cup orange juice
	2 oz dry, unsweetened cereal
	1 banana
Lunch	1 cheeseburger with lettuce, tomato, and onion
	1 small order French fries
	1 medium low-fat milk shake
Snack	1 peanut butter sandwich
	8 oz of 1% milk
	1 cup yogurt
Dinner	½ cup canned mixed fruit
	12 oz baked chicken breast
	1 slice whole wheat bread
	½ cup cooked rice
	1 serving corn on the cob
	1½ cup tossed green salad with low-fat dressing
	8 oz Snapple fruit drink
Snack	¾ cup vegetable juice (e.g., V8)
	2-3 graham crackers

Total Servings

Grain group	7
Vegetable group	5
Fruit group	4
Milk group	5
Meat group	2

Serving sizes are minimums for nutritional adequacy. Many children eat more.
*Use fats, oils, and sweets sparingly. Increase fluids with servings of water.
†Adolescents require increased portions in the milk, yogurt, and cheese group to meet the recommended 1200 mg calcium required for bone growth. This section may be photocopied and distributed to families.
From Wong DL, Hess CS: *Wong and Whaley's Clinical manual of pediatric nursing,* ed 5. Copyright © 2000, Mosby, St Louis.

IMMUNIZATIONS
Licensed Vaccines and Toxoids Available in the United States and Recommended Routes of Administration

VACCINE/ROUTE

Adenovirus*/oral
Anthrax/subcutaneous
Bacillus of Calmette and Guérin (BCG)/intradermal
    or subcutaneous
Cholera/subcutaneous, intramuscular, or intradermal†
Diphtheria-tetanus-pertussis (DTP)/intramuscular
DTP-*Haemophilus influenzae* type b conjugate (DTP-Hib)‡/
    intramuscular
DTaP-Hib conjugate‡/intramuscular
Diphtheria-tetanus-acellular pertussis (DTaP)/intramuscular
Hepatitis A/intramuscular
Hepatitis B/intramuscular§
Haemophilus influenzae type b conjugate (Hib)‡/
    intramuscular
Hib conjugate–Hepatitis B/intramuscular
Influenza/intramuscular
Japanese encephalitis/subcutaneous
Measles/subcutaneous
Measles-rubella/subcutaneous
Measles-mumps-rubella (MMR)/subcutaneous
Meningococcal/subcutaneous
Mumps/subcutaneous
Pertussis/intramuscular
Plague/intramuscular
Pneumococcal/intramuscular or subcutaneous
Poliovirus vaccine, inactivated (IPV)/subcutaneous
    or intramuscular‖
Poliovirus vaccine, oral (OPV)
Rabies/intramuscular or intradermal¶
Rotavirus/oral
Rubella/subcutaneous
Tetanus/intramuscular
Tetanus-diphtheria (Td or DT)/intramuscular
Typhoid (parenteral)/subcutaneous#
Typhoid (Ty21a)/oral
Varicella/subcutaneous
Yellow fever/subcutaneous

Modified from American Academy of Pediatrics: active and passive immunization. In Peter G, editor: *1997 Red Book: report of the Committee on Infectious Diseases*, ed 24, Elk Grove Village, IL, 1997, American Academy of Pediatrics.

*Available only to the U.S. Armed Forces.

†The intradermal dose is lower than the subcutaneous dose.

‡May be administered in combination products or as reconstituted products with DTP or DTaP if approved by the FDA for the child's age and if administration of other vaccine is justified.

§Not administered in dorsogluteal muscle (buttock) because of possible reduced immunologic response.

‖Routes according to package insert.

¶The intradermal dose of rabies vaccine, human diploid cell (HDCV), is lower than the intramuscular dose and is used only for preexposure vaccination. **Rabies vaccine, adsorbed (RVA) should not be used intradermally.** Another rabies vaccine, PCEC (purified chicken embryo cell culture), RabAvert, may be given by intramuscular route only for preexposure or postexposure prophylactic use in persons who are sensitive to the other rabies vaccines. (Availability of new rabies vaccine for human use, 1998.)

#Booster doses may be administered intradermally unless vaccine that is acetone-killed and dried is used.

Product Brand Names, Manufacturers/Distributors, and Routes of Administration for Principal Childhood Vaccine Types

DTaP Diphtheria and tetanus toxoids and acellular pertussis vaccine	ACEL-IMUNE® (WLV) Certiva™ (NAV, distributed by ALI) Infanrix® (SBB, distributed by SB) Tripedia® (CON, distributed by PMC)	**IM**
DTaP-Hib Diphtheria and tetanus toxoids and acellular pertussis and *Haemophilus influenzae* type b vaccine	TriHIBit®* (ActHIB® Hib reconstituted with Tripedia® DTaP; distributed by PMC)	**IM**
DTwP Diphtheria and tetanus toxoids and whole-cell pertussis vaccine	Tri-Immunol® (WLV)† (Generic products from other manufacturers)	**IM**
DTwP-Hib Diphtheria and tetanus toxoids and whole-cell pertussis and *Haemophilus influenzae* type b vaccine	ActHIB® Hib reconstituted with DTwP (CON; distributed by PMC) TETRAMUNE® (WLV)	**IM**
Hep A Hepatitis A vaccine	HAVRIX® (SBB, distributed by SB) VAQTA® (MRK)	**IM**
Hep B Hepatitis B vaccine	ENGERIX-B® (SBB, distributed by SB) RECOMBIVAX HB® (MRK)	**IM**

Hib
 	
Haemophilus influenzae type b conjugate vaccine
  HbOC—Oligosaccharides conjugated to diphtheria CRM_{197} toxin protein
  PRP-OMP—Polyribosylribitol phosphate polysaccharide conjugated to a meningococcal outer membrane protein
  PRP-T—Polyribosylribitol phosphate polysaccharide conjugated to tetanus toxoid
  PRP-D—Polyribosylribitol phosphate polysaccharide conjugated to diphtheria toxoid
	
	HibTITER® (WLV)
	
	PedvaxHIB® (MRK)
	
	ActHIB® (PMSV, distributed by CON, PMC)
	OmniHIB™ (PMSV, distributed by SB)
	ProHIBiT® (CON, distributed by PMC)
		IM

Hib-HepB *Haemophilus influenzae* type b and hepatitis B vaccine	COMVAX® (Hib component = PRP-OMP) (MRK)	**IM**
IPV Trivalent inactivated polio vaccine (killed Salk type)	IPOL® (PMSV, distributed by CON, PMC)	**IM** or **SUBQ**
MMR Measles-mumps-rubella vaccine	M-M-R® II (MRK)	**SUBQ**
OPV Trivalent oral polio vaccine (live Sabin type)	Orimune® (WLV)	**ORAL**
Rv Rotavirus vaccine (live, oral, tetravalent)	RotaShield® (WLV)	**ORAL**
Var Varicella (chickenpox) vaccine	VARIVAX® (MRK)	**SUBQ**

Modified from American Academy of Pediatrics: Combination vaccines for childhood immunization: recommendations of the Advisory Committee on Immunization Practices (ACIP), the American Academy of Pediatrics (AAP), and the American Academy of Family Physicians (AAFP), *Pediatrics* 103(5):1072, 1999. Copyright American Academy of Pediatrics. Used with permission.

ALI, Ross Products Division, Abbott Laboratories Inc.; *CON,* Connaught Laboratories, Inc.; *MRK,* Merck & Co., Inc.; *NAV,* North American Vaccine, Inc.; *PMC,* Pasteur Mérieux Connaught; *PMSV,* Pasteur Mérieux Sérums & Vaccins, S.A.; *SBB,* SmithKline Beecham Biologicals; *SB,* SmithKline Beecham Pharmaceuticals; *WLV,* Lederle Laboratories Division of American Cyanamid Company (marketed by Wyeth-Lederle Vaccines, Wyeth-Ayerst Laboratories); *IM,* intramuscular injection; *SUBQ,* subcutaneous injection.

*As of April 10, 1999, TriHIBit® was licensed only for the fourth dose recommended at age 15-18 months in the vaccination series.

†Manufacture discontinued.

COMMUNITY FOCUS

Improving Immunization Among Children and Adolescents

Strategies that may increase immunization compliance include giving parents vaccine information at the time of the newborn's discharge, mailing reminder cards, making immunization services readily available, removing barriers to vaccination (such as long waiting times and appointment-only systems), and taking every opportunity to immunize children when they enter a health care facility (such as emergency departments, clinics, private offices, and hospitals).

Despite improving vaccination rates among infants and young children, *adolescents* are often incompletely immunized.

An immunization update is an important part of adolescent preventive care, especially at 11 to 12 years of age. With the exception of pregnant teenagers, all adolescents should receive a second dose of the *measles-mumps-rubella (MMR) vaccine* unless they have documentation of two MMR vaccinations following the first 12 months of life. All adolescents who have not previously completed the three-dose series of the *hepatitis B (HBV) vaccine* should initiate or complete the series at age 11 to 12 years.

Adolescents ages 11 to 12 years and no older than 16 years should receive a booster dose of *tetanus diphtheria (Td) vaccine* if they have received the primary series of vaccinations and if no dose has been received during the previous 5 years. Unvaccinated adolescents who lack a reliable history of chickenpox should receive the *varicella virus vaccine* at age 11 to 12 years.

Hepatitis A vaccine should be given to adolescents who are traveling or living in countries where the hepatitis A virus is endemic, or in communities with high rates of hepatitis A, chronic liver disease, intravenous drug use, or males who have sex with other males.

Adolescents who have chronic disorders or underlying medical conditions that place them at high risk for complications associated with a disease, such as influenza, should receive the appropriate vaccines. (See p. 183.)

ATRAUMATIC CARE

Immunizations

To minimize local reactions from vaccines:
   Select a needle of adequate length (1 inch in infants) to deposit the antigen deep in the muscle mass
   Inject into the vastus lateralis or ventrogluteal muscle; the deltoid may be used in children 18 months or older or in infants receiving HBV vaccine
   Use an air bubble to clear the needle after injecting the vaccine (theoretically beneficial but unproved)
To minimize pain:
   Apply the topical anesthetic EMLA to the injection site and cover with an occlusive dressing for 2½ hours before the injection
   Apply a vapocoolant spray (e.g., ethyl chloride or Fluori-Methane) directly to the skin or to a cotton ball, which is placed on the skin for 15 seconds immediately before the injection*
   In preschool children use distraction, such as telling the child to "take a deep breath and blow and blow and blow until I tell you to stop."
NOTE: Changing the needle on the syringe after drawing up the vaccine and before injecting it has not been shown to decrease local reactions.
In children 4 to 6 years of age, the administration of sequential injections or simultaneous injections of vaccines did not alter their perceptions of distress, but parents preferred the simultaneous method.†

*Reis EC, Holubkov R: Vapocoolant spray is equally effective as EMLA cream in reducing immunization pain in school-aged children, *Pediatrics* 100(6): 1025, 1997.

†Horn MI, McCarthy AM: Children's responses to sequential versus simultaneous immunization injections, *J Pediatr Health Care* 13(1):18-23, 1999.

Recommended Childhood Immunization Schedule
United States, January–December 1999

Vaccines[1] are listed under routinely recommended ages. Bars *indicate range of recommended ages for immunization. Any dose not given at the recommended age should be given as a "catch-up" immunization at any subsequent visit when indicated and feasible.* Ovals *indicate vaccines to be given if previously recommended doses were missed or given earlier than the recommended minimum age.*

Age ▶ Vaccine ▼	Birth	1 mo	2 mos	4 mos	6 mos	12 mos	15 mos	18 mos	4-6 yrs	11-12 yrs	14-16 yrs
Hepatitis B[2]	Hep B		Hep B		Hep B					Hep B	
Diphtheria, Tetanus, Pertussis[3]			DTaP	DTaP	DTaP		DTaP[3]		DTaP	Td	
H. influenzae type b[4]			Hib	Hib	Hib	Hib					
Polio[5]			IPV	IPV		Polio[5]			Polio		
Rotavirus[6]			Rv[6]	Rv[6]	Rv[6]						
Measles, Mumps, Rubella[7]						MMR			MMR[7]	MMR[7]	
Varicella[8]							Var			Var[8]	

Approved by the Advisory Committee on Immunization Practices (ACIP), the American Academy of Pediatrics (AAP), and the American Academy of Family Physicians (AAFP).

[1] This schedule indicates the recommended ages for routine administration of currently licensed childhood vaccines. Combination vaccines may be used whenever any components of the combination are indicated and its other components are not contraindicated. Providers should consult the manufacturers' package inserts for detailed recommendations.

[2] *Infants born to HBsAg-negative mothers* should receive the second dose of hepatitis B vaccine at least 1 month after the first dose. The third dose should be administered at least 4 months after the first dose and at least 2 months after the second dose, but not before 6 months of age for infants.

Infants born to HBsAg-positive mothers should receive hepatitis B vaccine and 0.5 mL hepatitis B immune globulin (HBIG) within 12 hours of birth at separate sites. The second dose is recommended at 1-2 months of age and the third dose at 6 months of age.

Infants born to mothers whose HBsAg status is unknown should receive hepatitis B vaccine within 12 hours of birth. Maternal blood should be drawn at the time of delivery to determine the mother's HBsAg status; if the HBsAg test is positive, the infant should receive HBIG as soon as possible (no later than 1 week of age). All children and adolescents (through 18 years of age) who have not been immunized against hepatitis B may begin the series during any visit. Special efforts should be made to immunize children who were born in or whose parents were born in areas of the world with moderate or high endemicity of HBV infection. The manufacturer of Recombivax HB (Merck and Co, Inc, West Point, PA) has standardized the dose of this hepatitis vaccine to 5 μg for children from birth through 19 years of age regardless of maternal hepatitis B surface antigen carrier status. The change was made to avoid the confusion that occasionally occurred due to the availability of multiple dose formulations of this vaccine product. Children who have received a 2.5-μg dose of Recombivax for any or all the recommended doses are considered adequately immunized and no additional doses need to be administered. The other available hepatitis B vaccine, Engerix B (SmithKline Beecham, Pittsburgh, PA), also has a standard dose (10 μg) for all children from birth through 19 years of age. The vaccines are interchangeable when given in the doses recommended by the manufacturers.
NOTE: Because hepatitis B vaccines contain thimerosal, a mercury-containing compound, practitioners may consider giving the first dose of the vaccine not at birth, but at 2 to 6 months of age. This temporary schedule adjustment applies only to infants born to HbsAg-negative mothers. Vaccination just after birth is still needed by infants born to HbsAg-positive mothers. As of this writing, a thimerosal-free HBV vaccine is pending FDA approval. (Reference: Press release, AAP, July 14, 1999, www.aap.org/new/thimpublic.htm.)

[3] DTaP (diphtheria and tetanus toxoids and acellular pertussis vaccine) is the preferred vaccine for all doses in the immunization series, including completion of the series in children who have received 1 or more doses of whole-cell DTP vaccine. Whole-cell DTP is an acceptable alternative to DTaP. The fourth dose (DTP or DTaP) may be administered as early as 12 months of age, provided 6 months have elapsed since the third dose and if the child is unlikely to return at age 15-18 months. Td (tetanus and diphtheria toxoids) is recommended at 11-12 years of age if at least 5 years have elapsed since the last dose of DTP, DTaP, or DT. Subsequent routine Td boosters are recommended every 10 years.

[4] Three H. influenzae type b (Hib) conjugate vaccines are licensed for infant use. If PRP-OMP (PedvaxHIB and COMVAX [Merck]) is administered at 2 and 4 months of age, a dose at 6 months is not required. Because clinical studies in infants have demonstrated that using some combination products may induce a lower immune response to the Hib vaccine component, DTaP/Hib combination products should not be used for primary immunization in infants at 2, 4, or 6 months of age, unless FDA-approved for these ages.

[5] Two poliovirus vaccines currently are licensed in the United States: inactivated poliovirus vaccine (IPV) and oral poliovirus vaccine (OPV). The AAP and AAFP now recommend that the first two doses of poliovirus vaccine should be IPV. Use of IPV for all doses also is acceptable and is recommended for immunocompromised persons and their household contacts. OPV is no longer recommended for the first two doses of the schedule.
NOTE: **Recommendations of the Advisory Committee on Immunization Practices: Revised Recommendations for Routine Poliomyelitis Vaccination**—On June 17, 1999, to eliminate the risk for vaccine-associated paralytic polio (VAPP), the ACIP recommended an all-IPV schedule for routine childhood polio vaccination in the United States. As of January 1, 2000, all children should receive four doses of IPV at ages 2 months, 4 months, 6-18 months, and 4-6 years. OPV should be used only for the following special circumstances: 1. Mass vaccination campaigns to control outbreaks of paralytic polio. 2. Unvaccinated children who will be traveling in less than 4 weeks to areas where polio is endemic. 3. Children of parents who do not accept the recommended number of vaccine injections. These children may receive OPV only for the third or fourth dose or both; in this situation, health care providers should administer OPV only after discussing the risk for VAPP with parents or caregivers. (Reference: *MMWR 48*(27):590, 1999.)

[6] Rotavirus (Rv) vaccine is shaded and italicized to indicate: 1) health care providers may require time and resources to incorporate this new vaccine into practice; and 2) the AAFP feels that the decision to use rotavirus vaccine should be made by the parent or guardian in consultation with the physician or other health care provider. The first dose of Rv vaccine should not be administered before 6 weeks of age, and the minimum interval between doses is 3 weeks. The Rv vaccine series should not be initiated at 7 months of age or older, and all doses should be completed by the first birthday.
NOTE: Since the availability of the rotavirus vaccine and as of July 7, 1999, 15 cases of intussusception (a bowel obstruction in which one segment of bowel becomes enfolded within another segment) were reported to the Vaccine Adverse Event Reporting System (VAERS). Although available data suggest but do not establish a causal association between receipt of RV vaccine and intussusception, the ACIP of the Centers for Disease Control and Prevention (CDC) recommends postponing administration of RV vaccine to children scheduled to receive the vaccine before November 1999, including those who already have begun the RV vaccine series. As of this writing, it is not known if this recommendation will be extended beyond November 1999. (Reference: Intussusception among recipients of rotavirus vaccine—United States, 1998-1999, *MMWR 48*(27):577-581, July 16, 1999.)

[7] The second dose of measles, mumps, and rubella vaccine (MMR) is recommended routinely at 4-6 years of age but may be administered during any visit, provided at least 4 weeks have elapsed since receipt of the first dose and that both doses are administered beginning at or after 12 months of age. Those who have not previously received the second dose should complete the schedule by the 11- to 12-year-old visit.

[8] Varicella vaccine is recommended at any visit on or after the first birthday for susceptible children, i.e., those who lack a reliable history of chickenpox (as judged by a health care provider) and who have not been immunized. Susceptible persons 13 years of age or older should receive 2 doses, given at least 4 weeks apart.

From American Academy of Pediatrics, Committee on Infectious Diseases: **Recommended childhood immunization schedule—United States, January - December 1999**, *Pediatrics* 103(1):181-182, inset, 1999.

NOTE: Detailed recommendations for the use of the vaccines routinely indicated during infancy, childhood, and adolescence are given in the *1997 Red Book*, American Academy of Pediatrics (AAP) statements (www.aap.org); the Advisory Committee on Immunization Practices (ACIP) statements (www.cdc.gov/nip) on specific vaccines; and the respective manufacturers' package inserts. Updates are also available on the Web at www.mosby.com/WOW/.

Recommended Immunization Schedules for Children Not Immunized in First Year of Life in the United States[a]

Recommended Time/Age	Immunization(s)[b,c]	Comments
Younger Than 7 Years		
First visit	DTaP (or DTP), Hib, HBV, MMR, OPV[d]	If indicated, tuberculin testing may be done at same visit. If child is 5 years of age or older, Hib is not indicated in most circumstances.
Interval after first visit		
1 month (4 weeks)	DTaP (or DTP), HBV, Var[e]	The second dose of OPV may be given if accelerated poliomyelitis vaccination is necessary, such as for travelers to areas where polio is endemic.
2 months	DTaP (or DTP), Hib, OPV[d]	Second dose of Hib is indicated only if the first dose was received when younger than 15 months.
≥8 months	DTaP (or DTP), HBV, OPV[d]	OPV and HBV are not given if the third doses were given earlier.
Age 4-6 years (at or before school entry)	DTaP (or DTP), OPV[d], MMR[f]	DTaP (or DTP) is not necessary if the fourth dose was given after the fourth birthday; OPV is not necessary if the third dose was given after the fourth birthday.
Age 11-12 years	(See p. 186.)	
7-12 Years		
First visit	HBV, MMR, Td, OPV[d]	
Interval after first visit		
2 months (8 weeks)	HBV, MMR[f], Var[e], Td, OPV[d]	OPV also may be given 1 month after the first visit if accelerated poliomyelitis vaccination is necessary.
8-14 months	HBV[g], Td, OPV[d]	OPV is not given if the third dose was given earlier.
Age 11-12 years	(See p. 186.)	

From American Academy of Pediatrics Committee on Infectious Diseases, Peter G, editor. 1997 *Red Book: report of the Committee on Infectious Diseases*, ed 24, Elk Grove Village, IL, 1997, The Academy.

HBV, Hepatitis B virus vaccine; *Var*, varicella vaccine; *DTP*, diphtheria and tetanus toxoids and pertussis vaccine; *DTaP*, diphtheria and tetanus toxoids and acellular pertussis vaccine; *Hib, Haemophilus influenzae* type b conjugate vaccine; *OPV*, oral poliovirus vaccine; *IPV*, inactivated poliovirus vaccine; *MMR*, live measles-mumps-rubella vaccine; *Td*, adult tetanus toxoid (full dose) and diphtheria toxoid (reduced dose), for children ≥7 years and adults.

[a]Table is not completely consistent with all package inserts. For products used, also consult manufacturer's package insert for instructions on storage, handling, dosage, and administration. Biologics prepared by different manufacturers may vary, and package inserts of the same manufacturer may change from time to time. Therefore the physician should be aware of the contents of the current package insert.

[b]If all needed vaccines cannot be administered simultaneously, priority should be given to protecting the child against those diseases that pose the greatest immediate risk. In the United States, these diseases for children younger than 2 years usually are measles and *H. influenzae* type b infection; for children older than 7 years, they are measles, mumps, and rubella. Before 13 years of age, immunity against hepatitis B and varicella should be ensured.

[c]DTaP, HBV, Hib, MMR, and Var can be given simultaneously at separate sites if failure of the patient to return for future immunizations is a concern.

[d]IPV is also acceptable. However, for infants and children starting vaccination late (i.e., after 6 months of age), OPV is preferred in order to complete an accelerated schedule with a minimum number of injections.

[e]Varicella vaccine can be administered to susceptible children any time after 12 months of age. Unvaccinated children who lack a reliable history of chickenpox should be vaccinated before their thirteenth birthday.

[f]Minimal interval between doses of MMR is 1 month (4 weeks).

[g]HBV may be given earlier in a 0-, 2-, and 4-month schedule.

NOTE: For rotavirus, see footnote 6 on p.186.

Unit 2

Routine Immunization for Infants and Children—Provincial and Territorial Schedules, Canada, 1998

Province or Territory	DTaP (Months)	Polio-IPV (Months)	Hib (Months)	Td/Td-IPV (Years)	Hepatitis B (3 Doses)	MMR (First Dose) (Months)	MMR/MR (Second Dose)
Alberta	2, 4, 6, 18 and 4-6 years	2, 4, 6, 18 and 4-6 years	2, 4, 6, 18	Td, 14-16	Grade 5	12	MMR, 4-6 years
British Columbia	2, 4, 6, 18 and 4-6 years*	2, 4, 6, 18 and 4-6 years*	2, 4, 6,18	Td, 14-16	Grade 6	12	MMR, 18 months
Manitoba	2, 4, 6, 18 and 4-6 years	2, 4, 6, 18 and 4-6 years	2, 4, 6, 18	Td, 14-16	Not planned	12	MMR, 5 years
Newfoundland	2, 4, 6, 18 and 4-6 years	2, 4, 6, 18 and 4-6 years	2, 4, 6, 18	Td-IPV, 14-16	Grade 4	12	MMR, 18 months
New Brunswick	2, 4, 6, 18 and 4-6 years†	2, 4, 6, 18 and 4-6 years	2, 4, 6, 18	Td-IPV, 14-16‡	Infants 0, 2, 12 months or grade 4§	12	MMR, 18 months
Northwest Territories	2, 4, 6, 18 and 4-6 years‖	2, 4, 6, 18 and 4-6 years‖	2, 4, 6, 18	Td-IPV, 14-16¶	Infants 0, 1, 6 months or grade 4#	12	MMR, 18 months
Nova Scotia	2, 4, 6, 18 and 4-6 years	2, 4, 6, 18 and 4-6 years	2, 4, 6, 18	Td-IPV, 14-16	Grade 4	12	MMR, 4-6 years
Ontario	2, 4, 6, 18 and 4-6 years**	2, 4, 6, 18 and 4-6 years**	2, 4, 6, 18	Td-IPV, 14-16††	Grade 7	12	MMR, 4-6 years
Prince Edward Island	2, 4, 6, 18 and 4-6 years	2, 4, 6, 18 and 4-6 years	2, 4, 6, 18	Td-IPV, 14-16	Infants 2, 4, 15 months or grade 3‡‡	15	MMR, 18 months§§
Quebec	2, 4, 6, 18 and 4-6 years	2, 4, 6, 18 and 4-6 years‖‖	2, 4, 6, 18	Td-IPV, 14-16‖‖	Grade 4	12	MMR, 18 months
Saskatchewan	2, 4, 6, 18 and 4-6 years¶¶	2, 4, 6, 18 and 4-6 years¶¶	2, 4, 6, 18	Td, 14-16##	Grade 6	12	MR, 18 months
Yukon Territory	2, 4, 6, 18 and 4-6 years	2, 4, 6, 18 and 4-6 years	2, 4, 6, 18	Td-IPV, 14-16	Grade 4	12	MMR, 18 months

From Health Canada-Paediatrics & Child Health, Vol. 3, Supp. B-March/April 1998. Web site: http://www.hc-sc.gc.ca/main/lcdc/web/publicat/paediatr/vol3supb/pche_j.html#tab6

Hib, Haemophilus influenzae b vaccine. *MR,* Measles and rubella vaccine; *Td,* Tetanus diphtheria toxoid adult-type.

*In British Columbia, fifth dose of diphtheria, tetanus and acellular pertussis (DTaP) and inactived polio vaccine (IPV) at 4 to 6 years is not necessary if the fourth dose was given after the fourth birthday.

†In New Brunswick, whole-cell pertussis vaccine was used through 1997.

‡In New Brunswick, polio vaccine at 14 to 16 years is not required if the child has completed the primary series and received one or more doses of oral polio vaccine (OPV) in the past.

§In New Brunswick, hepatitis B vaccination is currently given to children in grade 4 who have not been vaccinated in infancy.

‖In Northwest Territories, fifth dose of DTaP and IPV at 4 to 6 years is not necessary if the fourth dose was given after the fourth birthday.

¶In Northwest Territories, polio vaccine at 14 to 16 years is not required if the child has completed the primary series and received one or more doses of OPV in the past.

#In Northwest Territories, hepatitis b vaccination is currently given to children in grade 4 who have not been vaccinated in infancy.

**In Ontario, fifth dose of DTaP and IPV at 4 to 6 years is not necessary if the fourth dose was given after the fourth birthday.

††In Ontario, polio vaccine at 14 to 16 years is not required if the child has completed the primary series and received one or more doses of OPV in the past (OPV was used routinely from January 1990 through March 1993).

‡‡In Prince Edward Island, hepatitis B vaccination is currently given to children in grade 3 who have not been vaccinated in infancy.

§§In Prince Edward Island, currently a second measles, mumps and rubella (MMR) vaccine dose is given to children 4 to 6 years of age who would not have received their second dose at 18 months.

‖‖In Quebec, polio vaccine doses at 4 to 6 years and at 14 to 16 years are omitted if OPV was used for earlier doses.

¶¶In Saskatchewan, fifth dose of DTaP and IPV fifth dose at 4 to 6 years are not necessary if the fourth dose was given after the fourth birthday.

##In Saskatchewan, polio vaccine at 14 to 16 years is given only if one dose of OPV was not received in the past.

Guide to Tetanus Prophylaxis in Routine Wound Management, 1991

History of Adsorbed Tetanus Toxoid (Doses)	Clean, Minor Wounds		All Other Wounds*	
	Td†	TIG	Td†	TIG
Unknown or <three	Yes	No	Yes	Yes
≥Three‡	No§	No	No‖	No

From Recommendations of the Immunization Practices Advisory Committee (ACIP): Diphtheria, tetanus, and pertussis: recommendations for vaccine use and other preventive measures, *MMWR 40*(RR-10):1-28, 1991.

*Such as, but not limited to, wounds contaminated with dirt, feces, soil, or saliva; puncture wounds; avulsions; and wounds resulting from missiles, crushing, burns, or frostbite.

†For children <7 years old; DTP (DT, if pertussis vaccine is contraindicated) is preferred to tetanus toxoid alone. For persons ≥7 years of age, Td is preferred to tetanus toxoid alone.

‡If only three doses of *fluid* toxoid have been received, then a fourth dose of toxoid, preferably an adsorbed toxoid, should be given.

§Yes, if >10 years since last dose.

‖Yes, if >5 years since last dose. (More frequent boosters are not needed and can accentuate side effects.)

Recommendations for Selected Nonmandated Vaccines

Description	Administration/Precautions
INFLUENZA VIRUS VACCINE (SEVERAL TRADE NAMES)	
Affords protection against strains of influenza Recommended for children age 6 months and older with chronic disorders of cardiovascular or pulmonary systems, including asthma, whose severity warranted regular medical care or hospitalization during preceding year; other eligible children include those with diabetes mellitus, renal dysfunction, anemia, immunosuppression, human immunodeficiency virus (HIV) infection, or those on long-term aspirin therapy (because aspirin increases the risk of developing Reye syndrome after influenza infection)	Administered in fall, preferably November; repeated yearly Intramuscular injection: two doses of split vaccine at least 4 weeks apart for children age 12 years or younger; one dose of split or whole vaccine for children over 12 years of age Contraindicated in persons with anaphylactic hypersensitivity to eggs May be given simultaneously with other childhood immunizations but at separate site
PNEUMOCOCCAL POLYSACCHARIDE VACCINE (PNEUMOVAX: PNU-IMUNE)	
Affords protection against 23 types of *Streptococcus pneumoniae* Recommended for children 2 years and older with sickle cell disease; functional or anatomic asplenia; nephrotic syndrome or chronic renal failure; conditions associated with immunosuppression, such as organ transplantation, drug therapy or cytoreduction therapy (including long-term systemic corticosteroid therapy); HIV infection; cerebrospinal fluid leaks; chronic cardiovascular disease (e.g., congestive heart failure or cardiomyopathy); chronic pulmonary disease (e.g., emphysema or cystic fibrosis, but not asthma); chronic liver disease (e.g., cirrhosis); or living in special environments or social settings in which the risk of invasive pneumococcal disease or its complications is very high (e.g., Alaskan Native and certain American Indian populations)	Subcutaneous or intramuscular injection Should be deferred during pregnancy Revaccination after 3 to 5 years is recommended for children 10 years or younger who are at high risk of severe pneumococcal infection. These children include those who have sickle cell disease; are functionally or anatomically asplenic; have conditions associated with a rapid antibody decline after initial immunization, such as from nephrotic syndrome, renal failure, or transplantation; or are at increased risk because of HIV infection or malignancy (e.g., leukemia, lymphoma, and Hodgkin's disease). Since most young children who are vaccinated are at continuing high risk of pneumococcal disease, routine vaccinations should be considered for any child who was originally vaccinated before 5 years of age. Reimmunization also is indicated for high-risk, older children who were initially immunized at least 5 years before. Revaccination once only is recommended.
MENINGOCOCCAL POLYSACCHARIDE VACCINE (MENOMUNE)	
Affords protection against *Neisseria meningitidis*; sero-groups A, C, Y, and W-135 Recommended for children 2 years and older with terminal complement deficiencies and anatomic or functional asplenia	Subcutaneous injection Duration of protection unknown Safety during pregnancy not established
HEPATITIS A (HAVRIX, VAQTA)	
Affords protection against hepatitis A infection Recommended for children 2 years and older in communities with high endemic rates and for preexposure prophylaxis	Intramuscular injection (not in gluteal region) Requires two doses, 6 months apart for children 2 to 18 years Duration of protection unknown May be administered with other vaccines in a separate syringe and at a different site
LYME DISEASE VACCINE (LYMERIX)	
Affords protection against infection with the spirochete, *Borrelia burgdorferi,* which causes Lyme disease (LD) Recommended for individuals 15 to 70 years at high risk for LD from significant exposure to tick habitats in endemic areas (northeast and north-central United States) and for those who have been infected with LD	Intramuscular injection in deltoid muscle Administered on 0-, 1-, and 12-month schedule; dose 2 and 3 should be given several weeks before *B. burgdorferi* season, which usually begins in April

Possible Side Effects of Recommended Childhood Immunizations and Related Nursing Responsibilities

Immunization	Reaction	Nursing Responsibilities
Hepatitis B virus	Well tolerated, few side effects	Explain to parents reason for this immunization Consider that cost for three injections may be a factor
Diphtheria	Fever usually within 24 to 48 hours Soreness, redness, and swelling at injection site Behavioral changes: drowsiness, fretfulness, anorexia, prolonged or unusual crying	Nursing responsibilities for DTP apply to immunizations for diphtheria, tetanus, and pertussis Instruction for DTP: advise parents of possible side effects
Tetanus	Same as for diphtheria but may include urticaria and malaise All may have delayed onset and last several days Lump at injection site may last for weeks or even months, but gradually disappears	Recommend prophylactic use of acetaminophen at time of DTP immunization and every 4 to 6 hours for a total of three doses Advise parents to notify practitioner *immediately* of any unusual side effects, such as those listed under pertussis on p. 192. Before administering next dose of DTP, inquire about reactions, especially those listed under pertussis on p. 192.
Pertussis	Same as for tetanus but may include loss of consciousness, convulsions, persistent inconsolable crying episodes, generalized or focal neurologic signs, fever (temperature at or above 40.5° C [105° F]), systemic allergic reaction	
***Haemophilus influenzae* type b**	Mild local reactions (erythema, pain) at injection site Low-grade fever	Advise parents of possible mild side effects
Poliovirus (OPV)*	Essentially no immediate side effects Vaccine-associated paralysis rarely occurs within 2 months of immunization (estimated risk 1:7.8 million doses); more likely to occur in close contact than in OPV recipient	Assess presence of family members at risk from trivalent OPV because of immune deficiency states
Measles	Anorexia, malaise, rash, and fever may occur 7 to 10 days after immunization Encephalitis may rarely occur (estimated risk 1:1 million doses)	Advise parents of more common side effects and use of antipyretics for fever If a persistent fever with other obvious signs of illness occurs, have parents notify physician immediately
Mumps	Essentially no side effects other than a brief, mild fever	See general comment to parents†
Rotavirus	Fever, decreased appetite, irritability, decreased activity	Advise parents of mild side effects Take latex allergy history because **RotaShield** packaging contains dry natural rubber Health care professionals with latex sensitivity who administer the vaccine should do so with caution Administer orally, never parenterally
Rubella	Fever, lymphadenopathy, or mild rash that lasts 1 or 2 days within a few days after immunization Arthralgia, arthritis, or paresthesia of the hands and fingers may occur approximately 2 weeks after vaccination and is more common in older children and adults	Advise parents of side effects, especially of time delay before joint swelling and pain; assure them that these symptoms will disappear May recommend use of acetaminophen for pain
Varicella	Pain, tenderness, or redness at the injection site Mild, vaccine-associated maculopapular or varicelliform rash at the vaccine site or elsewhere	Advise parents of possible side effects May recommend use of acetaminophen for pain

*Inactivated poliovirus vaccine (IPV)—no serious adverse effects have been associated with the currently available product; rare adverse reactions, however, cannot be excluded. Trace amounts of neomycin, streptomycin, and polymixin B may be present in IPV.

†General comment to parents: the benefit of being protected by each immunization is believed to greatly outweigh the risk from the disease.

The ***National Childhood Vaccine Injury Act*** requires the following information for childhood mandated vaccines to be documented in the child's permanent medical record: day, month, and year of administration; manufacturer and lot number of vaccine; and the name, address, and title of the person administering the vaccine. Additional data to record are the site and route of administration and evidence that the parent or legal guardian gave informed consent before the immunization was administered. Any adverse reaction after the administration of any vaccine is reported to the ***Vaccine Adverse Event Reporting System (VAERS).*** For information call (800) 822-7967; Web site: www.cdc.gov/nip/vaers.htm.

Contraindications and Precautions for Vaccinations*

True Contraindications and Precautions	Not Contraindications (Vaccines May Be Administered)

General for All Vaccines (DTP/DTAP, OPV, IPV, MMR, Hib, Hepatitis B, VZIG)

Contraindications

Anaphylactic reaction to a vaccine contraindicates further doses of that vaccine

Anaphylactic reaction to a vaccine constituent contraindicates the use of vaccines containing that substance

Moderate or severe illnesses with or without a fever

Not Contraindications

Mild to moderate local reaction (soreness, redness, swelling) following a dose of an injectable antigen

Mild acute illness with or without low-grade fever

Current antimicrobial therapy

Convalescent phase of illness

Prematurity (same dosage and indications as for normal, full-term infants)

Recent exposure to an infectious disease

History of penicillin or other nonspecific allergy or family history of such allergies

Diphtheria, Tetanus, Pertussis or Acellular Pertussis (DTP/DTAP)

Contraindication

Encephalopathy within 7 days of administration of previous dose of DTP

Precautions†

Fever of ≥40.5° C (105° F) within 48 hours after vaccination with a prior dose of DTP

Collapse or shocklike state (hypotonic-hyporesponsive episode) within 48 hours of receiving a prior dose of DTP

Seizures within 3 days of receiving a prior dose of DTP‡

Persistent, inconsolable crying lasting ≥3 hours within 48 hours of receiving a prior dose of DTP

Not Contraindications

Temperature of <40.5° C (105° F) following a previous dose of DTP

Family history of convulsions‡

Family history of sudden infant death syndrome

Family history of an adverse event following DTP administration

Oral Polio (OPV)§

Contraindications

Infection with HIV or a household contact with HIV

Known altered immunodeficiency (hematologic and solid tumors; congenital immunodeficiency; and long-term immunosuppressive therapy)

Immunodeficient household contact

Not Contraindications

Breast-feeding

Current antimicrobial therapy

Diarrhea

Precaution†

Pregnancy

Inactivated Polio (IPV)

Contraindication

Anaphylactic reaction to neomycin or streptomycin

Precaution†

Pregnancy

Based on recommendations of the American Academy of Pediatrics, Committee on Infectious Diseases, Peter G, editor: *1997 Red Book: report of the Committee on Infectious Diseases,* ed 24, Elk Grove Village, IL, 1997, The Academy.

*This information is based on the recommendations of the Advisory Committee on Immunization Practices (ACIP) and those of the Committee on Infectious Diseases (Red Book Committee) of the American Academy of Pediatrics (AAP). Sometimes these recommendations vary from those contained in the manufacturer's package inserts. For more detailed information, providers should consult the published recommendations of the ACIP, AAP, and the manufacturer's package inserts.

†The events or conditions listed as precautions, although not contraindications, should be carefully reviewed. The benefits and risks of administering a specific vaccine to an individual under the circumstances should be considered. If the risks are believed to outweigh the benefits, the vaccination should be withheld; if the benefits are believed to outweigh the risks (e.g., during an outbreak or foreign travel), the vaccination should be administered. Whether and when to administer DTP to children with proven or suspected underlying neurologic disorders should be decided on an individual basis. It is prudent on theoretic grounds to avoid vaccinating pregnant women.

‡Acetaminophen given before administering DTP and every 4 hours thereafter for 24 hours should be considered for children with a personal or family history of convulsions in siblings or parents.

§No data exist to substantiate the theoretic risk of a suboptimal immune response from the administration of OPV and MMR within 30 days of each other.

‖Measles vaccination may temporarily suppress tuberculin reactivity. If testing cannot be done the day of MMR vaccination, the test should be postponed for 4 to 6 weeks.

¶From American Academy of Pediatrics, Committee on Infectious Diseases: Prevention of rotavirus disease: guidelines for use of rotavirus vaccine, *Pediatrics* 102(6):1483-1491, 1998.

Unit 2

Contraindications and Precautions for Vaccinations—cont'd

True Contraindications and Precautions	Not Contraindications (Vaccines May Be Administered)

Measles, Mumps, Rubella (MMR)§

Contraindications

Pregnancy
Known altered immunodeficiency (hematologic and solid tumors, congenital immunodeficiency, and long-term immunosuppressive therapy)

Precautions†

Recent immune globulin administration
Immune globulin products and MMR should not be given simultaneously; if unavoidable, give at different sites and revaccinate or test for seroconversion in 3 months; if IG is given first, MMR should not be given for at least 3 to 6 months, depending on the dose; if MMR is given first, IG should not be given for 2 weeks
Thrombocytopenia/thrombocytopenia purpura

Not Contraindications§

Tuberculosis or positive PPD skin test
Simultaneous TB skin testing‖
Breast-feeding
Pregnancy of mother of recipient
Immunodeficient family member or household contact
Infection with HIV
Nonanaphylactic reactions to eggs or neomycin

Haemophilus Influenzae Type b (Hib)

Contraindication

Nonidentified

Not a Contraindication

History of Hib disease

Hepatitis B Virus (HBV)

Contraindication

Anaphylactic reaction to common baker's yeast

Not a Contraindication

Pregnancy

Rotavirus¶

Contraindications

Known or suspected immune deficiency diseases and conditions such as combined immunodeficiency, hypogammaglobulinemia, agammaglobulinemia, human immunodeficiency virus (HIV) infection, thymic abnormalities, malignancy, leukemia, lymphoma, or advanced debilitating conditions
Compromised immune status, such as those who are being treated with systemic corticosteroids, alkylating drugs, antimetabolites, radiation, or other immunosuppressive therapies
Ongoing diarrhea or vomiting; severe or even moderate febrile illness
Hypersensitivity to any component of the vaccine including aminoglycoside antibiotics, amphotericin B, or monosodium glutamate

Precautions

Immunodeficient household contact for up to 4 weeks after vaccine administration
Possible history of latex allergy because packaging for **RotaShield** contains dry natural rubber

Not Contraindications

Minor illness, such as a mild upper respiratory infection with or without low-grade fever
Breast-feeding

Varicella

Contraindications

Immunocompromised individuals (e.g., HIV, acute lymphocytic leukemia)
Pregnancy
Children receiving corticosteroids

Not a Contraindication

Breast-feeding

Unit 2

SAFETY AND INJURY PREVENTION
Child Safety Home Checklist

Safety: Fire, Electrical, Burns

- ☐ Guards in front of or around any heating appliance, fireplace, or furnace (including floor furnace)*
- ☐ Electrical wires hidden or out of reach*
- ☐ No frayed or broken wires; no overloaded sockets
- ☐ Plastic guards or caps over electrical outlets or furniture in front of outlets*
- ☐ Hanging tablecloths out of reach, away from open fires*
- ☐ Smoke detectors tested and operating properly
- ☐ Kitchen matches stored out of child's reach*
- ☐ Large, deep ashtrays throughout house (if used)
- ☐ Small stoves, heaters, and other hot objects (cigarettes, candles, coffee pots, slow cookers) placed where they cannot be tipped over or reached by children
- ☐ Hot water heater set at 49° C (120° F) or lower
- ☐ Pot handles turned toward back of stove or toward center of table
- ☐ No loose clothing worn near stove
- ☐ No cooking or eating hot foods or liquids with child standing nearby or sitting in lap
- ☐ All small appliances, such as iron, turned off, disconnected, and placed out of reach when not in use
- ☐ Cool, not hot, mist vaporizer used
- ☐ Fire extinguisher available on each floor and checked periodically
- ☐ Electrical fuse box and gas shutoff accessible
- ☐ Family escape plan in case of a fire practiced periodically; fire escape ladder available on upper-level floors
- ☐ Telephone number of fire or rescue squad and address of home with nearest cross street posted near phone

Safety: Suffocation and Aspiration

- ☐ Small objects stored out of reach*
- ☐ Toys inspected for small, removable parts or long strings*
- ☐ Hanging crib toys and mobiles placed out of reach
- ☐ Plastic bags stored away from young child's reach, large plastic garment bags discarded after tying in knots*
- ☐ Mattress or pillow not covered with plastic or in a way that is accessible to child*
- ☐ Crib designed according to federal regulations (crib slats less than 2⅜ inches [6 cm] apart) with snug-fitting mattress*†
- ☐ Crib positioned away from other furniture or windows*
- ☐ Portable playpen gates up at all times while in use*
- ☐ Accordion-style gates not used*
- ☐ Bathroom doors kept closed and toilet seats down or toilet lid fasteners used*
- ☐ Faucets turned off firmly*
- ☐ Pool fenced with locked gate
- ☐ Proper safety equipment at poolside
- ☐ Electric garage door openers stored safely and garage door adjusted to rise when door strikes object
- ☐ Doors of ovens, trunks, dishwashers, refrigerators, and front-loading clothes washers and dryers kept closed*

---

*Safety measures are specific for homes with young children. All safety measures should be implemented in homes where children reside and in homes they visit frequently, such as those of grandparents or babysitters.

†Federal regulations are available from U.S. Consumer Product Safety Commission, (800) 638-CPSC.

‡For Community and Home Care Instructions for infant cardiopulmonary resuscitation and infant/child choking see pp. 640-650.

This section may be photocopied and distributed to families.

From Wong DL, Hess CS: *Wong and Whaley's Clinical manual of pediatric nursing,* ed 5. Copyright © 2000, Mosby, St Louis.

- ☐ Unused appliances, such as refrigerators, securely closed with lock or doors removed*
- ☐ Food served in small, noncylindric pieces*
- ☐ Toy chests without lids or with lids that securely lock in open position*
- ☐ Buckets and wading pools kept empty when not in use*
- ☐ Clothesline above head level
- ☐ At least one member of household trained in basic life support (CPR) including first aid for choking‡

Safety: Poisoning

- ☐ Toxic substances, including batteries, placed on a high shelf, preferably in a locked cabinet
- ☐ Toxic plants hung or placed out of reach*
- ☐ Excess quantities of cleaning fluid, paints, pesticides, drugs, and other toxic substances not stored in home
- ☐ Used containers of poisonous substances discarded where child cannot obtain access
- ☐ Telephone number of local poison control center and address of home with nearest cross street posted near phone
- ☐ Syrup of ipecac in home, at least two doses per child
- ☐ Medicines clearly labeled in childproof containers and stored out of reach
- ☐ Household cleaners, disinfectants, and insecticides kept in their original containers, separate from food and out of reach
- ☐ Smoking only allowed in areas away from children

Safety: Falls

- ☐ Nonskid mats, strips, or surfaces in tubs and showers
- ☐ Exits, halls, and passageways in rooms kept clear of toys, furniture, boxes, or other items that could be obstructive
- ☐ Stairs and halls well lighted, with switches at both top and bottom
- ☐ Sturdy handrails for all steps and stairways
- ☐ Nothing stored on stairways
- ☐ Treads, risers, and carpeting in good repair
- ☐ Glass doors and walls marked with decals
- ☐ Safety glass used in doors, windows, and walls
- ☐ Gates on top and bottom of staircases and elevated areas, such as porch or fire escape*
- ☐ Guardrails on upstairs windows with locks that limit height of window opening and access to areas such as fire escape*
- ☐ Crib side rails raised to full height; mattress lowered as child grows*
- ☐ Restraints used in high chairs, walkers, or other baby furniture; preferably walkers not used*
- ☐ Scatter rugs secured in place or used with nonskid backing
- ☐ Walks, patios, and driveways in good repair

Safety: Bodily Injury

- ☐ Knives, power tools, and unloaded firearms stored safely or placed in locked cabinet
- ☐ Garden tools returned to storage racks after use
- ☐ Pets properly restrained and immunized for rabies
- ☐ Swings, slides, and other outdoor play equipment kept in safe condition
- ☐ Yard free of broken glass, nail-studded boards, other litter
- ☐ Cement birdbaths placed where young child cannot tip them over*

Injury Prevention During Infancy

Age: Birth-4 Months
Major Developmental Accomplishments

Involuntary reflexes, such as the crawling reflex, may propel infant forward or backward, and the startle reflex may cause the body to jerk

May roll over

Increasing eye-hand coordination and voluntary grasp reflex

Injury Prevention

Aspiration

Not as great a danger to this age-group, but should begin practicing safeguards early (see under Age: 4-7 Months)

Never shake baby powder directly on infant; place powder in hand and then on infant's skin; store container closed and out of infant's reach

Hold infant for feeding; do not prop bottle

Know emergency procedures for choking*

Use pacifier with one-piece construction and loop handle

Suffocation/Drowning

Keep all plastic bags stored out of infant's reach; discard large plastic garment bags after tying in a knot

Do not cover mattress with plastic

Use a firm mattress and loose blankets; no pillows

Make sure crib design follows federal regulations—crib slats less than 2⅜ in (6 cm) apart—and mattress fits snugly

Position crib away from other furniture, windows, and radiators

Do not tie pacifier on a string around infant's neck

Remove bibs at bedtime

Never leave infant alone in bath

Do not leave infant under 12 months alone on adult or youth mattress

Falls

Always raise crib rails

Never leave infant unguarded on a raised surface

When in doubt as to where to place child, use the floor

Restrain child in infant seat and never leave child unattended while the seat is resting on a raised surface

Avoid using a high chair until child can sit well with support

Poisoning

Not as great a danger to this age-group, but should begin practicing safeguards early (See under Age: 4-7 Months.)

Burns

Install smoke detectors in home

Use caution when warming formula in microwave oven; always check temperature of liquid before feeding

Check temperature of bathwater

Do not pour hot liquids when infant is close by, such as sitting on lap

Beware of cigarette ashes that may fall on infant

Do not leave infant in the sun for more than a few minutes; keep exposed skin covered

Wash flame-retardant clothes according to label directions

Use cool-mist vaporizers

Do not leave child in parked car

Check surface heat of restraint before placing child in car seat

Motor Vehicles

Transport infant in federally approved, rear-facing car seat,* preferably in backseat

Do not place infant on the seat or in lap

Do not place child in a carriage or stroller behind a parked car

Do not place infant or child in front passenger seat with an air bag

Bodily Damage

Avoid sharp, jagged objects

Keep diaper pins closed and away from infant

Age: 4-7 Months
Major Developmental Accomplishments

Rolls over

Sits momentarily

Grasps and manipulates small objects

Resecures a dropped object

Has well-developed eye-hand coordination

Can focus on and locate very small objects

Mouthing is very prominent

Can push up on hands and knees

Crawls backward

Injury Prevention

Aspiration

Keep buttons, beads, syringe caps, and other small objects out of infant's reach

Keep floor free of any small objects

Do not feed infant hard candy, nuts, food with pits or seeds, or whole or cylindrical pieces of hot dog

Exercise caution when giving teething biscuits because large chunks may be broken off and aspirated

Do not feed while infant is lying down

Inspect toys for removable parts

Keep baby powder, if used, out of reach

Avoid storing large quantities of cleaning fluid, paints, pesticides, and other toxic substances in home

Discard used containers of poisonous substances

Do not store toxic substances in food containers

Discard used button-sized batteries; store new batteries in safe area

---

*For home care instructions for care of the choking infant, see pp. 645-647; for use of child safety seats, see pp. 204-208.

†Information available from U.S. Consumer Product Safety Commission, (800) 638-CPSC.

This section may be photocopied and distributed to families.

From Wong DL, Hess CS: *Wong and Whaley's Clinical manual of pediatric nursing*, ed 5. Copyright © 2000, Mosby, St Louis.

Continued

Age: 4-7 Months—cont'd
Injury Prevention—cont'd

Know telephone number of local poison control center (usually listed in front of telephone directory) and post near phone

Suffocation

Keep all latex balloons out of reach

Remove all crib toys that are strung across crib or playpen when child begins to push up on hands or knees or is 5 months old

Falls

Restrain in a high chair

Keep crib rails raised to full height

Poisoning

Make sure that paint on walls, furniture, window sills, and toys does not contain lead

Place toxic substances on a high shelf or in locked cabinet

Hang plants or place them out of reach

Burns

Keep faucets out of reach

Place hot objects (e.g., cigarettes, candles, incense) on high surface

Limit exposure to sun; apply sunscreen

Motor Vehicles

(See under Age: Birth-4 Months.)

Bodily Damage

Give toys that are smooth and rounded, preferably made of wood or plastic; avoid long, pointed objects as toys

Avoid toys that are excessively loud

Keep sharp objects out of infant's reach

Age: 8-12 Months
Major Developmental Accomplishments

Crawls/creeps
Stands, holding onto furniture
Stands alone
Cruises around furniture
Walks
Climbs
Pulls on objects

Throws objects
Is able to pick up small objects; has pincer grasp
Explores by putting objects in mouth
Dislikes being restrained
Explores away from parent
Increasing understanding of simple words and phrases

Injury Prevention

Aspiration

Keep lint and small objects off floor, furniture, and out of reach of children

Take care in feeding solid table food to ensure that very small pieces are given

Do not use beanbag toys or allow child to play with dried beans

(See also under Age: 4-7 Months.)

Suffocation/Drowning

Keep doors of ovens, dishwashers, refrigerators, coolers, and front-loading clothes washers and dryers closed at all times

If storing an unused appliance, such as a refrigerator, remove the door

Supervise contact with inflated balloons; immediately discard popped balloons and keep uninflated balloons out of reach

Fence swimming pools; keep gate locked

Always supervise when near any source of water, such as cleaning buckets, drainage areas, and toilets

Keep bathroom doors closed

Eliminate unnecessary pools of water

Keep one hand on child at all times when in tub

Falls

Avoid walkers, especially near stairs*

Fence stairways at top and bottom if child has access to either end†

Dress infant in safe shoes and clothing (e.g., soles that do not "catch" on floor, tied shoelaces, pant legs that do not touch floor)

Ensure that furniture is sturdy enough for child to pull self to standing position and cruise

Poisoning

Do not describe medications as a candy

Do not administer medications unless so prescribed by a practitioner

Replace medications and poisons immediately after use; replace child-protector caps properly

Have syrup of ipecac in home; use only if advised

Burns

Place guards in front of or around any heating appliances, fireplaces, or furnace

Keep electrical wires hidden or out of reach

Place plastic guards over electrical outlets; place furniture in front of outlets

Keep hanging tablecloths out of reach (child may pull down hot liquids or heavy or sharp objects)

---

*Because there is a considerable risk of major and minor injuries and even death from the use of walkers, and because there is no clear benefit from their use, the American Academy of Pediatrics recommends a ban on the manufacture and sale of mobile infant walkers in the United States. The particular risk of walkers in households with stairs is falls. (American Academy of Pediatrics, Committee on Injury and Poison Prevention: Injuries associated with infant walkers, *Pediatrics* 95(5):778-780, 1995.)

†Information available from U.S. Consumer Product Safety Commission; (800) 638-CPSC.

Injury Prevention During Early Childhood (1-5 Years of Age)

Developmental Abilities Related to Risk of Injury	Injury Prevention
Walks, runs, and climbs Able to open doors and gates Can ride tricycle Can throw ball and other objects	**Motor Vehicles** Use federally approved car restraint; if restraint is not available, use lap belt Supervise child while playing outside Do not allow child to play on curb or behind a parked car Do not permit child to play in piles of leaves, snow, or in large cardboard container in trafficked areas Supervise tricycle riding Lock fences and doors if children not directly supervised Teach child to obey pedestrian safety rules: 　Obey traffic regulations; walk only in crosswalks and when traffic signal indicates it is safe to cross 　Stand back a step from curb until it is time to cross 　Look left, right, and left again and check for turning cars before crossing street 　Use sidewalks; when there is no sidewalk, walk on left, facing traffic 　At night, wear clothing in light colors and with fluorescent material attached
Able to explore if left unsupervised Has great curiosity Helpless in water, unaware of its danger; depth of water has no significance	**Drowning** Supervise closely when near any source of water, including buckets Keep bathroom door and lid on toilet closed Have fence around swimming pool; lock gate Teach swimming and water safety (not a substitute for protection)
Able to reach heights by climbing, stretching, standing on toes, and using objects as a ladder Pulls objects Explores any holes or openings Can open drawers and closets Unaware of potential sources of heat or fire Plays with mechanical objects	**Burns** Turn pot handles toward back of stove Place electric appliances, such as coffee maker, frying pan, and popcorn popper, toward back of counter Place guardrails in front of radiators, fireplaces, or other heating elements Store matches and cigarette lighters in locked or inaccessible area; discard carefully Place burning candles, incense, hot foods, ashes, embers, and cigarettes out of reach Do not let tablecloth hang within child's reach Do not let electric cord from iron or other appliance hang within child's reach Cover electrical outlets with protective devices Keep electrical wires hidden or out of reach Do not allow child to play with electrical appliances, wires, or lighters Stress danger of open flames; explain what "hot" means Always check bathwater temperature; set hot water heater at 48.9° C (120° F) or lower; do not allow children to play with faucets Apply a sunscreen with SPF 15 or higher when child is exposed to sunlight (See Community Focus box, p. 199.)
Explores by putting objects in mouth Can open drawers, closets, and most containers Climbs Cannot read warning labels Does not know safe dose or amount	**Poisoning** Place all potentially toxic agents (including plants) in a locked cabinet or out of reach Replace medications and poisons immediately; replace child-resistant caps properly Do not refer to medications as candy Do not store large supplies of toxic agents Promptly discard empty poison containers; never reuse to store a food item Teach child not to play in trash containers Never remove labels from containers of toxic substances Have syrup of ipecac in home; use only if advised Know number and location of nearest poison control center (usually listed in front of telephone directory) and post near phone

Continued

This section may be photocopied and distributed to families.
From Wong DL, Hess CS: *Wong and Whaley's Clinical manual of pediatric nursing,* ed 5. Copyright © 2000, Mosby, St Louis.

Injury Prevention During Early Childhood (1-5 Years of Age)—cont'd

Developmental Abilities Related to Risk of Injury	Injury Prevention
Able to open doors and some windows Goes up and down stairs Depth perception unrefined	**Falls** Keep screen in window, nail securely, and use guardrail Place gates at top and bottom of stairs Keep doors locked or use child-resistant doorknob covers at entry to stairs, high porch, or other elevated area, such as laundry chute Remove unsecured or scatter rugs Apply nonskid mats in bathtubs or showers Keep crib rails fully raised and mattress at lowest level Place carpeting under crib and in bathroom Keep large toys and bumper pads out of crib or playpen (child can use these as "stairs" to climb out); move to youth bed when child is able to crawl out of crib Avoid using walkers, especially near stairs Dress in safe clothing (e.g., soles that do not "catch" on floor, tied shoelaces, pant legs that do not touch floor) Keep child restrained in vehicles; never leave unattended in shopping cart or stroller Supervise at playgrounds; select play areas with soft ground cover and safe equipment (Community Focus box)
Puts things in mouth May swallow hard or nonedible pieces of food	**Choking and Suffocation** Avoid large, round chunks of meat, such as whole hot dogs (slice lengthwise, then into short pieces) Avoid fruit with pits, fish with bones, dried beans, hard candy, chewing gum, nuts, popcorn, grapes, and marshmallows Choose large, sturdy toys without sharp edges or small, removable parts Discard old refrigerators, ovens, and other appliances; if storing old appliance, remove doors Keep automatic garage door transmitter in inaccessible place Select toy boxes or chests without heavy, hinged lids Keep venetian blind cords out of child's reach Remove drawstrings from clothing

Still clumsy in many skills
Easily distracted from tasks
Unaware of potential danger from strangers or other people
	Bodily Damage
	Avoid giving sharp or pointed objects (such as knives, scissors, or toothpicks), especially when walking or running
	Do not allow lollipops or similar objects in mouth when walking or running
	Teach safety precautions (e.g., to carry fork or scissors with pointed ends away from face)
	Store all dangerous tools, garden equipment, and firearms in locked cabinets
	Be alert to danger from animals, including household pets
	Use safety glass and decals on large glassed areas, such as sliding glass doors
	Teach personal safety
	    Teach name, address, and phone number and to ask for help from appropriate people (cashier, security guard, policeman) if lost; have identification on child (e.g., sewn in clothes or inside shoe)
	    Avoid letting child wear personalized clothing in public places
	    Teach child to never go with a stranger
	    Teach child to tell parents if anyone makes child feel uncomfortable in any way
	    Always listen to child's concerns regarding behavior of others
	    Teach child to say "no" when confronted with uncomfortable situations

Unit 2

COMMUNITY FOCUS

Reducing Sun Exposure

Remember that tanning indicates sun injury, and the risk of skin cancer begins in childhood.

Keep infants and children out of the sun as much as possible.

Use carriage with hood when taking infants outdoors.

Use stroller with canopy for older infants.

Schedule activities to avoid child's sun exposure between 10 AM and 3 PM whenever possible.

Take increased precautions when living or vacationing in the mountains or the tropics.

Protect child with clothing (e.g., sun hat, long-sleeved shirt, long pants) when outdoors; avoid sandals (wear closed shoes).

Avoid sheer clothing or bathing suits that allow the sun's rays to penetrate the fabric.

Use sunscreen with SPF of at least 15.

Apply sunscreen liberally to exposed areas:

Before every exposure

On cloudy as well as sunny days

Even when child plays in shade (sun reflects from sand, snow, cement, and water)

Reapply liberally every 2 to 3 hours and after child goes in the water or sweats heavily.

Check with child's practitioner regarding any medications the child is taking which may cause photosensitivity and observe for any evidence of side effects (rash, redness, swelling).

Examine skin regularly for signs of any change in pigmented nevi (rapid growth, crusting, ulceration, bleeding, change in pigmentation, development of inflamed satellite lesions, loss of normal skin lines) or subjective symptoms (tenderness, pain, itching).

Prohibit child from using sun lamps or tanning parlors.

Set a good example by following the above guidelines.

Modified from *For every child under the sun,* New York, Undated, The Skin Cancer Foundation.

COMMUNITY FOCUS

Playground Safety

Be certain that playground equipment has no sharp edges, corners, or projections.

Make sure that concrete footings are not exposed.

Examine area to make sure that there is a safe, resilient surface under equipment (such as sand or wood chips) to reduce the impact from a fall.

Be certain that the size of the equipment matches child.

Make sure there are no holes or other places where fingers, arms, legs, and necks could get caught.

Slides should not have an incline of more than 30 degrees, and should have evenly spaced rungs for climbing and protective "tunnels."

S-hooks on swings must be closed.

Check for litter, broken glass, exposed wires, electrical outlets, or animal excreta.

Unit 2

Injury Prevention During School-Age Years

Developmental Abilities Related to Risk of Injury	Injury Prevention
	Motor Vehicles
Is increasingly involved in activities away from home Is excited by speed and motion Is easily distracted by environment Can be reasoned with	Educate child regarding proper use of seat belts while riding in a vehicle Maintain discipline while in a vehicle (e.g., children must keep arms inside, not lean against doors, or interfere with driver) Remind parents and children that no one should ride in the bed of a pickup truck Emphasize safe pedestrian behavior Insist on wearing safety apparel (e.g., a helmet) where applicable, such as when riding a bicycle, motorcycle, moped, or all-terrain vehicle (See Fig. 2-3.)
	Drowning
Is apt to overdo May work hard to perfect a skill Has cautious, but not fearful, gross motor actions Likes swimming	Teach child to swim Teach basic rules of water safety Select safe and supervised places to swim Check sufficient water depth for diving Teach child to swim with a companion Make sure child wears an approved flotation device in water or while boating Advocate for legislation requiring fencing around pools Learn CPR
	Burns
Has increasing independence Is adventuresome Enjoys trying new things	Make sure smoke detectors are in home Set hot-water heater temperature at 48.9° C (120° F) to avoid scald burns Instruct child in behavior involving contact with potential burn hazards (e.g., gasoline, matches, bonfires or barbecues, lighter fluid, firecrackers, cigarette lighters, cooking utensils, and chemistry sets); and to avoid climbing or flying kites around high-tension wires Instruct child in proper behavior in the event of fire (e.g., fire drills at home and school) Teach child safe cooking methods (use low heat, avoid frying, be careful of steam burns, scalds, or exploding food, especially from microwaving) Apply a sunscreen with SPF 15 or higher when child is exposed to sunlight
	Poisoning
Adheres to group rules May be easily influenced by peers Has strong allegiance to friends	Educate child regarding hazards of taking nonprescription drugs and chemicals, including aspirin and alcohol Teach child to say "no" if offered illegal or dangerous drugs or alcohol Keep potentially dangerous products in properly labeled receptacles—preferably locked and out of reach
	Bodily Damage
Has increased physical skills Needs strenuous physical activity Is interested in acquiring new skills and in perfecting attained skills Is daring and adventurous, especially with peers Frequently plays in hazardous places Confidence often exceeds physical capacity Desires group loyalty and has strong need for friends' approval Attempts hazardous feats Accompanies friends to potentially hazardous facilities Is likely to overdo Growth in height exceeds muscular growth and coordination	Help provide facilities for supervised activities Encourage playing in safe places Keep firearms safely locked up except during adult supervision Teach proper care of, use of, and respect for devices with potential danger (e.g., power tools, firecrackers) Teach children animal safety (Community Focus box) Stress eye, ear, and mouth protection when using potentially hazardous objects or devices or when engaged in potentially hazardous sports (e.g., baseball) Teach safety regarding use of corrective devices (glasses); if child wears contact lenses, monitor duration of wear to prevent corneal damage Stress careful selection, use, and maintenance of sports and recreation equipment such as skateboards and in-line skates (See Community Focus boxes on p. 202.) Emphasize proper conditioning, safe practices, and use of safety equipment for sports or recreational activities Caution against engaging in hazardous sports, such as those involving trampolines Use safety glass and decals on large glassed areas, such as sliding glass doors Use window guards to prevent falls

Injury Prevention During School-Age Years—cont'd

Developmental Abilities Related to Risk of Injury	Injury Prevention
	Bodily Damage—cont'd
	Teach name, address, and phone number, and how to ask for help from appropriate people (cashier, security guard, policeman) if lost; have identification on child (sewn in clothes, inside shoe)
	Teach stranger safety:
	Don't let child wear personalized clothing in public places
	Caution child to never go with a stranger
	Have child tell parents if anyone makes child feel uncomfortable in any way
	Always listen to child's concerns regarding behavior of others
	Teach child to say "no" when confronted with uncomfortable situations

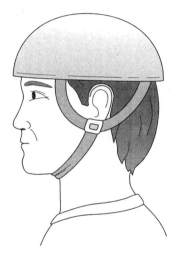

Fig. 2-3 Proper bicycle helmet fit. A helmet should sit on top of the head in a level position and not rock back and forth or from side to side. If the child can't see the edge of the brim at the extreme upper range of vision, the helmet is probably out of place. Adjust the chinstraps so that, when buckled, they hold the helmet firmly in place. Try to remove the helmet without undoing the chinstrap. If the helmet comes off or shifts over the eyes, readjust and try again. If no adjustment seems to work, this helmet is not a good fit; try another. Make sure child *always* fastens the strap when wearing the helmet.

COMMUNITY FOCUS

Animal Safety

Teach children to avoid all strange animals, especially wild, sick, or injured ones, who may be carriers of rabies. (Use the same techniques employed in teaching children not to talk to strangers.)

Teach children to avoid dangerous and nervous animals in their neighborhood.

Vaccinate your own dog against rabies.

Never permit children to break up an animal fight, even when their own pet is involved. Adults must use a rake, broom, or garden hose to separate fighting animals.

Teach children the danger of mistreating or teasing pets (i.e., that animals will bite if mauled, annoyed, or frightened).

Spay or neuter your pets. (Spaying or neutering reduces aggression, not protectiveness.)

Avoid direct eye contact with a threatening dog; remain motionless until the threatening dog leaves the area.

Teach children to never put their face close to an animal.

Teach children not to disturb an animal that is eating, sleeping, or caring for its young.

Teach children to never tease, pull the tail, or take away food, bones, or toys from an animal.

Never approach a strange dog that is confined or restrained; do not keep animals confined with short ropes or chains. (This can make them aggressive or vicious, especially when teased.)

Teach children to not run, ride a bicycle, or skate in front of a dog (it will startle the dog); teach children the importance of avoiding bike routes where dogs are known to chase vehicles.

Do not allow an inexperienced child or adult to feed a dog. (If the person pulls back when the animal moves to take the food, this can frighten the animal.)

If a dog has not seen you approach, speak to the animal to make it aware of your presence and avoid startling the animal.

Allow a dog to see and sniff a child before allowing the child to pet the animal.

Do not permit a child to lead a large dog.

Train or socialize a dog for appropriate behavior; avoid aggressive play with pets.

Do not adopt pets for children until children demonstrate their maturity and ability to handle and care for pets.

From The Humane Society of the United States: *Preventing and avoiding dog bites,* Washington, DC, 1998, The Society.

COMMUNITY FOCUS

Bicycle Safety

Always wear properly fitted bicycle helmet that is Snell or American National Standards Institute (ANSI) approved (see Fig. 2-3); replace damaged helmet.

Ride bicycles with traffic and away from parked cars.

Ride single file.

Walk bicycles through busy intersections using crosswalks only.

Give hand signals well in advance of turning or stopping.

Keep as close to the curb as practical.

Watch for drainage grates, potholes, soft shoulders, and loose dirt or gravel.

Keep both hands on handlebars, except when signaling.

Never ride with more than one person on a bicycle.

Do not carry packages that interfere with vision or control; do not drag objects behind bike.

Watch for and yield to pedestrians.

Watch for cars backing up or pulling out of driveways; be especially careful at intersections.

Look left, right, then left again before turning into traffic or onto a roadway.

Never hitch a ride by grabbing onto a truck or other vehicle.

Learn rules of the road and show respect for traffic officers.

Obey all local ordinances.

Wear shoes that fit securely while riding.

Wear light colors at night and attach fluorescent material to clothing and bicycle.

Be certain the bicycle is the correct size for the rider.

Equip bicycle with proper lights and reflectors.

Have the bicycle inspected to ensure good mechanical condition.

Children passengers must wear appropriate-size helmets and ride in specially designed protective seats.

From American Academy of Pediatrics, Committee on Injury and Poison Prevention: Bicycle helmets, *Pediatrics* 95(4):609-610, 1995.

COMMUNITY FOCUS

Skateboard and In-line Skate Safety

Children younger than 5 years of age should not use skateboards or in-line skates. They are not developmentally prepared to protect themselves from injury.

Children who ride skateboards or in-line skates should wear helmets and protective equipment, especially on knees, wrists, and elbows, to prevent injury.

Skateboards and in-line skates should never be used near traffic, and should be prohibited on streets and highways. Activities that bring motor vehicles and skateboards together (e.g., "catching a ride") are especially dangerous.

Some types of use, such as riding homemade ramps on hard surfaces, can be particularly hazardous.

Modified from American Academy of Pediatrics, Committee on Injury and Poison Prevention: Skateboard injuries, *Pediatrics* 95(4):611-612, 1995.

COMMUNITY FOCUS

Safe Use of All-Terrain Vehicles

Children under the age of 16 years should not operate an ATV.

Vehicles should be sturdy and stable; quality construction is essential.

Riders should receive instruction from a mature, experienced cyclist or from a certified instructor.

Riding should be supervised and allowed only after the rider has demonstrated competence in handling the machine on familiar terrain (preferably require licensing).

Riders should wear approved helmets and protective clothing (e.g., trousers, boots, and gloves).

Riders should avoid public roadways.

Riding should be restricted to familiar terrain.

Nighttime riding should not be allowed.

Vehicles should not carry more than one person.

Modified from American Academy of Pediatrics, Committee on Accident and Poison Prevention: All-terrain vehicles: two-, three-, and four-wheeled unlicensed motorized vehicles, *Pediatrics* 79:306-308, 1987.

Injury Prevention During Adolescence

Developmental Abilities Related to Risk of Injury	Injury Prevention

Developmental Abilities Related to Risk of Injury

Need for independence and freedom
Testing independence
Age permitted to drive a motor vehicle (varies)
Inclination for risk taking
Feeling of indestructibility
Need for discharging energy, often at expense of logical thinking and other control mechanisms
Strong need for peer approval
May attempt hazardous feats
Peak incidence for practice and participation in sports
Access to more complex tools, objects, and locations
Can assume responsibility for own actions (Community Focus box)

COMMUNITY FOCUS

Steps for Condom Use*

1. Be careful when opening the package; handle the condom gently, and check for breaks or holes in the condom.
2. Squeeze a dab of contraceptive jelly or cream with nonoxynol-9 into the tip of the condom.
3. Put on the condom as soon as erection occurs and before any vaginal, anal, or oral contact with the penis.
4. Unroll the condom on the erect penis, leaving about ½ inch of space at the tip of the condom.
5. Apply some of the contraceptive cream or jelly around the vagina or anus before entry.
6. Hold the rim of the condom in place when withdrawing the penis.
7. Take the condom off when away from the partner's genitalia.
8. Throw the used condom away. **Never reuse a condom.**

Modified from *Entering adulthood: preventing sexually transmitted diseases,* Santa Cruz, CA, 1989, Network Publications.

*For additional information on AIDS/HIV, contact **CDC National AIDS Clearinghouse,** PO Box 6003, Rockville, MD 20849, (800) 458-5231, e-mail: hivmail@cdc.gov; **CDC National AIDS Hotline,** (800) 342-AIDS, Spanish, (800) 344-7432, hearing impaired (800) 243-7889; and **National Center for HIV, STD, and TB Prevention (NCHSTP),** Web site: www.cdc.gov, e-mail: hivmail@cidhivl.em.cdc.gov.

Injury Prevention

Motor/Nonmotor Vehicles

Pedestrian—Emphasize and encourage safe pedestrian behavior
　At night, walk with a friend
　If someone is following you, go to nearest place with people
　Do not walk in secluded areas; take well-traveled walkways
Passenger—Promote appropriate behavior while riding in a motor vehicle
Driver—Provide competent driver education; encourage judicious use of vehicle, discourage drag racing, "playing chicken"; maintain vehicle in proper condition (brakes, tires, and so on)
　Teach and promote safety and maintenance of motorcycles; promote and encourage wearing of safety apparel such as a helmet and long trousers
　Reinforce teaching about the dangers of drugs, including alcohol, when operating a motor vehicle

Drowning

Teach nonswimmers to swim
Teach basic rules of water safety
　Judicious selection of place to swim
　Sufficient water depth for diving
　Swimming with companion

Burns

Reinforce proper behavior involving contact with burn hazards (gasoline, electric wires, fires)
Advise regarding excessive exposure to natural or artificial sunlight (ultraviolet burn)
Discourage smoking
Encourage use of sunscreen

Poisoning

Educate in hazards of drug use, including alcohol

Falls

Teach and encourage general safety measures in all activities

Bodily Damage

Promote proper instruction in sports and safe use of sports equipment
Instruct in safe use of and respect for firearms and other devices with potential danger (e.g., power tools, firecrackers)
Provide and encourage use of protective equipment when using potentially hazardous devices
Promote access to and/or provision of safe facilities for sports and recreation
Be alert for signs of depression (potential suicide)
Discourage use and/or availability of hazardous sports equipment (e.g., trampoline, surfboards)
Instruct regarding proper use of corrective devices such as glasses, contact lenses, and hearing aids
Encourage judicious application of safety principles and prevention

Unit 2

COMMUNITY AND HOME CARE INSTRUCTIONS

Guidelines for Automobile Safety Seats*

This important information is provided because automobile crashes are the number one preventable cause of death in infants and young children. All states now have laws that require children to be buckled up in cars. For more information about your laws, contact your state highway safety office.

Remember that the most dangerous place for an infant or child to ride is in the arms or on the lap of another person.

SEAT SELECTION

If you are buying or borrowing a used safety seat, make sure that the seat meets or exceeds Federal Motor Vehicle Safety Standard 213 and is not more than 10 years old. A manufacture date after January 1, 1981, should be stamped on the seat. Problems with a used safety seat include the possibility of missing parts and instructions, and that the seat may have been in a crash or may have been recalled by the manufacturer. ***Be cautious: buy or borrow a used seat only if you are sure it is safe.*** If you are purchasing a new safety seat, make sure to fill out and send in the registration card attached to the seat. The card allows the manufacturer to contact you if the seat is recalled.†

Make sure that the safety seat can be used with your make of car and type of seats and seat belts. Look for and read labels on seat belts and sun visors and follow instructions. Door-mounted seat belts should not be used to anchor child restraints. Auto dealers can install a special lap belt to lock child restraints in place. Some safety seats are too large for compact cars. Choose a seat that is simple to use. Practice with harness straps, shields, or other seat features. Ask yourself: "How many steps are involved in using the safety seat? Will it be easy to get

the child into and out of the seat?" Try the seat before you buy it, or make certain that you can return the seat if it does not fit or is not easy to use in your car.

Shop around: There are many safety seats for sale and costs vary. Watch for sales.‡

Some areas have low-cost rental or loan programs that are worth checking. Possible places to check for these services are local and state health departments, hospitals, American Red Cross chapters, or library reference desks.

Special needs restraints may be required for very small children or for those with medical conditions, such as prematurity, breathing problems, or casts.

For older children a special vest is available that secures the child in a lying-down position to the back seat.§ Children in wheelchairs present special challenges because the wheelchair should be anchored with four points of attachment to the vehicle (two in front and two behind) and should always face forward. The family should consult the wheelchair manufacturer for specific instructions regarding safe vehicle transportation.

SAFETY SEATS FOR NEWBORNS AND INFANTS

Choose a safety seat before the birth of an infant (a gift certificate for a safety seat is a good idea for a baby gift because it lets parents choose a seat that works well with their car). Take the seat and its instructions to the hospital. Before the baby is discharged, practice putting the infant into the seat and adjust the straps. Adjust straps snugly so that only one finger fits between strap and child. *Use the seat starting with the first ride home from the hospital.*

You can choose from infant-only seats or convertible seats. Infant-only seats (Fig. 1) are designed for babies from birth to about 18 to 22 pounds (or 26 inches). An infant's head should be at least an inch below the top of the shell. The seat must be installed in a rear-facing position to protect the infant's fragile neck and chest. Advantages of infant-only seats are that the size is right for an infant (particularly during the first 3 months) and that the seat is easy to get in and out of a car. There are now convertible child safety seats that can be used rear-facing for large infants (up to 30 pounds).

When installing an infant-only or convertible child safety seat (used rear-facing) recline the seat to 45 degrees to keep the baby's head from slumping forward and blocking its airway. Some child safety seats have a level or a line on the seat to help parents know when the seat is properly reclined.

For infants, provide lateral support by placing rolled receiving blankets in the seat on either side of the baby. A rolled wash cloth placed between the crotch strap and crotch can prevent the infant from sliding forward. Avoid using safety seat accessories such as thick car seat liners or pads; these can compress during a crash and cause the seat's harness to loosen.

Dress the infant comfortably. Some types of clothing (such as buntings) do not let the straps go between the infant's legs and should not be used. If blankets are needed, place them over the infant after the harness is buckled.

Although some safety seats may double as infant carriers, remember that lightweight household infant carriers and beds do not provide the protection given by a safety seat that meets federal

---

*Judith G. Sheese, PhD, Director, and Judith Talty, BA, BS, LPN, Occupant Protection Manager, Automotive Safety for Children Program, Indiana University Medical Center, Indianapolis, IN, assisted in revising this section.

†As of this writing, a new federal plan has just been initiated to create a universal, easy-to-use child restraint system in which a top tether strap will help restrict head movement in a crash. For questions about these new guidelines, or to check if a car seat has been recalled by the manufacturer, call the Auto Safety Hotline of the National Highway Traffic Safety Administration (NHTSA) at (800) 424-9393; Web site www.nhtsa.dot.gov. Also available from NHTSA is an excellent resource, *Are You Using it Right?* (Item #1P0040), 1995. Other resources are Safety Belt Safe USA, (800) 745-SAFE; (Spanish) (800) 747-SANO. Web site, www.carseat.org; and The National SAFE Kids Campaign, (800) 441-1888; Web site www.safekids.org. Booklets entitled *The What to Expect Guide to Car Seat Safety* can be ordered from The Nissan "Quest for Safety" helpline at (800) 955-4500.

‡A shopping guide for different models of seats, and information on car seats for premature infants, may be obtained from: American Academy of Pediatrics, 141 Northwest Point Blvd., Elk Grove Village, IL 60007-1098; (800) 433-9016. Information on restraints for children with special needs is available from the Automotive Safety for Children Program, Riley Hospital for Children, Indiana University Medical Center, 575 West Drive, Room 004, Indianapolis, IN 46202-5109; (317) 274-2977 or (800) KID-N-CAR (in Indiana).

§E-Z-On Vest is available from E-Z-On Products, 605 Commerce Way West, Jupiter, FL 33458; (561) 747-6920, or (800) 323-6598 (outside Florida).

This section may be photocopied and distributed to families.

COMMUNITY AND HOME CARE INSTRUCTIONS

Guidelines for Automobile Safety Seats—cont'd

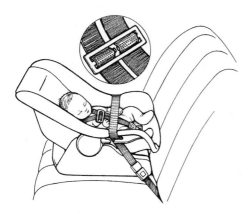

Fig. 1 Rear-facing, infant-only safety seat.

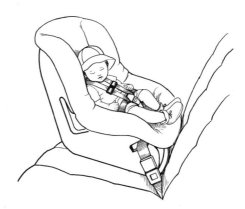

Fig. 2 Convertible seat in rear-facing position for use with infants.

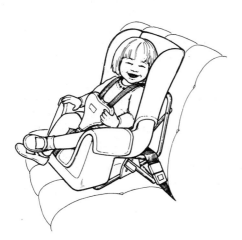

Fig. 3 Convertible seat in forward-facing position for older infants and children.

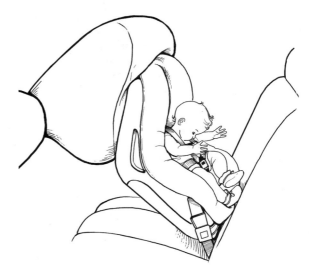

Fig. 4 An air bag can strike a child safety seat, seriously injuring or even killing the infant.

Continued

Unit 2

Guidelines for Automobile Safety Seats—cont'd

safety standards. These carriers and beds are unsafe if used as car safety seats.

Convertible seats (Figs. 2 and 3) are designed for children up to approximately 40 pounds or 40 inches. They must be used rear-facing for infants and forward-facing for children over 20 pounds. Convertible seats with shields or trays should not be used with newborns or small infants because of their proximity to the infant's face and neck.

Regardless of whether you choose an infant-only or convertible' safety seat for your infant, rear-facing safety seats must not be placed in the front seats of cars equipped with a passenger side airbag. Because rear-facing seats extend closer to the dashboard, the infant could be seriously injured or killed if the air bag is released (Fig. 4).

SAFETY SEATS FOR TODDLERS AND YOUNG CHILDREN

A child who weighs 20 pounds and is 1 year old can use a forward-facing seat. Appropriate safety seats include the convertible models mentioned previously, seats designed for use in a forward-facing position only, and integrated seats available in some vehicles. Some of these models can be adjusted (semi-reclining to upright) so that the child can nap comfortably. Follow the manufacturer's instructions for safe travel positions and for adjusting the harness system as the child grows.

The safety seat should be used until the child outgrows it (at about 40 pounds or 40 inches tall), at which time the child can be moved into a booster seat. Because safety belts are made to fit an adult's body, booster seats help position children properly until they are large enough to use a safety belt alone. Boosters also allow the child to see out of the car more easily.

Two types of boosters are available. The belt-positioning booster is used in combination with a lap/shoulder belt (Fig. 5). A small shield booster is used with a lap belt only. Although a booster may be certified for use at weights as low as 30 pounds, it will not provide the level of protection offered by a forward-facing child safety seat. Children who weigh between 30 and 40 pounds should continue to use a convertible

seat. Use of a booster seat with a shield, once recommended when no shoulder belt was available, does not provide upper body support and may contribute to a child being ejected in a crash. For all booster seats, the center of the child's head must not be higher than the back of the seat. If it is, the child is too big for the booster seat.

Children are ready for an adult safety belt (without a booster) when: they can sit without slouching against the back of the seat with knees bent over the edge; the lap belt makes good contact low over the hips (doesn't slide over abdomen); and a shoulder belt fits comfortably. Some children may not meet these criteria until 8 years of age or older.

If a safety belt can be used, it must be properly positioned on the child. The lap portion of the belt should go across the lap below the hips, as low as possible, and the belt should fit snugly. The shoulder portion should fit snugly across the chest, not across the neck or face (Fig. 6). Never tuck the shoulder belt under the child's arm or behind the child's back. Using the belt incorrectly can cause serious injuries in the event of a crash. The vehicle's seat back should be upright, not reclined.

RESTRAINING THE INFANT OR CHILD IN THE SEAT

Always follow the seat manufacturer's instructions about how to harness the child and position the seat belt. Seat models manufactured since 1981 come with instructions attached to the seat. Refer also to the car owner's guide for placement of or special changes required for seat belts with safety seats.

Apply all harness straps snugly so that only one finger fits between strap and child. Many models have a harness retainer or clip that keeps shoulder straps from slipping off. (See inset, Fig. 1.) The clip should be placed at armpit level and not near the neck or stomach.

The safest place for the car seat is in the middle of the back seat. Anchor all safety seats with the car's standard seat belt so that the safety seat cannot be moved. The seat belt is placed through the frame or shell, or across the front of the safety seat (follow the manufacturer's instructions). The belt is then pulled

tight so that the safety seat is securely fastened and cannot be moved. If it can be moved, the safety seat cannot be used with the seat belt. Tty another seat belt location within the car; in some cases, the seat belts must be replaced for the safety seat to be buckled in properly. If the car is equipped with automatic seat belts, it may be necessary for the dealer to install special equipment to properly secure the safety seat. For information regarding your car, refer to the car manufacturer's instruction booklet.

Remember: Never install a rear-facing safety seat in front of a passenger-side airbag.

Emergency locking seat belt systems allow the passenger freedom of movement but lock into place upon braking or impacts. With this system, a safety seat may seem loose or slide around after it has been buckled in. Belts that have a sliding emergency-locking latchplate require use of a locking clip to prevent this movement (Fig. 7). Locking clips are available through safety seat manufacturers, car dealers' parts departments, or retailers of safety seats.

When a rear-facing seat is secured against a soft car seat, the safety seat may tilt into the car seat, causing the infant to slump forward. To correct this forward tilt, roll a small blanket or towel and place it beneath the safety seat base until the safety seat is level.

Some safety seats for children with special needs, and selected older seat models, require the use of a tether (anchor) strap that must be bolted to a sturdy metal panel of the car (Fig. 8). Optional tethers may be added to some seat models as an extra measure of protection for the child's head. If using a tethered seat in more than one car, keep in mind that a tether strap and bolt system must be in place in each car in order to use the seat properly. The car dealer's service department or a knowledgeable mechanic can install a tether. Choose a different seat if you cannot anchor it on every ride.

Make it a rule: Do not start the car until everyone is buckled up.

GENERAL TIPS

Seats with vinyl covering and metal pieces can become very hot and burn a

COMMUNITY AND HOME CARE INSTRUCTIONS

Guidelines for Automobile Safety Seats—cont'd

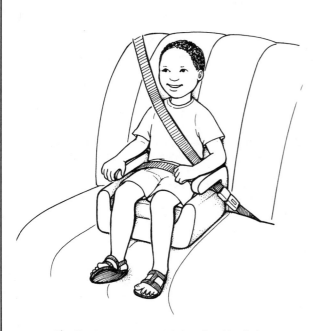

Fig. 5   Booster seat with lap-shoulder belt.

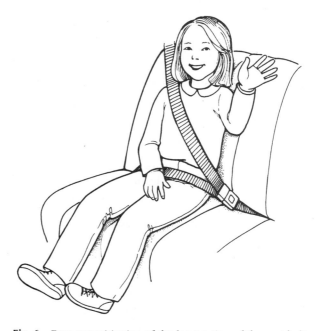

Fig. 6   Proper positioning of the lap portion of the seat belt below the hip bones and of the shoulder belt across the chest.

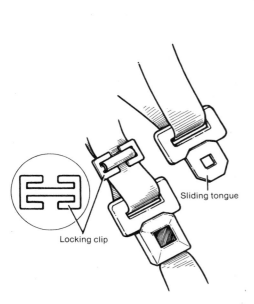

Locking clip   Sliding tongue

Fig. 7   Use of a locking clip.

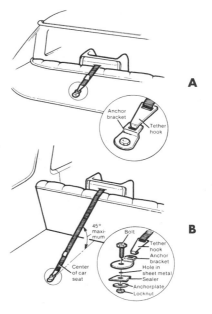

A

Anchor bracket   Tether hook

B

45° maximum   Bolt   Tether hook   Anchor bracket   Hole in sheet metal   Sealer   Anchorplate   Locknut   Center of car seat

Fig. 8   Tether straps. **A,** Rear window shelf installation for sedans. **B,** Floor mount installation for hatchback, station wagon, or van.

Unit 2

COMMUNITY AND HOME CARE INSTRUCTIONS

Guidelines for Automobile Safety Seats—cont'd

child's skin. Place a cloth cover over the seat; a "homemade" cover, such as a towel or blanket with slip openings for harness straps, works just as well as those that can be bought. Cool the seat's metal pieces before use (a damp cloth works well).

When two vehicles are used to transport the child, having a safety seat for each car is more convenient than having to move one safety seat between cars.

Always keep the safety seat buckled properly in the car when it is not being used to transport a child. In a quick stop or crash, the seat can become a deadly object inside the car. For the same reason, avoid "loose" objects in the car, such as toys or groceries, and use the trunk for these whenever possible. Soft toys can be attached to the car seat with plastic links, Velcro, or cords shorter than 6 inches.

If the safety seat is involved in a crash, it must be replaced. Even low mile-per-hour crashes can damage seat belts. Check harness straps for wear. Some manufacturers will replace seats free in order to study their products. Check with your insurance agent regarding replacement of a safety seat involved in a crash because most policies cover this loss.

TIPS FOR GOOD BEHAVIOR

Besides safety, another benefit of always using safety seats is that children who ride buckled up behave better and are less likely to distract the driver. To make safety seats a habit, try the following tips:

- Praise children often for good behavior while riding in the seat.
- Insist that others who transport children (babysitters, grandparents) also follow safety rules and keep children in proper child safety restraints.
- Never allow children to ride unbuckled or to climb out of their seats. If this happens, stop the car and say, "You must put on your seat belt." Be firm.

To help a young child use a safety seat when he has not previously been required to do so, follow these hints:

- Give the seat as a special present.
- Let the child help put the seat in the car, then try it out for a ride around the block.
- Let the child pretend being an astronaut, pilot, or firefighter while in the seat.
- Be firm and patient when teaching a child this new seat habit.

Remember: A good example helps children learn—buckle your seat belt.

TRIP TIPS

Expect that infants and young children will need to stop more often for feeding, changing, stretching, and play. Plan frequent travel breaks.

Dress the child comfortably and for convenience. Take along disposable diapers, wash cloths, and tissues.

Plan ahead to have activities ready. For infants, secure pictures and toys to the seat with Velcro or tape for the child to look at. Small, soft teething toys, stuffed animals, and pacifiers are helpful. For young children, books, toys (new ones provide greater diversion and interest), and games (counting, finding numbers or colors in the scenery) ease the monotony of long trips.

Sing or listen to stories on a tape recorder. The child will enjoy recording and listening to his or her own sounds.

Prepare small snacks (cereal, crackers, fresh fruit) and drinks (cups with lids are handy). Avoid hard candies, candy on sticks, raisins, carrots, or other foods that could cause injury or result in choking in a crash.

When making an airline trip, check the safety seat label to see if the seat may be used inflight, or check with the airline company regarding the airline's policies.

PARENTAL GUIDANCE
Guidance During Infancy

First 6 Months

Teach car safety with use of federally approved car seat, facing rearward, in the middle of the backseat—not in a seat with an air bag.

Understand each parent's adjustment to newborn, especially mother's postpartal emotional needs.

Teach care of infant; assist parents to understand infant's individual needs and temperament and that the infant expresses wants through crying.

Reassure parents that infant cannot be spoiled by too much attention during the first 4 to 6 months.

Encourage parents to establish a schedule that meets needs of child and themselves.

Help parents understand infant's need for stimulation in environment.

Support parents' pleasure in seeing child's growing friendliness and social responses, especially smiling.

Plan anticipatory guidance for safety.

Stress need for immunization.

Prepare for introduction of solid foods.

Second 6 Months

Prepare parents for child's "stranger anxiety."

Encourage parents to allow child to cling to them and avoid long separation from either parent.

Guide parents concerning discipline because of infant's increasing mobility.

Encourage use of negative voice and eye contact rather than physical punishment as a means of discipline.

Encourage showing most attention when infant is behaving well, rather than when infant is crying.

Teach injury prevention because of child's advancing motor skills and curiosity.

Encourage parents to leave child with suitable caregiver to allow themselves some free time.

Discuss readiness for weaning.

Explore parents' feelings regarding infant's sleep patterns.

Guidance During Toddler Years

Ages 12 to 18 Months

Prepare parents for expected behavioral changes of toddler, especially negativism and ritualism.

Assess present feeding habits and encourage gradual weaning from bottle and increased intake of solid foods.

Stress expected feeding changes of physiologic anorexia, presence of food fads and strong taste preferences, need for scheduled routine at mealtimes, inability to sit through an entire meal, and lack of table manners.

Assess sleep patterns at night, particularly habit of a bedtime bottle, which is a major cause of dental caries, and procrastination behaviors that delay hour of sleep.

Prepare parents for potential dangers of the home, particularly motor vehicle, poisoning, and falling injuries; give appropriate suggestions for childproofing the home.

Discuss need for firm but gentle discipline and ways in which to deal with negativism and temper tantrums; stress positive benefits of appropriate discipline.

Emphasize importance for both child and parents of brief, periodic separations.

Discuss new toys that use developing gross and fine motor, language, cognitive, and social skills.

Emphasize need for dental supervision, types of basic dental hygiene at home, and food habits that predispose children to caries; stress importance of supplemental fluoride.

Ages 18 to 24 Months

Stress importance of peer companionship in play.

Explore need for preparation for additional sibling; stress importance of preparing child for new experiences.

Discuss present discipline methods, their effectiveness, and parents' feelings about child's negativism; stress that nega-

tivism is important aspect of developing self-assertion and independence and is not a sign of spoiling.

Discuss signs of readiness for toilet training; emphasize importance of waiting for physical and psychologic readiness.

Discuss development of fears, such as darkness or loud noises, and of habits, such as security blanket or thumb sucking; stress normalcy of these transient behaviors.

Prepare parents for signs of regression in time of stress.

Assess child's ability to separate easily from parents for brief periods under familiar circumstances.

Allow parents opportunity to express their feelings of weariness, frustration, and exasperation; be aware that it is often difficult to love toddlers at times when they are not asleep!

Point out some of the expected changes of the next year, such as longer attention span, somewhat less negativism, and increased concern for pleasing others.

Ages 24 to 36 Months

Discuss importance of imitation and domestic mimicry and need to include child in activities.

Discuss approaches toward toilet training, particularly realistic expectations and attitude toward toileting accidents.

Stress uniqueness of toddlers' thought processes, especially regarding their use of language, poor understanding of time, causal relationships in terms of proximity of events, and inability to see events from another's perspective.

Stress that discipline must still be quite structured and concrete and that relying solely on verbal reasoning and explanations leads to confusion, misunderstanding, and even injuries.

Discuss investigation of preschool or daycare center toward completion of second year.

Unit 2

Guidance During Preschool Years

Age 3 Years

Prepare parents for child's increasing interest in widening relationships.

Encourage enrollment in preschool.

Emphasize importance of setting limits.

Prepare parents to expect exaggerated tension-reduction behaviors, such as need for "security blanket."

Encourage parents to offer choices when child vacillates.

Prepare parents to expect marked changes at 3½ years, when child becomes less coordinated, becomes insecure, and exhibits emotional extremes.

Prepare parents for normal dysfluency in speech, and advise them to avoid focusing on the pattern.

Prepare parents to expect extra demands on their attention as a reflection of child's emotional insecurity and fear of loss of love.

Warn parents that equilibrium of 3-year-old will change to the aggressive, out-of-bounds behavior of 4-year-old.

Inform parents to anticipate a more stable appetite with wider food selections.

Stress need for protection and education of child to prevent injury.

Age 4 Years

Prepare parents for more aggressive behavior, including motor activity and offensive language.

Prepare parents to expect resistance to their authority.

Explore parental feelings regarding child's behavior.

Suggest some type of respite for primary caregivers, such as placing child in preschool for part of the day.

Prepare parents for child's increasing sexual curiosity.

Emphasize importance of realistic limit-setting on behavior and appropriate discipline techniques.

Prepare parents for highly imaginative 4-year-old who indulges in "tall tales" (to be differentiated from lies) and who has imaginary playmates.

Prepare parents to expect nightmares or an increase in nightmares and suggest they make sure child is fully awakened from a frightening dream.

Provide reassurance that a period of calm begins at 5 years of age.

Age 5 Years

Inform parents to expect tranquil period at 5 years.

Help parents to prepare child for entrance into school environment.

Make sure immunizations are up-to-date before entering school.

Suggest that nonemployed mothers (or fathers if appropriate) consider own activities when child begins school.

Suggest swimming lessons for child.

Guidance During School-Age Years

Age 6 Years

Prepare parents to expect child's strong food preferences and frequent refusals of specific food items.

Prepare parents to expect increasingly ravenous appetite.

Prepare parents for emotionality as child experiences erratic mood changes.

Help parents anticipate continued susceptibility to illness.

Teach injury prevention and safety, especially bicycle safety.

Encourage parents to respect child's need for privacy and to provide a separate bedroom for child, if possible.

Prepare parents for child's increasing interests outside the home.

Help parents understand the importance of encouraging child's interactions with peers.

Ages 7 to 10 Years

Prepare parents to expect improvement in child's health and fewer illnesses, but warn them that allergies may increase or become apparent.

Prepare parents to expect an increase in minor injuries.

Emphasize caution in selecting and maintaining sports equipment and reemphasize safety.

Prepare parents to expect increased involvement with peers and interest in activities outside the home.

Emphasize the need to encourage independence while maintaining limit-setting and discipline.

Prepare mothers to expect more demands when child is 8 years of age.

Prepare fathers to expect increasing admiration at 10 years of age; encourage father-child activities.

Prepare parents for prepubescent changes in girls.

Ages 11 to 12 Years

Help parents prepare child for body changes of pubescence.

Prepare parents to expect a growth spurt in girls.

Make certain child's sex education is adequate with accurate information.

Prepare parents to expect energetic but stormy behavior at 11, to become more even tempered at 12.

Encourage parents to support child's desire to "grow up" but to allow regressive behavior when needed.

Prepare parents to expect an increase in masturbation.

Instruct parents that the amount of rest child needs may increase.

Help parents educate child regarding experimentation with potentially harmful activities.

Health Guidance

Help parents understand the importance of regular health and dental care for child.

Encourage parents to teach and model sound health practices, including diet, rest, activity, and exercise.

Stress the need to encourage children to engage in appropriate physical activities.

Emphasize providing a safe physical and emotional environment.

Encourage parents to teach and model safety practices.

COMMUNITY FOCUS

Collaboration Between School Nurses and Teachers

Have complete health cards for all students.

Give all teachers a list of students who have health problems.

Designate in teacher grade books those students who have health problems so that substitute teachers can recognize these students and intervene appropriately if problems occur.

If possible, provide adaptive physical education classes for students who cannot attend the regular classes.

Have metered dose inhalers available to all students with asthma for their emergency use in physical education and other classes.

Supervise selection of teams for physical education so that one team is not stacked with all the best players.

Give students an opportunity to redo a skill or activity in physical education if they have not performed well because every child has good and bad days.

Avoid questioning a child's ability in front of other students.

Provide privacy for height/weight checks and vision/hearing screening.

Suggestions submitted by Linda L. Smith, Health/Physical Education Teacher

COMMUNITY FOCUS

Violence in Schools

In recent years, reports of abuse and violence by some children have raised concern for early identification of these individuals. In particular, concern has focused on sudden acts of fatal violence in schools.* In assessing both adults and children, look for a history of animal abuse, torment, or torture. Look also for childhood or adolescent acts of violence toward other children and, possibly, adults. A history of destructiveness to property, such as fire setting, is also significant.

Cruelty to animals and cruelty to humans should be viewed as a continuum of abuse. These acts are not harmless ventings of emotions in healthy individuals; they are warning signs that these individuals need professional intervention. Abusing animals does not dissipate violent emotions; rather, the abuse may fuel them.

*An excellent resource is Dwyer K, Osher D, Warger C: *Early warning, timely response: a guide to safe schools,* Washington, DC, 1998, U.S. Department of Education. Available from U.S. Department of Education, Special Education and Rehabilitative Services, Room 3131, Mary E. Switzer Building, Washington, DC 20202-2524; telephone (877) 433-7827 or (202) 205-9043; Telecommunication Devices for the Deaf (TDD): (202) 205-5465 or Federal Information Relay Service (FIRS): (800) 877-8339; e-mail David_Summers@ed.gov; Web site: www.ed.gov/offices/OSERS/OSEP/earlywrn.html

Another useful pamphlet is *Raising children to visit violence:what you can do,* (1995) by the American Psychological Association and the American Academy of Pediatrics. Available from American Academy of Pediatrics, Division of Publications, 141 Northwest Point Blvd, PO Box 747, Elk Grove Village, IL 60009-0747; (800) 433-9016; fax (847) 228-1281; Web site: www.aap.org.

Guidance During Adolescence

Encourage Parents to:

Accept adolescent as a unique individual.

Respect adolescent's ideas, likes and dislikes, and wishes.

Be involved with school functions and attend adolescent's performances, whether they be sporting events or a school play.

Listen and try to be open to adolescent's views, even when they differ from parental views.

Avoid criticism about no-win topics.

Provide opportunities for choosing options and to accept the natural consequences of these choices.

Allow young person to learn by doing, even when choices and methods differ from those of adults.

Provide adolescent with clear, reasonable limits.

Clarify house rules and the consequences for breaking them.

Let society's rules and the consequences teach responsibility outside the home.

Allow increasing independence within limitations of safety and well-being.

Be available but avoid pressing teen too far.

Respect adolescent's privacy.

Try to share adolescent's feelings of joy or sorrow.

Respond to feelings as well as to words.

Be available to answer questions, give information, and to provide companionship.

Try to make communication clear.

Avoid comparisons with siblings.

Assist adolescent in selecting appropriate career goals and in preparing for adult role.

Welcome adolescent's friends into the home and treat them with respect.

Provide unconditional love.

Be willing to apologize when mistaken.

Be Aware That Adolescents:

Are subject to turbulent, unpredictable behavior.

Are struggling for independence.

Are extremely sensitive to feelings and behaviors that affect them.

May receive a different message than what was sent.

Consider friends extremely important.

Have a strong need "to belong."

PLAY
Functions of Play

Sensorimotor Development

Improves fine and gross motor skills and coordination
Enhances development of all the senses
Encourages exploration of the physical nature of the world
Provides for release of surplus energy

Intellectual Development

Provides multiple sources of learning:
  Exploration and manipulation of shapes, sizes, textures, and colors
  Experience with numbers, spatial relationships, and abstract concepts
  Opportunity to practice and expand language skills
Provides opportunity to rehearse past experiences to assimilate them into new perceptions and relationships
Helps children to comprehend the world in which they live and to distinguish between fantasy and reality

Socialization and Moral Development

Teaches adult roles, including sex role behavior
Provides opportunities for testing relationships
Develops social skills
Encourages interaction and development of positive attitudes toward others
Reinforces approved patterns of behavior and moral standards

Creativity

Provides an expressive outlet for creative ideas and interests
Allows for fantasy and imagination
Enhances development of special talents and interests

Self-Awareness

Facilitates the development of self-identity
Encourages regulation of own behavior
Allows for testing of own abilities (self-mastery)
Provides for comparison of own abilities with those of others
Allows opportunities to learn how own behavior affects others

Therapeutic Value

Provides for release from tension and stress
Allows expression of emotions and release of unacceptable impulses in a socially acceptable fashion
Encourages experimentation and testing of fearful situations in a safe manner
Facilitates nonverbal and indirect verbal communication of needs, fears, and desires

General Trends During Childhood

Age	Social Character of Play	Content of Play	Most Prevalent Type of Play	Characteristics of Spontaneous Activity	Purpose of Dramatic Play	Development of Ethical Sense
Infant	Solitary	Social-affective	Sensorimotor	Sense-pleasure	Self-identity	
Toddler	Parallel	Imitative	Body movement	Intuitive judgment	Learning gender role	Beginning of moral values
Preschool	Associative	Imaginative	Fantasy Informal games	Concept formation Reasonably constant ideas	Imitating social life Learning social roles	Developing concern for playmates Learning to share and cooperate
School-age	Cooperative	Competitive games and contests Fantasy	Physical activity Group activities Formal games Play acting	Testing concrete situations and problem solving Adding fresh information	Vicarious mastery	Peer loyalty Playing by the rules Hero worship
Adolescent	Cooperative	Competitive games and contests Daydreaming	Social interaction	Abstract problem solving	Presenting ideas	Causes and projects

Guidelines for Toy Safety*

Selection

Select toys that suit the skills, abilities, and interests of children.

Select toys that are safe for the specific child; look for a label that indicates the intended age-group. Toys that are safe for one age may not be safe for another.

For infants, toddlers, and all children who still mouth objects, avoid toys with small parts that may pose a fatal choking hazard or aspiration hazard. Toys in this category are usually labeled as "Not recommended for children under 3 years."

For infants, avoid toys with strings or cords that are 6 inches or longer because they may cause strangulation.

For all children under 8 years, avoid electric toys with heating elements.

For children under 5 years, avoid arrows or darts.

Check for safety labels such as "flame retardant" or "flame resistant."

Select toys durable enough to survive rough play; look for sturdy construction such as tightly secured eyes and nose on stuffed animals, or any small parts.

Select toys light enough that they will not cause harm if one falls on a child.

Look for toys with smooth, rounded edges. Avoid toys with sharp edges that can cut or that have sharp points. Points on the inside of the toy can puncture if the toy is broken.

Avoid toys with any shooting or throwing objects that can injure eyes.

This includes toys with which other missiles, such as sticks or pebbles, might be used as substitutes for the intended projectiles.

Arrows and darts used by children should have soft tips such as rubber suction cups and be manufactured from resilient materials; make certain the tips are securely attached.

Make certain that materials in toys are nontoxic.

Avoid toys that make loud noises that might be damaging to a child's hearing.

Even some squeaking toys are too loud when held close to the ear.

If selecting caps for cap guns, look for the label required by federal law to be on boxes or packages of caps, which states: "Warning—Do not fire closer than 1 foot to the ear. Do not use indoors."

If selecting a toy gun, be certain that the barrel or the entire gun is brightly colored to avoid being mistaken for a real gun.

Check toy instructions for clarity. They should be clear to an adult and, when appropriate, to the child.

Supervision

Maintain a safe play environment:

Remove and discard plastic wrappings on toys immediately; they could suffocate a child.

Remove large toys, bumper pads, and boxes from playpens; an adventuresome child can use such items as a means of climbing or falling out.

Set "ground rules" for play.

Supervise young children closely during play.

Teach children how to use toys properly and safely.

Instruct older children to keep their toys away from younger brothers, sisters, and friends.

Keep children who are playing with riding toys away from stairs, hills, traffic, and swimming pools.

Establish and enforce rules regarding protective gear:

Insist that children wear helmets when using bicycles, skateboards, or in-line skates.

Insist that children wear gloves and wrist, elbow, and knee pads when using skateboards or in-line skates.

Instruct children on electrical safety:

Teach children the proper way to unplug an electric toy—pull on the plug, not the cord.

Teach children to beware of electrical appliances and even electrically operated playthings; often children are unfamiliar with the hazards of electricity in association with water.

Teach children the safe use of items that under certain circumstances can cause injury—scissors, knives, needles, heating elements, loops, long strings, and cords.

Maintenance

Regularly inspect old and new toys for breakage, loose parts, and other potential hazards.

Look for jagged or sharp edges, or broken parts that might constitute a choking hazard.

Check movable parts to make certain they are attached securely to the toys; sometimes pieces that are safe when attached to the toy become a danger when detached.

Examine outdoor toys for rust and weak or sharp parts that could be a danger to children.

Check electrical cords and plugs for cracked or fraying parts.

Maintain toys in good repair, without possible hazards such as sharp edges, splinters, weak seams, or rust.

Make repairs immediately, or discard the toy out of reach of children.

Sand sharp or splintered surfaces on wooden toys so they are smooth.

Only use paint labeled "nontoxic" to repaint toys, toy boxes, or children's furniture.

Storage

Provide a safe place for children to store toys:

Select a toy chest or toy box that is ventilated, free of self-locking devices that could trap a child inside. Make sure it has a lid designed not to pinch a child's fingers or fall on a child's head.

To avoid entrapment and suffocation, containers other than toy chests used for storage purposes should be fitted with spring-loaded support devices if they have a hinged lid.

Teach children to store toys safely in order to prevent accidental injury from stepping, tripping, or falling on them.

Playthings meant for older children and adults should be safely stowed away on high shelves, in locked closets, or in other areas unavailable to young children.

---

*Another helpful resource is *Toy safety: guidelines for parents* from **American Academy of Pediatrics,** Division of Publications, 141 Northwest Point Blvd., Elk Grove Village, IL 60007-1098; (800) 433-9016.

This section may be photocopied and distributed to families.

From Wong DL, Hess CS: *Wong and Whaley's Clinical manual of pediatric nursing,* ed 5. Copyright © 2000, Mosby, St Louis.

Play During Infancy

Age (Months)	Visual Stimulation	Auditory Stimulation	Tactile Stimulation	Kinetic Stimulation
SUGGESTED ACTIVITIES				
Birth-1	Look at infant at close range Hang bright, shiny object within 20-25 cm (8-10 inches) of infant's face and in midline Hang mobiles with black-and-white designs	Talk to infant; sing in soft voice Play music box, radio, television Have ticking clock or metronome nearby	Hold, caress, cuddle Keep infant warm May like to be swaddled	Rock infant; place in cradle Use carriage for walks
2-3	Provide bright objects Make room bright with pictures or mirrors Take infant to various rooms while doing chores Place in infant seat for vertical view of environment	Talk to infant Include in family gatherings Expose to various environmental noises other than those of home Use rattles, wind chimes	Caress infant while bathing, at diaper change Comb hair with a soft brush	Use infant swing Take in car for rides Exercise body by moving extremities in swimming motion Use cradle gym
4-6	Place infant in front of safety (unbreakable) mirror Give brightly colored toys to hold (small enough to grasp)	Talk to infant; repeat sounds infant makes Laugh when infant laughs Call infant by name Crinkle different papers by infant's ear Place rattle or bell in hand	Give infant soft squeeze toys of various textures Allow to splash in bath Place nude on soft, furry rug and move extremities	Use swing or stroller Bounce infant in lap while holding in standing position Support infant in sitting position; let infant lean forward to balance self Place infant on floor to crawl, roll over, sit
6-9	Give infant large toys with bright colors, movable parts, and noisemakers Place unbreakable mirror where infant can see self Play peekaboo, especially hiding face in a towel Make funny faces to encourage imitation	Call infant by name Repeat simple words such as "dada," "mama," "bye-bye" Speak clearly Name parts of body, people, and foods Tell infant what you are doing Use "no" only when necessary Give simple commands Show how to clap hands, bang a drum	Let infant play with fabrics of various textures Have bowl with foods of different sizes and textures to feel Let infant "catch" running water Encourage "swimming" in large bathtub or shallow pool Give wad of sticky tape to manipulate	Hold upright to bear weight and bounce Pick up, say "up" Put down, say "down" Place toys out of reach, encourage infant to get them Play pat-a-cake
9-12	Show infant large pictures in books Take infant to places where there are animals, many people, different objects (shopping center) Play ball by rolling it to child, demonstrate "throwing" it back Demonstrate building a two-block tower	Read infant simple nursery rhymes Point to body parts and name each one Imitate sounds of animals	Give infant finger foods of different textures Let infant mess up and squash food Let infant feel cold (ice cube) or warm (bath water); say what temperature each is Let infant feel a breeze (fan blowing)	Give large push-pull toys Place furniture in a circle to encourage cruising Turn in different positions

Play During Infancy—cont'd

Age (Months)	Visual Stimulation	Auditory Stimulation	Tactile Stimulation	Kinetic Stimulation
SUGGESTED TOYS				
Birth-6	Nursery mobiles Unbreakable mirrors See-through crib bumpers Contrasting colored sheets	Music boxes Musical mobiles Crib dangle bells Small-handled clear rattle	Stuffed animals Soft clothes Soft or furry quilt Soft mobiles	Rocking crib/cradle Weighted or suction toy Infant swing
6-12	Various colored blocks Nested boxes or cups Books with rhymes and bright pictures Strings of big beads Simple take-apart toys Large ball Cup and spoon Large puzzles Jack-in-the-box	Rattles of different sizes, shapes, tones, and bright colors Squeaky animals and dolls Recordings of light, rhythmic music	Soft, different-textures animals and dolls Sponge toys, floating toys Squeeze toys Teething toys Books with textures and objects, such as fur and zippers	Activity box for crib Push-pull toys Wind-up swing

Unit 2

Play During Toddlerhood

Physical Development	Social Development	Mental Development and Creativity
SUGGESTED ACTIVITIES		
Provide spaces that encourage physical activity Provide sandbox, swing, and other scaled-down playground equipment	Provide replicas of adult tools and equipment for imitative play Permit child to "help" with adult tasks Encourage imitative play Provide toys and activities that allow for expression of feelings Allow child to play with some actual items used in the adult world; for example, let child help wash dishes or play with pots and pans and other utensils (check for safety)	Provide opportunities for water play Encourage building, drawing, and coloring Provide various textures in objects for play Provide large boxes and other safe containers for imaginative play Read stories appropriate to age Monitor TV viewing
SUGGESTED TOYS		
Push-pull toys Rocking horse, stick horse Riding toy Balls (large) Blocks (unpainted) Pounding board Low gym and slide Pail and shovel Containers Play dough	Record player or tape recorder Purse Housekeeping toys (broom, dishes) Toy telephone Dishes, stove, table and chairs Mirror Puppets, dolls, stuffed animals (check for safety [e.g., no button eyes])	Wooden puzzles Cloth picture books Paper, finger paint, thick crayons Blocks Large beads to string Wooden shoe for lacing Appropriate TV programs

This section may be photocopied and distributed to families.
From Wong DL, Hess CS: *Wong and Whaley's Clinical manual of pediatric nursing,* ed 5. Copyright © 2000, Mosby, St Louis.

Play During Preschool Years

Physical Development	Social Development	Mental Development and Creativity
SUGGESTED ACTIVITIES		
Provide spaces for the child to run, jump, and climb	Encourage interactions with neighborhood children	Encourage creative efforts with raw materials
Teach child to swim	Intervene when children become destructive	Read stories
Teach simple sports and activities	Enroll child in preschool	Monitor TV viewing
		Attend theater and other cultural events appropriate to child's age
		Take short excursions to park, seashore, museums
SUGGESTED TOYS		
Medium-height slide	Child-sized playhouse	Books
Adjustable swing	Dolls, stuffed toys	Jigsaw puzzles
Vehicles to ride	Dishes, table	Musical toys (xylophone, piano, drum, horns)
Tricycle	Ironing board and iron	Picture games
Wading pool	Cash register, toy typewriter, computer	Blunt scissors, paper, glue
Wheelbarrow	Trucks, cars, trains, airplanes	Newsprint, crayons, poster paint, large brushes, easel, finger paint
Sled	Play clothes for dress-up	Flannel board and pieces of felt in colors and shapes
Wagon	Doll carriage, bed, high chair	Records, tapes
Roller skates, speed graded to skill	Doctor and nurse kits	Blackboard and chalk (colored and white)
	Toy nails, hammer, saw	Wooden and plastic construction sets
	Grooming aids, play makeup or shaving kits	Magnifying glass, magnets

This section may be photocopied and distributed to families.
From Wong DL, Hess CS: *Wong and Whaley's Clinical manual of pediatric nursing,* ed 5. Copyright © 2000, Mosby, St Louis.

Unit 2

Pediatric Variations of Nursing Interventions

Symbol ■ indicates material that may be photocopied and distributed to families.

Related Topics

Unit 3

GUIDELINES FOR PREPARING CHILDREN FOR PROCEDURES
General Guidelines

Determine the details of the exact procedure to be performed.

Review the parents' and child's present levels of understanding.

Plan the actual teaching based on the child's developmental age and existing level of knowledge.

Incorporate parents in the teaching if they so desire, and especially if they plan to participate in the care.

Inform parents of their role during the procedure, such as standing near child's head or in line of vision and talking softly to child.

While preparing the child and family, allow for ample discussion to prevent information overload and ensure adequate feedback.

Use concrete, not abstract, terms and visual aids to describe the procedure. For example, use a simple line drawing of a boy or girl (Fig. 3-1, *A* or *B*), and mark the body part that will be involved in the procedure. Anatomically correct manikens are also available for preparing children and families for procedures and as teaching models for technical instruction, such as caring for a central venous access device. The soft-sculpture dolls and adapters and overlays customized for several medical conditions and procedures are available from Legacy Products, Inc., PO Box 267, Cambridge City, IN 47327; 1-800-238-7951; e-mail, Legacyez2b@aol.com; or visit the Web site at www.amis.cba.bgsu.edu/p/pbarton/legacy/index.htm.

Emphasize that no other body part will be involved.

If the body part is associated with a specific function, stress the change or noninvolvement of that ability (e.g., following tonsillectomy, the child can still speak).

Use words appropriate to the child's level of understanding (a rule of thumb for number of words is the age in years plus 1).

Avoid words/phrases with dual meanings unless the child understands such words.

Clarify all unfamiliar words (e.g., "Anesthesia is a *special sleep*").

Emphasize the sensory aspects of the procedure—what the child will feel, see, smell, and touch and what the child can do during the procedure (e.g., lie still, count out loud, squeeze a hand, hug a doll).

Allow the child to practice those procedures that will require cooperation (e.g., turning, deep breathing, using an incentive spirometer or mask).

Introduce anxiety-laden information last (e.g., the preoperative injection).

Be honest with the child about the unpleasant aspects of a procedure but avoid creating undue concern. When discussing a procedure that may be uncomfortable, state that it feels differently to different people. After the procedure, have the child describe how it felt.

Emphasize the end of the procedure and any pleasurable events afterward (e.g., going home, seeing the parent). Stress the positive benefits of the procedure (e.g., "After your tonsils are fixed, you won't have as many sore throats").

Unit 3

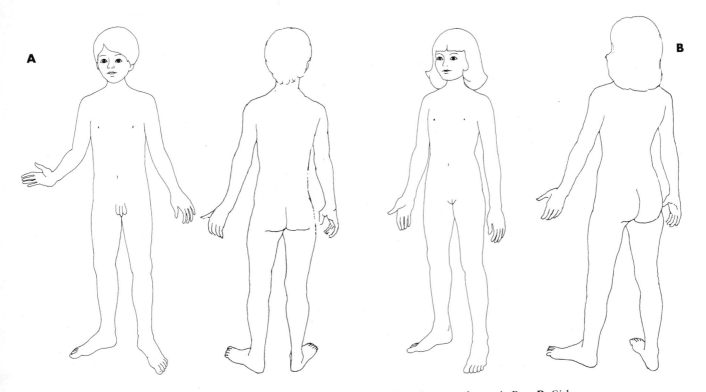

Fig. 3-1   Human figure drawings for preparing children for procedures. **A,** Boy. **B,** Girl.

Fig. 3-1. **A** and **B** may be photocopied and distributed to staff for their use. From Wong DL, Hess CS: *Wong and Whaley's Clinical manual of pediatric nursing,* ed 5. Copyright 2000, Mosby, St Louis.

Preparing Children for Procedures Based on Developmental Characteristics

INFANCY: DEVELOPING A SENSE OF TRUST AND SENSORIMOTOR THOUGHT

Attachment to Parent

*Involve parent in procedure if desired.
Keep parent in infant's line of vision.
If parent is unable to be with infant, place familiar object with infant (e.g., stuffed toy).

Stranger Anxiety

*Have usual caregivers perform or assist with procedure.
Make advances slowly and in nonthreatening manner.
*Limit number of strangers entering room during procedure.

Sensorimotor Phase of Learning

Use sensory soothing measures during procedure (e.g., stroking skin, talking softly, giving pacifier).
*Use analgesics (e.g., local anesthetic, intravenous opioid) to control discomfort.
Cuddle and hug child after stressful procedure; encourage parent to comfort child.

Increased Muscle Control

Expect older infants to resist.
Restrain adequately.
Keep harmful objects out of reach.

Memory for Past Experiences

Realize that older infants may associate objects, places, or persons with prior painful experiences and will cry and resist at the sight of them.
*Keep frightening objects out of view.
*Perform painful procedures in a separate room (not in crib or bed).
*Use nonintrusive procedures whenever possible (e.g., axillary or tympanic temperatures, oral medication).

Imitation of Gestures

Model desired behavior (e.g., opening mouth).

TODDLER: DEVELOPING A SENSE OF AUTONOMY AND SENSORIMOTOR TO PREOPERATIONAL THOUGHT

Use same approaches as for infant in addition to the following:

Egocentric Thought

Explain procedure in relation to what child will see, hear, taste, smell, and feel.
Emphasize those aspects of procedure that require cooperation (e.g., lying still).
Tell child it's OK to cry, yell, or use other means to express discomfort verbally.

---

*Applies to any age.

Negative Behavior

Expect treatments to be resisted; child may try to run away.
Use firm, direct approach.
Ignore temper tantrums.
Use distraction techniques (e.g., singing a song *with* child).
Restrain adequately.

Animism

Keep frightening objects out of view. (Young children believe objects have lifelike qualities and can harm them.)

Limited Language Skills

Communicate using behaviors.
Use a few simple terms familiar to child.
Give one direction at a time (e.g., "Lie down," then "Hold my hand").
Use small replicas of equipment; allow child to handle equipment.
Use play; demonstrate on doll but avoid child's favorite doll, since child may think doll is really "feeling" procedure.
Prepare parents separately to avoid child's misinterpreting words.

Limited Concept of Time

Prepare child shortly or immediately before procedure.
Keep teaching sessions short (about 5 to 10 minutes).
Have preparations completed before involving child in procedure.
Have extra equipment nearby (e.g., alcohol swabs, new needle, adhesive bandages) to avoid delays.
Tell child when procedure is completed.

Striving for Independence

Allow choices when they exist but realize that child may still be resistant and negative.
Allow child to participate in care and to help whenever possible (e.g., drink medicine from a cup, hold a dressing).

PRESCHOOLER: DEVELOPING A SENSE OF INITIATIVE AND PREOPERATIONAL THOUGHT

Egocentric

Explain procedure in simple terms and in relation to how it affects child (as with toddler, stress sensory aspects).
Demonstrate use of equipment.
Allow child to play with miniature or actual equipment.
Encourage "playing out" experience on a doll both before and after procedure to clarify misconceptions.
Use neutral words to describe the procedure (Guidelines box).

Increased Language Skills

Use verbal explanation but avoid overestimating child's comprehension of words.
Encourage child to verbalize ideas and feelings.

Concept of Time and Frustration Tolerance Still Limited

Implement same approaches as for toddler but may plan longer teaching session (10 to 15 minutes); may divide information into more than one session.

GUIDELINES

Selecting Nonthreatening Words or Phrases

Words/Phrases to Avoid	Suggested Substitutions	Words/Phrases to Avoid	Suggested Substitutions
Shot, bee sting, stick	Medicine under the skin	Deaden	Numb, make sleepy
Organ	Special place in body	Cut, fix	Make better
Test	See how [specify body part] is working	Take (as in "take your temperature or blood pressure")	See how warm you are; check your pressure; hug your arm
Incision	Special opening	Put to sleep, anesthesia	Special sleep
Edema	Puffiness, swelling	Catheter	Tube, straw
Stretcher, gurney	Rolling bed	Monitor	TV screen
Stool	Child's usual term	Electrodes	Stickers, ticklers
Dye	Special medicine	Specimen	Sample
Pain	Hurt, discomfort, "owie," "boo-boo"		

Illness and Hospitalization May Be Viewed as Punishment

Clarify why each procedure is performed; a child will find it difficult to understand how medicine can taste bad and make him or her feel better at the same time.

Ask for child's thoughts regarding why a procedure is performed.

State directly that procedures are never a form of punishment.

Animism

Keep equipment out of sight, except when shown to or used on child.

Fears of Bodily Harm, Intrusion, and Castration

Point out on drawing, doll, or on child where procedure will be performed.

Emphasize that no other body part will be involved.

Use nonintrusive procedures whenever possible (e.g., axillary temperatures, oral medication).

Apply an adhesive bandage over puncture site.

Encourage parental presence.

Realize that procedures involving genitalia produce anxiety.

Allow child to wear underpants with gown.

Explain unfamiliar situations, especially noises or lights.

Striving for Initiative

Involve child in care whenever possible (e.g., to hold equipment, remove dressing).

Give choices when they exist but avoid excessive delays.

Praise child for helping and for attempting to cooperate; never shame child for lack of cooperation.

SCHOOL-AGE CHILD: DEVELOPING A SENSE OF INDUSTRY AND CONCRETE THOUGHT

Increased Language Skills; Interest in Acquiring Knowledge

Explain procedures using correct scientific/medical terminology.

Explain reason for procedure using simple diagrams of anatomy and physiology.

Explain function and operation of equipment in concrete terms.

Allow child to manipulate equipment; use doll or another person as model to practice using equipment whenever possible (doll play may be considered "childish" by older school-age child).

Allow time before and after procedure for questions and discussion.

Improved Concept of Time

Plan for longer teaching sessions (about 20 minutes).

Prepare in advance of procedure.

Increased Self-Control

Gain child's cooperation.

Tell child what is expected.

Suggest ways of maintaining control (e.g., deep breathing, relaxation, counting).

Striving for Industry

Allow responsibility for simple tasks (e.g., collecting specimens).

Include in decision-making (e.g., what time of day to perform procedure, the preferred site).

Encourage active participation (e.g., removing dressings, handling equipment, opening packages).

Developing Relationships with Peers

May prepare two or more children for same procedure or encourage one peer to help prepare another.

Provide privacy from peers during procedure to maintain self-esteem.

ADOLESCENT: DEVELOPING A SENSE OF IDENTITY AND ABSTRACT THOUGHT

Increasingly Capable of Abstract Thought and Reasoning

Supplement explanations with reasons why procedure is necessary or beneficial.

Explain long-term consequences of procedures.

Realize that adolescent may fear death, disability, or other potential risks.

Encourage questioning regarding fears, options, and alternatives.

Continued

Unit 3

Preparing Children for Procedures Based on Developmental Characteristics—cont'd

ADOLESCENT: DEVELOPING A SENSE OF IDENTITY AND ABSTRACT THOUGHT—cont'd

Conscious of Appearance

Provide privacy.

Discuss how procedure may affect appearance (e.g., scar) and what can be done to minimize it.

Emphasize any physical benefits of procedure.

Concerned More with Present than with Future

Realize that immediate effects of procedure are more significant than future benefits.

Striving for Independence

Involve in decision-making and planning (e.g., choice of time and place; individuals present during procedure, such as parents; what clothing to wear).

Impose as few restrictions as possible.

Suggest methods of maintaining control.

Accept regression to more childish methods of coping.

Realize that adolescent may have difficulty in accepting new authority figures and may resist complying with procedures.

Developing Peer Relationships and Group Identity

Same as for school-age child but assumes even greater significance.

Allow adolescents to talk with other adolescents who have had the same procedure.

PLAY DURING HOSPITALIZATION
Functions of Play in the Hospital

Facilitates mastery over an unfamiliar situation

Provides opportunity for decision-making and control

Helps to lessen stress of separation

Provides opportunity to learn about parts of body, their functions, and own disease/disability

Corrects misconceptions about the use and purpose of medical equipment and procedures

Provides diversion and brings about relaxation

Helps the child feel more secure in a strange environment

Provides a means to release tension and express feelings

Encourages interaction and development of positive attitudes toward others

Provides an expressive outlet for creative ideas and interests

Provides a means for accomplishing therapeutic goals

Using Play in Procedures
*Projects Involving Hospital Routines and Environment**

LANGUAGE GAMES

State or list nouns found in the hospital and what they do or how they are used; recognize pictures and names of hospital equipment and/or match them.

Sort hospital nouns (words on cards) into people, places, and things.

List on board the equipment found in hospital. One child gives description of its use, and other children guess which equipment is being described.

Have children write and illustrate stories such as: "Sounds at Night," "Advice to Doctors," "Hospitals in the Future," "Things I Like and Don't Like in the Hospital."

Keep ongoing journals with pictures (captioned only or with stories) such as: "Me in the Hospital," "The Part of Me That Is Sick," "My Doctor," "My Nurse," "My Room," "Me at Home with My Family," "My Roommate," "Before I Got Sick," "After I Got Sick."

SCIENCE

Learn about body systems: list them and put in alphabetical order; draw pictures; make organs out of clay or play dough;

have children identify which of their body systems is involved in their medical problem.

Learn about nutrition in general and reasons for special diets.

Discuss how medicines, traction, and casts work, and how healing takes place.

MATHEMATICS

Use hospital material to discuss the metric system and become familiar with weights, lengths, and volumes. Measure routine and hospital objects in appropriate units.

Word problems: use hospital situations (e.g., If each nurse works 8-hour shifts, and you need six nurses on each shift, how many nurses do you need for 1 day?).

SOCIAL SCIENCES

How many different jobs are there in a hospital? Older children can be more detailed about the skills and education required for each job.

Talk about each child's neighborhood attractions.

GEOGRAPHY

Make map of unit or of hospital.

Make map of what is seen from hospital windows—locate on map of the city/county/state.

---

*From *Ideas and activities with hospitalized children,* Washington, DC, 1982, The Association for the Care of Children's Health.

HISTORY

Research the hospital's history, the history of a branch of medical science or a medical profession, find out more about famous people in medicine's history (Hippocrates, Florence Nightingale, Clara Barton, Wilhelm Roentgen) or of medical discoveries and progress (the first corrective lenses, the discovery of penicillin).

INTERACTION WITH HOSPITAL DEPARTMENTS AND PERSONNEL

Take field trips to the cafeteria, kitchen, animal labs, historical places within the hospital, or offices (medical records, etc.).

Have personnel talk about their professions (e.g., electrical engineering, security guards, housekeeping, nurses, doctors, technicians, public relations, social workers, pharmacists, occupational and physical therapists).

Have staff teach part of lesson (e.g., have nurse or doctor discuss how medicine works, technician explain x-rays, or a dietitian talk about an aspect of nutrition).

Play Activities for Specific Procedures

Fluid Intake

Make freezer pops using child's favorite juice.

Cut gelatin into fun shapes.

Make game of taking sip when turning page of book or during games such as "Simon says."

Use small medicine cups; decorate the cups.

Color water with food coloring or powdered drink mix.

Have a tea party; pour at small table.

Let child fill a syringe and squirt it into mouth or use it to fill small, decorated cups.

Cut straws in half and place in small container (much easier for child to suck liquid).

Decorate straw; cut out small design with two holes and pass straw through; place small sticker on straw.

Use a "crazy" straw.

Make a "progress poster"; give rewards for drinking a predetermined quantity.

Deep Breathing

Blow bubbles with bubble blower.

Blow bubbles with straw (no soap).

Blow on pinwheel, feathers, whistle, harmonica, balloons, toy horns, or party noise makers.

Practice on band instruments.

Have blowing contest using balloons, boats, cotton balls, feathers, marbles, Ping-Pong balls, pieces of paper; blow such objects over a table top goal line, over water, through an obstacle course, up in the air, against an opponent, or up and down a string.

Move paper or cloth from one container to another using suction from a straw.

Use blow bottles with colored water to transfer water from one side to the other.

Dramatize scenes, such as "I'll huff and puff and blow your house down" from the "Three Little Pigs."

Do straw-blowing painting.

Take a deep breath and "blow out the candles" on a birthday cake.

Use a little paint brush to "paint" nails with water, then blow nails dry.

Range of Motion and Use of Extremities

Throw beanbags at fixed or movable target; toss wadded paper into a wastebasket.

Touch or kick Mylar balloons held or hung in different positions (if child is in traction, hang balloon from trapeze).

Play "tickle toes"; have child wiggle them on request.

Play games such as Twister or "Simon says."

Play pretend and guess games (e.g., imitate a bird, butterfly, horse).

Have tricycle or wheelchair races in safe area.

Play kick or throw ball with soft foam ball in safe area.

Position bed so that child must turn to view television or doorway.

Have child climb wall with fingers like a "spider."

Pretend to teach "aerobic" dancing or exercise; encourage parents to participate.

Encourage swimming if feasible.

Play video games or pinball (fine motor movement).

Play "hide and seek" game; hide toy somewhere in bed (or room, if ambulatory) and have child find it using specified hand or foot.

Provide clay to mold with fingers.

Have child paint or draw on large sheets of paper placed on floor or wall.

Encourage combing own hair; play "beauty shop" with "customer" in different positions.

Soaks

Play with small toys or objects (cups, syringes, soap dishes) in water.

Wash dolls or toys.

Bubbles may be added to bathwater if permissible; more bubbles to create shapes or "monsters."

Pick up marbles or pennies* from bottom of bath container.

Make designs with coins on bottom of container.

Pretend a boat is a submarine by keeping it immersed.

During soaks, read to child, sing with child, or play game such as cards, checkers, or other board game (if both hands are immersed, move the board pieces for the child).

Sitz bath: give child something to listen to (music, stories) or look at (Viewmaster, book).

Punch holes in bottom of plastic cup, fill with water, and let it "rain" on child.

Injections

Let child handle syringe (without needle), vial, and alcohol swab and pretend to give an injection to doll or stuffed animal.

Use syringes to decorate cookies with frosting, squirt paint, or target shoot into a container.

Draw a "magic circle" on area before injection; draw smiling face in circle after injection, but avoid drawing on puncture site.

Allow child to have a "collection" of syringes (without needles); make "wild" creative objects with syringes.

---

*Small objects such as marbles or coins, as well as gloves or balloons, are unsafe for young children because of possible aspiration. Latex products also present the risk of an allergic reaction.

Continued

Unit 3

Injections—cont'd

If child is receiving multiple injections or venipunctures, make a "progress poster"; give rewards for predetermined number of injections.

Have child count to 10 or 15 during injection or "blow the hurt away."

Ambulation

Give child something to push:
Toddler, push-pull toy
School-age child, wagon or decorated IV stand
Adolescent, a doll in a stroller or wheelchair
Have a parade; make hats, drum, etc.

Extending Environment (Patients in Traction, etc.)

Make bed into a pirate ship or airplane with decorations.
Put up mirrors so patient can see around room.
Move patient's bed frequently, especially to playroom, hallway, or outside.

INFORMED CONSENT TO TREAT CHILD

Children are considered minors (usually until 18 years of age) and, except under special circumstances, the parent or the person designated as legal guardian for the child is required to give informed consent before medical treatment is implemented or any procedure is performed on the child. Separate permission is also required for the following:
Major surgery
Minor surgery, for example, cutdown, biopsy, dental extraction, suturing a laceration (especially one that may have a cosmetic effect), removal of a cyst, and closed reduction of a fracture
Diagnostic tests with an element of risk, for example, bronchoscopy, needle biopsy, angiography, electroencephalogram, lumbar puncture, cardiac catheterization, ventriculography, and bone marrow aspiration
Medical treatments with an element of risk, for example, blood transfusion, thoracentesis or paracentesis, radiation therapy, and shock therapies
Other hospital situations that require written parental permission include the following:
Taking photographs for medical, educational, or other public use
Removal of the child from the hospital against medical advice
Postmortem examinations, except in unexplained deaths such as sudden infant death, violent death, or suspected suicide

Release of medical information
Exceptions to the previously mentioned regulations include the following:
Informed consent of persons in loco parentis (in place of the parent) permission granted by the person responsible for the child during parents' absence
Oral informed consent—Telephone consent or oral consent from a parent who is unable to sign permit (have witness to verbal consent)
Mature or emancipated minor—A person who is legally underage but who is recognized as having the legal capacity of an adult such as an unmarried pregnant minor, a minor who is married, or a minor who lives apart from the parents and is self-supporting
Treatment without parental consent—Situations in which children need prompt medical or surgical treatment and a parent is not readily available to give consent
Parental negligence—When children need protection from their parents, such as when parents neglect or impose improper punishment on a child or refuse needed treatment; or when parents' refusal is a direct violation of the law

GENERAL HYGIENE AND CARE
Skin Care
General Guidelines

Cleanse skin with gentle soap (e.g., Dove) or cleanser (e.g., Cetaphil). Rinse well with plain, warm water.
Provide daily cleansing of eyes, oral area, and diaper or perianal area, and any areas of skin breakdown.
Apply moisturizing agents after cleansing to retain moisture and rehydrate skin.
Use minimum tape/adhesive. On very sensitive skin, use a protective, pectin-based or hydrocolloid skin barrier between skin and tape/adhesives.
Use adhesive remover (if skin is not fragile) or water when removing tape/adhesives.
Place pectin-based or hydrocolloid skin barriers directly over excoriated skin. Leave barrier undisturbed until it begins to peel off. With wet, oozing excoriations, place a small amount of stoma powder (as used in ostomy care) on site, remove excess powder, and apply skin barrier. Hold barrier in place for several minutes to allow barrier to soften and mold to skin surface.

Alternate electrode placement sites and thoroughly assess skin underneath electrodes at least every 24 hours.
Be certain fingers or toes are visible whenever extremity is used for IV or arterial line.
Reduce friction by keeping skin dry (may apply absorbent powder such as cornstarch) and using soft, smooth bed linen and clothes.
Use a draw sheet to move a child in bed or onto a gurney to reduce friction and shearing injuries; do not drag the child from under the arms.
Identify children who are at risk for skin breakdown before it occurs. Employ measures such as *pressure-reducing devices* (reduce pressure more than would usually occur on a regular hospital bed or chair) or *pressure-relieving devices* (maintains pressure below that which would cause capillary closing) to prevent breakdown.

Unit 3

Do not massage reddened, bony prominences because this can cause deep tissue damage; provide pressure relief to these areas instead.

Keep skin free of excess moisture (e.g., urine or fecal incontinence, wound drainage, excessive perspiration).

Routinely assess the child's nutritional status. A child who is NPO for several days and who is only receiving IV fluids is nutritionally at risk. This can also affect the skin's ability to maintain its integrity. Hyperalimentation should also be considered for these children before they are at risk.

Neonatal Guidelines

General Skin Care

Cleanse skin with plain, warm water. Use bland, nonalkaline soaps or cleansers only when necessary, such as for removal of stool.

Provide daily cleansing of eye, oral, and diaper areas, as well as any areas of skin breakdown.

Apply moisturizing agents to skin, after cleansing it with warm water, to retain moisture and rehydrate skin. Cleanse skin gently of any old oil or cream before applying a new layer, except in diaper area.

Use pressure-reducing mattress to prevent pressure areas.

Use of Adhesives on Skin

Use minimal tape/adhesive or minimal zinc oxide base adhesive such as HyTape. Evaluate need for all tape/adhesive used.

Use a protective pectin-based or hydrocolloid skin barrier between skin and all tape/adhesives. Place on all areas where tape/adhesives are used, such as for securing chest tubes, nasogastric tubes, dressings, extremities to IV board, monitor leads, endotracheal tubes, and temperature probe (cut "keyhole" for temperature probe in barrier or place circular patch of skin barrier over probe).

Place pectin-based or hydrocolloid skin barrier directly over excoriated skin. Leave barrier undisturbed until it begins to peel off. With wet, oozing excoriations, dust site with a small amount of stoma powder (as used in ostomy care), brush excess away, and apply skin barrier. Hold barrier in place for several minutes to allow barrier to soften and mold to the skin surface.

Use transparent elastic film dressings to secure and protect central lines and peripheral arterial line insertion sites, as well as over open skin lesions. Leave dressing in place until it begins to peel off, usually within 5 to 7 days.

Alternate electrode placement sites and avoid standard adhesive electrode. Use limb electrodes rather than chest electrodes or use hydrogel electrodes. Assess skin thoroughly underneath electrodes. Remove and rotate electrodes at a minimum of every 24 hours, or more frequently if skin injury is noted.

Remove adhesives with warm water–soaked gauze or a small amount of bland, diluted soap, rather than alcohol or adhesive removers. To remove a skin barrier, slowly and gently peel away from skin, holding barrier in one hand and supporting skin underneath with other hand. If needed, soak off with warm water. Do not use bonding agents such as tincture of benzoin or commercial swabs.

Avoid using scissors to remove tape or dressings; this prevents cutting skin or amputating digits.

Use of Substances on Skin

Evaluate all substances that come in contact with the infant's skin.

Avoid or limit use of the following substances that have the potential for percutaneous absorption and systemic effects:

Adhesive removers	Isopropyl alcohol
Boric acid	Neomycin ointment
Chlorhexidine	Povidone iodine
Chlorophenol	Salicylic acid
Epinephrine	Silver sulfadiazine cream
Estrogen	Steroids
Hexachlorophene	Tincture of benzoin
Hydrogen peroxide	

If any of these agents is used, chart the amount and frequency of application.

Before using any topical agent, analyze components of preparation and:

Use sparingly and only when necessary.

Confine use to smallest possible area.

Whenever possible and appropriate, wash off with water.

Monitor infant carefully for signs of toxicity and systemic effects.

Use of Thermal Devices

Avoid heat lamps because of increased potential for burns. If needed, measure actual temperature of exposed skin every 15 minutes.

When using heating pads (Aqua-K pads):

Change infant's position every 1 to 2 hours or as needed according to skin condition and developmental level.

Preset temperature of heating pads <40° C (104° F).

When using preheated transcutaneous electrodes:

Avoid use on infants <1000 g.

Set at lowest possible temperature (<44° C [111.2° F]) and secure with plastic wrap.

Use pulse oximetry rather than transcutaneous monitoring whenever possible.

When prewarming heels before phlebotomy, avoid temperatures >40° C.

Warm ambient humidity, direct away from infant; use aerosolized sterile water and maintain ambient temperature so as not to exceed 40° C.

Document use of all heating devices.

Use of Fluid Therapy/Hemodynamic Monitoring

Be certain fingers or toes are visible whenever extremity is used for IV or arterial line.

Secure catheter or needle with transparent dressing/tape to promote easy visualization of site.

Assess site hourly for signs of ischemia, infiltration, and inadequate perfusion (check capillary refill).

Avoid use of restraints (e.g., armboards); if used, check that they are secured safely and are not restricting circulation or movement (check for pressure areas).

Use commercial IV protector (e.g., IV House) with minimal tape.

Modified from Malloy MB, Perez-Woods R: Neonatal skin care: prevention of skin breakdown, *Pediatr Nurs* 17(1):41-48, 1991.

Unit 3

Pressure Reduction/Relief Devices

Description	Advantages	Disadvantages	Examples*
Overlay†			
Foam: Varying density; 2- to 4-inch convoluted and non-convoluted	Primarily pressure reduction, although in children may have pressure relief advantages; can be cut to fit cribs	Can be soiled by incontinent patient; inability to reduce skin moisture because of lack of airflow	Aerofoam, BioGard, Dura-Pedic, GeoMatt, Ultra Form Pediatric (does not include ordinary convoluted foam mattresses)
Gel/water filled: Pressure reduction; water or gel conforms to patient's contours	One-time charge; low cost for water; gels are expensive Relieves pressure and shear; nonpowered, easy cleaning	Mattress is a dense collection of viscous fluid cells; there have been reports that the mattress is cold to the touch; patients may have to spare vital calories to warm the mattress Heavy	Aqua-Pedics (water and gel), Tender Gel and Water, Theracare (water and gel), RIK mattress
Alternating-pressure mattress: An overlay with rows of air cells and pump; pump cycles air to provide inflation and deflation over pressure points	The intent is to relieve pressure points to create pressure gradients that enhance blood flow	Studies show inconsistent results; some have reported very low deflation interface pressures, but only the deflation pressures were used for analysis; tissue interface pressures during inflation are consistently higher and must be incorporated into the statistical analysis; clinical trials indicate higher pressure ulcer incidence rates when compared with other products	AeroPulse, AlphaBed, AlphaCare, BetaBed, Bio Flote, Dyna-CARE, Lapidus, PCA Systems, Pillo-Pump, Tenderair
Static air: Designed with interlocking air cells that provide dry flotation; inflated with a blower	Mattress overlays that are designed with multiple chambers, allowing air exchange between the compartments	Pressure reduction depends on adequate air volume and periodic reinflation	DermaGard, K-Soft, Koala-Kair, Roho, Sof-Care, Tenderair
Low–air-loss specialty overlay: Multiple airflow cushions that cover the entire bed; pressures can be set and controlled by a blower	Surface materials are constructed to reduce friction and shear and to eliminate moisture; pressure relief; can be used for prevention and/or treatment of ulcers	Surface mattress and pump are a rental item; cost of electricity used is incurred by family; not available for cribs	Acucair, Bio Therapy, CLINICARE, CRS 4000, RibCor Therapeutic Mattress Pad, TheraPulse, Select Firstep®, Dynapulse®
Specialty Beds‡			
Low–air-loss beds: Bed surface consists of inflated air cushions; each section is adjusted for optimum pressure relief for patient's body size; some models have built-in scales	Provides pressure relief in any position; treatment for stages III and IV pressure ulcers; available in pediatric crib sizes	Bed is more bulky than a hospital bed, and some homes may not be able to accommodate its size; reimbursement is questionable; family incurs electric bill	Air Plus, Flexicair, KinAir III® Mediscus For cribs: Pedcare, PNEU-CARE/PEDI, Clinitron, TheraPulse,® KCI's PediDyne,™ BariKare,® with FirstStep,® Select Heavy Duty™

Modified from Hagelgans NA: Pediatric skin care issues for the home care nurse, *Pediatr Nurs* 19(5):499-507, 1993. Material revised by Ivy Razmus, MSN, RN.
*This list is a representative sampling of products and is not intended to be all inclusive. No endorsement of any product is intended. Within each category, products must be individually evaluated on their efficacy as comfort, pressure-reducing, or pressure-relieving devices. All products within a category do not necessarily perform equally.
†A device that is made to fit over a regular hospital mattress.
‡"High-tech" beds used in place of the standard hospital bed. These are normally used on a rental basis and are intended for short-term use. They usually provide pressure relief and eliminate shear, friction, and maceration.

Unit 3

Pressure Reduction/Relief Devices—cont'd

Description	Advantages	Disadvantages	Examples*
Low–air-loss mattress replacements	Provides pressure relief in any position; fits on hospital frame	Requires mattress storage	Flexicair Eclipse SilkAir— home use
Air-fluidized beds: Air is blown through beads to "float" patient	Provides pressure relief for oncology patients and for treatment of full thickness pressure ulcers, postoperative flaps, burns; lighter weight home care units available	Can be difficult to transfer patient	Clinitron At Home, Clinitron Elexis, Clinitron Fluid Air, Skytron, Elite,™ Clinitron Uplift Fluid Air
Kinetic Therapy: Therapy surfaces that provide continuous gentle side-to-side rotation of 40 degrees or more on each side; table based or cushion based	Has been demonstrated to improve mucous transport, redistribute pulmonary blood flow, and mobilize pulmonary interstitial fluid; has been utilized for trauma victims and unstable spinal cord injuries (should use table based; once stabilized, may use cushion based)	Used in acute care setting	***Cushion Based*** **With air loss:** BioDyne II, Effica CC, Pulmonex, Triadyne,™ Pro-Turn, Synergy, Pneu-Care Plus, Pediadyne™ ***Table Based*** **Without air loss:** RotoRest,® Delta, Keane Mobility bed
Continuous Lateral Rotation Beds (CLRT): Less than 40 degrees side-to-side rotation	Helps reposition unstable spinal cord injury patient; promotes comfort and shifts pressure points		BariAir™, Q2Plus,® Effica Pulmonex

Bathing

Unless contraindicated, bathe infant or child in a tub at the bedside, on the bed, or in a standard bathtub.
Never leave infant or small child unattended in a bathtub.
Hold infant who is unable to sit alone.
  Support infant's head securely with one hand or grasp the infant's farther arm firmly and rest the head comfortably on your wrist.
Closely supervise the infant or child who is able to sit without assistance.
Place a pad in the bottom of the tub to prevent slipping and loss of balance.
Offer older children the option of a shower, if available.
Use judgment regarding the amount of supervision older children require.
  Children with mental and/or physical limitations such as severe anemia or leg deformities, and suicidal or psychotic children (who may commit bodily harm) require close supervision.
Clean the ears, between skinfolds, the neck, the back, and the genital area carefully.
  Retract the foreskin of uncircumcised boys gently (usually those over 3 years of age), clean the exposed surfaces, and replace the foreskin. Never forcefully retract the foreskin.
Provide more extensive assistance with bathing and other aspects of hygienic care to children who are ill or debilitated:
  Encourage them to perform as much as they are capable of without overtaxing their energies.
  Expect increasing involvement with improved strength and endurance.

Hair Care

Brush and comb hair or help children with hair care at least once daily.
Style hair for comfort and in a manner pleasing to the child and parents.
  Do not cut hair without parental permission. although shaving hair to provide access to scalp vein for intravenous needle insertion is permissible.
Shampoo the hair in the tub or shower or transport the child by gurney to an accessible sink or washbasin.
  Wash the hair of the newborn daily as part of the bath if this is the institution's policy.
  Wash the hair and scalp as needed in later infancy and childhood.
  Teenagers may need more frequent hair care and shampoos.

Continued

Hair Care—cont'd

If the child is unable to be transported, shampoo in the bed with adequate protection and/or with specially adapted equipment or positioning.

Use commercial "dry shampoo" products on a short-term basis.

Provide appropriate hair care for black children:

Avoid using most standard combs, which cause hair breakage and discomfort.

Use a special comb with widely spaced teeth.

Combing hair wet causes less breakage.

Remind parents to bring a comb (if possible) if one is not available on the unit.

Apply special hair dressing or pomade.

Consult the child's parents regarding the preparation they wish to be used and ask if they can provide some.

Do not use petroleum jelly.

Rub the preparation on the hair to make it more pliable and manageable.

If braiding or plaiting the hair is desired, loosely weave damp hair.

Mouth Care

Perform mouth care for infants and debilitated children.

Assist small children to brush teeth, although many can manage a toothbrush satisfactorily and should be encouraged to do so.

Remind older children to brush and floss.

Provide a toothbrush or toothpaste for those children who do not have their own, or ask parents to bring these from home. (See p. 585 for specific oral hygiene techniques.)

PROCEDURES RELATED TO MAINTAINING SAFETY

Ensure that environmental safety measures are in operation, such as the following:

Nonsmoking policy

Good illumination

Floors clear of fluid or objects that might contribute to falls

Nonskid surfaces in showers and tubs

Electrical equipment maintained in good working order, used only by personnel familiar with their use, and not in contact with moisture or near tubs

Beds of ambulatory patients locked in place and at a height that allows easy access to the floor

Proper care and disposal of small, breakable items, such as thermometers and bottles

A well-organized fire plan known to all staff members

All windows securely screened

Electrical outlets covered to prevent burns

Be sure the child is wearing a proper identification band.

Check bathwater carefully before placing the child in the bath

Use furniture scaled to the child's proportions and sturdy and well balanced to prevent tipping over.

Securely strap infants and small children into infant seats, feeding chairs, and strollers.

Do not leave infants, young children, and youngsters who are agitated or cognitively impaired unattended on treatment tables, on scales, or in treatment areas.

Keep portholes in incubators securely fastened when not attending the infant.

Prevent child's access to tubs, laundry bags or chutes, medication rooms/carts, and elevators.

Keep crib sides up and fastened securely unless an adult is at the bedside.

Leave crib sides up regardless of child's ability to get out, and even when the crib is unoccupied, to remove the temptation for the child to climb in.

Never turn away from an infant or small child in a crib that has the sides down without maintaining contact with the child's back or abdomen to prevent rolling, crawling, or jumping from the open crib.

Place the child who may climb over the side of the crib in a specially constructed crib with a cover or one that has a safety net placed over the top.

Tie net to the frame in such a manner that there is ready access to the child in case of emergency.

Never tie nets to the movable crib sides, or use knots that do not permit quick release.

Do not place cribs within reach of heating units, appliances, dangling cords, outlets, or other objects that can be reached by curious hands.

Assess the safety of toys brought to the hospital for children and determine whether they are appropriate to the child's age and condition.

Inspect toys to make certain they are allergy-free, washable, and unbreakable and that they have no small, removable parts that can be aspirated or swallowed.

Set limits for the child's safety.

Make sure children understand where they are permitted to go and what they are permitted to do in the hospital.

Enforce the limitations consistently and repeat them as frequently as necessary to make certain that they are understood.

Transporting

Carry infants and small children for short distances within the unit:

In the horizontal position, hold or carry small infants with the back supported and the thighs grasped firmly by the carrying arm.

In the football hold, support the infant on the nurse's arm with the head supported by the hand and the body held securely between the body and elbow.

In the upright position, hold the infant with the buttocks on the nurse's forearm and the front of the body resting against the chest. Support the infant's head and shoulders with the other arm to allow for any sudden movement by the infant.

For more extended trips, use a suitable conveyance:

Determine the method of transporting children by considering their age, condition, and destination.

Use appropriate safety belts and/or raised sides to secure child.

Transport infants in their incubators, cribs, baby buggies, strollers, wheeled feeding chairs, and tables or in wagons with raised sides.

Use wheelchairs or gurneys with side rails for older children.

Restraining Methods and "Therapeutic Hugging"
General Guidelines

Understand the purpose of restraints:
  Provide safety
  Maintain desired position only as long as needed
  Facilitate examination
  Aid in performing diagnostic tests and therapeutic procedures (Practice Alert)

PRACTICE ALERT

Physical restraint should never be used as a substitute for good nursing care (such as adequate preparation of the child or pain management/use of sedation), for punishment, or as a convenience to the staff.

Prepare child for needed restraints:
  Explain the restraint and the reason for the restraint.
  Repeat information as often as needed to gain cooperation.
  Have child verbalize understanding of need for restraint.
  Explain how the child can help (e.g., "Your job is to keep your arm as still as a tree").
  Reassure child that the restraint is not a punishment.

Explain restraints and their purpose to parents:
  Explain purpose and function of restraints.
  Document parental consent for restraints.
  Show parents how to remove and reapply them (if feasible).
  Teach signs of complications.
  Explain ways in which parents can help to ensure maximal benefit and minimal stress (e.g., have the parent emotionally support the child by staying near the child, such as at the head of the bed [provide a chair for the parent] and soothe/calm the child by talking softly, singing, and stroking the skin).

Employ comfort measures:
  Use "therapeutic hugging" rather than mechanical restraints (Practice Alert).
  Release restraints periodically to allow the child to move extremities when this practice does not interfere with therapy.
  Pad rigid or constricting devices for comfort and to reduce possibility of injury.
  Raise head of bed 30 degrees unless contraindicated.
  Provide range of motion as appropriate.
  Offer food, fluids, and toileting as appropriate; give infant a pacifier.
  Administer analgesics and sedatives if ordered or request them if needed.
  Provide distraction and touch.

Obtain practitioner order for restraints used for other than diagnostic tests or procedures.

Discuss criteria for removal of restraints.

Select the most appropriate and least restrictive type of restraint (e.g., arm boards are less restrictive than 4 point extremity restraints); consider assigning a "sitter" (assistant or volunteer) to stay with child.

Use ***therapeutic hugging***—a secure, comfortable holding position that provides close physical contact with the parent or other trusted caregiver.

Assess restraining devices every 1 to 2 hours and document findings for the following:
  Correctly applied
  Accomplishing the purpose for which applied
  Do not impair circulation or cause damage to nerves or tissues

Make certain that all restraints allow for easy access to the child in case of emergency:
  Restraints with ties are secured to bed or crib frame, not side rails; do not interfere with raising and lowering crib sides or bedrails.
  Restraints are tied with a slipknot for easy removal.

PRACTICE ALERT

Some believe the parents should not hold the child because children cannot understand why parents would participate in a painful procedure. Others have found that children are more relaxed when parents hold them. Before deciding on how and who should immobilize, consult the parents and the child, if old enough.

Of note, when school-age children were asked what would help most if they were in pain, 99.2% answered having their parents present, even though most realized that the parents could not alleviate the pain.

Ross DM, Ross SA: Childhood pain: the school-aged child's viewpoint, *Pain* 29(2):179-191, 1984.

Unit 3

Types of Mechanical Restraints

Type	Function	Description
Jacket restraint	To prevent child from climbing out of crib or bed	Waist-length, sleeveless jacket with back closure fastened with ties Long ties on bottom of jacket secure child to crib, chair, or bed

Mummy restraint ("swaddle")	To control child's movements
	To immobilize extremities
	To provide temporary restraining device for short procedures
		Place opened sheet or blanket on flat surface with one corner folded to the center
		Place infant on blanket with shoulders at blanket fold and feet toward opposite corner
		Place infant's right arm straight against side of body
		Pull side of blanket on right side firmly across right shoulder and chest
		Secure beneath left side of body
		Place left arm straight against side
		Bring remaining side of blanket across left shoulder and chest
		Secure beneath body
		Fold lower corner and bring up to shoulders and secure ends beneath body
		Fasten in place with safety pins or tape
		Modification for chest examination:
		    Left and right corners are brought over arms only to, but not including, chest and secured under body
		    Bottom corner is secured at waist rather than at shoulders

Papoose board	Same as mummy restraint	Solid board with attached straps that secure infant or small child to the board, similar to a mummy restraint Pad board for comfort

Arm and leg restraints	To immobilize one or more extremities:
	    For treatments
	    For procedures
	    To facilitate healing
		Soft, padded commercial restraints
		Clove-hitch restraint (Fig. 3-2)
		Folded towel, pinned around extremity
		Gauze or cotton bandage, padded well

Elbow restraint	To prevent child from bending elbow To prevent child from reaching head, face, neck, or chest	Muslin square with vertical pockets to contain tongue depressors that supply vertical rigidity and horizontal flexibility; ties secure the device around the arm Padded large-diameter towel roller Tubular plastic container with top and bottom removed and suitably padded for comfort and safety

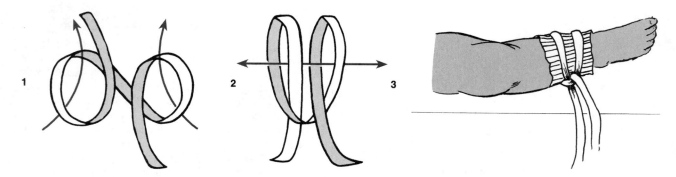

Fig. 3-2 Clove hitch restraint.

POSITIONING FOR PROCEDURES

(See Atraumatic Care box.)

Extremity Venipuncture or Dermal Injection

Place child on parent's (or assistant's) lap, with the child facing toward the parent and in the straddle position (Fig. 3-3).

For venipuncture, place child's arm on a firm surface such as the treatment table (for support) and on top of a soft cloth or towel.

Have assistant or parent immobilize child's arm for venipuncture.

Have parent hug the child around the chest to hold the child's free arm; or,

Place child on parent's (or assistant's) lap, with the child facing away from the parent (Fig. 3-4).

To hold the child's legs still, place them between the parent's legs. This position is appropriate for an injection into the thigh; or, for an injection into the arm, place child in parent's (or assistant's) lap, with the child facing sideward (Fig. 3-5).

Place the child's arm closest to the parent under the parent's arm and wrap toward the back.

Have the parent hold the arm receiving the injection against the child's body.

ATRAUMATIC CARE

Analgesia and Sedation

For painful procedures, the child should receive adequate analgesia and conscious sedation to minimize pain and the need for excessive restraint. (See p. 329.) For local anesthesia, use buffered lidocaine to reduce stinging sensation or apply EMLA or Numby Stuff. (See p. 335.)

Some painful procedures, such as bone marrow tests, can be performed without restraint using unconscious sedation (e.g., propofol [Diprivan]).

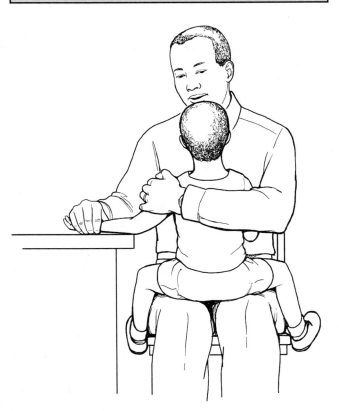

Fig. 3-3 Chest-to-chest straddle sitting position.

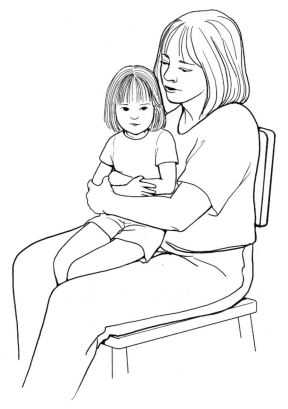

Fig. 3-4 Chest-to-back sitting position with legs secured.

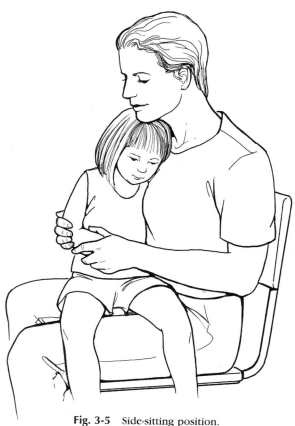

Fig. 3-5   Side-sitting position.

Jugular Venipuncture

Place child in mummy restraint.

Alternate procedure may be used.

The arms and legs of an infant or small child can be restrained with the nurse's forearms at the same time the child's head is positioned and restrained.

Facing the child, position child with head and shoulders extended over the edge of a table or small pillow with neck extended and turned sharply to the side.

Take care that excessive pressure does not compromise circulation or breathing and that the nose and mouth are not covered by the restrainer's hand.

Femoral Venipuncture

Place infant supine with legs in frog position to provide extensive exposure of the groin.

Restrain legs in frog position with hands while controlling the child's arm and body movements with downward and inward pressure of forearms.

Cover genitalia to protect the operator and the venipuncture site from contamination if the child urinates during the procedure.

Site is not advisable for long-term venous access in mobile child because of risk of infection and trauma to flexion area.

Subdural Puncture (Through Fontanel or Bur Holes)

Place active infant in mummy restraint.

Position supine with head accessible to examiner.

Control head movement with firm hold on each side of the head.

Nose and/or Throat Access

Position supine with face accessible to examiner.

Control head and arms by holding child's extended arms over and close to the head, thus immobilizing both head and arms.

Ear Access

Place child in parent's (or assistant's) lap with the child's body sideways and the ear to be examined away from the parent (Fig. 3-6).

Place the child's arm closest to the parent under the parent's arm and wrap toward the back.

Have the parent hold the other arm against the child's body and use the free arm to hold the head against the parent's chest.

To hold the child's legs still, place them between the parent's legs.

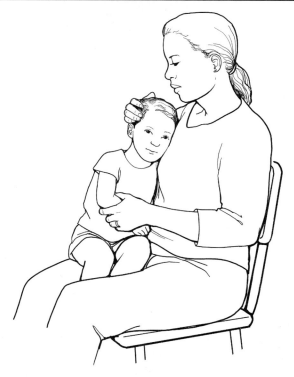

Fig. 3-6   Side-sitting position with head and legs secured.

Lumbar Puncture

INFANT

Place infant in sitting position with buttocks extended over the edge of the table and head flexed on chest.

In neonates, use side-lying position with modified head extension to decrease respiratory distress during procedure. Pulse oximetry and heart rate monitoring are advisable.

Immobilize arms and legs with nurse's hands.

Observe child for difficulty in breathing.

OLDER INFANT OR YOUNG CHILD

While standing, hold child upright against the nurse's (or parent's) chest with child's legs wrapped around the adult's waist (Fig. 3-7).

Use arms to hug and restrain child.

Place a small pillow or folded towel between child's abdomen and adult to help arch the child's back

Use side-lying position as described for neonate.

CHILD

Place child on side with back close to or extended over the edge of examining table, head flexed, and knees drawn up toward the chest.

Reach over the top of the child and place one arm behind child's neck and the other behind the knees.

Stabilize this position by clasping own hands in front of the child's abdomen.

Take care that excessive pressure does not compromise circulation or breathing and that the nose and mouth are not covered by the restrainer's body.

Bone Marrow Examination

For posterior iliac site:
Position child prone.
Place a small pillow or folded towel under the hips to raise them slightly.
Apply restraint at upper body and lower extremities, preferably with two persons.

For anterior iliac site or tibia:
Position child supine.
Apply restraint at upper body and lower extremities, preferably with two persons.

Urinary Catheterization

Have the parent sit in a chair or on an examining table with a back support. Place the child leaning back in the parent's lap with the parent's arms hugging the child's upper body (Fig. 3-8).

Place the child's legs in the frog position, with the parent's legs over the child's to stabilize them. In this comfortable position the perineum is exposed for the procedure.

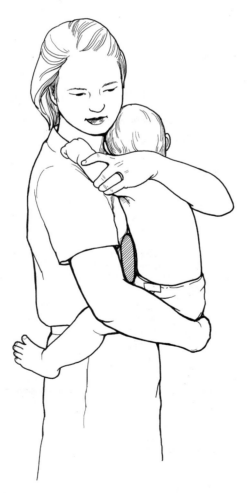

Fig. 3-7   Chest-to-chest straddle standing position.

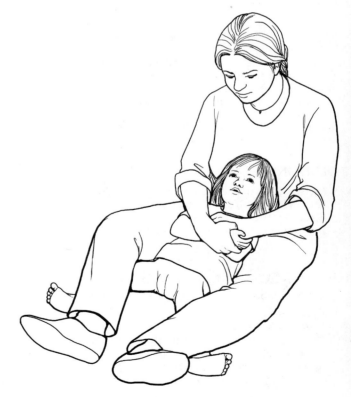

Fig. 3-8   Semi-reclining position with legs secured.

COLLECTION OF SPECIMENS
Urine

(See Practice Alert.)

NON–TOILET-TRAINED CHILD*

Use a collection bag; cut a small slit in the diaper and pull the bag through to allow room for urine to collect and to facilitate checking the contents. To obtain small amounts of urine, use a syringe without a needle to aspirate urine directly from the diaper; if diapers with absorbent gelling material that trap urine are used, place a small gauze dressing, some cotton balls, or a urine collection device† inside the diaper to collect urine, then aspirate the urine with a syringe.
Check bag frequently and remove as soon as specimen is available.
Urine collected for culture should either be tested within 30 minutes, refrigerated, or placed in a sterile container with a preservative.

TOILET-TRAINED YOUNG CHILD

May not be able to urinate on request.
May be more successful if potty chair or bedpan is placed on the toilet.

---

*See Community and Home Care Instructions, p. 591.
†The Bard Infant Urine Collector is available from Bard Urological Division, C.R. Bard, Inc., 8195 Industrial Blvd. Covington, GA 30014; (800) 526-4455.

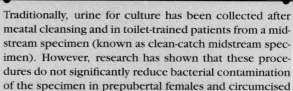

PRACTICE ALERT

Traditionally, urine for culture has been collected after meatal cleansing and in toilet-trained patients from a midstream specimen (known as clean-catch midstream specimen). However, research has shown that these procedures do not significantly reduce bacterial contamination of the specimen in prepubertal females and circumcised or uncircumcised males.*

*MacDonald N and others: Efficacy of chlorhexidine cleansing in reducing contamination of bagged urine specimens, *Can Med Assoc J* 133:1211-1213, 1985; Lohr J, Donowitz L, and Dudley S: Bacterial contamination rates in voided urine collection in girls, *J Pediatr* 114(1):91-93, 1989; Saez-Llorens X, Umana M, Odio C, and Lohr J: Bacterial contamination rates for non–clean-catch and clean-catch midstream urine collection in uncircumcised boys, *J Pediatr* 114(1):93-95, 1989; and Leisure MK, Dudley SM, Donowitz LG: Does a clean-catch urine sample reduce bacterial contamination? *N Engl J Med* 328(4):289-290, 1993.

Use familiar terms, such as "pee pee," "wee wee," or "tinkle." Enlist parent's assistance.

TOILET-TRAINED OLDER CHILD

Cooperative but appreciates explanation of what specimen is for.
Provide privacy and a receptacle, preferably with some means of concealing it, such as a paper bag.

Unit 3

Bladder Catheterization

Bladder catheterization is employed for the following reasons:
Collection of a urine specimen
Diagnostic testing
Continuous urinary drainage
Intravesical instillation of medications or chemotherapeutic agents

Materials needed

Sterile gloves (See Practice Alert.)

PRACTICE ALERT

Non-latex catheters and sterile gloves should be used for all infants and children with known latex allergy, latex sensitivity, or those on latex precautions (i.e., children with conditions associated with frequent exposure to latex-containing products).

Catheter:
(See Practice Alert.)
Select a catheter based on the purpose of the procedure, the age and gender of the child, and any history of prior urologic surgery.

When collecting a urine specimen or completing a diagnostic test requiring catheterization for a brief period, use:
A soft, 4 to 5 French, 15-inch feeding tube for the infant, toddler, or school-aged child.
A soft, 8 French, 15-inch feeding tube or an 8 to 12 French in and out catheter for the adolescent girl.
An 8 to 12 French straight-tipped or coudé-tipped in and out catheter for the adolescent boy.
When placing an indwelling catheter, use:
A 5 French feeding tube or a 6-8 French Foley catheter with a 3 ml retention balloon for the infant.
A 6-8 French Foley catheter with a 3 to 5 ml retention balloon for the toddler or school-aged child.
An 8 to 12 French Foley catheter with a 5 ml retention balloon for the adolescent girl.
An 8 to 16 French Foley catheter with a 5 ml retention balloon for the adolescent boy. Larger French sizes (14 to 16) are reserved for older adolescents with more fully developed prostates. A coudé-tipped catheter is selected for the adolescent boy with a history of urologic surgery.
Catheter tray:
Catheter insertion trays are available that provide a cost-effective alternative to gathering individual supplies for catheterization. These kits may come with or without a catheter, and both should be available for use with chil-

Bladder Catheterization—cont'd

Materials Needed—cont'd

dren. When a tray is not accessible, the following materials are needed in addition to the catheter: Betadine cleanser with cotton balls, sterile draping, a syringe with 5 ml of sterile water, and sterile, water-soluble lubricating jelly.
Xylocaine jelly:
(See Atraumatic Care box.)

ATRAUMATIC CARE

Reducing Catheterization Discomfort

Xylocaine jelly can reduce or eliminate the burning and discomfort associated with catheterization in children. In addition, instillation a 2% Xylocaine jelly preparation into the urethra assists in the task of advancing the catheter into the bladder in boys.*

*Gray ML: Atraumatic urethral catheterization of children, *Pediatr Nurs* 22(4):306-309, 1996.

A 5 ml, 2% Xylocaine sterile lubricating jelly should be used for all catheterization procedures, unless the child is allergic to Xylocaine or has absent pelvic sensations. Individual packages designed for injecting into the urethral lumen are available.*
Container for urine collection:
When collecting a specimen or completing a diagnostic test, an appropriate urine specimen container and 500 ml basin is used; when inserting an indwelling catheter, a bedside drainage bag is obtained prior to the procedure. When inserting a Foley catheter, it is preferable to use a pre-connected (closed) system containing catheter and bedside drainage bag.

Procedure

1. Explain procedure to child and parents.
    Give a careful and thorough explanation of the procedure, according to the developmental level of the child, before preparation of the perineum. Include an explanation of the purpose of the catheterization and reassure child that it is not punishment.
    Reassure parents that catheterization will not harm their child or damage the urethra or hymen.
    Reassure child that insertion of the catheter will not feel like having a sharp object inserted, but will produce a feeling of pressure and desire to urinate.
2. Give instruction on pelvic muscle relaxation whenever possible.
    Young child is taught to blow (using a pinwheel is helpful) and to press the hips against the bed or procedure table during catheterization in order to relax the pelvic and periurethral muscles.
    Older child or adolescent is taught to contract and relax the pelvic muscles, and the relaxation procedure is repeated during catheter insertion. If the youngster vigorously contracts the pelvic muscles when the

catheter reaches the striated sphincter (proximal urethra in boys and mid-urethra in girls), catheter insertion is temporarily stopped. The catheter is neither removed nor advanced; instead the child is assisted to press the hips against the bed or examining table and relax the pelvic muscles. The catheter is then gently advanced into the bladder.
3. Assemble necessary equipment.
4. Place the infant or child in a supine position with the perineum adequately exposed. Girls may bend the knees and abduct the legs in a "frog-like" position; boys should lie with the penis lying above the upper thighs. For a young child, have the parent sit on the bed or examining table with a back support. Place the child leaning back in the parent's lap with the parent's arms hugging the child's upper body. When the child's legs are in the frog position, the parent's legs can be placed over the child's to stabilize them. In this comfortable position the perineum is exposed for the procedure and the child is helped to lie still.
5. Put on a pair of sterile gloves. (See Practice Alert, p. 235.)
6. Place a sterile drape over the perineum of girls, ensuring that the vagina, labia, and urethral meatus remain exposed. Most catheter insertion kits provide a sterile drape with a diamond-shaped hole in the middle to assist with this. For boys, the sterile drape is placed over the upper aspect of the thighs so that the penis lies over its upper border.
7. Place 5 ml of sterile lubricating jelly on the sterile drape. When catheterizing an adolescent or child accustomed to the procedure, the catheter may be placed on the sterile drape laid over the perineum. When catheterizing an anxious child, the catheter should remain on a sterile field that will not be upset should the child move during the procedure.
8. Cleanse the perineum of girls, including the labia, vaginal introitus, and urethral meatus. Use a new cotton ball for each wipe, moving in a front-to-back motion along each side of the labia minora, along the sides of the urinary meatus, and finally straight down over the urethral opening. For boys, the entire glans penis is cleansed, in an outward circular fashion, using one cotton ball for each wipe. The foreskin is retracted in the uncircumcised boy to ensure adequate exposure. If the foreskin cannot be easily retracted, particular care is taken to ensure that the glans penis is adequately cleaned prior to catheter insertion.
9. Wipe the cleanser from the skin using sterile cotton balls.
10. Use 2% Xylocaine jelly urethral injecting system. For girls, apply 2 to 3 ml around the mucosa immediately adjacent to the urethral meatus, then inject the remaining 2 to 3 ml directly into the urethra. Allow the lubricant to remain in place 2 to 5 minutes before inserting the catheter. For boys, insert the entire 5 ml into the urethral lumen and gently compress the glans penis so the 2% Xylocaine jelly remains in place; wait 2 to 5 minutes before catheter insertion.
11. *Girls:* Spread the labia (if necessary) using one hand in order to clearly visualize the urethral meatus. With the other hand, grasp the catheter and apply a small amount of sterile lubricant from the sterile field onto the tip of the catheter. (It is rarely necessary to spread the labia in infants; instead, locate the urethra, which often appears as a dimple above the hymen.) Gently insert the catheter until urine return is seen. If inserting an indwelling catheter, insert approximately one half the length of the catheter before attempting to fill the retention balloon.
12. *Boys:* Maintain gentle compression of the glans penis using one hand (Step 10). Grasp the catheter with the other hand

*International Medication Systems, Ltd. (IMS), South El Monte, CA 91733; and Astra USA, Inc., Westborough, MA 01581-4500.

and apply a small amount of sterile lubricant from sterile field onto the tip of the catheter. Insert the catheter by briefly relaxing the compression of the glans penis so that a small amount of 2% Xylocaine jelly exits the meatus, but ensuring that the majority remains within the urethra. Insert the catheter until urine return occurs; this may take several seconds longer because of the additional lubricant present in the urethra. If inserting an indwelling catheter, advance until urine return is noted, then advance to the bifurcation of the filling port before filling the retention balloon.

13. When catheterizing for specimen collection, allow 15 to 30 ml for urinalysis and urine culture. Drain bladder and record post-void urinary volume if collected soon after urination. Cap the specimen, label, and send it to the lab.
14. When inserting an indwelling catheter, gently pull catheter back until resistance is met; this ensures that the retention balloon lies just above the bladder neck. Tape tubing to the leg to avoid pulling. Hang drainage apparatus to bed frame (avoid bed rails to prevent pulling on catheter).

24-Hour Urine Collection

Begin and end collection with an empty bladder:
    At time collection begins, instruct child to void and discard specimen.
    Twenty-four hours after that specimen was discarded, instruct child to void for last specimen.
Save all voided urine during the 24 hours in a refrigerated container marked with date, total time, and child's name.

*See Community and Home Care Instructions, p. 591.

NON–TOILET-TRAINED CHILD*

Prepare skin with thin coating of skin sealant (unless contraindicated, such as in premature infant or on irritated and/or nonintact skin) and apply a urine collection bag with a collection tube that allows urine to drain into a large receptacle.*
If a collection tube is not available, insert a small feeding tube through a puncture hole at the top of the bag; use a syringe without needle to aspirate urine through the feeding tube.

Stool

Collect stool without urine contamination, if possible.

NON–TOILET-TRAINED CHILD

Apply a urine collection bag.
Apply diaper over bag.
After bowel movement, use tongue blade to collect stool.
Place specimen in appropriate covered container.

TOILET-TRAINED CHILD

Have child urinate, then flush toilet.
Have child defecate into bedpan or toilet.
To facilitate collecting specimen, place a sheet of plastic wrap over toilet seat, or use a commercial potty hat.
After bowel movement, use tongue blade to collect stool.
Place in appropriate covered container.

Respiratory (Nasal) Secretions

To obtain nasal secretions using a nasal washing:
    Place child supine.
    Instill 1 to 3 cc sterile normal saline with a sterile syringe (without needle or with 2 inches of 18- or 20-gauge tubing) into one nostril.

Aspirate contents with a small, sterile bulb syringe.
Place in sterile container.

Sputum

Older children and adolescents are able to cough as directed and supply specimens when given proper direction.
Specimens can sometimes be collected from infants and young children who have an endotracheal tube or tracheostomy by means of tracheal aspiration with a mucous trap or suction apparatus.

Blood
Heel or Finger

Puncture should be no deeper than 2.4 mm.

Explain procedure to child as developmentally appropriate and provide atraumatic care (Atraumatic Care box).

Obtain necessary equipment, including appropriate specimen container(s).

Maintain strict asepsis and standard precautions.

To increase blood flow, warm heel by placing towel soaked in warm (39° to 44° C) water on puncture site for 10 to 15 minutes or hold finger under warm water for a few seconds before puncture.

Prepare area for puncture with bacteriostatic agent.

Perform puncture on heel or finger in proper location:

Usual site for heel puncture is outer aspects of heel (Fig. 3-9, *A*). Boundaries can be marked by an imaginary line extending posteriorly from a point between the fourth and fifth toes and running parallel to the lateral aspect of the heel and another line extending posteriorly from the middle of the great toe and running parallel to the medial aspect of the heel.

ATRAUMATIC CARE

Guidelines for Atraumatic Skin/Vessel Punctures

To reduce the pain associated with heel, finger, venous, or arterial punctures:[*]

- Apply EMLA topically over site if time permits (need at least 60 minutes). To remove the Tegaderm dressing atraumatically, grasp opposite sides of the film and pull sides away from each other to stretch and loosen the film. After the film begins to loosen, grasp the other two sides of the film and pull. Use Numby Stuff (iontophoresis) over site if time permits (need 8 to 20 minutes, depending on amount of current); a vapocoolant spray; or use buffered lidocaine (injected intradermally near vein with 30-gauge needle) to numb skin. (See p. 335.)
- Use nonpharmacologic methods of pain and anxiety control (e.g., ask child to take a deep breath when the needle is inserted and again when the needle is withdrawn; have child exhale a large breath or blow bubbles to "blow hurt away"; ask child to count slowly and then faster and louder if pain is felt).
- Keep all equipment out of sight until used.
- Enlist parent's presence and/or assistance if they wish to participate.
- Restrain child *only as needed* to perform the procedure safely; use "therapeutic hugging"—the use of a secure, comfortable holding position, usually a sitting position, that provides close physical contact with the parent or other trusted caregiver.
- Allow skin preparation to dry completely before penetrating skin.
- Use smallest gauge needle (i.e., 25 gauge) that permits free flow of blood; 27 gauge can be used for obtaining 1 to 1.5 ml of blood and for prominent veins (needle length is only ½ inch).

- Avoid placing IV in dominant hand or in the hand child uses to suck thumb.
- Use automatic lancet device for precise puncture depth of finger or heel; press device lightly against skin and avoid steadying finger against a hard surface.
- Emphasize that blood entering syringe or tube does not hurt; reassure young children that you did not "take their blood" away and that they have a lot more inside.
- Place small bandage over puncture site to make removal easy and less painful and to reassure young children that "their blood will not leak out."
- Have a "two-try" only policy to reduce excessive insertion attempts (two operators each have two insertion attempts; if not successful after four punctures, consider alternative venous access, such as peripherally inserted central catheter [PICC]). Have policy for identifying children with difficult access and appropriate interventions (e.g., most experienced operator for first attempt)[†]

For multiple blood samples:

- Use an intermittent infusion device ("saline or heparin lock") to collect additional samples from existing intravenous line; consider peripherally inserted central catheters (PICC) lines early, not as a last resort. Preferably, use saline flush for catheter larger than 24 gauge (less painful, compatible with drugs, and less costly).
- Coordinate care to allow several tests to be performed on one blood sample using micromethods of testing.
- Anticipate tests (e.g., drug levels, chemistry, immunoglobulin levels) and ask laboratory to save blood for additional testing.

[*]Contrary to popular belief, a study of children ages 3 to 6 years found that asking them not to look at the "finger stick" to avoid the sight of blood, or applying a decorated bandage, did not lessen their rating of pain intensity (Johnston CC, Stevens B, Arbess G: The effect of the sight of blood and use of decorative adhesive bandages on pain intensity ratings by preschool children, *J Pediatr Nurs* 8(3):147-151, 1993).

[†]For an example of one hospital's guidelines for reducing excessive IV insertion attempts, see Catudal, J: Pediatric IV therapy: actual practice, *J Venous Access Devices* 4(1):27-29, Spring 1999.

Usual site for finger puncture is just to the side of the finger pad (Fig. 3-9, *B*), which has more blood vessels and fewer nerve endings).

Collect blood sample in appropriate specimen container.

Apply pressure to puncture site with a dry, sterile gauze pad until bleeding stops.

Clean area of prepping agent with water to avoid absorption in neonate.

Praise child for cooperation.

Discard lancet or puncture device in puncture-resistant container near site of use.

Document site and amount of blood withdrawn as well as type of test obtained.

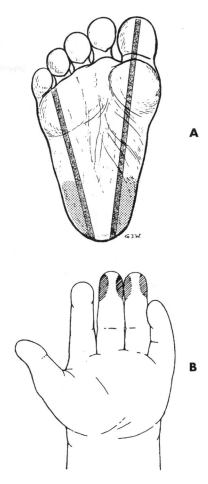

Fig. 3-9 A, Puncture sites (stippled areas) on infant's heel. **B,** Puncture sites on fingers. (**B** from Smith DP and others: *Comprehensive child and family nursing skills,* St Louis, 1991, Mosby.)

Vein

Explain procedure to child as developmentally appropriate and provide atraumatic care. (See Atraumatic Care box.)

Obtain necessary equipment, including appropriate specimen container(s).

Maintain strict asepsis and standard precautions.

Restrain child only as needed to prevent injury.

Prepare area for puncture with bacteriostatic agent.

Apply tourniquet; optional tourniquet for neonate is a rubber band.

Visualize or palpate vein.

Insert needle with bevel up; a slight pop may be felt when entering a child's vein; in small and preterm infants this may not occur.

Withdraw required amount of blood and place in appropriate container.

Release tourniquet, if used.

Withdraw needle from site and apply dry, sterile gauze or cotton ball to site with firm pressure until bleeding stops. If antecubital site is used, keep arm extended to reduce bruising.

Clean area of prepping agent with water to decrease absorption in neonate.

Praise child for cooperation.

Discard syringe and uncapped, uncut needle in puncture-resistant container near site of use.

Document site and amount of blood withdrawn as well as type of test obtained.

Artery

Explain procedure to child as developmentally appropriate and provide atraumatic care. (See Atraumatic Care box.) Arterial blood samples from punctures are painful and often cause crying and breathholding, which affect the accuracy of blood gas values (decreased PO_2).

Obtain necessary equipment, including appropriate specimen container(s).

Maintain strict asepsis and standard precautions.

Prepare area for puncture with bacteriostatic agent.

Arterial punctures may be performed using the radial, brachial, or femoral arteries.

Palpate artery for puncture.

Perform *Allen test* to determine adequacy of collateral circulation:

Elevate extremity distal to puncture site and blanch by squeezing gently (such as making a fist); two arteries supplying blood flow to the extremity (such as radial and ulnar arteries of the wrist) are then occluded.

Lower extremity and remove pressure from one artery (such as ulnar); color return to the blanched extremity in less than 5 seconds indicates collateral circulation.

Prepare area for puncture with bacteriostatic agent.

Insert needle at a 60- to 90-degree angle.

Withdraw required amount of blood into syringe (or specimen container, as appropriate).

Withdraw needle and apply pressure to site with a dry, sterile gauze pad for 5 to 10 minutes until bleeding stops. NOTE: Pressure must be applied at the site to prevent a hematoma.

Place specimen in appropriate container (this may have to be done by a second person to prevent specimen from clotting while pressure is being applied by first person performing puncture).

Clean area of prepping agent with water to decrease absorption in neonate.

Praise child for cooperation.

Discard syringe and uncapped, uncut needle in puncture-resistant container near site of use.

Document site and amount of blood withdrawn as well as type of test obtained.

Implanted Venous Access Device

Explain procedure to child as developmentally appropriate and provide atraumatic care, especially for implanted port. (See Atraumatic Care box.)

Obtain necessary equipment, including appropriate specimen container(s).

Maintain strict asepsis and standard precautions.

Prepare injection port with bacteriostatic agent.

Palpate skin over port to locate diaphragm.

Insert sterile small-gauge needle (e.g., 25-gauge) into port in center of diaphragm.

To obtain a blood specimen from a central venous line or peripheral lock when infusion solution may interfere with test results, first aspirate a minimum quantity of blood equal to the volume of fluid in the catheter and discard; then aspirate the blood sample. For a blood culture, use the first sample of blood, since organisms are most likely to collect within catheter itself.

Withdraw the required amount of blood. (If blood volume is crucial, reinstill first amount withdrawn containing heparinized IV solution; otherwise, discard.)

Remove needle and aspiration device (usually a syringe) from injection port.

Follow institution protocol for administering a heparin or saline flush after blood sampling (if ordered).

Praise child for cooperation.

Discard syringe and uncapped, uncut needle in puncture-resistant container near site of use.

Document access device function, specimen obtained, and type and amount of flush solution used after procedure.

PROCEDURES RELATED TO ADMINISTRATION OF MEDICATIONS
General Guidelines
Estimating Drug Dosage

Body surface area as a basis: estimated from height and weight by use of West nomogram (Fig. 3-10)

Body surface area related to adult dose:

$$\frac{\text{Body surface area of child}}{\text{Body surface area of adult}} \times \frac{\text{Average}}{\text{adult dose}} = \frac{\text{Estimated}}{\text{child's dose}}$$

Body surface area related to average dose per square meter (m^2):

Body surface area of child (m^2) $\times$ Dose/m^2 = Estimated child's dose

WEST NOMOGRAM

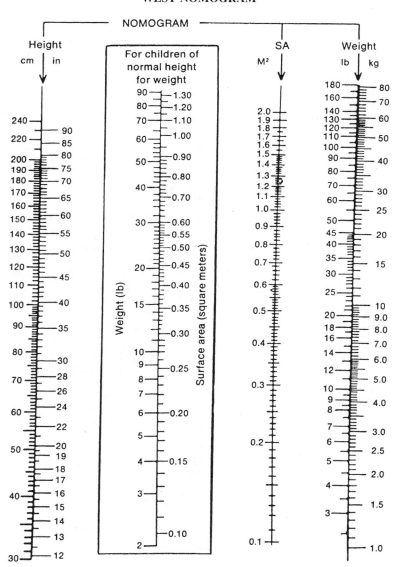

Fig. 3-10 West nomogram (for estimation of surface areas). The surface area is indicated where a straight line connecting the height and weight intersects the surface area (SA) column; or, if the patient is approximately of normal proportion, from the weight alone (boxed area). (Nomogram modified from data of E. Boyd by C.D. West. In Behrman RE, Vaughan VC, editors: *Nelson textbook of pediatrics*, ed 14, Philadelphia, 1992, WB Saunders.)

Unit 3

Approaches to Pediatric Patients

Children's reactions to treatments are affected by the following:
  Developmental characteristics, such as physical abilities and cognitive capabilities
  Environmental influences
  Past experiences
  Current relationship with the nurse
  Perception of the present situation
Expect success: use a positive approach.
Provide an explanation appropriate to the child's developmental level.

Allow the child choices whenever they exist.
Be honest with the child.
Involve the child in the treatment in order to gain cooperation.
Provide distraction for a frightened or uncooperative child.
Allow the child the opportunity to express his/her feelings.
Praise the child for doing his/her best.
Spend some time with the child after administering the medication.
Let the child know he/she is accepted as a person of value.
(See also Preparing children for procedures, p. 219.)

Safety Precautions

Take a drug allergy history.
Check the following 5 "Rs" for correctness:
  Right drug
  Right dosage
  Right time
  Right route
  Right child (always check identification band)
Double-check drug and dosage with another nurse.
  Always double-check the following:
    Digoxin
    Insulin
    Heparin

    Blood
    Chemotherapy
    Cardiotoxic drugs
  May also double-check the following:
    Epinephrine
    Opioids (narcotics)
    Sedatives
Be aware of drug/drug or drug/food interactions.
Document all drugs administered.
Monitor child for side effects.
Be prepared for serious side effects (e.g., respiratory depression or anaphylaxis).

Teaching Family to Administer Medication

Family needs to know the following:
  Name of the drug
  Purpose for which the drug is given
  Amount of the drug to be given
  Length of time to be administered (e.g., for intravenous or inhaled medication)
  Anticipated effects of the drug (therapeutic effects and possible side effects)
  Signs that might indicate an adverse reaction to the drug
  Time(s) to give the drug
  Safe storage of drug (Practice Alert)
Assess the family's level of understanding.
Explain the administration procedure. Instruction needed varies markedly with the intellectual level of the learner and the type and route of medication to be administered.
Demonstrate and have family return the demonstration (if appropriate).

Give written instructions. (See Community and Home Care Instructions related to administering medication beginning on p. 597.)
Assist family in scheduling the time for administration around the family routine.
Be certain family knows what to do and whom to contact if any side effects occur.

 PRACTICE ALERT

Dispose of any plastic covers that may be on the ends of syringes. These covers are small enough to be aspirated by young children.*

*Botash SA: Syringe caps: an aspiration hazard, *Pediatrics* 90(1):92-93, 1992.

Oral Administration*

1. Follow safety precautions for administration.
2. Select appropriate vehicle, for example, calibrated cup, syringe, dropper, measuring spoon, or nipple (Practice Alert).
3. Prepare medication:
    Measure into appropriate vehicle.
    Crush tablets (except when contraindicated, e.g., time-released or enteric-coated preparations) for children who will have difficulty swallowing; mix with syrup, juice, and so on (Atraumatic Care box).
    Avoid mixing medications with essential food items such as milk and formula.
4. Employ safety precautions in identification and administration (Practice Alert).

INFANTS

Hold in semireclining position.
Place syringe, measuring spoon, or dropper in mouth well back on the tongue or to the side of the tongue.
Administer slowly to reduce likelihood of choking or aspiration.
Allow infant to suck medication placed in a nipple.

OLDER INFANT OR TODDLER

Offer medication in cup or spoon.
Administer with syringe, measuring spoon, or dropper (as with infants).
Use mild or partial restraint with reluctant children.
Do not force actively resistive children because of danger of aspiration; postpone 20 to 30 minutes and offer medication again.

PRESCHOOL CHILDREN

Use straightforward approach.
For reluctant children, use the following:
    Simple persuasion
    Innovative containers
    Reinforcement, such as stars, stickers, or other tangible rewards for compliance

---

*See Community and Home Care Instructions, p. 598.

ATRAUMATIC CARE

Encouraging a Child's Acceptance of Oral Medications

Give the child a flavored ice pop or a small ice cube to suck to numb the tongue before giving the drug.
Mix the drug with a small amount (about 1 tsp) of sweet-tasting substance such as honey (except in infants because of the risk of botulism), flavored syrup, jam, fruit puree, sherbet, or ice cream; avoid essential food items, such as formula or milk, because the child may later refuse to eat them.
Give a "chaser" of water, juice, soft drink, flavored ice pop, or frozen juice bar after the drug.
If nausea is a problem, give a carbonated beverage poured over finely crushed ice before or immediately after the medication.
When medication has an unpleasant taste, have the child pinch the nose and drink the medicine through a straw. (Much of what we taste is associated with smell.)
Another alternative is to have the pharmacist prepare the drug in a flavored, chewable troche or lozenge.*
Infants will suck medicine from a needleless syringe or dropper in small increments (0.25 to 0.5 ml) at a time. Use a nipple or special pacifier with a reservoir for the drug.

*For information about compounding drugs, contact Technical Staff, Professional Compounding Centers of America (PCCA), PO Box 368, Sugarland, TX 77487, (800) 331-2498; Web site: www.thecompounders.com.

PRACTICE ALERT

Many pediatric medications are given by drops or dropper. A misunderstanding of these terms by parents can result in a potential overdose.* In addition, many droppers that come with medications are marked in tenths of cubic centimeters. If a parent were to use a syringe instead of the dropper, 0.4 cc may be thought to be the same as 4 cc. Educate parents about the correct methods for giving medication and demonstrate the proper techniques.

*Rudy C: A drop or a dropper: the risk of overdose, *J Pediatr Health Care* 6(1):40, 51-52, 1992.

PRACTICE ALERT

When a dose is ordered that is outside the usual range, or if there is some question regarding the preparation or the route of administration, the nurse always checks with the practitioner before proceeding with the administration, since the nurse is legally liable for any drug administered.

 Unit 3

Intramuscular Administration*

Explain procedure to child as developmentally appropriate and provide atraumatic care (Atraumatic Care box).

Use safety precautions in administering medications. (See p. 242.)

Obtain necessary equipment.

Select needle and syringe appropriate to the following:
Amount of fluid to be administered (syringe size)
Viscosity of fluid to be administered (needle gauge)
Amount of tissue to be penetrated (needle length)

Maximum volume to be administered in a single site is 1 ml for older infants and small children.

If withdrawing medication from an ampule, use a needle equipped with a filter that removes glass particles; then use a new, nonfilter needle for injection.

Maintain strict asepsis and standard precautions.

Determine the site of injection (See pp. 245-246.); make certain muscle is large enough to accommodate volume and type of medication.
Older children—select site as with the adult patient; allow child some choice of site, if feasible.
Following are acceptable sites for infants and small or debilitated children:
Vastus lateralis muscle
Ventrogluteal muscle
Dorsogluteal muscle is insufficiently developed to be a safe site for infants and small children.

Administer the medication:
Provide for sufficient help in restraining the child; children are often uncooperative, and their behavior is usually unpredictable.
Explain briefly what is to be done and, if appropriate, what the child can do to help.
Expose injection area for unobstructed view of landmarks.
Select a site where the skin is free of irritation and danger of infection; palpate for and avoid sensitive or hardened areas. With multiple injections, rotate sites.
Place the child in a lying or sitting position; the child is not allowed to stand for the following reasons:
Landmarks are more difficult to assess.
Restraint is more difficult.
The child may faint and fall.
Grasp the muscle firmly between the thumb and fingers to isolate and stabilize the muscle for deposition of the drug in its deepest part; in obese children spread the skin with the thumb and index finger to displace subcutaneous tissue and grasp the muscle deeply on each side.
Prepare area for puncture with bacteriostatic agent.
Insert needle quickly using a dartlike motion.
Avoid tracking any medication through superficial tissues:
Replace needle after withdrawing medication.
Use the Z track and/or air-bubble technique as indicated.
Avoid any depression of the plunger during insertion of the needle.
Aspirate for blood.
If blood is found, remove syringe from site, change needle, and reinsert into new location.
If no blood is found, inject into a relaxed muscle:
Dorsogluteal—Place child on abdomen with legs and toes rotated inward.
Ventrogluteal—Place child on side with upper leg flexed and placed in front of lower leg.
Inject medication slowly over several seconds.
Remove needle quickly; hold gauze sponge firmly against skin near needle when removing it to avoid pulling on tissue.

*See Community and Home Care Instructions, p. 600, for intramuscular injection; and p. 603 for subcutaneous injection.

ATRAUMATIC CARE

Parenteral Injections

Select a method to anesthetize the puncture site:
Apply EMLA on site 2½ hours before 1M injection.
Use a vapocoolant spray (e.g., Fluori-Methane or ethyl chloride)* just before injection

Allow skin preparation to dry completely before skin is penetrated.

Have medication at room temperature.

Use a new, sharp needle with smallest gauge that permits free flow of the medication and safe penetration of muscle.

Decrease perception of pain:
Distract child with conversation.
Give child something on which to concentrate (e.g., squeezing a hand or bed rail, pinching own nose, humming, counting, yelling "ouch!").
Say to child, "If you feel this, tell me to take it out."
Have child hold a small bandage and place it on puncture site after IM injection is given.

Enlist parents' presence if they wish to participate and/or assist.

Restrain child *only as needed* to perform procedure safely. (See restraining methods and "therapeutic hugging," p. 229.)

Insert needle quickly using a dartlike motion.

Avoid tracking any medication through superficial tissues:
Replace needle after withdrawing medication, or wipe medication from needle with sterile gauze.
If withdrawing medication from an ampule, use a needle equipped with a filter that removes glass particles; then use a new, nonfilter needle for injection.

Use the Z track and/or air-bubble technique as indicated.

Avoid any depression of the plunger during insertion of the needle.

Place a small bandage on puncture site (unless skin is compromised, e.g., in low-birth-weight infant); with young children decorate bandage by drawing a smiling face or other symbol of acceptance.

Hold and cuddle young child and encourage parents to comfort child; praise older child.

*Abbott K, Fowler-Kerry S: The use of a topical refrigerant anesthetic to reduce injection pain in children, *J Pain Symptom Manage* 10(8):584-590, 1995; Cohen Reis E, Holubkov R: Vapocoolant spray is equally effective as EMLA cream in reducing immunization pain in school-aged children, *Pediatrics* 100(6):E5, 1997.

Apply firm pressure with dry, sterile gauze to the site after injection; massage the site to hasten absorption unless contraindicated (e.g., with heparin, iron, dextran).

Clean area of prepping agent with water to decrease absorption of agent in neonate.

Praise child for cooperation.

Discard syringe and uncapped, uncut needle in puncture-resistant container near site of use.

Record date, time, dose, drug, and site of injection.

Unit 3

Intramuscular Injection Sites in Children

Site	Discussion

Vastus Lateralis

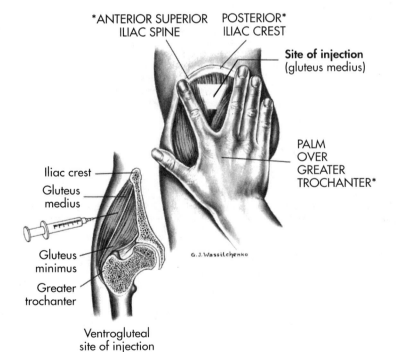

GREATER TROCHANTER*
Sciatic nerve
Femoral artery
Site of injection
(vastus lateralis)
Rectus femoris
KNEE JOINT*

Location*

Palpate to find greater trochanter and knee joints; divide vertical distance between these two landmarks into thirds; inject into middle one third

Needle insertion and size

Insert needle at 90-degree angle between syringe and upper thigh in infants and in young children
22 to 25 gauge, ⅝ to 1 inch†

Advantages

Large, well-developed muscle that can tolerate larger quantities of fluid (0.5 ml [infant] to 2.0 ml [child])
Easily accessible if child is supine, side lying, or sitting

Disadvantages

Thrombosis of femoral artery from injection in midthigh area (rectus femoris muscle)
Sciatic nerve damage from long needle injected posteriorly and medially into small extremity
More painful than deltoid or gluteal sites

Ventrogluteal

ANTERIOR SUPERIOR ILIAC SPINE   POSTERIOR ILIAC CREST

Site of injection (gluteus medius)

PALM OVER GREATER TROCHANTER*

Iliac crest
Gluteus medius
Gluteus minimus
Greater trochanter

G.J.Wassilchenko

Ventrogluteal site of injection

Location*

Palpate to locate greater trochanter, anterior superior iliac tubercle (found by flexing thigh at hip and measuring up to 1 to 2 cm above crease formed in groin), and posterior iliac crest; place palm of hand over greater trochanter, index finger over anterior superior iliac tubercle, and middle finger along crest of ilium posteriorly as far as possible; inject into center of V formed by fingers

Needle insertion and size

Insert needle perpendicular to site but angled slightly toward greater trochanter
22 to 25 gauge, ½ to 1 inch

Advantages

Free of important nerves and vascular structures
Easily identified by prominent bony landmarks
Thinner layer of subcutaneous tissue than in dorsogluteal site, thus less chance of depositing drug subcutaneously rather than intramuscularly
Can accommodate larger quantities of fluid (0.5 ml [infant] to 2.0 ml [child])
Easily accessible if child is supine, prone, or side lying
Less painful than vastus lateralis

Disadvantages

Health professionals' unfamiliarity with site

---

*Locations of landmarks are indicated by asterisks on illustrations.
†Research has shown that a 1-inch needle is needed for adequate muscle penetration in infants 4 months old, and possibly in infants as young as 2 months (Hick J and others: Optimum needle length for diphtheria-tetanus-pertussis inoculation of infants, *Pediatrics* 84(1):136-137, 1989). One of the most important features of injecting vaccines is adequate penetration of the muscle for the deposition of the drug intramuscularly and not subcutaneously. Based on ultrasonography, two injection techniques have been studied to determine the best needle length for the deltoid and vastus lateralis sites. If the muscle is grasped or bunched, a needle length of 25 mm (1 inch) is recommended. If the muscle is stretched or flattened, a needle length of 16 mm (⅝ inch) is adequate (Groswasser J and others: Needle length and injection technique for efficient intramuscular vaccine delivery in infants and children evaluated through an ultrasonographic determination of subcutaneous and muscle layer thickness, *Pediatrics* 99(3, pt 1):400-402, 1997). Unfortunately, the conclusions of the study fail to address whether these lengths apply to both muscles. From the data, it appears more likely that the recommendations apply to the thigh muscle only. Other recommendations for needle size and volume of fluid are based on traditional practice and have not been verified by research.

Continued

Unit 3

Intramuscular Injection Sites in Children—cont'd

Site	Discussion

Dorsogluteal

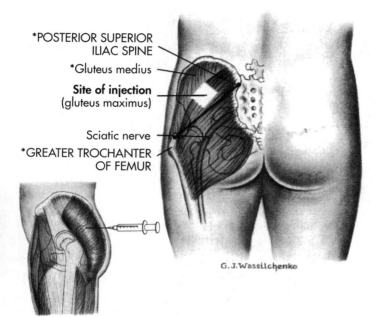

G.J.Wassilchenko

Location*

Locate greater trochanter and posterior superior iliac spine; draw imaginary line between these two points and inject lateral and superior to line into gluteus maximus or medius muscle

Needle insertion and size

Insert needle perpendicular to surface on which child is lying when prone

20 to 25 gauge, ½ to 1½ inches

Advantages

In older child, large muscle mass; well-developed muscle can tolerate greater volume of fluid (up to 2.0 ml)

Child does not see needle and syringe

Easily accessible if child is prone or side lying

Disadvantages

Contraindicated in children who have not been walking for at least 1 year

Danger of injury to sciatic nerve

Thick, subcutaneous fat, predisposing to deposition of drug subcutaneously rather than intramuscularly

Inaccessible if child is supine

Exposure of site may cause embarrassment in older child

Labels on illustration: *POSTERIOR SUPERIOR ILIAC SPINE; *Gluteus medius; **Site of injection** (gluteus maximus); Sciatic nerve; *GREATER TROCHANTER OF FEMUR

Deltoid

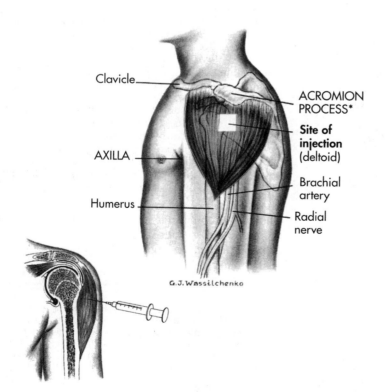

G.J.Wassilchenko

Location*

Locate acromion process; inject only into upper third of muscle that begins about two fingerbreadths below acromion but is above axilla

Needle insertion and size

Insert needle perpendicular to site with syringe angled slightly toward elbow

22 to 25 gauge, ½ to 1 inch

Advantages

Faster absorption rates than gluteal sites

Easily accessible with minimum removal of clothing

Less pain and fewer local side effects from vaccines as compared with vastus lateralis

Disadvantages

Small muscle mass; only limited amounts of drug can be injected (0.5 to 1.0 ml)

Small margins of safety with possible damage to radial nerve and axillary nerve (not shown, lies under deltoid at head of humerus)

Labels on illustration: Clavicle; ACROMION PROCESS*; **Site of injection** (deltoid); AXILLA; Brachial artery; Humerus; Radial nerve

---

*Locations of landmarks are indicated by asterisks on illustrations.

Unit 3

Subcutaneous and Intradermal Administration

Explain procedure to child as developmentally appropriate and provide atraumatic care. (See Atraumatic Care box on p. 244.)

Obtain necessary equipment.

Maintain strict asepsis and standard precautions.

Any site may be used where there are relatively few sensory nerve endings, and large blood vessels and bones are relatively deep.

Suggested sites:

Center third of lateral aspect of upper arm

Abdomen

Center third of anterior thigh

(Avoid the medial side of arm or leg, where skin is more sensitive.)

After injection:

Clean area of prepping agent with water to decrease absorption of agent in neonate.

Praise child for cooperation.

Discard syringe and uncapped, uncut needle in puncture-resistant container near site of use.

Record date, time, dose, drug, and site of injection.

NEEDLE SIZE AND INSERTION

Use 26- to 30-gauge needle; change needle before skin puncture if it pierced a rubber stopper on a vial.

Prepare area for puncture with bacteriostatic agent.

Inject small volumes (up to 0.5 ml).

SUBCUTANEOUS ADMINISTRATION (FIG. 3-11)

Pinch tissue fold with thumb and index finger.

Using a dartlike motion, insert needle at a 90-degree angle. (Some practitioners use a 45-degree angle on children with little subcutaneous tissue or those who are dehydrated. However, the benefit of using the 45-degree angle rather than the 90-degree angle remains controversial.)

Aspirate for blood. (Some practitioners believe it is not necessary to aspirate before injecting subcutaneously; however, this is not universally accepted. Automatic injector devices do not aspirate before injecting.)

Inject medication slowly without tracking through tissues.

INTRADERMAL ADMINISTRATION

Spread skin site with thumb and index finger if needed for easier penetration.

Insert needle with bevel up and parallel to skin.

Aspirate for blood.

Inject medication slowly.

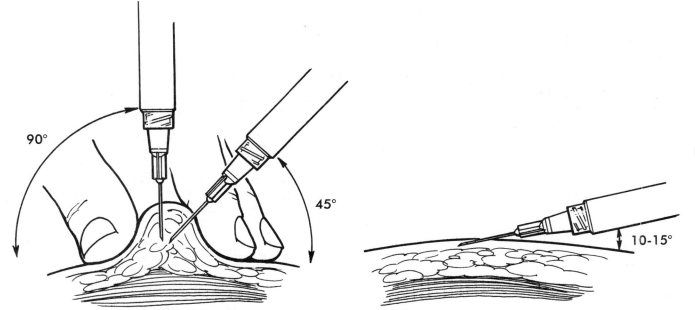

Fig. 3-11 A, Comparison of the angles of insertion for injections. **A,** Subcutaneous (90 or 45 degrees); **B,** intradermal (10 to 15 degrees).

Intravenous Administration*

Explain procedure to child as developmentally appropriate and provide atraumatic care. (See Atraumatic Care box on p. 244.)

Obtain necessary equipment.

Maintain strict asepsis and standard precautions (Community Focus box).

Prepare area for puncture with bacteriostatic agent.

To establish venous access:

Apply tourniquet; optional tourniquet for neonate is a rubber band.

Visualize or palpate vein.

Insert needle with bevel up; a slight pop may be felt when entering child's vein; in small and preterm infants this may not occur.

Release tourniquet, if used.

To access existing IV device:

Assess the status of IV infusion to determine that it is functioning properly.

Inspect injection site to make certain the catheter or needle is secure.

See also implanted venous access device, p. 240.

Dilute the drug in an amount of solution in a syringe or graduate chamber of buret (such as a Volutrol) according to the following:

Compatibility with infusion fluids or other intravenous drugs child is receiving

Size of the child

Size of the vein being used for infusion

Length of time over which the drug is to be administered (e.g., 30 minutes, 1 hour, or 2 hours)

Rate at which the drug is to be infused

---

*Directions for care of intermittent infusion device and central venous catheter are in Community and Home Care Instructions on pp. 605-610.

Strength of the drug or the degree to which it is toxic to subcutaneous tissues

Need for fluid restriction

Monitor until medication has been infused. Medication is not completely administered until solution in tubing between buret chamber and needle site has infused also (amount of solution depends on tubing length).

Withdraw needle from device or site.

Apply dry, sterile gauze or cotton ball to site with firm pressure until bleeding stops.

If antecubital site is used, keep arm extended to reduce bruising.

Clean area of prepping agent with water to decrease absorption of agent in neonate.

Praise child for cooperation.

Discard syringe and uncapped, uncut needle in puncture-resistant container near site of use.

Record date, time, dose, drug, and site of infection.

COMMUNITY FOCUS

Preventing IV Site Infections

With the increasing use of IV therapy in the community, preventing infection is essential. The most effective ways to prevent infection of an IV site are to wash hands between each patient, wear gloves when inserting an IV catheter, closely monitor the date of IV placement, and inspect the insertion site and physical condition of the IV dressing. Proper education of the patient and family regarding signs and symptoms of an infected IV site can help prevent infections from going unnoticed.

Rectal Administration
*Suppository**

Medications may need to be administered rectally if the oral route is not available (Practice Alert).

---

*See Community and Home Care Instructions, p. 611.

Retention Enema

1. Dilute drug in smallest amount of solution possible.
2. Insert well into rectum. Depending on volume, may use

PRACTICE ALERT

Rectal suppositories are usually inserted with the apex (pointed end) first. One study demonstrated easier insertion and a lower expulsion rate when the suppository was inserted with the base (blunt end) first.* Reverse contractions or the pressure gradient of the anal canal may help the suppository to slip higher into the canal. This study, however, did not consider the issue of comfort on insertion.

*Abd-el-Maeboud K and others: Rectal suppository: common sense and mode of insertion, *Lancet* 338(8770):798-800, 1991.

syringe with rubber tubing, enema bottle, or enema bag. (See Fig. 1-6, p. 33.)

3. Hold or tape buttocks together for 5 to 10 minutes.

Eye, Ear, and Nose Administration

(See Atraumatic Care box.)

Unit 3

*Eye Medication**

Eye drops are administered in the same manner as to adults. Children, however, require additional preparation (Practice Alert).

———

*See Community and Home Care Instructions, p. 612.

*Ear Medication**

Depending on the child's age, the pinna is pulled differently. Such variations are discussed in the Community and Home Care Instructions.

———

*See Community and Home Care Instructions, p. 613.

*Nose Drops**

Nose drops are administered in the same manner as to adults. Different positions may be used, depending on the child's age.

———

*See Community and Home Care Instructions, p. 614.

Nasogastric, Orogastric, or Gastrostomy Administration

Use elixir or suspension preparations of medication (rather than tablets) whenever possible (Practice Alert).

Dilute viscous medication or syrup with a small amount of water if possible.

If administering tablets, crush them to a very fine powder and dissolve drug in a small amount of warm water.

Never crush enteric-coated or sustained-release tablets or capsules.

Avoid oily medications because they tend to cling to the sides of the tube.

Do not mix medication with enteral formula unless fluid is restricted. If adding a drug:

Check with pharmacist for compatibility.

Shake formula well and observe for any physical reaction (e.g., separation or precipitation).

Label formula container with name of medication, dosage, date, and time infusion started.

Have medication at room temperature.

Measure medication in calibrated cup or syringe.

Check for correct placement of nasogastric or orogastric tube.

Attach syringe (with adaptable tip but without plunger) to tube.

Pour medication into syringe.

Unclamp tube and allow medication to flow by gravity.

Adjust height of container to achieve desired flow rate (e.g., increase height for faster flow).

 PRACTICE ALERT

Sprinkle-type medications should be avoided. However, if there is no other option and the tube is large gauge (18 French or greater), but usually not a Foley catheter, it may be given by mixing the sprinkles with a small amount of pureed fruit and thinning with water. The fruit keeps the sprinkles suspended so they do not float to the top. Flush well. This procedure is not recommended for skin-level gastrostomy devices.

As soon as syringe is empty, pour in water to flush tubing.

Amount of water depends on length and gauge of tubing.

Determine amount before administering any medication by using a syringe to completely fill an unused nasogastric or orogastric tube with water. The amount of flush solution is usually 1½ times this volume.

With certain drug preparations (e.g., suspensions), more fluid may be needed.

If administering more than one drug at the same time, flush the tube between each medication with clear water.

Clamp tube after flushing, unless tube is left open.

PROCEDURES RELATED TO MAINTAINING FLUID BALANCE OR NUTRITION
Intravenous Fluid Administration

Intravenous therapy is employed for infants and children for the following reasons:

Fluid replacement

Fluid maintenance

A route for administration of medications or other therapeutic substances (e.g., blood, blood products, and immunoglobulin)

Characteristics of pediatric administration sets are as follows:

Calibrated volume and control chamber with a limited capacity and an automatic cutoff mechanism

Drip chamber with microdropper delivering 60 drops/minute or 60 cc/hour

Small-gauge (23 to 25) butterfly (winged) needle, flexible plastic over-the-needle catheter (22 to 24 gauge) or polyethylene tube via surgical cutdown procedure

For longer-term administration, an intermittent infusion device (peripheral or PRN adapter), midline catheter, peripherally inserted central catheter (PICC, p. 251), central venous catheter,* or implanted port (p. 251.)

Injection sites are as follows:

Superficial veins of hand, foot, or arm

Scalp veins (infants)

A site is chosen that restricts the child's movements as little as possible (e.g., avoid a site over a joint).

For extremity veins, start with most distal site, especially if irritating or sclerosing agents are to be used.

Maintain integrity of intravenous site:

Maintain strict asepsis and standard precautions.

Use small, padded armboard.

Use restraints for infants and small children *only as needed.* (See p. 229.)

Provide adequate protection of site.

Observe for signs of infiltration, which may include erythema, pain, edema, blanching, streaking on the skin along the vein, and darkened area at the insertion site.

Change IV tubing and solution at regular intervals (usually every 72 hours) according to institution's policy.

Electronic infusion devices may be used:

Types

Pumps—Have mechanisms to propel the solution at the desired rate under pressure; more accurate than controllers, especially for small infusion rates, but increase the risk of infiltration because of pressure used to infuse fluid; may employ a syringe pump (prefilled syringe is placed in a chamber) or volumetric pump (fluid is pulled from a container by a special disposable cassette)

Controllers—Regulate gravity flow by counting drops with a sensor; are less accurate than pumps; are affected by patient movement but are less likely to cause an infiltration than pumps

Precautions

Excess buildup of pressure:

Drip rate faster than vein can accommodate

Needle out of vein lumen

Apparatus infusing an incorrect amount of fluid:

Assess drip rate by assessing amount infused in a given length of time

Time drip rate if a discrepancy between amount infused and rate set on machine (applies primarily to controllers)

---

*See Community and Home Care Instructions, pp. 605 and 607.

Peripherally Inserted Central Catheters

Description	Benefits	Care Considerations
Made of Silastic or polyurethane material Single or double lumen available Inserted into antecubital fossa and passed through basilic or cephalic vein into superior vena cava (SVC) Positioning of tip in SVC maximizes hemodilution and reduces likelihood of vessel wall damage, phlebitis, or thrombus formation Can be placed as a "midline" catheter, also known as a halfway catheter, ending near axillary vein (Not suitable for total parenteral nutrition [TPN], hyperosmolar solutions, or vesicant chemotherapy)	Do not require operating room placement Can be inserted by specially trained RNs Can use small insertion needles Fast placement Sepsis rates are ≤2%	Sometimes difficult to thread into SVC Reports of resistance to removal Not suitable for rapid fluid replacement because of small lumen size 5- to 10-ml syringe is used for flushing to prevent catheter wall rupture

Long-Term Central Venous Access Devices

Description	Benefits	Care Considerations
TUNNELED CATHETER (E.G., HICKMAN/BROVIAC CATHETER)		
Silicone, radiopaque, flexible catheter with open ends One or two Dacron Cuffs or Vitacuffs (biosynthetic material impregnated with silver ions) on catheter(s) enhance tissue ingrowth May have more than one lumen	Reduced risk of bacterial migration after tissue adheres to Dacron cuff or Vitacuff Easy to use for self-administered infusions	Requires daily heparin flushes Must be clamped or have clamp nearby at all times Must keep exit site dry Heavy activity restricted until tissue adheres to cuff Risk of infection still present Protrudes outside body; susceptible to damage from sharp instruments and may be pulled out; may affect body image More difficult to repair Patient/family must learn catheter care
GROSHONG CATHETER		
Clear, flexible, silicone, radiopaque catheter with closed tip and two-way valve at proximal end Dacron cuff or Vitacuff on catheter enhances tissue ingrowth May have more than one lumen	Reduced time and cost for maintenance care; no heparin flushes needed Reduced catheter damage—no clamping needed because of two-way valve Increased patient safety because of minimum potential for blood backflow or air embolism Reduced risk of bacterial migration after tissue adheres to Dacron cuff or Vitacuff Easily repaired Easy to use for self-administered infusions	Requires weekly irrigation with normal saline Must keep exit site dry Heavy activity restricted until tissue adheres to cuff Risk of infection still present Protrudes outside body; susceptible to damage from sharp instruments and may be pulled out; may affect body image Patient/family must learn catheter care
IMPLANTED PORTS (PORT-A-CATH, INFUS-A-PORT, MEDIPORT, NORPORT, GROSHONG PORT)		
Totally implantable metal or plastic device that consists of self-sealing injection port with top or side access with pre-connected or attachable silicone catheter that is placed in large blood vessel	Reduced risk of infection Placed completely under the skin; therefore cannot be pulled out or damaged No maintenance care and reduced cost for family Heparinized monthly and after each infusion to maintain patency (Groshong port only requires saline) No limitations on regular physical activity, including swimming Dressing only needed when port accessed with Huber needle that is not removed No or only slight change in body appearance (slight bulge on chest)	Must pierce skin for access; pain with insertion of needle; can use local anesthetic (EMLA) or intradermal buffered lidocaine before accessing port Special noncoring needle (Huber) with straight or angled design must be used to inject into port Skin preparation needed before injection Hard to manipulate for self-administered infusions Catheter may dislodge from port, especially if child "plays" with port site (Twiddler syndrome) Vigorous contact sports generally not allowed

Tube Feeding

The purpose of tube feeding is to supply gastrointestinal feeding for the child who is unable to take nourishment by mouth because of anomalies of the throat or esophagus, impaired swallowing capacity, severe debilitation, respiratory distress, or unconsciousness.

Gavage (Nasogastric or Orogastric Tube) Feeding*
Materials Needed

A suitable tube selected according to the size of the child and the viscosity of the solution being fed. Feeding tubes are available in silicone rubber, polyurethane, polyethylene, or polyvinylchloride. Polyurethane and silicone rubber tubes are smaller in diameter and more flexible than the others and are often referred to as small bore tubes.

A receptacle for the fluid: for small amounts a 10- to 30-ml syringe barrel or Asepto syringe is satisfactory; for larger amounts a 50 ml syringe with a catheter tip is more convenient

A syringe to aspirate stomach contents and/or to inject air after the tube has been placed

Water or water-soluble lubricant to lubricate the tube (sterile water is used for infants)

Paper or nonallergenic tape to mark the tube and to attach the tube to the infant's or child's cheek (and nose, if placed in nares)

A stethoscope to determine the correct placement in the stomach

The solution for feeding

*See Community and Home Care Instructions, p. 618.

Procedure: Placement of the Tube

1. Place the child supine with the head slightly hyperflexed or in a sniffing position (nose pointed toward ceiling).
2. Measure the tube for approximate length of insertion and mark the point with a small piece of tape. Two standard methods of measuring length are as follows:
   Measuring from the nose to the earlobe and then to the end of the xiphoid process, or
   Measuring from the nose to the earlobe and then to a point midway between the xiphoid process and umbilicus (Practice Alert)
3. Lubricate the tube with sterile water or water-soluble lubricant and insert through either the mouth or one of the nares to the predetermined mark. Since most young infants are obligatory nose breathers, insertion through the mouth causes less distress and also helps to stimulate sucking. In older infants and children the tube is passed through the nose and the position alternated between nostrils. An indwelling tube is almost always placed through the nose.
   When using the nose, slip the tube along the base of the nose and direct it straight back toward the occiput.
   When entering through the mouth, direct the tube toward the back of the throat.
   If the child is able to swallow on command, synchronize passing the tube with swallowing.
4. Check the position of the tube by using *both* of the following:
   Attach the syringe to the feeding tube and apply negative pressure. Aspiration of stomach contents indicates proper placement, but aspiration of respiratory secretions may be mistaken for stomach contents. However, absence of fluid is not necessarily evidence of improper placement. The stomach may be empty or the tube may not be in contact with stomach contents. Note the amount and character of any fluid aspirated and return the fluid to the stomach.
   With the syringe, inject a small amount of air (0.5 to 1 ml in premature or very small infants to 5 ml in larger children) into the tube while simultaneously listening with a stethoscope over the stomach area. Sounds of gurgling or growling will be heard if the tube is properly situated in the stomach, although it is possible to hear the air entering the stomach even when the tube is positioned above the gastroesophageal sphincter.

If in doubt about placement, consult with the practitioner; radiography may be necessary.

5. Stabilize the tube by holding or taping it to the cheek, not to the forehead because of possible damage to the nostril. To maintain correct placement, measure and record the amount of tubing extending from the nose or mouth to the distal port when the tube is first positioned. Recheck this measurement before each feeding (Table 3-1).

PRACTICE ALERT

Two standard methods for measuring length for tube insertion are described in the text. However, research on using these methods in preterm infants has found both placements to be too high (in the esophagus), although the latter method provided better placement.*

*Weibley TT and others: Gavage tube insertion in the premature infant, *MCN* 12:24-27, 1987; Welch JA and others: Staff nurses' experiences as co-investigators in a clinical research project, *Pediatr Nurs* 16(4):364-367, 396, 1990.

TABLE 3-1 Recommended Minimum Insertion Lengths for Orogastric Tubes in Very-Low-Birth-Weight Infants

	Daily Weight (g)			
	<750	750-999	1000-1249	1250-1499
Insertion length (cm)	13	15	16	17

From Gallaher KJ and others: Orogastric tube insertion length in very-low-birth-weight infants (<1500 grams), *J Perinatol* 13(2):128-131, 1993. Used with permission.

Procedure: Feeding Through the Tube

1. Whenever possible, hold the infant or young child during the feeding to associate the comfort of physical contact with the procedure. When this is not possible, place the infant or child supine or slightly toward the right side with head and chest slightly elevated.

   Use a folded blanket under the head and shoulders for infants and a pillow for small children.

   Raise the head of the bed for larger children.

   If possible, allow infant to suck on a pacifier during feeding for association of suck and satiation (feeling satisfied).

2. Warm the formula to room temperature. Do not microwave. Pour formula into the barrel of the syringe attached to the feeding tube. To start the flow, give a gentle push with the plunger, but then remove the plunger and allow the fluid to flow into the stomach by gravity. To prevent nausea and regurgitation, the rate of flow should not exceed 5 ml every 5 to 10 minutes in preterm and very small infants and 10 ml/minute in older infants and children. The rate is determined by the diameter of the tubing and the height of the reservoir containing the feeding. The rate is regulated by adjusting the height of the syringe. A typical feeding may take 15 to 30 minutes to complete.

3. Flush the tube with sterile water (1 or 2 ml for small tubes; 5 to 15 ml or more for large ones; see discussion of flushing after administering medication through nasogastric tubes on p. 250) to clear it of formula.

4. Cap or clamp indwelling tubes to prevent loss of feeding. If the tube is to be removed, first pinch it firmly to prevent escape of fluid as the tube is withdrawn; then withdraw the tube quickly.

5. Position the child on the right side for at least 1 hour in the same manner as following any infant feeding to minimize the possibility of regurgitation and aspiration. If the child's condition permits, bubble the youngster after the feeding.

6. Record the feeding, including the type and amount of residual, the type and amount of formula, and the manner in which it was tolerated. For most infant feedings, any amount of residual fluid aspirated from the stomach is re-fed to prevent electrolyte imbalance. The amount is subtracted from the prescribed amount of feeding. For example, if the infant/child is to receive 30 ml, and 10 ml is aspirated from the stomach before the feeding, the 10 ml of aspirated stomach contents is re-fed plus 20 ml of feeding. Another method in children: if residual is more than one fourth of the last feeding, return aspirate and recheck in 30 to 60 minutes. When residual is less than one fourth of last feeding, give scheduled feeding. If high aspirates persist and the child is due for another feeding, notify the practitioner.

7. Between feedings give infants pacifiers to satisfy oral needs.

*Gastrostomy Feeding**

The gastrostomy tube is placed under general anesthesia or percutaneously using an endoscope under local anesthesia (typically known as PEG). The tube used can be a Foley, wing-tip, or a mushroom catheter. For children on long-term gastrostomy feeding, a skin-level device may be placed after the initial tube. This device is a small, flexible silicone device that protrudes slightly from the abdomen. It is cosmetically pleasing in appearance, affords increased comfort and mobility to the child, is easy to care for, is fully immersible in water, and has a one-way valve that minimizes reflux and eliminates the need for clamping.

Positioning and feeding of water, formula, and pureed foods is carried out in the same manner and rate as gavage feeding. A mechanical pump may be used to regulate the volume and rate of feeding. With some skin-level devices that do not lock, the child must remain fairly still, because the tubing may easily disconnect from the device if the child moves. Some devices require an additional tube other than the feeding tube to be used for stomach decompression; some do not.

After feedings, the infant or child is positioned on the right side or in Fowler position; the tube may be clamped or left open and suspended between feedings, depending on the child's condition. If the skin-level device is used, insert the extension tube (or decompression tube, in some devices) to remove air in the stomach.

If a Foley catheter is used as the gastrostomy tube, very slight tension is applied and the tube securely taped to maintain the balloon at the gastrostomy opening. This prevents leakage of gastric contents and the tube's progression toward the pyloric sphincter, where it may occlude the stomach outlet. As a precaution, the length of the tube should be measured postoperatively and then remeasured each shift to be sure it has not slipped. A mark can be made above the skin level to further ensure its placement.

*See Community and Home Care Instructions, p. 620.

PROCEDURES RELATED TO MAINTAINING CARDIORESPIRATORY FUNCTION
Respiratory Therapy

Inhalation therapy involves changing the composition, volume, or pressure of inspired gases.

Oxygen Therapy

Methods include use of a mask, hood, hut, nasal cannula, face tent, or oxygen tent.

Method is selected on the basis of the following:
Concentration of inspired oxygen needed
Ability of the child to cooperate in its use

Oxygen is a drug and is only administered as prescribed by dose.

Concentration is regulated according to the needs of the child (usually 40% to 50%, or 4 to 6 liters flow).

Oxygen is dry; therefore, it must be humidified.

Use the following precautions with an oxygen hood:
Do not allow oxygen to blow directly on the infant's face.
Position hood to avoid rubbing against the infant's neck, chin, or shoulders.

Use the following precautions with an oxygen tent:
Plan nursing activities so tent is opened as little as possible.

Tuck open edges of tent carefully to reduce oxygen loss (oxygen is heavier than air).

Check temperature inside tent frequently.

Make certain cooling mechanism is functioning.

Keep child warm and dry.

Examine bedding and clothing periodically and change as needed.

Inspect any toys placed in the tent for safety and suitability. Any source of sparks (e.g., from mechanical or electrical toys) is a potential fire hazard.

Monitor child's color, respirations, and O_2 saturation.

Periodically analyze oxygen concentration at a point near the child's head and adjust oxygen flow rate to maintain desired concentration.

Provide comfort and reassurance to the child, Make sure the child is able to see someone nearby.

Invasive and Noninvasive Oxygen Monitoring

An essential goal in managing sick or injured children is to ensure the continuous delivery of adequate oxygen to vital organs. Although life-saving, oxygen therapy can cause a number of serious sequelae. To monitor oxygen therapy, blood oxygen levels are routinely measured.

Arterial Blood Gas

Direct sampling of the blood's oxygen content (measured as partial pressure of oxygen [Po_2]) can be done on blood obtained from an indwelling arterial catheter or from arterial puncture (Atraumatic Care box).

Arterial blood gases may also be drawn via an umbilical arterial catheter in neonates; a pulmonary arterial catheter may be used in infants and children after heart surgery; and a radial arterial catheter is sometimes utilized for blood sampling. These arterial catheters have inherent dangers, and sampling for arterial blood gases must follow stringent institutional policy to minimize complications.*

ATRAUMATIC CARE

Blood Gas Monitoring

For continuous monitoring of blood gases, noninvasive measurements are used whenever possible. Oximetry should be used before arterial punctures are performed when information about O_2 saturation is sufficient to evaluate the child's condition. (See also p. 238.)

---

*For specific guidelines, see Webster HF: Bioinstrumentation: principles and techniques. In Hazinski MF: *Nursing care of the critically ill child,* St Louis, 1992, Mosby.

Pulse Oximetry

Measures arterial hemoglobin oxygen saturation (Sao_2) by passage of two different wavelengths of light through blood-perfused tissues to a photodetector. Sao_2 and heart rate are displayed on digital readout.

Attach sensor to earlobe, finger, or toe (Fig. 3-12); make certain light source and photodetector are in opposition.

Avoid sites with restricted bloodflow (e.g., distal to a blood pressure cuff or indwelling arterial catheter).

Secure sensor with tape or self-adhering wrap to avoid interference by patient movement. Shield sensor from bright light. Keep extremity warm (e.g., use a sock over foot or hand if extremity is cool).

Avoid intravenous dyes; green, purple, or black nail polish; nonopaque synthetic nails; and possibly footprint ink, which may cause erroneous readings.

Change placement of sensor every 4 to 8 hours. Inspect skin at sensor site in compromised children and change sensor more frequently if needed to prevent pressure necrosis.

Advantages:
    Noninvasive technique
    No complicated preparation or calibration of sensor
    No special skin care needed
    Convenient sites can be used

Disadvantages:
    Requires peripheral arterial pulsation
    Limited use in hypotention or with vasoconstricting drugs
    Sensor affected by movement (Practice Alert).

Sao_2 is related to Po_2, but the values are not the same. As a rule of thumb, an Sao_2 of:
    98% = Po_2 of 100 mm Hg or greater
    90% = Po_2 of 60 mm Hg
    80% = Po_2 of 45 mm Hg
    60% = Po_2 of 30 mm Hg
    (See Fig. 3-13.)

In general, normal range is 95% to 99%. A consistent Sao_2 less than 95% should be investigated, and an Sao_2 of 90% signifies developing hypoxia.

! PRACTICE ALERT !

For the infant: Tape the sensor securely to the great toe and tape the wire to the sole of the foot (or use a commercial holder that fastens with a self-adhering closure). Place a snugly fitting sock over the foot.

For the child: Tape the sensor securely to the index finger and tape the wire to the back of the hand. Use self-adhering Ace-type wrap (e.g., Coban) around the finger and/or hand to further secure the sensor and wire.

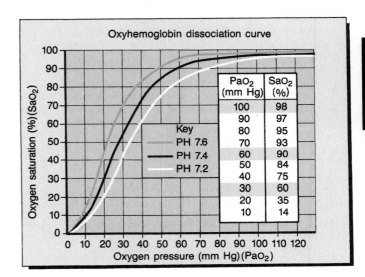

	PaO$_2$ (mm Hg)	SaO$_2$ (%)
	100	98
	90	97
	80	95
	70	93
	60	90
	50	84
	40	75
	30	60
	20	35
	10	14

Key
PH 7.6
PH 7.4
PH 7.2

Fig. 3-13 Oxyhemoglobin dissociation curve. Changes in the affinity of hemoglobin for oxygen shift the position of the oxyhemoglobin dissociation curve. ***Standard curve*** (middle curve): Assumes normal pH (7.4), temperature, Pco_2, and 2,3-DPG levels. ***Shift to left*** (left curve): Increases O_2 affinity of Hb; decreased pH; and increased temperature, Pco_2, and 2,3-DPG. ***Shift to right*** (right curve): Decreases O_2 affinity of Hb; decreased pH; and increased temperature, Pco_2, and 2,3-DPG.

Unit 3

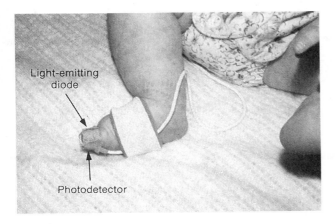

Fig. 3-12 Oximeter sensor on great toe. Note that sensor is positioned with light-emitting diode opposite photodetector. Cord is secured to foot with self-adhering band (not tape) to minimize movement of sensor. (From Wong DL et al: *Whaley and Wong's Nursing care of infants and children,* ed 6, St Louis, 1999, Mosby.)

Transcutaneous Oxygen Monitoring

Measures transcutaneous partial pressure of oxygen in arterial blood (tcPao$_2$) (amount of oxygen dissolved in blood). An electrode attached to the skin causes local hyperemia and arterialization of blood within the capillaries beneath the electrode. A current, created as oxygen diffuses from the capillaries through the skin and a semipermeable membrane, is measured and converted to partial pressure of oxygen (Po$_2$). This is displayed on digital readout. Place electrode on an area with good blood flow but thin subcutaneous skin:
Children—Place on chest

Newborns and young infants—Place on chest, abdomen, or back
Thin infants—Place center of sensor over an intercostal space on chest
Avoid any pressure on electrode (e.g., infant lying on sensor).
Keep temperature of electrode at 44° or 45° C for term infants.
Change placement of electrode every 3 to 4 hours; change more frequently if needed to prevent superficial burns.
Recalibrate electrode each time it is moved.

Aerosol Therapy

The purpose is the inhalation of a solution in droplet (particle) form for direct deposition in the tracheobronchial tree.
Aerosols consist of liquid medications (e.g., bronchodilators, steroids, mucolytics, decongestants, antibiotics, and antiviral agents) suspended in a particulate form in air.
Aerosol generators propelled by air or air-oxygen mixtures generally fall into three categories:
Small-volume jet nebulizers or hand-held nebulizers
Ultrasonic nebulizers for sterile water or saline aerosol only
Metered-dose inhalers (sometimes with a "spacer" device that acts as a reservoir and simplifies use of the inhaler; newer devices, such as the *rotohaler* or *turbuhaler;* eliminate the need for a spacer device and are easier for young children to use)

Deposition of aerosol is maximized by instructing the child to breathe through the mouth with slow, deep inhalations, followed by holding the breath for 5 to 10 seconds, then slow exhalations while in an upright position.
Using an incentive spirometer can help a cooperative child learn this ventilatory pattern.
For infants and young children, activities to produce deep breathing and coughing include feet tapping, tactile stimulation, and crying. The infant must be held upright.
Assessment of breath sounds and work of breathing is performed before and after treatments.

*Bronchial (Postural) Drainage**

The purpose is to facilitate drainage and expectoration of lung and bronchial secretions from specific areas by correct positioning of the patient, using gravity as an aid.

*See Community and Home Care Instructions, p. 632.

Aids to Facilitate Drainage

Consistency of lung secretions is changed from viscid to more liquid by use of the following:
Maintenance of adequate fluid balance (oral or intravenous)
Medication (mucolytics)

Percussion and vibration
Cough stimulation
Breathing exercises

Indications

Pulmonary conditions: bronchitis, cystic fibrosis, pneumonia, asthma, lung abscess, obstructive lung disease
Postoperative prophylaxis: thoracotomy, stasis pneumonia

Prophylaxis in:
Prolonged artificial ventilation
Paralytic conditions
Unconscious patient

Cardiopulmonary Resuscitation (CPR)*
One-rescuer CPR

	Objectives	ACTIONS		
		Adult (over 8 yr)	Child (1 to 8 yr)	Infant (under 1 yr)
A. AIRWAY	1. Assessment: Determine unresponsiveness.	Tap or gently shake shoulder.		
		Say, "Are you okay?"		Speak loudly.
	2. Get help.	Activate EMS.	Shout for help. If second rescuer available, have person activate EMS.	
	3. Position the victim.	Turn on back as a unit, supporting head and neck if necessary (4-10 seconds).		
	4. Open the airway.	Head-tilt/chin-lift.		
B. BREATHING	5. Assessment: Determine breathlessness.	Maintain open airway. Place ear over mouth, observing chest. Look, listen, feel for breathing (3-5 seconds).*		
	6. Give 2 rescue breaths.	Maintain open airway.		
		Seal mouth to mouth.		Mouth to nose/mouth.
		Give 2 slow breaths. Observe chest rise. Allow lung deflation between breaths.		
		1½ to 2 seconds each	1 to 1½ seconds each	
	7. Option for obstructed airway.	a. Reposition victim's head. Try again to give rescue breaths.		
			b. Activate EMS.	
		c. Give 5 subdiaphragmatic abdominal thrusts (the Heimlich maneuver).		c. Give 5 back blows.
				c. Give 5 chest thrusts.
		d. Tongue-jaw lift and finger sweep.	d. Tongue-jaw lift, but finger sweep only if you see a foreign object.	
		If unsuccessful, repeat a, c, and d until successful.		
C. CIRCULATION	8. Assessment: Determine pulselessness.	Feel for carotid pulse with one hand; maintain head-tilt with the other (5-10 seconds).		Feel for brachial pulse: keep head-tilt.
CPR	Pulse absent: Begin chest compressions: 9. Landmark check.	Run middle finger along bottom edge of rib cage to notch at center (top of sternum).		Imagine a line drawn between the nipples.
	10. Hand position.	Place index finger next to finger on notch:		Place 2-3 fingers on sternum. 1 finger's width below line. Depress ½ -1 in.
		Two hands next to index finger. Depress 1½-2 in.	Heel of one hand next to index finger. Depress 1-1½ in.	
	11. Compression rate.	80-100 per minute	100 per minute	At least 100 per minute
	12. Compressions to breaths.	2 breaths to every 15 compressions	1 breath to every 5 compressions	
	13. Number of cycles.	4	20 (approximately 1 minute)	
	14. Reassessment.	Feel for carotid pulse.		Feel for brachial pulse.
		If no pulse, resume CPR, starting with compressions.	If alone, activate EMS. If no pulse, resume CPR, starting with compressions.	
	Pulse present; not breathing: Begin rescue breathing.	1 breath every 5 seconds (12 per minute)	1 breath every 3 seconds (20 per minute)	

Fig. 3-14 One-rescuer CPR. (Modified from Chandra NC, Hazinski MF, editors: *Textbook of basic life support for healthcare providers,* Dallas, 1997, American Heart Association.)
*If victim is breathing or resumes effective breathing, place in recovery position: (1) move head, shoulders, and torso simultaneously; (2) turn onto side; (3) leg not in contact with ground may be bent and knee moved forward to stabilize victim; (4) victim should not be moved in any way if trauma is suspected and should not be placed in recovery position if rescue breathing or CPR is required.

*For a more detailed discussion of CPR in infants, children 1 to 8 years, and children over 8 years, see Community and Home Care Instructions, pp. 640-644.

Two-rescuer CPR for Children Over 8 Years of Age

Step	Objective	Actions
1. AIRWAY	**One rescuer (ventilator):** Assessment: Determine unresponsiveness.	Tap or gently shake shoulder.
		Shout, "Are you okay?"
	Call for help.	Activate EMS.
	Position the victim.	Turn on back if necessary (4-10 sec).
	Open the airway.	Use a proper technique to open airway.
2. BREATHING	Assessment: Determine breathlessness.	Look, listen, and feel (3-5 sec).
	Ventilate twice.	Observe chest rise: 1-1.5 sec/inspiration.
3. CIRCULATION	Assessment: Determine pulselessness.	Feel for carotid pulse (5-10 sec).
	State assessment results.	Say "No pulse."
	Other rescuer (compressor): Get into position for compressions.	Hand, shoulders in correct position.
	Locate landmark notch.	Landmark check.
4. COMPRESSION/ VENTILATION CYCLES	**Compressor:** Begin chest compressions.	Correct ratio compressions/ventilations: 5/1
		Compression rate: 80-100/min (5 compressions/3-4 sec).
		Say any helpful mnemonic.
		Stop compressing for each ventilation.
	Ventilator: Ventilate after every 5th compression and check compression effectiveness. (Minimum of 10 cycles.)	Ventilate 1 time (1.5-2 sec/inspiration).
		Check pulse occasionally to assess compressions.
5. CALL FOR SWITCH	**Compressor:** Call for switch when fatigued.	Give clear signal to change.
		Compressor completes 5th compression.
		Ventilator completes ventilation after 5th compression.
6. SWITCH	Simultaneously switch:	
	Ventilator: Move to chest.	Move to chest.
		Become compressor.
		Get into position for compressions.
		Locate landmark notch.
	Compressor: Move to head.	Move to head.
		Become ventilator.
		Check carotid pulse (5 sec).
		Say "No pulse."
		Ventilate once (1.5-2 sec/inspiration).
7. CONTINUE CPR	Resume compression/ventilation cycles.	Resume Step 4.

Fig. 3-15   Two-rescuer CPR for children over 8 years of age. NOTE: Two-rescuer CPR for children ages 1 to 8 years can be performed similarly to that for adults, with appropriate changes in chest compressions and ventilations. (Modified from Chandra NC, Hazinski MF, editors: *Textbook of basic life support for healthcare providers,* Dallas, 1997, American Heart Association.)

Unit 3

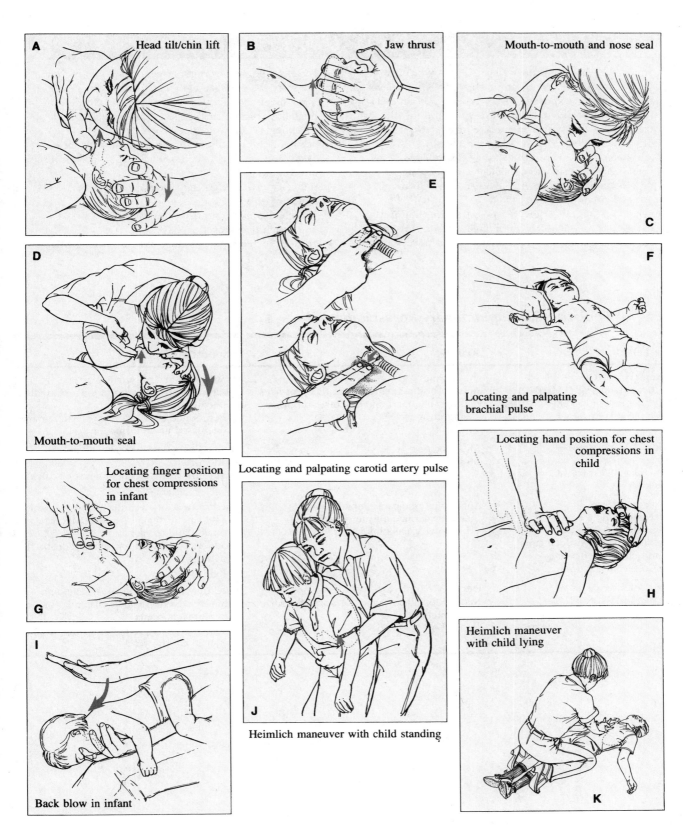

Fig. 3-16 Procedures for cardiopulmonary resuscitation, **A** to **H**; and airway obstruction, **I** to **K**. (From Chandra NC, Hazinski MF, editors: *Textbook of basic life support for healthcare providers*, Dallas, 1997, American Heart Association.)

PRACTICE ALERT

Rescuers who have infections (regardless of type) that may be transmitted by blood or saliva, or who believe they have been exposed to such an infection, should not perform mouth-to-mouth resuscitation if the circumstances allow other immediate or effective methods of ventilation (e.g., use of a bag-valve-mask).

The volume of air in an infant's lungs is small and the air passages are considerably smaller, with resistance to flow potentially higher than in adults. Therefore small puffs of air are delivered.

When a child requires CPR, consider the size, not just the age, of the child, since the guidelines for infants and for children ages 1 to 8 years may not always apply.

For example, young children who can be placed on the rescuer's thigh should receive infant CPR. Since many older children with severe chronic illnesses or disabilities remain small in size, pediatric, not adult CPR, may be appropriate.

When administering drugs during CPR (or a "code"), use a saline flush between medications to prevent drug interactions.

In a conscious, choking child, attempt to relieve the obstruction *only* if:

The child is unable to make any sounds.

The cough becomes ineffective.

These is increasing respiratory difficulty with stridor.

Drugs for Pediatric Cardiopulmonary Resuscitation

Drug/Dose	Action	Implications
Epinephrine HCl IV/IO: 0.01 mg/kg (1:10,000) ET: 0.1 mg/kg (1:1000) (Volume of all doses = 0.1 ml/kg)	Adrenergic Acts on both alpha and beta receptor sites, especially heart and vascular and other smooth muscle	Most useful drug in cardiac arrest Disappears rapidly from bloodstream after injection May produce renal vessel constriction and decreased urine formation
Sodium bicarbonate IV/IO: 1 mEq/kg Newborn: 0.5 mEq/ml 2 mg/kg	Alkalinizer Buffers pH	Infuse slowly and only when ventilation is adequate Don't mix with catecholamines or calcium
Atropine sulfate 0.02 mg/kg/dose Minimum dose: 0.1 mg Maximum single dose: infants and children, 0.5 mg; adolescents, 1.0 mg	Anticholinergic-parasympatholytic Increases cardiac output, heart rate by blocking vagal stimulation in heart	Used to treat bradycardia after ventilatory assessment; always provide adequate ventilation and oxygenation Produces pupil dilation, which constricts with light
Calcium chloride 10% 20 mg/kg IV 0.2 mg/kg/dose q 10 min	Electrolyte replacement Needed for maintenance of normal cardiac contractility	Used only for hypocalcemia, calcium blocker overdose, hyperkalemia, or hypermagnesemia Administer slowly, very sclerosing, administer in central vein

Unit 3

Drugs for Pediatric Cardiopulmonary Resuscitation—cont'd

Drug/Dose	Action	Implications
Lidocaine HCl 1 mg/kg/dose	Antidysrhythmic Inhibits impulses from sensory nerves	Used for ventricular dysrhythmias only
Bretylium 5 mg/kg; may be increased to 10 mg/kg/dose	Antidysrhythmic Inhibits release of norepinephrine in post- ganglionic nerve endings that control ventricular tachycardia	Not a first-line drug for ventricular tachy- cardia; used if lidocaine is not effective Administer rapidly
Adenosine 0.1 to 0.2 mg/kg Maximum single dose: 12 mg Follow with 2 to 3 ml normal saline flush	Antidysrhythmic, for supraventricular tachy- cardia (SVT) Causes a temporary block through the atrioventricular (AV) node and interrupts the reentry circuits	Administer rapidly Very effective Minimal side effects
Naloxone (Narcan) 0.1 mg/kg/dose* May repeat q2 to 3 min	Reverses respiratory arrest due to excessive opiate administration	Evaluate level of pain following administra- tion because analgesic effects of opioids are reversed with large dose of naloxone

Infusions

Drug/Dose	Action	Implications
Epinephrine HCl infusion 0.1 to 1.0 µg/kg/min	Adrenergic (See p. 260.)	Titrated to desired hemodynamic response
Dopamine HCl infusion 2 to 20 µg/kg/min	Agonist Acts on alpha receptors, causing vasocon- striction Increases cardiac output	Titrated to desired hemodynamic response
Dobutamine HCl infusion 2.5 to 15 µg/kg/min	Adrenergic direct-acting β_1-agonist Increases contractility and heart rate	Titrated to desired hemodynamic response Little vasoconstriction, even at high rates
Lidocaine HCl infusion 20 to 50 µg/kg/min	Antidysrhythmic Increases electrical stimulation threshold of ventricle	(See above.) Lower infusion dose used in shock Used for ventricular tachycardia
Isoproterenol 0.1 to 2 µg/kg/min	Relaxes bronchial smooth muscle, increases cardiac contractility and heart rate	Used for emergency treatment of atropine- resistant bradycardia and shock Increased effects with epinephrine

IV, Intravenous route; *IO,* intraosseous route; *ET,* endotracheal route.
*Dose of naloxone to reverse respiratory depression without reversing analgesia from opioids is 0.5 µg/kg in children <40 kg (American Pain Society,
1992).

Unit 3

Foreign Body Airway Obstruction Management
Signs of Life-threatening Obstruction

The truly choking child *cannot speak, becomes cyanotic,* and *collapses*				
	Objectives	**Actions**		
		Adult (over 8 yr)	Child (1 to 8 yr)	Infant (under 1 yr)
CONSCIOUS VICTIM	1. Assessment: Determine airway obstruction.	Ask, "Are you choking?" Determine if victim can cough or speak.		Observe breathing difficulty, ineffective cough, no strong cry.
	2. Act to relieve obstruction.	Perform up to 5 subdiaphragmatic abdominal thrusts (Heimlich maneuver).		Give 5 back blows.
				Give 5 chest thrusts.
	Be persistent.	Repeat Step 2 until obstruction is relieved or victim becomes unconscious.		
VICTIM WHO BECOMES UNCONSCIOUS	3. Position the victim: call for help.	Turn on back as a unit, supporting head and neck, face up, arms by sides. Call out, "Help!" Activate EMS. If second rescuer available, have person activate EMS.		
	4. Check for foreign body.	Perform tongue-jaw lift and finger sweep.	Perform tongue-jaw lift. Remove foreign object only if you actually see it.	
	5. Give rescue breaths.	Open the airway with head-tilt/chin-lift. Try to give rescue breaths. If airway is obstructed, reposition head and try to ventilate again.		
	6. Act to relieve obstruction.	Perform up to 5 subdiaphragmatic abdominal thrusts (Heimlich maneuver).		Give 5 back blows.
				Give 5 chest thrusts.
	7. Be persistent.	Repeat steps 4-6 until obstruction is relieved.		
UNCONSCIOUS VICTIM	1. Assessment: Determine unresponsiveness.	Tap or gently shake shoulder. Shout, "Are you okay?"	Tap or gently shake shoulder.	
		If unresponsive, activate EMS.		
	2. Call for help: position the victim.	Turn on back as a unit, supporting head and neck, face up, arms by sides.		
			Call out for help.	
	3. Open the airway.	Head-tilt/chin-lift.		Head-tilt/chin-lift, but do not tilt too far.
	4. Assessment: Determine breathlessness.	Maintain an open airway. Ear over mouth; observe chest. Look, listen, feel for breathing (3-5 seconds).		
	5. Give rescue breaths.	Make mouth-to-mouth seal.		Make mouth-to-nose-and-mouth seal.
		Try to give rescue breaths.		
	6. If chest is not rising, try again to give rescue breaths.	Reposition head. Try rescue breaths again.		
	7. Activate the EMS system.		If airway obstruction not relieved after about 1 minute, activate EMS as rapidly as possible.	
	8. Act to relieve obstruction.	Perform up to 5 subdiaphragmatic abdominal thrusts (Heimlich maneuver).		Give 5 back blows.
				Give 5 chest thrusts.
	9. Check for foreign body.	Perform tongue-jaw lift and finger sweep.	Perform tongue-jaw lift. Remove foreign object only if you actually see it.	
	10. Rescue breaths.	Open the airway with head-tilt/chin-lift. Try again to give rescue breaths. If airway is obstructed, reposition head and try to ventilate again.		
	11. Be persistent.	Repeat steps 8-10 until obstruction is relieved.		

Fig. 3-17   Foreign body airway obstruction management. (Modified from Chandra NC, Hazinski MF, editors: *Textbook of basic life support for healthcare providers,* Dallas, 1997, American Heart Association.)

Nursing Care Plans

Unit 4

THE PROCESS OF NURSING INFANTS AND CHILDREN

The care of hospitalized children and their families requires the same systematic decision-making approach that is applied to nursing care for all patients. This problem-solving process involves both cognitive and operational skills and consists of five phases:

1. **Assessment**—The analysis and synthesis of collected data
2. **Problem identification**—The determination of the actual or potential problem or need stated as a *nursing diagnosis*
3. **Plan formulation**—A design of action sometimes stated as nursing orders, nursing interventions, or nursing functions
4. **Implementation**—The performance or execution of the plan
5. **Evaluation**—A measure of the outcome of nursing action(s) that either completes the nursing process or serves as a basis for reassessment

Nursing Diagnoses

The nursing diagnosis is the naming of the cue clusters that are obtained during the assessment phase. The North American Nursing Diagnosis Association's (NANDA) currently accepted definition of the term **nursing diagnosis** is: "a clinical judgment about individual, family, or community responses to actual and potential health problems/life processes. Nursing diagnoses provide the basis for selection of nursing interventions to achieve outcomes for which the nurse is accountable."

Nursing diagnoses do *not* describe everything that nursing does. Nursing practice consists of three types of activity: dependent, interdependent, and independent. The differences reside in the source of authority for the action. **Dependent activities** are those areas of nursing practice that hold the nurse accountable for implementing the prescribed medical regimen. **Interdependent activities** are those areas of nursing practice in which medical and nursing responsibility and accountability overlap and require collaboration between the two disciplines. **Independent activities** are those areas of nursing practice that are the direct responsibility of the individual nurse. Nursing diagnoses should reflect the *interdependent* and *independent* dimensions of nursing. In the nursing care plans that follow, dependent activities are identified by an asterisk (*) or a dagger (†).

The nursing diagnoses used in this segment are those compiled and approved by NANDA and organized according to priority. Those selected for inclusion in this unit represent only one interpretation (Box 4-1). Some diagnoses are closely related, and it is often difficult to determine which diagnostic category best represents any given goal. The diagnoses selected for inclusion and nursing interventions serve as a general guide for nursing care of children with health problems; therefore others must be added by the user to individualize care for a specific child or family.

Both NANDA and Marjory Gordon have developed frameworks for nursing diagnoses. NANDA bases its framework on 9 human response patterns; and Gordon bases hers on 11 functional health patterns (Box 4-2). In clinical practice, the classification systems, especially Gordon's patterns, serve as a framework for organizing a nursing assessment and standardizing data collection. Additional research is needed to broaden the list of nursing diagnoses, especially for specialty areas such as pediatrics, and to define a universally accepted taxonomy.

Unit 4

BOX 4-1

NANDA-Approved Nursing Diagnoses 1999-2000

Activity intolerance
Activity intolerance, risk for
Adaptive capacity, decreased: intracranial
Adjustment, impaired
Airway clearance, ineffective
Anxiety
Anxiety, death
Aspiration, risk for
Body image disturbance
Body temperature, altered, risk for
Bowel incontinence
Breastfeeding, effective
Breastfeeding, ineffective
Breastfeeding, interrupted
Breathing pattern, ineffective
Cardiac output, decreased
Caregiver role strain
Caregiver role strain, risk for
Communication, impaired verbal
Community coping, ineffective
Community coping, potential for enhanced
Confusion, acute
Confusion, chronic
Constipation
Constipation, perceived
Constipation, risk for
Coping, defensive
Coping, family: potential for growth
Coping, ineffective family: compromised
Coping, ineffective family: disabling
Coping, ineffective individual
Decisional conflict (specify)
Denial, ineffective
Dentition, altered
Development, altered, risk for
Diarrhea
Disuse syndrome, risk for
Diversional activity deficit
Dysreflexia
Dysreflexia, autonomic, risk for
Energy field disturbance
Environmental interpretation syndrome, impaired
Failure to thrive, adult
Family processes, altered
Family processes, altered: alcoholism
Fatigue
Fear
Fluid volume deficit
Fluid volume deficit, risk for
Fluid volume excess
Fluid volume imbalance, risk for
Gas exchange, impaired
Grieving, anticipatory
Grieving, dysfunctional
Growth, altered, risk for

Growth and development, altered
Health maintenance, altered
Health-seeking behaviors (specify)
Home maintenance management, impaired
Hopelessness
Hyperthermia
Hypothermia
Incontinence, stress
Incontinence, total
Incontinence, urge
Incontinence, urinary, functional
Incontinence, urinary, reflex
Incontinence, urinary urge, risk for
Infant behavior, disorganized
Infant behavior, disorganized: risk for
Infant behavior, organized: potential for enhanced
Infant feeding pattern, ineffective
Infection, risk for
Injury, perioperative positioning: risk for
Injury, risk for
Knowledge deficit (specify)
Latex allergy
Latex allergy, risk for
Loneliness, risk for
Management of therapeutic regimen, community: ineffective
Management of therapeutic regimen, families: ineffective
Management of therapeutic regimen, individual, effective
Management of therapeutic regimen, individuals: ineffective
Memory, impaired
Mobility, impaired bed
Mobility, impaired physical
Mobility, impaired wheelchair
Nausea
Noncompliance (specify)
Nutrition, altered: less than body requirements
Nutrition, altered: more than body requirements
Nutrition, altered: risk for more than body requirements
Oral mucous membrane, altered
Pain
Pain, chronic
Parent/infant/child attachment, altered: risk for
Parental role conflict
Parenting, altered
Parenting, altered, risk for
Peripheral neurovascular dysfunction, risk for
Personal identity disturbance
Poisoning, risk for

Posttrauma syndrome
Posttrauma syndrome, risk for
Powerlessness
Protection, altered
Rape-trauma syndrome
Rape-trauma syndrome: compound reaction
Rape-trauma syndrome: silent reaction
Relocation stress syndrome
Role performance, altered
Self-care deficit, bathing/hygiene
Self-care deficit, dressing/grooming
Self-care deficit, feeding
Self-care deficit, toileting
Self-esteem, chronic low
Self-esteem disturbance
Self-esteem, situational low
Self-mutilation, risk for
Sensory/perceptual alterations (specify) (visual, auditory, kinesthetic, gustatory, tactile, olfactory)
Sexual dysfunction
Sexuality patterns, altered
Skin integrity, impaired
Skin integrity, impaired, risk for
Sleep deprivation
Sleep pattern disturbance
Social interaction, impaired
Social isolation
Sorrow, chronic
Spiritual distress (distress of the human spirit)
Spiritual distress, risk for
Spiritual well-being, potential for enhanced
Suffocation, risk for
Surgical recovery, delayed
Swallowing, impaired
Thermoregulation, ineffective
Thought processes, altered
Tissue integrity, impaired
Tissue perfusion, altered (specify type) (renal, cerebral, cardio-pulmonary, gastrointestinal, peripheral)
Trauma, risk for
Unilateral neglect
Urinary elimination, altered
Urinary retention
Ventilation, inability to sustain spontaneous
Ventilatory weaning response, dysfunction (DVWR)
Violence, risk for: directed at others
Violence, risk for: self-directed
Walking, impaired
Wheelchair transfer ability, impaired

North American Nursing Diagnosis Association: *Nursing diagnoses: definitions and classification 1999-2000*, Philadelphia, 1999, NANDA.

BOX 4-2

Classification Systems for Nursing Diagnoses

Human Response Patterns*

Exchanging—Involves mutual giving and receiving
Communicating—Involves sending messages
Relating—Involves establishing bonds
Valuing—Involves the assigning of relative worth
Choosing—Involves the selection of alternatives
Moving—Involves activity
Perceiving—Involves the reception of information
Knowing—Involves the meaning associated with information
Feeling—Involves the subjective awareness of sensation or affect

Functional Health Patterns†

Health perception-health management pattern—Perceptions related to general health management and preventive practices
Nutritional-metabolic pattern—Intake of food and fluids related to metabolic requirements

Elimination pattern—Regularity and control of excretory functions, bowel, bladder, skin, and wastes
Activity-exercise pattern—Activity patterns that require energy expenditure and provide for rest
Sleep-rest pattern—Effectiveness of sleep and rest periods
Cognitive-perceptual pattern—Adequacy of language, cognitive skills, and perception related to required or desired activities; includes pain perception
Self-perception–self-concept pattern—Beliefs and evaluation of self-worth
Role-relationship pattern—Family and social roles, especially parent-child relationships
Sexuality-reproductive pattern—Problems or potential problems with sexuality or reproduction
Coping-stress tolerance pattern—Stress tolerance level and coping patterns, including support systems
Value-belief patterns—Values, goals, or beliefs that influence health-related decisions and actions

*Modified from the North American Nursing Diagnosis Association: *Nursing diagnoses: definitions and classifications,* 1999-2000, Philadelphia, 1999, NANDA.

†Modified from Gordon M: *Manual of nursing diagnosis,* 1999-2000, St Louis, 1999, Mosby.

NURSING CARE OF THE CHILD AND FAMILY DURING STRESS AND ILLNESS

Illness and hospitalization constitute crisis in the life of the child. Hospitalized children must deal with a strange environment, a number of unfamiliar caregivers, and a general disruption of their usual lifestyle. Often, they must submit to painful procedures, the loss of independence, and an endless series of unknowns. Their interpretation of events, their responses to the experience, and the significance they place on these experiences are directly related to their developmental level (Table 4-1). Therefore to meet the needs of hospitalized children, it is essential that the pediatric nurse has a knowledge of normal growth and development, including some understanding of children's cognitive processes and the meaning that hospitalization has for children of any age. (See Box 4-3, p. 270; and Table 4-2, p. 271.)

NURSING CARE PLAN

The Child in the Hospital

TABLE 4-1   Overview of Children's Reactions to Stress*

Development Achievement and Major Fears	Behavior Reactions	Interventions
INFANT **Trust vs Mistrust**		
Separation	**Protest**—Cries, screams, searches with eyes for parent, clings to parent, avoids and rejects contact with strangers Behaviors may last from hours to days Protest, such as crying, may be continuous, ceasing only with physical exhaustion Approach of stranger may precipitate increased protest **Despair**—Inactive, withdraws from others, depressed, sad, uninterested in environment Behaviors may last for variable length of time; physical condition may deteriorate from refusal to eat, drink, or move **Detachment**—Shows increased interest in surroundings, interacts with strangers or familiar caregivers, forms new but superficial relationships, appears happy Behaviors represent a superficial adjustment; detachment usually occurs after prolonged separation from parent; rarely seen in hospitalized children	Meet physical needs promptly Encourage parents to stay with infant and assist with care Interview parents to determine their customary means for comforting the infant and meeting the child's needs; apply this knowledge in the role of caregiver Provide consistency in staff to allow for continuity of care; assign a primary nurse and associates (primary care) Employ pain reduction techniques Employ comfort measures
Pain	Neonate—Total body reaction, easily distracted Later infancy—Localized reaction, uncooperative, offers physical resistance	
TODDLER **Autonomy vs Shame and Doubt**		
Separation	**Protest**—Verbal cries for parent; verbal attack on others; physically attacks others (e.g., kicks, bites, hits, pinches); tries to escape to find parent; clings to parent and tries to physically force parent to stay **Despair**—Inactive, sad, depressed, uninterested in environment, uncommunicative; regresses to earlier behaviors (e.g., thumb sucking, bed-wetting); loss of language skills **Detachment**—Similar to infants, less regressive behaviors	Encourage parents to room-in whenever possible Allow child to express feelings of protest Accept regressive behaviors without comment Encourage child to talk about family members Encourage parents to leave comfort objects (e.g., a favorite blanket and toy) Interpret child's behaviors to the parents

*For more specific developmental characteristics of children's responses to pain, see p. 321; for additional interventions, see Nursing Care Plan: The Child in Pain, p. 315.

The Child in the Hospital—cont'd

TABLE 4-1 Overview of Children's Reactions to Stress*—cont'd

Development Achievement and Major Fears	Behavior Reactions	Interventions
TODDLER—cont'd		
Autonomy vs Shame and Doubt—cont'd		
Loss of control—Physical constriction, loss of routine and rituals, dependency	Resistance Physical aggression Verbal uncooperativeness	Incorporate home routines important to the child's care as much as possible (e.g., bedtime and bath rituals) Allow child as much mobility as possible
Bodily injury and pain	Regression Negativism Temper tantrums	Employ pain reduction techniques Employ comfort measures
PRESCHOOL		
Initiative vs Guilt		
Separation	**Protest**—Less direct and aggressive than toddler, may displace feelings on others **Despair**—Similar to toddler **Detachment**—Similar to toddler	Encourage parents to visit often Encourage rooming-in whenever possible Allow child to express protest and anger
Loss of control—Sense of own power Bodily injury and pain—Intrusive procedures, mutilation	Aggression—Physical and verbal Regression—Dependency; withdrawal; feelings of fear, anxiety, guilt, shame; physiologic responses	Encourage the child to discuss home and family Accept regressive behaviors Assist child in moving from regressive responses to behaviors appropriate to age (if extended hospitalization) Provide play and diversional activities Encourage child to "play out" feelings and fears Allow as much mobility as possible Encourage parents to leave the child's favorite toys and some tangible evidence of their love Acknowledge the child's fears and anxieties Avoid intrusive procedures when possible (e.g., rectal temperature measurement) Employ appropriate interventions to alleviate pain
SCHOOL-AGE		
Industry vs Inferiority		
Separation (parents as well as peers) Loss of control—Enforced dependency, altered family roles Bodily injury and pain—Fear of illness itself, disability, and death; intrusive procedures in genital area	Usually do not see the behaviors of protest, despair, or detachment associated with earlier stages Any of following may indicate separation as well as other fears—loneliness, boredom, isolation, withdrawal, depression, displaced anger, hostility, frustration Seeks information May passively accept pain Groans or whines Holds rigidly still Tries to act brave Communicates about pain May try to postpone painful event	Encourage parents to visit or room-in whenever possible Allow expression of feelings, both verbally and nonverbally Acknowledge child's fears and concerns and encourage discussion Involve child in activities appropriate to developmental level and condition Encourage peer contacts Continue with child's schooling Employ appropriate interventions to alleviate pain

Continued

The Child in the Hospital—cont'd

TABLE 4-1   Overview of Children's Reactions to Stress*—cont'd

Development Achievement and Major Fears	Behavior Reactions	Interventions
ADOLESCENT		
Identity vs Role Diffusion		
Loss of control—Loss of identity, enforced dependency	Rejection	Explore feelings regarding the hospital and the significance specific illness might have on relationships, identity formation, and future plans
	Uncooperativeness	
Bodily injury and pain—Mutilation, sexual changes	Withdrawal	
	Self-assertion	
	Self-control	Explain procedures, therapies, and routines
	Cooperativeness	Help develop positive coping mechanisms
	Fear, anxiety	Encourage family members to stay or visit often; discuss any preferences with family and adolescent
	Overconfidence	
		Encourage maintaining contact with peer group
Separation (especially peer group)	Depression	Provide privacy
	Loneliness	Provide individualized schooling and recreation
	Boredom	Employ appropriate intervention to alleviate pain

*For more specific developmental characteristics of children's responses to pain, see p. 321; for additional interventions, see Nursing Care Plan: The Child in Pain, p. 315.

BOX 4-3

Meaning of Illness and Hospitalization to the Child

Infant

Change in familiar routine and surroundings; responds with global reaction

Separation from love-object

Toddler

Fear of separation, desertion; separation anxiety highest in this age-group

Relates illness to a concrete condition, circumstance, or behavior

Preschool

Fear of bodily harm or mutilation, castration, intrusive procedures

Separation anxiety less intense than toddler but strong

Causation same as toddler; often considers own role in causation (e.g., illness as a punishment for wrongdoing)

School-age

Fears physical nature of illness

Concern about separation from age-mates and ability to maintain position in peer group

Perceives an external cause for illness, although illness located in body

Adolescent

Anxious regarding loss of independence, control, identity

Concern about privacy

Perceives malfunctioning organ or process as cause of illness

Able to explain illness

The Child in the Hospital—cont'd

TABLE 4-2   **Children's Developmental Concepts of Illness and Pain***

Cognitive Stage (Age)	Concept of Illness†	Concept of Pain‡
Preoperational Thought (2 to 7 years)	*Phenomenism*—Perceives an external, unrelated, concrete phenomenon as the cause of illness (e.g., "being sick because you don't feel well") *Contagion*—Perceives cause of illness as proximity between two events that occurs by "magic" (e.g., "getting a cold because you are near someone who has a cold")	Conceives of pain primarily as physical, concrete experience Thinks in terms of magical disappearance of pain May view pain as punishment for wrongdoing Tends to hold someone accountable for own pain and may strike out at that person
Concrete Operational Thought (7 to 10+ years)	*Contamination*—Perceives cause as a person, object, or action external to the child that is "bad" or "harmful" to the body (e.g., "getting a cold because you didn't wear a hat") *Internalization*—Perceives illness as having an external cause but as being located inside the body (e.g., "getting a cold by breathing in air and bacteria")	Conceives of pain physically (e.g., headache, stomachache) Able to perceive psychologic pain (e.g., someone dying) Fears bodily harm and annihilation (body destruction and death) May view pain as punishment for wrongdoing
Formal Operational Thought (13 years and older)	*Physiologic*—Perceives cause as malfunctioning or nonfunctioning organ or process; can explain illness in sequence of events *Psychophysiologic*—Realizes that psychologic actions and attitudes affect health and illness	Able to give reason for pain (e.g., fell and hit nerve) Perceives several types of psychologic pain Has limited life experiences to cope with pain as adult might cope despite mature understanding of pain Fears losing control during painful experience

*Note: Yoos suggests that children with chronic illness, because of their experiences, may have an understanding of illness beyond that suggested by their developmental stage. (Yoos HL: Children's illness concepts: old and new paradigms, *Pediatr Nurs* 20(2):134-140, 145, 1994.)

†Data from Bibace R, Walsh ME: Development of children's concepts of illness, *Pediatrics* 66(6):912-917, 1980.

‡Data from Hurley A, Whelan EG: Cognitive development and children's perception of pain, *Pediatr Nurs* 14(1):21-24, 1988.

ASSESSMENT

Perform a nursing admission history (Box 4-4), especially regarding clues to child's past experiences with hospitalization, illness, and factors related to reason for hospitalization (e.g., emergency treatment, diagnosis, etc.); determine type of preparation for hospitalization.

Perform a physical assessment. (See Unit 1.)

Observe for manifestations of specific disorder for which child is admitted.

Observe for evidence of stress reactions to the illness and/or hospitalization. (See Table 4-1.)

Continued

Unit 4

The Child in the Hospital—cont'd

BOX 4-4

Nursing Admission History According to Functional Health Patterns*

Health Perception-Health Management Pattern

Why has your child been admitted?

How has your child's general health been?

What does your child know about this hospitalization?

　Ask the child why he or she came to the hospital.

　If answer is, "for an operation or for tests," ask the child to tell you about what will happen before, during, and after the operation or tests.

Has your child ever been in the hospital before?

　How was that hospital experience?

　What things were important to you and your child during that hospitalization? How can we be most helpful now?

What medications does your child take at home?

　Why are they given?

　When are they given?

　How are they given (if a liquid, with a spoon; if a tablet, swallowed with water; or other)?

　Does your child have any trouble taking medication? If so, what helps?

　Is your child allergic to any medications?

What, if any, forms of alternative or complementary medicine are being used?

Nutrition-Metabolic Pattern

What are the family's usual mealtimes?

Do family members eat together or at separate times?

What are your child's favorite foods, beverages, and snacks?

　What are the average amounts consumed or usual size of portions?

　Any special cultural practices, such as eating only ethnic food?

What foods and beverages does your child dislike?

What are your child's feeding habits (bottle, cup, spoon, eats by self, needs assistance, any special devices)?

How does your child like food served (warmed, cold, one item at a time)?

How would you describe your child's usual appetite (hearty eater, picky eater)?

　Has being sick affected your child's appetite?

Are there any known or suspected food allergies? Is your child on a special diet?

Are there any feeding problems (excessive fussiness, spitting up, colic); any dental or gum problems that affect feeding?

What do you do for these problems?

Elimination Pattern

What are your child's toilet habits (diaper, toilet-trained [day only or day and night], words used to communicate urination or defecation, potty chair, regular toilet, other routines)?

What is your child's usual patterns of elimination (bowel movements)?

Do you have any concerns about elimination (bed-wetting, constipation, diarrhea)?

　What do you do for these problems?

Have you ever noticed that your child sweats a lot?

Sleep-Rest Pattern

What are your child's usual hours of sleep and awakening?

What is your child's schedule for naps; length of naps?

Is there a special routine before sleeping (bottle, drink of water, bedtime story, nightlight, favorite blanket or toy, prayers)?

Is there a special routine during sleep time, such as waking to go to the bathroom?

What type of bed does your child sleep in?

Does your child have a separate room or share a room; if shared, with whom?

What are the home sleeping arrangements (alone or with others [e.g., sibling, parent, other person])?

What is your child's favorite sleeping position?

Are there any sleeping problems (falling asleep, waking during night, nightmares, sleep walking)?

Are there any problems awakening and getting ready in the morning?

What do you do for these problems?

Activity-Exercise Pattern

What is your child's schedule during the day (preschool, daycare center, regular school, extracurricular activities)?

What are your child's favorite activities or toys (both active and quiet interests)?

What is your child's usual television viewing schedule at home?

　What are your child's favorite programs?

　Are there any television restrictions?

Does your child have any illness or disabilities that limit activity?

　If so, how?

What are your child's usual habits and schedule for bathing (tub bath or shower, sponge bath, shampoo)?

What are your child's dental habits (brushing, flossing, fluoride supplements or rinses, favorite toothpaste); schedule of daily dental care?

*The focus of the admission history is the child's psychosocial environment. Most of the questions are worded in terms of parental responses. Depending on the child's age, they should be addressed directly to the child when appropriate.

Unit 4

The Child in the Hospital—cont'd

BOX 4-4

Nursing Admission History According to Functional Health Patterns*—cont'd

Activity-Exercise Pattern—cont'd

Does your child need help with dressing or grooming, such as hair combing?

Are there any problems with the above (dislike of or refusal to bathe, shampoo hair, or brush teeth)? What do you do for these problems?

Are there special devices that your child requires help in managing (eyeglasses, contact lenses, hearing aid, orthodontic appliances, artificial elimination appliances, orthopedic devices)?

NOTE: Use the following code to assess functional self-care level for feeding, bathing/hygiene, dressing/grooming, toileting:

O: Full self-care

I: Requires use of equipment or device

II: Requires assistance or supervision from another person

III: Requires assistance or supervision from another person and equipment or device

IV: Is dependent and does not participate

Cognitive-Perceptual Pattern

Does your child have any hearing difficulty?

Does the child use a hearing aid?

Have "tubes" been placed in your child's ears?

Does your child have any vision problems?

Does the child wear glasses or contact lenses?

Does your child have any learning difficulties?

What is the child's grade in school?

Self-Perception–Self-Concept Pattern

How would you describe your child (e.g., takes time to adjust, settles in easily, shy, friendly, quiet, talkative, serious, playful, stubborn, easygoing)?

What makes your child angry, annoyed, anxious, or sad? What helps?

How does your child act when annoyed or upset?

What has been your child's experience with and reaction to temporary separation from you (the parent)?

Does your child have any fears (e.g., of places, objects, animals, people, situations)? How do you handle them?

Do you think your child's illness has changed the way he or she thinks about self (e.g., more shy, embarrassed about appearance, less competitive with friends, stays at home more)?

Role-Relationship Pattern

Does your child have a favorite nickname?

What are the names of other family members or others who live in the home (relatives, friends, pets)?

Who usually takes care of your child during the day/night (especially if other than parent, such as baby-sitter or relative)?

Which members of your family/extended family participate in childrearing/health decisions? To what extent?

What are the parents' occupations and work schedules?

Are there any special family considerations (adoption, foster child, stepparent, divorce, single parent)?

Have any major changes in the family occurred lately (death, divorce, separation, birth of a sibling, loss of a job, financial strain, mother beginning a career, other)? Describe child's reaction.

Who are your child's play companions or social groups (peers, younger or older children, adults, prefers to be alone)?

Do things generally go well for your child in school and with friends?

Does your child use "security" objects at home (pacifier, thumb, bottle, blanket, stuffed animal, or doll)? Did you bring any of these to the hospital?

How do you handle discipline problems at home? Are these methods always effective?

Does your child have any condition that interferes with communication? If so, what are your suggestions for communicating with your child?

Will your child's hospitalization affect the family's financial support or care of other family members (e.g., other children)?

What concerns do you have about your child's illness and hospitalization?

Who will be staying with your child while hospitalized?

How can we contact you or another close family member outside of the hospital?

Sexuality-Reproductive Pattern

(Answer questions that apply to your child's age-group.)

Has your child begun puberty (developing physical sexual characteristics, menstruation)? Have you or your child had any concerns?

Does your daughter know how to do breast self-examination?

Does your son know how to do testicular self-examination?

How have you introduced topics of sexuality with your child?

Do you feel you might need some help with some topics?

Has your child's illness affected the way he or she feels about being a boy or a girl? If so, how?

Do you have any concerns with behaviors in your child, such as masturbation, asking many questions or talking about sex, not respecting others' privacy, or wanting too much privacy?

Continued

The Child in the Hospital—cont'd

BOX 4-4

Nursing Admission History According to Functional Health Patterns*—cont'd

Sexuality-Reproductive Pattern—cont'd

Initiate a conversation about an adolescent's sexual concerns using open-ended to more direct questions and using the terms "friends" or "partners" rather than "girlfriend" or "boyfriend":

"Tell me about your social life."

"Who are your closest friends?" (If one friend is identified, consider asking more about that relationship, such as how much time they spend together, how serious they are about each other, if the relationship is going the way the teenager hoped.)

Consider asking about dating and sexual issues, such as the teenager's views on sex education, "going steady," "living together," and premarital sex.

"Which friends would you like to have visit in the hospital?"

Coping-Stress Tolerance Pattern

(Answer questions that apply to your child's age-group.)

What does your child do when tired or upset?

If upset, does your child want a special person or object? If so, explain.

If your child has temper tantrums, what causes them and how do you handle them?

Whom does your child talk to when worried about something?

How does your child usually handle problems or disappointments?

Have there been any big changes or problems in your family recently?

How did you handle them?

Has your child ever had a problem with drugs or alcohol or attempted suicide?

Do you think your child is "accident prone"? If so, explain.

Value-Belief Pattern

Do you have religious beliefs? If so, what religion?

How is religion or faith important in your child's life?

What religious practices would you like continued in the hospital (e.g., prayers before meals/bedtime; visit by minister, priest, or rabbi; prayer group)?

What religious practices do you follow that affect child-rearing/health practice (e.g., fasting/herbal remedies)?

What do you believe caused your child's illness/condition?

When illness/injury occurs, do you use any herbs, medicines, healer, rituals, or ceremonies?

What are your family's prior health care experiences?

What are your concerns with this health care system?

What do you do when your child is sick? What person do you go to first?

What generation immigrant are you—first? Second? Third?

What languages does your child speak/understand? What languages do you and other family members speak/understand?

With whom do you discuss child-related concerns or problems?

*The focus of the admission history is the child's psychosocial environment. Most of the questions are worded in terms of parental responses. Depending on the child's age, they should be addressed directly to the child when appropriate.

The Child in the Hospital—cont'd

NURSING DIAGNOSIS: Anxiety/fear related to separation from accustomed routine and support system; unfamiliar surroundings

---

■ **PATIENT GOAL 1:** Will experience minimized separation

NURSING INTERVENTIONS/*RATIONALES*

Assign same nursing personnel as much as possible and a primary nurse *to provide the consistency that builds trust*

Arrange workload and schedule to allow personal contact with child

Encourage parents to room-in whenever possible *to prevent separation*

Provide an atmosphere of warmth and acceptance for both child and parents

Encourage parents and others to cuddle, hug, and otherwise demonstrate affection for child

Recognize child's separation behaviors as normal

    Allow child to cry, *since this is a normal response to separation*

    Provide support through physical presence

Maintain child's contact with parents and siblings and home

    Talk frequently about child's family

    Encourage child to talk about and remember family members, pets

    Stress significance of parents' and siblings' visits, telephone calls, and letters

Help parents understand the behaviors of separation anxiety and suggest ways of supporting the child

    Explain to child when parents leave and when they will return

    Tell hospitalized child the reason for leaving

    Convey the expected time of return in terms of anticipated events. For example, if the parents will return in the morning, they can say they will see the child, "After the sun comes up," or, "When (a favorite program) is on television"

    Use a clock or calendar for an older child *so child can anticipate next family visit*

    Encourage family to visit for short but frequent periods, rather than one long time; encourage parents and relatives to take turns visiting

    Encourage visits from siblings, grandparents, and other significant persons in child's life

    Leave favorite articles from home, such as a blanket, toy, bottle, feeding utensil, or article of clothing, with child *since this helps child tolerate separation*

    Respect treasured objects of older children, such as a stuffed animal

    Encourage family to provide photographs of family members and recordings of the parents' voices (e.g., reading a story, singing a song, saying prayers before bedtime, or relating events at home) *to familiarize child with the unfamiliar environment and to provide comfort during times of separation*

    Play family recordings at lonely times, such as before sleep

    Suggest that the family leave small gifts for the child to open each day: if the parents know when their next visit will be, have them leave the number of packages that correspond to the days between visits

Assign a "foster grandparent" or consistent volunteer to be with child if available

EXPECTED OUTCOMES

Child has consistent caregivers

Parents visit as much as possible

Parents cooperate in care (specify)

Child accepts and responds positively to comforting measures

Child discusses the family, including pets

Parents demonstrate an understanding of separation behaviors

Siblings, grandparents, and other significant persons visit as much as possible

Family provides child with familiar and/or cherished articles from home

Assigned person spends time with child (specify amount)

■ **PATIENT GOAL 2:** Will express feelings

NURSING INTERVENTIONS/*RATIONALES*

Accept expression of feelings *so that child continues these expressions*

Provide an atmosphere that encourages free expression of feelings

Provide opportunities for the child to verbalize, "play out," or otherwise express feelings without fear of punishment

Encourage drawing and other expressive activities *because children often find it easier to express themselves in images rather than words*

Encourage keeping a journal or diary *to allow child to express feelings and review progress and changes in feelings*

EXPECTED OUTCOME

Child verbalizes or plays out feelings or concerns

■ **PATIENT GOAL 3:** Will remain calm

NURSING INTERVENTIONS/*RATIONALES*

Do nothing to make child more anxious; remember that what may not provoke anxiety in an adult may make a child very anxious

Maintain calm, relaxed, and reassuring manner

Spend time with child and family *to establish rapport*

Give competent, consistent nursing care *to instill confidence in both parents and child*

Try to avoid intrusive procedures

EXPECTED OUTCOMES

Child exhibits no signs of apprehension

Child rests quietly and calmly

■ **PATIENT GOAL 4:** Will exhibit trusting behaviors

NURSING INTERVENTIONS/*RATIONALES*

Be positive in approach to child

Be honest with child *to encourage child to trust*

Convey to the child the behavior expected

Be consistent in expectations and relationships with child *because consistency is an important component of the development of trust*

Treat child fairly and help child to feel this

Encourage parents to maintain a truthful relationship with the child

Make certain child has call light or other signal device within reach

Unit 4

Continued

The Child in the Hospital—cont'd

EXPECTED OUTCOMES
Child develops rapport with primary nurse
Child maintains trusting feelings toward family

■ **PATIENT GOAL 5:** Will experience feelings of security

NURSING INTERVENTIONS/*RATIONALES*
Maintain child's identity
  Address child by name or usual nickname
  Avoid assigning a nickname to child or converting a given name to its counterpart in another language (e.g., using Joe instead of José)
Avoid communicating any signals of rejection, distaste, or other negative feelings to child
When necessary, communicate disapproval of unacceptable *behavior,* not disapproval of the *child*
Communicate (verbally and nonverbally) that the child is a valued person
Discourage treatments or procedures in the child's room or playroom *to maintain these areas as "safe places"*

EXPECTED OUTCOMES
Child interacts with staff
*Staff demonstrates respect for child

■ **PATIENT GOAL 6:** Will experience reduction of or no fear

NURSING INTERVENTIONS/*RATIONALES*
Explain routines, items, procedures, and events in a language and method appropriate to the child's developmental level; use simple language, drawings, and play *to facilitate understanding and mastery*
Reassure child and repeat reassurance as necessary
Ask child to explain reason for hospitalization and correct if necessary *to help absolve child from any guilt about being hospitalized*
Encourage parent(s) to participate in child's care
Encourage child to handle items that may seem strange or threatening *to reduce fear of the unknown*
Give encouragement and positive feedback for cooperation in care

EXPECTED OUTCOMES
Child exhibits understanding of information presented (specify information and means of demonstration)
Child discusses procedures and activities without evidence of anxiety

■ **PATIENT GOAL 7:** Will be allowed to regress

NURSING INTERVENTIONS/*RATIONALES*
Inform parents that regressive behavior is a feature of illness *so that it is not viewed as abnormal*
Accept regressive behavior and help child with dependency
Assist child in reconquering the negative counterpart of the psychosocial stage to which child has regressed (e.g., overcome mistrust; facilitate development of trust)

EXPECTED OUTCOME
*Staff and parents exhibit an attitude of acceptance of regressive behaviors

■ **PATIENT GOAL 8:** Will experience adequate comfort level

NURSING INTERVENTIONS/*RATIONALES*
Provide pacifier, if appropriate, *to meet oral needs and to provide comfort*
Hold infant or young child when this does not interfere with therapy
Touch, talk, and otherwise comfort child who cannot be held
Provide sensory stimulation and diversion appropriate to child's level of development and need for rest
Encourage family members to visit and allow them to comfort and care for child to the extent possible

EXPECTED OUTCOMES
Infant or young child engages in nonnutritive sucking
Child exhibits no signs of distress
Family is involved in care

NURSING DIAGNOSIS: Anxiety/fear related to distressing procedures, events

■ **PATIENT GOAL 1:** Will be prepared for hospitalization

NURSING INTERVENTIONS/*RATIONALES*
Prepare child as needed *to reduce fear of the unknown and to promote cooperation*
Select appropriate preparatory materials
Involve parents *to enable them to serve as effective resources for their child*
Modify preparation in special situations (e.g., day hospital, emergency admission, ICU) (Guidelines box)

EXPECTED OUTCOME
Child is prepared for hospital experience

■ **PATIENT GOAL 2:** Will exhibit decreased fear of bodily injury

NURSING INTERVENTIONS/*RATIONALES*
Recognize developmental fears associated with illness and procedures *to ensure appropriate intervention*
Provide age-appropriate explanations for procedures, especially those that are intrusive or involve the genitals, and include information about what body parts will not be affected, as well as those that will
Provide age-appropriate explanations for procedures the child may see or hear performed on other patients *to decrease child's fears*
Reassure child that certain body parts can be removed without producing harm (e.g., blood, tonsils, appendix)
Provide privacy for any procedure that exposes the body
Protect child from seeing unclothed patients
Use interventions that preserve child's concept of body integrity (e.g., bandages over puncture sites)

EXPECTED OUTCOME
Child displays minimum fear of bodily injury

■ **PATIENT GOAL 3:** Will receive support during tests and procedures

*Nursing outcome.

Supporting the Child and Family During Hospital Admission

Preadmission

Assign a room based on developmental age, seriousness of diagnosis, communicability of illness, and projected length of stay.

Prepare roommate(s) for the arrival of a new patient; when children are too young to benefit from this consideration, prepare parents.

Prepare room for child and family, with admission forms and equipment nearby to eliminate need to leave child.

Admission

Introduce primary nurse to child and family.

Orient child and family to inpatient facilities, especially to assigned room and unit; emphasize positive areas of pediatric unit.

Room—Explain call light, bed controls, television; direct to bathroom, telephone

Unit—Direct to playroom, desk, dining area, other areas

Introduce family to roommate and roommate's parents.

Apply identification band to child's wrist, ankle, or both (if not done).

Explain hospital regulations and schedules (e.g., visiting hours, mealtimes, bedtime, limitations); give written information if available

Perform nursing admission history. (See Box 4-4.)

Take vital signs, blood pressure, height, and weight.

Obtain specimens as needed and order needed laboratory work.

Support child and perform or assist practitioner with physical examination (for purposes of nursing assessment).

Emergency Admission

Lengthy preparatory admission procedures are often impossible and inappropriate for emergency situations.

Unless an emergency is life-threatening, children need to participate in their care to maintain a sense of control.

Focus on essential components of admission counseling, including:

Appropriate introduction to the family

Use of child's name, not terms such as "honey" or "dear"

Determination of child's age and some judgment about developmental age (e.g., if the child is of school age, asking about the grade level will offer some evidence for concurrent intellectual ability)

Information about child's general state of health, any problems that may interfere with medical treatment (e.g., sensitivity to medication), and previous experience with hospital facilities

Information about the chief complaint from both the parents and the child

Admission to Intensive Care Unit (ICU)

Prepare child and parents for elective ICU admission, such as for postoperative care after cardiac surgery.

Prepare child and parents for unanticipated ICU admission by focusing primarily on the sensory aspects of the experience and on usual family concerns (e.g., persons in charge of child's care, schedule for visiting, area where family can stay).

Prepare parents regarding child's appearance and behavior before they first visit child in ICU.

Accompany family to bedside to provide emotional support and answer questions.

Prepare siblings for their visit; plan length of time for sibling visitation; monitor siblings' reactions during visit to prevent them from becoming overwhelmed.

Encourage parents to stay with their child.

If visiting hours are limited, allow flexibility in schedule to accommodate parental needs.

Give family members a written schedule of visiting times.

If visiting hours are liberal, be aware of family members' needs and suggest periodic respites.

Assure family they can call the unit at any time.

Prepare parents for expected role changes and identify ways for parents to participate in child's care without overwhelming them with responsibilities, such as:

Help with bath or feeding

Touch and talk to child

Help with procedures

Provide information about child's condition in understandable language.

Repeat information often.

Seek clarification of understanding.

During bedside conferences, interpret information for family members and child or, if appropriate, conduct report outside room.

Prepare child for procedures, even if this involves explanation while procedure is performed.

Assess and manage pain; recognize that a child who cannot talk, such as an infant or child in a coma or on a ventilator, can be in pain.

Establish a routine that maintains some similarity to daily events in child's life whenever possible.

Organize care during normal waking hours.

Keep regular bedtime schedules, including quiet times when TV or radio is lowered or turned off.

Provide uninterrupted sleep cycles (60 minutes for infant, 90 minutes for older child).

Close and open drapes and dim lights to keep day/night orientation.

Place curtain around bed for privacy.

Orient child to day and time; have clocks or calendars in easy view for older children.

Schedule a time when child is left undisturbed (e.g., during naps, visit with family, playtime, or favorite program).

Provide opportunities for play.

Reduce stimulation in environment.

Refrain from loud talking or laughing.

Keep equipment noise to a minimum:

Turn alarms as low as safely possible.

Perform treatments requiring equipment at one time.

Turn off bedside equipment, such as suction and oxygen, when not in use.

Avoid loud, abrupt noises, such as clattering bedpans or slamming doors.

Unit 4

NURSING INTERVENTIONS/*RATIONALES*

Prepare child for procedures according to age and level of
understanding, including strategies for coping

Remain with child *to provide support by physical presence*

Prepare child and family for surgery if appropriate

Answer questions and explain purposes of activities

Keep child (and family) informed of progress

EXPECTED OUTCOME

Child remains calm and cooperative during procedures

Child feels supported by others during procedure

NURSING DIAGNOSIS: Pain related to (specify)

- **PATIENT GOAL 1:** Will perceive less pain by using
appropriate strategies

NURSING INTERVENTIONS/*RATIONALES*

Employ nonpharmacologic strategies to help child manage
pain *because techniques such as relaxation, rhythmic
breathing, and distraction can make pain more tolerable*

Use strategy that is familiar to child or describe several
strategies and let child select one (See Guidelines box,
p. 339.) *to facilitate child's learning and use of strategy*

Involve parent in selection of strategy *because parent knows
child best*

Select appropriate person(s), usually parent, to assist child
with strategy

Teach child to use specific nonpharmacologic strategies
before pain occurs or before it becomes severe *since
these approaches appear to be most effective for
mild pain*

Assist or have parent assist child with using strategy during
actual pain *because coaching may be needed to help
child focus on required actions*

EXPECTED OUTCOMES

Child exhibits acceptable pain level

Child learns and implements effective coping strategies

Parent learns coping skills and is effective in assisting child
to cope

- **PATIENT GOAL 2:** Will experience either no pain or a
reduction of pain to level acceptable to child when
receiving analgesics

NURSING INTERVENTIONS/*RATIONALES*

Plan to administer prescribed analgesic before procedure *so
that its peak effect coincides with painful event*

Plan preventive schedule of medication around the clock
(ATC) or "PRN (as needed) to prevent pain" when pain is
continuous and predictable (e.g., postoperatively) *to maintain steady blood levels of analgesic*

Administer analgesia by least traumatic route whenever possible *to avoid causing additional pain;* avoid intramuscular
or subcutaneous injections

Prepare child for administration of analgesia by using supportive statements (e.g., "This medicine I am putting in the IV
will make you feel better in a few minutes.")

Reinforce effect of analgesic by saying that child will begin to
feel better in (fill in appropriate amount of time, according
to drug used; use clock or timer to measure onset of relief
with child; reinforce cause and effect of pain and analgesic *so that child becomes conditioned to expecting relief*

If injection must be given, avoid saying, "I am going to give
you an injection for pain," *since this is another pain in
addition to the existing pain;* if child refuses injection,
explain that the little hurt from the needle wil take away
the bigger hurt for a long time

Avoid statements such as "This is enough medicine to take
away anyone's pain" or "By now you shouldn't need so
much pain medicine," *because they convey a judgmental
and belittling attitude*

Give child control whenever possible (e.g., using patient-
controlled analgesia, choosing which arm for a venipuncture, taking bandages off, holding tape or other
equipment)

*Administer prescribed analgesic; nonopioids, including acet-
aminophen (Tylenol, paracetamol) and nonsteroidal antiinflammatory drugs (NSAIDs), are suitable for mild to
moderate pain (See Table 4-9, p. 332.); opioids are needed
for moderate to severe pain (See Table 4-10, p. 333.); combination of the two analgesics (See Box 4-14, p. 334.) attacks
pain at peripheral nervous system and at central nervous
system and provides increased analgesia without increased
side effects

Titrate (adjust) dosage for maximum pain relief

Begin with recommended dosage for age and weight

Increase dosage and/or decrease interval between dosages
if pain relief is inadequate

If using parenteral route, change to oral route as soon as possible using equianalgesic dosages *because of first-pass effect
(oral opioid is rapidly absorbed from gastrointestinal
tract and enters portal circulation, where it is partially
metabolized before reaching central circulation; therefore
oral dosages must be larger)*

*Avoid combining opioids with so-called "potentiators" *since
combining drugs such as promethazine (Phenergan) and
chlorpromazine (Thorazine) adds risk of sedation and
respiratory depression without increasing analgesia*

Do not use placebos in the assessment or treatment of pain
*since deceptive use of placebos does not provide useful
information about presence or severity of pain, can cause
side effects similar to those of opioids, can destroy child's
and family's trust in health care staff, and raises serious
ethical and legal questions*

EXPECTED OUTCOMES

Child exhibits absence or minimal evidence of pain

Child accepts administration of analgesia with minimal distress

---

**NURSING DIAGNOSIS: Risk for poisoning or injury
from medications related to sensitivity, excessive
dose, decreased gastrointestinal motility**

- **PATIENT GOAL 1:** Will exhibit normal respiratory
function

NURSING INTERVENTIONS/*RATIONALES*

Monitor rate and depth of respirations and level of sedation
because depression of these functions can lead to apnea

Have emergency drugs and equipment ready to begin therapy
as soon as needed in case of respiratory depression from
opioids

EXPECTED OUTCOME

Child's respirations and sedation level remain within acceptable limits (See inside front cover for normal variations.)

*Dependent nursing action.

The Child in the Hospital—cont'd

■ **PATIENT GOAL 2:** Will not develop constipation and will receive treatment for other opioid-related side effects

NURSING INTERVENTIONS/*RATIONALES*

*Administer stool softener or laxative *to prevent constipation*
Stop or decrease medication if evidence of rash
*Administer antipruritic *for itching*
*Administer antiemetic *for nausea and vomiting*
Encourage child to lie quietly *because movement increases nausea and vomiting*
Recognize signs of tolerance: decreasing pain relief, decreasing duration of pain relief
Recognize signs of withdrawal after discontinuing drug (physical dependence) (See Box 4-15, p. 337.)
†Help treat tolerance and physical dependence appropriately *because these are involuntary physiologic responses that occur from prolonged use of opioids*
Never refer to child who is tolerant or physically dependent as "addicted"

EXPECTED OUTCOMES

Child has regular bowel movements
Child exhibits no evidence of rash or itching
Child receives appropriate therapy for tolerance/dependency (See also Preparation for procedures, p. 219.)

> **NURSING DIAGNOSIS:** Powerlessness related to the health care environment

■ **PATIENT GOAL 1:** Will experience "homelike" atmosphere in the hospital environment

NURSING INTERVENTIONS/*RATIONALES*

Determine from parents or other caregiver the child's customary routine and the usual manner of handling the child
Maintain a routine similar to the one the child is accustomed to at home
Minimize a hospital-like environment as much as possible; allow child to sit at table to eat and wear own pajamas or street clothes
Use terms familiar to child, such as those for body functions
Encourage patients with extended hospitalizations or their parents to decorate room (e.g., with pictures, bedspread from home) *to make it more "homelike"*
Encourage sibling visitation
Explore the possibility of pet visitation for children with extended hospitalizations
Advocate for appropriate hospital signs that assist the child to move freely throughout the unit and hospital with confidence

EXPECTED OUTCOME

Child's routine and environment are similar to those at home (specify)
Child feels relatively at ease in hospital environment

■ **PATIENT GOAL 2:** Will experience opportunities to exert control

NURSING INTERVENTIONS/*RATIONALES*

Allow child choices whenever possible, such as food selection, clothing, options for time of basic care (bath, play, bedtime), selection of television channels, choice of activities *to give child some measure of control*
Use time structuring with older child (a jointly planned and written schedule of daily activities)
Permit freedom on the unit within defined and enforced limitations
Explain the reason for physically restraining a child to both child and parents
Encourage self-care according to child's abilities
Assign tasks to an older child, especially in extended hospitalization (e.g., making the bed, supervising younger children, distributing menus, collating charts)
Respect child's need for privacy

EXPECTED OUTCOMES

Child participates in planning care (specify)
Child moves about the unit but respects limits
Child participates in care activities (specify activities)
Child assumes responsibility for tasks (specify)
Child's need for privacy is maintained

> **NURSING DIAGNOSIS:** Diversional activity deficit related to impaired mobility, musculoskeletal impairment, confinement to hospital, effects of illness

■ **PATIENT GOAL 1:** Will have opportunity to participate in activities

NURSING INTERVENTIONS/*RATIONALES*

Schedule therapies and periods of rest to allow for activities
Involve child in planning care to the extent of capabilities *to reduce feelings of passivity*
Arrange for and encourage interaction with others as feasible *to promote socialization*
Encourage visits from family and friends
Provide opportunity to socialize with noninfectious children

EXPECTED OUTCOMES

Child helps plan care and schedule
Child interacts with family and other children

■ **PATIENT GOAL 2:** Will have opportunity to participate in diversional activities

NURSING INTERVENTIONS/*RATIONALES*

Spend time with child
Query child and parents regarding child's favorite diversional activities
Change position of bed in room periodically (if child is confined to bed) *to alter sensory stimuli*
Provide activities appropriate to child's condition, physical limitations, and developmental level

---

*Dependent nursing action.

†Nursing outcome.

Continued

Unit 4

The Child in the Hospital—cont'd

Encourage family to caress and hold infant or child

Maintain accustomed routine when possible

Consult with a child-life specialist *to provide diversional activities*

Encourage interaction with other children

Choose a roommate compatible in age, sex, and physical abilities

Monitor time spent watching television or playing electronic games vs interactive or creative activities

Allow ample time for play

Make play, art, music, and other expressive materials available to child

Encourage play activities and diversions appropriate to child's age, condition, and capabilities

Facilitate an activity by acting under the child's instructions to perform tasks the child is unable to do

Use play as a teaching strategy and anxiety-reducing technique

Promote the use of a separate activity room or area for adolescents

EXPECTED OUTCOMES

Child engages in activities appropriate for age, interests, and physical limitations (specify activities)

Child receives attention and comfort

Child engages in age-appropriate play (specify)

NURSING DIAGNOSIS: Activity intolerance related to generalized weakness, fatigue, imbalance between oxygen supply and demand, pain or discomfort

■ **PATIENT GOAL 1:** Will maintain adequate energy levels

NURSING INTERVENTIONS/*RATIONALES*

Assess child's level of physical tolerance

Anticipate child's need for rest, as evidenced by irritability, short attention span, and fretfulness; assist child in those activities of daily living that may be beyond tolerance

Provide entertainment and quiet diversional activities appropriate to child's age and interest *to conserve energy*

Provide diversional play activities *that promote rest and quiet but prevent boredom and withdrawal*

Choose an appropriate roommate of similar age and interests and one who requires the same level of restricted activity *to decrease feelings of loneliness and sadness*

Instruct child to rest when feeling tired

Balance rest and activity (when ambulatory)

EXPECTED OUTCOMES

Child plays and rests quietly and engages in activities appropriate to age and capabilities (specify)

Child tolerates increasing activity

■ **PATIENT GOAL 2:** Will receive optimum rest

NURSING INTERVENTIONS/*RATIONALES*

Provide quiet environment *to promote rest*

Organize activities for maximum sleep time

Schedule visiting to allow for sufficient rest

Keep visiting periods with friends and family short

Encourage parents to remain with child *to decrease separation and anxiety*

*Administer sedatives and analgesics as indicated if ordered for restlessness and pain

Encourage frequent rest periods

Enforce regular sleep times

Follow child's usual routine for bedtime, nap time

Implement measures to ensure sleep, such as quiet, darkened room

Be alert to signs that child is tired or overstimulated *to allow flexibility in scheduling or enforcing rest and sleep periods*

EXPECTED OUTCOMES

Child remains calm, quiet, and relaxed

Child gets a sufficient amount of rest (specify)

NURSING DIAGNOSIS: Risk for injury/trauma related to unfamiliar environment, therapies, hazardous equipment

■ **PATIENT GOAL 1:** Will experience no injury

NURSING INTERVENTIONS/*RATIONALES*

Employ environmental safety measures *to prevent injuries*

Report any potential hazards (e.g., slippery floors, poor illumination, electrical hazards, damaged or malfunctioning furniture or equipment, unprotected windows or stairwells)

Dispose of small, breakable items appropriately (e.g., thermometers, bottles)

Keep potentially hazardous articles out of child's reach

Check bathwater for temperature before bathing infant or child *to prevent burns*

Maintain surveillance of children in bathtub/shower

Keep crib sides up and securely fastened; use siderails for children who may fall out of bed

Use safety restraints only when absolutely necessary

  Remove as often as possible

  Discontinue as soon as possible

  Check that restraint is applied properly and regularly check for adequate circulation to the restrained area and any pressure points

Maintain hand contact while caring for a child in a crib with siderails down *to prevent falls*

Transport infants and children appropriately

  Hold with proper support

  Fasten safety belt on gurney, wheelchair

Alert parents and ancillary hospital personnel regarding child's physical tolerance and need for assistance during activity

Fasten safety belts in high chairs, swings

EXPECTED OUTCOME

Child remains free of injury

NURSING DIAGNOSIS: Bathing/hygiene and dressing/grooming self-care deficit related to physical or cognitive disability, mechanical restrictions

■ **PATIENT GOAL 1:** Will engage in self-help activities

NURSING INTERVENTIONS/*RATIONALES*

Allow child to help plan own daily routine and choose from alternatives when appropriate *to promote sense of control*

*Dependent nursing action.

Unit 4

The Child in the Hospital—cont'd

Encourage participation in self-care activities according to developmental level and capabilities *to promote mastery and decrease regression*

Provide devices, equipment, and methods to assist child in self-care

Advocate for child-sized features *that foster independence* (e.g., bathroom door handles that children can reach)

Assist with dressing, grooming, bathing as indicated

EXPECTED OUTCOME
Child engages in self-help activities to maximum capabilities

---

NURSING DIAGNOSIS: Toileting self-care deficit related to physical or cognitive disability, mechanical restrictions

---

■ **PATIENT GOAL 1:** Will exhibit normal elimination patterns

NURSING INTERVENTIONS/*RATIONALES*
Solicit information from child and parents regarding child's normal patterns and procedures of elimination

Sit child in upright position when possible *to encourage elimination*

Employ special devices where appropriate (e.g., fracture pan, commode, elevated toilet seat)

Carry out bowel-training program with hydration, high-fiber diet, stool softeners, and mild laxatives if needed

Provide privacy *to promote relaxation needed for elimination*

EXPECTED OUTCOME
Child has daily bowel movement

NURSING DIAGNOSIS: Altered urinary elimination related to discomfort, positioning

---

■ **PATIENT GOAL 1:** Will exhibit normal voiding

NURSING INTERVENTIONS/*RATIONALES*
Solicit information from child and parents regarding child's normal patterns and procedures of elimination

Position child as upright as possible to void

Hydrate child *to ensure adequate urinary output for age*

Stimulate bladder emptying with warm water, running water, stroking suprapubic area

Catheterize as indicated

EXPECTED OUTCOMES
Child exhibits normal frequency and volume of urinary voiding with minimal discomfort

(See also:
Nursing Care Plan: The Child with Chronic Illness or Disability, p. 287.)
Nursing Care Plan: The Child Undergoing Surgery, p. 304.)
Nursing Care Plan: The Child Who Is Terminally Ill or Dying, p. 296.)
Nursing Care Plan for specific health problem.)

Unit 4

NURSING CARE PLAN

The Family of the Child Who Is Ill or Hospitalized

Friedman defines family as "two or more persons who are joined together by bonds of sharing and emotional closeness and who identify themselves as being part of the family."*

To further acknowledge the variety of cultural styles, values, and alternative family structures that exist today, an even more inclusive definition allows the individual family to define itself.† These important people in the family's life may be related, unrelated, immediate family, or extended family members.

The understanding or perception of "family" is uniquely meaningful to an individual and is based on that person's experience and interpretation. This perception is held to be accurate until an experience leads to expansion or reinterpretation of the initial concept.‡ Whatever form the family takes, children need to feel that their family is acceptable and valuable.§

Throughout this book the term *family* is used to indicate the relationships between dependent children and one or more protective adults. It also implies relationships among siblings.

Factors that influence parental responses to illness of a child:
The seriousness of the threat to their child
Previous experience with illness or hospitalization
Medical procedures involved in diagnosis and treatment
Available support systems
Personal ego strengths
Previous coping abilities
Additional stresses on the family system
Cultural and religious beliefs
Communication patterns among family members

Factors that influence sibling responses to illness/hospitalization of the child:
Fear of contracting the illness
Younger age
Close relationship to sick sibling
Out-of-home residence during period of hospitalization
Minimal explanation of the sick child's illness
Perceived changes in parenting, such as increased parental anger

---

ASSESSMENT
(See Family Assessment, p. 69.)
Observe behavior of family members.

NURSING DIAGNOSIS: Anxiety/fear related to situational crisis, threat to role functioning, change in environment

■ **FAMILY GOAL 1:** Will adjust to hospital environment

NURSING INTERVENTIONS/*RATIONALES*
Introduce family to staff members
Describe hospital routine that affects child
Acclimate family to the new and strange surroundings (e.g., show them physical layout of unit, including playroom, unit kitchen, toilet, telephone, where they can stay, where they can store their belongings)
Direct family to areas they may need to use outside the unit (e.g., dining room, chapel)
Direct family to any places within the hospital that are interesting to look at or talk about
Provide an atmosphere that promotes questioning and expression of doubts and feelings
Be available to family *to facilitate their adjustment*
Be alert to signs of tension in family members
Provide for privacy

EXPECTED OUTCOMES
Family demonstrates familiarity with hospital environment
Family members ask questions

■ **FAMILY GOAL 2:** Will feel a part of the health care team

NURSING INTERVENTIONS/*RATIONALES*
Employ a polite, respectful approach and demeanor
Greet family by name when they arrive on the unit
Encourage family's presence
Include family in planning patient care
Encourage family to select and assume specific roles in child's care, as comfortable for them
Offer encouragement for their efforts
Ask family to share with staff what they know about child's care and needs
Convey an attitude of collegiality, not competition, with family

EXPECTED OUTCOME
Family becomes involved in planning and carrying out care for the child to extent they desire

■ **FAMILY GOAL 3:** Will experience reduced apprehension

NURSING INTERVENTIONS/*RATIONALES*
Allow for expression of feelings about child's hospitalization and illness
Provide needed information *to alleviate fear of the unknown*
Prepare family for what to expect (e.g., procedures, behaviors)
Explore family's expectations
Explore family's concerns and feelings of irritation, guilt, anger, disappointment, inadequacy

---

*Friedman M: *Family nursing: theory and practice,* ed 3, Norwalk, CT, 1992, Appleton-Century-Crofts.

†McGonigel M: Philosophy and conceptual framework. In McGonigel M, Kaufman R, Johnson B, editors: *Guidelines and recommended practices for the Individualized Family Service Plan,* ed 2, Bethesda, MD, 1991, Association for the Care of Children's Health.

‡Cody A: Helping the vulnerable or condoning control within the family: where is nursing? *J Adv Nurs* 23:882-886, 1996.

§Visher E, Visher J: Beyond the nuclear family: resources and implications for pediatricians, *Fam Focused Pediatr* 42(1):31-43, 1995.

Unit 4

The Family of the Child Who Is Ill or Hospitalized—cont'd

Explore family's fears and anxieties regarding child's status and expectations of results of procedures or therapy

Introduce parents to other families who have a child in the hospital, especially a child who is similarly affected, *to facilitate family-to-family support*

Provide something constructive and meaningful for family to focus on (e.g., keeping record of intake and output, pain relief record, ensuring a specified amount of fluid intake, collecting a specimen)

EXPECTED OUTCOMES

Family members verbalize feelings and concerns

Family demonstrates an understanding of procedures and behaviors (specify manner of demonstration and learning)

Family interacts with other families, as desired

■ **FAMILY GOAL 4:** Will be prepared for special procedures (e.g., radiology, diagnostic tests, surgery)

NURSING INTERVENTIONS/*RATIONALES*

Assess family's understanding of the procedure and its purpose

Provide needed information; clarify misconceptions

Explain special preparation needed (e.g., nothing by mouth [NPO], shaving, preprocedure medication or equipment)

Describe:

Where child will be during the procedure

Whether family can be with child

Where family can wait

Approximate length of time procedure requires

Reassure family that they will be notified regarding progress of the procedure

EXPECTED OUTCOME

Family demonstrates an understanding of procedures and tests (specify)

■ **FAMILY GOAL 5:** Will receive support during child's absence

NURSING INTERVENTIONS/*RATIONALES*

Provide a comfortable place for family to wait

Suggest activities to help reduce anxiety (e.g., go to the coffee shop or dining room, take a short walk [specify activity])

Be available to family *for support*

Make contact with family at frequent intervals *to relay information and provide comfort*

EXPECTED OUTCOME

Family feels a sense of support

■ **FAMILY GOAL 6:** Will adjust to child's appearance and behavior following procedure(s) or placement in special care unit

NURSING INTERVENTIONS/*RATIONALES*

Remain calm *to decrease family's anxiety*

Describe the environment, if appropriate (e.g., ICU)

Apply principles of learning to explanations

Begin with small amounts of information

Begin with very general information

Allow ample time for family to absorb information and to ask questions

Use age-appropriate explanations and techniques for siblings

Explain how child will look and the reasons for the child's appearance and equipment

Explain what child is experiencing

Prepare child and surroundings *to lessen the impact of the first impression*

Tidy the bed

Personalize the bed and bedside with a toy or other item(s)

Provide chairs for family

Be prepared for possible adverse reaction (e.g., fainting)

Convey an attitude of caring *about*, as well as *for*, the child

Accompany the family to the child's bedside

Allow time for follow-up discussion of questions and concerns

EXPECTED OUTCOME

Family feels prepared before coming to child's bedside

■ **FAMILY GOAL 7:** Will experience either reduction in or no fear

NURSING INTERVENTIONS/*RATIONALES*

Help family distinguish between realistic and unfounded fears

Help eliminate unfounded fears

Discuss with family their fears regarding:

Child's signs and symptoms

Child's anxiety

Consequences of disease or therapy

Deterioration of child's condition

Tests and procedures

Death

Answer questions honestly and compassionately

EXPECTED OUTCOME

Family members verbalize fears and explore nature and ramifications of these fears

---

NURSING DIAGNOSIS: Powerlessness related to health care environment

---

■ **FAMILY GOAL 1:** Will experience a sense of control

NURSING INTERVENTIONS/*RATIONALES*

Encourage family's presence at times convenient for them; consider variations (e.g., cultural, occupational) in visiting

Encourage expression of concerns regarding child's care and progress

Explore family's feelings regarding prescribed therapies

Encourage family to assume as much control as possible in child's management

Encourage participation in child's care

Include family in setting goals for care

Continued

Unit 4

The Family of the Child Who Is Ill or Hospitalized—cont'd

Involve family in scheduling and other aspects of care
Explain what family can do for child and how to handle child to maintain therapy (e.g., how to pick up the child who has an IV line)
Employ family's suggestions regarding child's care whenever possible

EXPECTED OUTCOMES

Family schedules time to be with child
Family readily discusses feelings and concerns
Family contributes to care and management of child, as desired
*Family's suggestions are incorporated into plan of care

NURSING DIAGNOSIS: Altered family processes related to situational crisis (threat to role functioning, hospitalization of a child)

■ **FAMILY GOAL 1:** Will demonstrate knowledge of child's illness

NURSING INTERVENTIONS/*RATIONALES*

Recognize family's concerns and need for information, support
Assess family's understanding of diagnosis and plan of care
Reinforce and clarify health professional's explanation of child's condition, suggested procedures and therapies, and the prognosis
Use every opportunity to increase family's understanding of the disease and its therapies
Repeat information as often as necessary *to facilitate understanding*
Interpret technical information *since family may not understand*
Help family interpret infant's or child's behaviors and responses
Do not appear rushed; if time is inappropriate, set a time for discussion as soon as feasible
Keep appointment faithfully

EXPECTED OUTCOME

Family demonstrates an understanding of the disease and its therapies (specify knowledge)

■ **FAMILY GOAL 2:** Will experience either reduction in or no guilt feelings

NURSING INTERVENTIONS/*RATIONALES*

Acknowledge feelings of guilt as normal
Provide accurate and specific information regarding the cause of the illness
Clarify misconceptions and false assumptions

EXPECTED OUTCOME

Family verbalizes understanding of the cause of the illness (specify)

■ **FAMILY GOAL 3:** Will receive adequate support

NURSING INTERVENTIONS/*RATIONALES*

Respect parental rights
Convey an attitude of respectful caring for both child and family
Support and emphasize family's strengths and abilities
Provide feedback and praise
Refer to other professionals (e.g., social service, clergy) *for additional interpersonal and concrete support*

EXPECTED OUTCOMES

Family exhibits behaviors that indicate a feeling of self-respect
Family uses supportive services

■ **FAMILY GOAL 4:** Will demonstrate positive coping behaviors toward child

NURSING INTERVENTIONS/*RATIONALES*

Determine family's understanding of the normal childhood responses to the stress of illness and hospitalization
Explain child's regression, magical thinking, egocentricity, separation anxiety, fears
Explain behavioral reactions generally expected of child (specify according to age and developmental level)
Reinforce family's endeavors to support child

EXPECTED OUTCOME

Family demonstrates an understanding of child's unfamiliar behaviors (specify manner of demonstration—verbalization, physical attitude, behaviors with child)

■ **FAMILY GOAL 5:** Will assist child in coping effectively with hospitalization

NURSING INTERVENTIONS/*RATIONALES*

Help parents determine the best way to prepare child for hospitalization, procedures
Provide family with precise information about what will take place so they know what child is likely to experience
Encourage family to trust child's capacity to cope
Impress on family the need for honesty in relating to child
Encourage family to use play as a coping strategy
Suggest appropriate items to bring to child (e.g., pajamas, favorite toys)
(See also Nursing Care Plan: The Child in the Hospital, p. 268.)

EXPECTED OUTCOMES

Family helps in planning strategies
Family is honest with child
Family uses play as a tool for relating with child

■ **FAMILY GOAL 6:** Will experience positive relationships

NURSING INTERVENTIONS/*RATIONALES*

Recognize that family members know child best and are "cued in" to child's needs
Welcome unlimited family presence *to promote family relationships*

---

*Nursing outcome.

The Family of the Child Who Is Ill or Hospitalized—cont'd

Encourage family to bring other significant family members to visit (e.g., siblings, grandparents, and pets [where permitted])

Encourage family to provide child with significant, but manageable, items from home *to provide security*

Arrange for family members to have a meal together

EXPECTED OUTCOMES

Child and family exhibit behaviors that indicate positive coping

Family is with child as often as desired

Child demonstrates an attitude of security with familiar persons and things

■ **FAMILY GOAL 7:** Will exhibit evidence of optimum health

NURSING INTERVENTIONS/*RATIONALES*

Stress importance of maintaining family members' health during child's illness and hospitalization

Encourage adequate rest *to promote health of family*

Provide sleeping facilities where possible

Encourage members to alternate visiting with child to allow some time at home

Explore means for respite care of dependent family members

Assure family that child will receive optimum care in their absence

Provide relief for family from direct care of child as needed

Promote adequate nutrition

Provide meals for parents if possible

Direct family to nutritious resources for meals

Encourage regular mealtimes

Provide access to unit kitchen to store and prepare snacks

EXPECTED OUTCOMES

Family shows no evidence of illness

Family members appear well rested

Family members eat regularly

■ **FAMILY GOAL 8:** Will experience smooth transition from hospital to home

NURSING INTERVENTIONS/*RATIONALES*

Assess family's learning needs

Outline and carry out a teaching plan

Determine services needed and make necessary referrals

Include family in planning and problem solving

Maintain open communication between family and heath care providers

EXPECTED OUTCOMES

Child and family demonstrate the ability to provide needed care in the home

Family has support during transition to home care

■ **FAMILY GOAL 9:** Will demonstrate knowledge of home care

NURSING INTERVENTIONS/*RATIONALES*

Assess family's knowledge to facilitate planning

Teach family the skills needed to carry out the therapeutic program (specify)

Allow ample time for preparation

Teach necessary techniques and observations

Help family by demonstration

Distribute appropriate home care instructions and/or other educational materials

Encourage questions and expression of feelings and concerns

Allow sufficient time for family to perform procedures under supervision

Inform parents of:

Signs of progress to observe for

Any unfavorable signs to be alert for

Problems that can be anticipated (e.g., care of equipment or devices)

Behaviors that indicate special needs (e.g., use of pain medication, imminent seizures)

A course of action to follow (e.g., seizure care)

Make certain family knows how to contact appropriate persons if or when needed

Prepare family for possible posthospital behaviors of the child (Box 4-5)

Ensure family's comprehension of child's needs before discharge

EXPECTED OUTCOMES

Family demonstrates procedures needed to care for child in the home (specify learning and method of demonstration)

Family is aware of how to seek help

■ **FAMILY GOAL 10:** Will demonstrate understanding of continuity of care

NURSING INTERVENTIONS/*RATIONALES*

Inform family of community resources available

Refer to agencies as appropriate (specify)

Help identify support group(s) for family, as desired

Be available to family by telephone or other means

Schedule follow-up appointments as needed

Ensure coordination of home care, if needed

EXPECTED OUTCOMES

Family seeks appropriate assistance

Family keeps appointments

(See also:

Nursing Care Plan: The Child in the Hospital, p. 268.)

Nursing Care Plan: The Child with Chronic Illness or Disability, p. 287.)

Nursing Care Plan: The Child Who Is Terminally Ill or Dying, p. 296.)

Unit 4

Continued

The Family of the Child Who Is Ill or Hospitalized—cont'd

BOX 4-5

Posthospital Behaviors in Children

Young Children

Some initial aloofness toward parents, which may last from a few minutes (most common) to a few days.

Frequently followed by dependency behaviors:

Tendency to cling to parents

Demand parents' attention

Vigorously oppose any separation (e.g., staying at preschool or with a baby-sitter)

Other negative behaviors include the following:

New fears (e.g., nightmares)

Resistance to going to bed, night waking

Withdrawal and shyness

Hyperactivity

Temper tantrums

Food finickiness

Attachment to blanket or toy

Regression in newly learned skills (e.g., self-toileting)

Older Children

Negative behaviors include the following:

Emotional coldness, followed by intense, demanding dependence on parents

Anger toward parents

Jealousy toward others (e.g., siblings)

NURSING CARE PLAN

The Child with Chronic Illness or Disability

Chronic illness—A condition that interferes with daily functioning for more than 3 months in a year, causes hospitalization of more than 1 month in a year, or (at time of diagnosis) is likely to do either of these

Congenital disability—A disability that has existed since birth but is not necessarily hereditary

Developmental delay—A maturational lag; an abnormal, slower rate of development in which a child demonstrates a functioning level below that observed in normal children of the same age

Developmental disability—Any mental and/or physical disability that is manifested before age 22 years and is likely to continue indefinitely

Disability—Typically defined as a physical or mental impairment substantially limiting one or more major life activities

(e.g., walking, seeing, speaking, breathing, learning), a new legal definition was incorporated in a change in the SSI program as part of welfare reform in PL 104-193: "a medically determinable physical or mental impairment which results in marked and severe functional limitations, which can be expected to result in death or which has lasted or can be expected to last for at least 12 months."

Handicap—A condition or barrier imposed by society, the environment, or one's own self; not a synonym for disability

Impairment—A loss or abnormality of structure or function

Technology-dependent child—A child between the ages of birth and 21 years with a chronic disability that requires the routine use of a medical device to compensate for the loss of a life-sustaining bodily function; daily ongoing care and/or monitoring is required by trained personnel

ASSESSMENT

Perform a physical assessment with special emphasis on specific condition.

Take a careful history of possible causative factors (initial assessment), progress and management of condition, child and family coping.

Observe for manifestations of specific condition.

Assist with diagnostic procedures and tests appropriate to specific condition.

NURSING DIAGNOSIS: Altered growth and development related to chronic illness or disability, parental reactions (overbenevolence), repeated hospitalization.

■ **PATIENT GOAL 1:** Will attain maximum expected growth and developmental potential

NURSING INTERVENTIONS/*RATIONALES*
(See Table 4-3.)

EXPECTED OUTCOME

Child attains appropriate physical, psychosocial, and cognitive development for age and abilities

---

NURSING DIAGNOSIS: Risk for altered family processes related to situational crisis (child with a chronic disease or disability)

■ **PATIENT (FAMILY) GOAL 1:** Will exhibit positive adjustment to the diagnosis

NURSING INTERVENTIONS/*RATIONALES*

Provide opportunity for family to adjust to discovery of diagnosis

Anticipate grief reaction to loss of the "perfect" child *because this usually occurs in the adjustment process*

Explore family's feelings regarding child and their ability to cope with the disorder

Encourage family to express their concerns

Repeat information as often as necessary *to reinforce family's understanding*

Serve as a role model regarding attitudes and behavior toward child

EXPECTED OUTCOMES

Parents verbalize feelings and concerns regarding implications of the disease or disability

Family demonstrates an attitude of acceptance and adjustment

■ **PATIENT (FAMILY) GOAL 2:** Will demonstrate understanding of disorder and treatment options

NURSING INTERVENTIONS/*RATIONALES*

Help family to understand the disorder, its therapies, and implications

Reinforce information given by others *to promote better understanding*

Clarify misconceptions

Provide accurate information at a rate family can absorb *because information given too rapidly will not be learned*

Discuss advantages and limitations of therapeutic plan

Encourage family to ask questions and express concerns

EXPECTED OUTCOME

Family demonstrates an understanding of the disease (specify) and treatment options

■ **PATIENT (FAMILY) GOAL 3:** Will experience reduction of fear and anxiety

NURSING INTERVENTIONS/*RATIONALES*

Explore family's concerns and feelings of irritation, guilt, anger, disappointment, inadequacy, and other feelings

Modified from Research and Training Center on Independent Living (RTC/IL): *Guidelines for reporting and writing about people with disabilities,* ed 3, Lawrence, KS, 1990; Hobbs N, Perrin J, editors: *Issues in the care of children with chronic illness,* San Francisco, 1985, Jossey-Bass; *Report to Congress and the Secretary by the Task Force on Technology-Dependent Children: fostering home and community-based care for technology-dependent children,* vol 2, HCFA Pub No 88-02171, 1988, US Department of Health and Human Services, Health Care Financing Administration; and Americans with Disabilities Act (ADA), cited in Siegel RD: Child care and the ADA, *Except Parent,* 25(2):34, 1995.

Continued

Unit 4

The Child with Chronic Illness or Disability—cont'd

TABLE 4-3   Developmental Aspects of Chronic Illness or Disability in Children

Developmental Tasks	Potential Effects of Chronic Illness or Disability	Supportive Interventions
Infancy		
Develop a sense of trust	Multiple caregivers and frequent separations, especially if hospitalized Deprived of consistent nurturing	Encourage consistent caregivers and care by parent in hospital or other care setting Encourage parents to visit frequently or room-in during hospitalization and to participate in care
Attach to parent	Delayed because of separation, parental grief for loss of "dream" child, parental inability to accept the condition (especially a visible defect)	Emphasize healthy, perfect qualities of infant Help parents learn special care needs of infant so they can feel competent
Learn through sensorimotor experiences	Increased exposure to painful experiences over pleasurable ones Limited contact with environment from restricted movement or confinement	Expose infant to pleasurable experiences through all senses (touch, hearing, sight, taste, movement) Encourage age-appropriate developmental skills (e.g., holding bottle, finger feeding, crawling)
Begin to develop a sense of separateness from parent	Increased dependency on parent for care Overinvolvement of parent in care	Encourage all family members to participate in care to prevent overinvolvement of one member Encourage periodic respite from demands of care responsibilities
Toddlerhood		
Develop autonomy	Increased dependency on parent	Encourage independence in as many areas as possible (e.g., toileting, dressing, feeding)
Master locomotor and language skills	Limited opportunity to test own abilities and limits	Provide gross motor skill activity and modification of toys or equipment, such as modified swing or rocking horse
Learn through sensorimotor experience, beginning preoperational thought	Increased exposure to painful experiences	Give choices to allow simple feeling of control (e.g., choice of what book to look at or what kind of sandwich to eat) Institute age-appropriate discipline and limit-setting Recognize that negative and ritualistic behavior are normal Provide sensory experiences (e.g., water play, sandbox, finger paint)
Preschool		
Develop initiative and purpose Master self-care skills Begin to develop peer relationships	Limited opportunities for success in accomplishing simple tasks or mastering self-care skills Limited opportunities for socialization with peers; may appear "like a baby" to age-mates Protection within tolerant and secure family may cause child to fear criticism and withdraw	Encourage mastery of self-help skills Provide devices that make task easier (e.g., Velcro for self-dressing) Encourage socialization, such as inviting friends to play, daycare experience, trips to park Provide age-appropriate play, especially associative play opportunities Emphasize child's abilities; dress appropriately to enhance desirable appearance
Develop sense of body image and sexual identification	Awareness of body may center on pain, anxiety, and failure Sex-role identification focused primarily on mothering skills	Encourage relationships with same-sex and opposite-sex peers and adults Help child deal with criticisms; realize that too much protection prevents child from mastering realities of world

Unit 4

The Child with Chronic Illness or Disability—cont'd

TABLE 4-3   Developmental Aspects of Chronic Illness or Disability in Children—cont'd

Developmental Tasks	Potential Effects of Chronic Illness or Disability	Supportive Interventions
Preschool—cont'd		
Learn through preoperational thought (magical thinking)	Guilt (thinking he or she caused the illness/disability or is being punished for wrongdoing)	Clarify that cause of child's illness or disability is not his or her fault or a punishment
School Age		
Develop a sense of accomplishment	Limited opportunities to achieve and compete (e.g., many school absences or inability to join regular athletic activities)	Encourage school attendance; schedule medical visits at times other than school; encourage to make up missed school work Educate teachers and classmates about child's condition, abilities, and special needs
Form peer relationships	Limited opportunities for socialization	Encourage sports activities (e.g., Special Olympics) Encourage socialization (e.g., Girl Scouts, Campfire, Boy Scouts, 4-H Clubs, having a best friend or joining a club)
Learn through concrete operations	Incomplete comprehension of the imposed physical limitations or treatment of the disorder	Provide child with knowledge about his or her condition Encourage creative activities (e.g., Very Special Arts)
Adolescence		
Develop personal and sexual identity	Increased sense of feeling different from peers and less able to compete with peers in appearance, abilities, special skills	Realize that many of the difficulties the teenager is experiencing are part of normal adolescence (rebelliousness, risk taking, lack of cooperation, hostility toward authority)
Achieve independence from family	Increased dependency on family; limited job/career opportunities	Provide instruction on interpersonal and coping skills Provide instruction on decision-making, assertiveness, and other skills necessary to manage personal plans Encourage increased responsibility for care and management of the disease or condition, such as assuming responsibility for making and keeping appointment (ideally, alone), sharing in the assessment and planning stages of health care delivery, contacting resources
Form heterosexual relationships	Limited opportunities for heterosexual friendships; less opportunity to discuss sexual concerns with peers	Encourage socialization with peers, including peers with and without special needs Encourage activities appropriate for age, such as attending mixed-gender parties, sports activities, driving a car Emphasize good appearance and wearing stylish clothes, use of makeup
Learn through abstract thinking	Increased concern with issues such as why did he or she get the disorder, and whether he or she can marry and have a family Decreased opportunity for earlier stages of cognition may impede achieving level of abstract thinking	Be alert to cues that signal readiness for information regarding implications of condition on sexuality and reproduction Understand that adolescent has same sexual needs and concerns as any other teenager Discuss planning for future and how condition can affect choices

Unit 4

The Child with Chronic Illness or Disability—cont'd

Help family distinguish between realistic fears and unfounded fears; address unfounded fears

Discuss with parents their fears regarding:

Dealing with child's anxiety about condition

Fear of dreadful developments

Fear of death

Fear of tests and procedures

Child's ability to compete with peers

Explore family's feelings regarding prescribed therapies

EXPECTED OUTCOME

Family members discuss their fears and concerns

■ **PATIENT (FAMILY) GOAL 4:** Will exhibit positive adaptation to child's condition

NURSING INTERVENTIONS/*RATIONALES*

Explore family's reaction to child and the disorder

Assess family's coping skills, abilities, and resources *so that these can be reinforced*

Help family to achieve a realistic view of child's capabilities and limitations

Foster positive family relationships *so that members' ability to cope is maximized*

Assess interpersonal relationships within family, especially behaviors that reflect family's attitudes toward affected child

Intervene appropriately if there is evidence of maladaptation; refer for counseling if appropriate

Encourage parents in their attemps to promote child's development

Emphasize positive aspects of child's abilities or attributes

Help family gain confidence in their ability to cope with child, the disorder, and the disorder's impact on other family members

EXPECTED OUTCOMES

Family verbalizes feelings and concerns regarding special needs of child and their effect on the family process

Family members demonstrate an attitude of confidence in their ability to cope

■ **PATIENT (FAMILY) GOAL 5:** Will exhibit ability to care for child

NURSING INTERVENTIONS/*RATIONALES*

Help family develop a thorough plan of care

Teach skills needed *to provide optimum care*

Interpret child's behavior to parents (e.g., anger, depression, regression, physical modifications as a result of disorder) *to prevent any unwarranted negative reaction to child (e.g., punishment)*

Help family plan for the future

EXPECTED OUTCOME

Family members set realistic goals for themselves, child, and others

■ **PATIENT (FAMILY) GOAL 6:** Will have needs as family unit met

NURSING INTERVENTIONS/*RATIONALES*

With family, identify family support systems (immediate family, extended family, friends, health service providers, parent-to-parent support groups)

Wiith family, assess the number, affiliation, and interrelationships (if any) of persons the family sees as important

Help family to assign specific tasks to specific people *so that family members receive support they need*

Reinforce positive coping mechanisms

Encourage family members to discuss their feelings with each other

Impress on parents the importance of providing the most normal life possible for the affected child

Emphasize the growth and developmental progress of their child *to help parents feel adequate in their maternal-paternal roles*

Help family foster child's development by stimulating child to achieve age-appropriate goals consistent with activity tolerance

EXPECTED OUTCOMES

Family demonstrates positive, growth-promoting behaviors

Family avails itself of support

■ **PATIENT (FAMILY) GOAL 7:** Will receive adequate support

NURSING INTERVENTIONS/*RATIONALES*

Be available to family *to provide support*

Listen to family members—singly or collectively

Allow for expression of feelings, including feelings of guilt, helplessness, and their perceptions about the impact that the condition may have (or does have) on the family

Refer to community agencies or special organizations that provide assistance—financial, social, and support

Refer to genetic counseling if appropriate

Help family members learn to expect feelings of frustration and anger toward child; reassure parents that it is not a reflection on their parenting

Assist family in problem solving

Encourage interaction with other families who have a similarly affected child

Introduce families

Provide information regarding support groups

Help families learn when to accept conditions and when to "fight" for the care and services they feel are needed

Inform families of legislation for services and how to advocate for services when they feel they are needed (See Community Focus box, p. 292.)

EXPECTED OUTCOMES

Family maintains contact with health providers

Family demonstrates an understanding of the needs of the child and the impact the condition will have on them

The Child with Chronic Illness or Disability—cont'd

Problems are dealt with early

Family becomes involved with local agencies and support groups as needed

■ **PATIENT (FAMILY) GOAL 8:** Will be prepared for home care

NURSING INTERVENTIONS/*RATIONALES*

Teach skills needed *to ensure optimum home care*

With family, assess home situation, including family's strengths, weaknesses, and support systems

Help device an individualized plan of care based on assessment of family's needs and resources

Encourage family involvement in care while still in the hospital *so that they are better prepared to assume child's care*

Encourage family to ask questions regarding posthospital care

Explore family's attitudes toward child's entry (or reentry) into the home

Help family acquire needed drugs, supplies, and equipment

Refer to special agencies, based on needs assessment, *for ongoing support and assistance*

Arrange for regular follow-up care *to assess effectiveness of home management*

EXPECTED OUTCOMES

Family demonstrates competence with needed skills (specify skills and method of demonstration)

Family members avail themselves of resources within their community (specify)

Family complies with home care program

■ **PATIENT (FAMILY) GOAL 9:** Will participate in ongoing care

NURSING INTERVENTIONS/*RATIONALES*

Participate in follow-up care *to ensure continuity of care*

Coordinate team management of child and family

Be alert to comments by child or family members that indicate possible problems *so that problems are identified early*

Assess interpersonal relationships within family, especially behaviors that reflect family's attitudes toward child

Be alert for cues that signal undue anxiety and guilt (e.g., preoccupation with causative factors, constant analysis of effects of therapies, experimentation with diets and folk remedies, seeking magical cures)

Be alert for overprotective behaviors such as assuming self-care activities for child or restricting child's activities or interactions with peers

Allow family to express discouragement at interference with activities and what appears to be slow progress

EXPECTED OUTCOMES

Family participates in follow-up care

Family expresses both positive and negative reactions to child's progress

*Signs that may indicate family's difficulty in adjusting to child's condition are identified early

■ **PATIENT (SIBLINGS) GOAL 10:** Will exhibit positive attachment behaviors with child

NURSING INTERVENTIONS/*RATIONALES*

Assess siblings *to identify areas of concern*

Communicate honestly with siblings about child's disease or disability in accord with parental wishes

Provide opportunity for siblings to ask questions and express feelings, but avoid lengthy explanations before they ask *so that they are not overwhelmed*

Help parents talk to siblings about child's condition and interpret siblings' needs and questions

Encourage parents to spend special time with their children who are not ill or disabled

Help siblings and family understand that it is normal for them to sometimes have negative feelings about child

Prepare siblings in advance for any household changes, *since preparation encourages coping*

Encourage parents to allow siblings to participate in child's care and therapy as appropriate

Help siblings learn how to explain child's condition to their peers and others

Acknowledge siblings' strengths and abilities to cope

Refer to sibling groups and networks composed of siblings of children with the same or similar conditions *for ongoing support*

Assess siblings periodically *to determine their adjustment to the family situation*

EXPECTED OUTCOMES

Siblings verbalize or otherwise demonstrate their feelings and concerns

Parents include siblings in discussions about affected child

Parents make an effort to spend time with other children

Siblings exhibit an understanding of household changes

Siblings assist with affected child's care (specify)

Siblings become involved in support groups (specify)

> **NURSING DIAGNOSIS:** Anxiety/fear related to tests, procedures, hospitalization, etc. (specify)

■ **PATIENT GOAL 1:** Will demonstrate understanding of hospitalization, procedures, etc. (specify)

NURSING INTERVENTIONS/*RATIONALES*

(See Preparation for procedures, p. 219.)

(See also Nursing Care Plan: The Child in the Hospital, p. 268.)

EXPECTED OUTCOME

Child copes with stresses of procedures, tests, etc. (specify)

*Nursing outcome.

Continued

Unit 4

The Child with Chronic Illness or Disability—cont'd

COMMUNITY FOCUS

Key Terms to Know in Special Education and Early Intervention

ADA—Americans with Disabilities Act (PL 101-336) prohibits discrimination against individuals with disabilities. The act applies to adults and children and affects many businesses and services, including stores, hotels, public transportation terminals, parks, museums, employers, schools, and daycare centers.

IDEA—Individuals with Disabilities Education Act (PL 101-476) is based on the Education for All Handicapped Children Act (PL 94-142). Children enrolled in special education (criteria vary by state) may be eligible to receive special education and related services mandated by IDEA. Covered disabilities range widely and include severe visual and hearing impairments, speech impairment, mental retardation, emotional problems, learning disabilities, physical disabilities, and other health impairments.

IEP—Individualized Education Plan is required under IDEA. Based on a multidisciplinary evaluation and shared with parents, the IEP outlines special education and other related services to be received by the child with special needs. Related services can include transportation, developmental services (speech, audiology, physical therapy, occupational therapy, and others), support-

ive services (psychologic services, social work), and medical services as required to assist a child in benefitting from special education.

IFSP—Individualized Family Service Plan, called for in PL 99-457, is based on the IEP concept but has components including a developmental assessment, identification of family strengths, plan for supporting the child's development, early intervention services to be provided for the child and the family, expected outcomes, a designated case manager, and a plan for transition to school services.

Part H—Title I (Part H) of PL 99-457 addresses early intervention services for children with special needs from birth to age 2 years, 11 months.

PL 99-457 (The Education of the Handicapped Act Amendments of 1986)—PL 99-457 was passed to address the needs of young children with disabilities. Title I (Part H) asks states to coordinate early intervention services for children from birth through age 2 years, 11 months. Title II extends the provisions of PL 94-142, a special education law, to children 3 to 5 years of age and notes that the services can be provided in the home or in other settings.

The Child with Chronic Illness or Disability—cont'd

> **NURSING DIAGNOSIS:** Risk for injury (specify)

- **PATIENT GOAL 1:** Will experience no injury

NURSING INTERVENTIONS/*RATIONALES*

Assess environment for hazards if indicated
Teach safety precautions *to decrease risk of injury*
Encourage activities that are compatible with the disease or disability

EXPECTED OUTCOME

Child remains free of injury and complications

- **PATIENT GOAL 2:** Will cope with limitations positively

NURSING INTERVENTIONS/*RATIONALES*

Help devise alternatives for restricted activities and help child cope with physical limitations *so that child's ability to cope is maximized*

EXPECTED OUTCOME

Child demonstrates appropriate adaptation to limitations (specify)

- **PATIENT GOAL 3:** Will experience no complications

NURSING INTERVENTIONS/*RATIONALES*

Stress importance of sound health practices and frequent health supervision *so that complications are less likely to develop*
Make certain child and family understand the therapeutic measures prescribed *to promote optimum health*
Encourage older child to choose activities but take responsibility for own safety
Plan appropriate activities with allied personnel (e.g., teachers, coaches, counselors)
Confer with school nurse (or other person) regarding any special needs of child
Discuss with parents any indicated limit-setting

EXPECTED OUTCOME

Child maintains optimum health

> **NURSING DIAGNOSIS:** Diversional activity deficit related to environmental lack of diversion, physical limitations (specify), hospitalization

- **PATIENT GOAL 1:** Will have opportunity to participate in diversional activities

NURSING INTERVENTIONS/*RATIONALES*

Provide appropriate stimulation
Encourage activities appropriate to age, interests, and capabilities of child

Encourage physical exercise that does not overtax child (if indicated)
Incorporate therapeutic needs in play activities as appropriate
Supervise and encourage activities of daily living
Encourage child's natural tendency to be active
Encourage interaction with family and peers
Include child in planning and scheduling care *to ensure adequate time for diversional activities*

EXPECTED OUTCOME

Child engages in age-appropriate activities within limits of capabilities

- **PATIENT GOAL 2:** Will engage in appropriate exercise

NURSING INTERVENTIONS/*RATIONALES*

Encourage child to participate in normal childhood activities commensurate with interests and capabilities
Encourage and reinforce age-appropriate behaviors, experiences, and socialization with peers
Discourage physical inactivity *so that child receives needed exercise*

EXPECTED OUTCOME

Child engages in nonsedentary activities within limits of disability or condition

> **NURSING DIAGNOSIS:** Impaired social interaction related to hospitalization, confinement to home, frequent illness, activity intolerance, fatigue (specify)

- **PATIENT GOAL 1:** Will experience positive interpersonal relationships

NURSING INTERVENTIONS/*RATIONALES*

Encourage child to maintain usual activities
Arrange for continued interpersonal contacts while hospitalized or otherwise confined
Provide opportunities for interaction with others, especially peers, *for optimum growth and development*
Encourage regular school attendance (including daycare, beginning school, return to school)
  Arrange for rest periods at school if needed *so that child is better able to attend school*
Promote peer contact whenever possible *so that relationships can develop and be maintained*
Encourage recreational outlets and after-school activities appropriate to child's interests and capabilities
Discourage activities that increase isolation from others

EXPECTED OUTCOMES

Child engages in appropriate activities
Child associates with peers and family
Child attends school with reasonable regularity

Continued

Unit 4

The Child with Chronic Illness or Disability—cont'd

NURSING DIAGNOSIS: Self-care deficit (specify) related to specific impairment (specify)

■ **PATIENT GOAL 1:** Will engage in self-care activities

NURSING INTERVENTIONS/*RATIONALES*

Teach child about the diseases and therapies *to ensure optimum understanding, cooperation, and safety*

Encourage child to assist in own care as age and capabilities permit

Provide and/or help devise methods to facilitate maximum functioning

Incorporate play that encourages desired behavior *to encourage cooperation and compliance*

Select toys and activities that allow maximum participation by child

Modify environment if needed (specify) *so that child can assume self-care activities*

Assist with self-care activities where needed (specify)

Avoid undue persistence to accomplish a goal

Provide incentives *to achieve desired behavior*

Instruct when to seek assistance from family or health care providers

EXPECTED OUTCOME

Child engages in self-help activities commensurate with capabilities (specify activities and extent of involvement)

■ **PATIENT GOAL 2:** Will achieve sense of competence and mastery

NURSING INTERVENTIONS/*RATIONALES*

Capitalize on child's assets; help child compensate for liabilities

Praise child for accomplishments and "near" accomplishments, such as partial completion of a task, *to encourage sense of competency*

Ensure adequate rest before attempting energy-expending activities

Emphasize child's abilities and focus on realistic endeavors

Emphasize positive coping behaviors

Discourage activities that are beyond child's capabilities; promote and reinforce successful endeavors

Encourage participation in own care to the extent that child is able

Teach and encourage responsibility for use of equipment, appliances, testing, medications (specify)

Help child become adept at self-management to maximum capabilities

EXPECTED OUTCOMES

Child takes responsibility for self-care according to age and capabilities (specify)

Child engages in appropriate activities without undue fatigue

NURSING DIAGNOSIS: Body image disturbance related to perception of disability (self and others), feeling of being different, inability to participate in specific activities (specify)

■ **PATIENT GOAL 1:** Will maintain positive attitude

NURSING INTERVENTIONS/*RATIONALES*

Convey an attitude of understanding, caring, and acceptance *to encourage positive attitude and self-image*

Maintain open communications with child

Relate to child on appropriate cognitive level

Serve as a role model for others *so that they are more accepting*

EXPECTED OUTCOME

Child maintains a positive attitude (specify behaviors)

■ **PATIENT GOAL 2:** Will express feelings and concerns

NURSING INTERVENTIONS/*RATIONALES*

Encourage verbalization of feelings and perceptions, especially feelings of "differentness"

Explore feelings concerning disease or disability and its implications: stress of being different, physical limitations, difficulty competing, relationships with peers, self-image

Encourage child to discuss feelings about how he or she thinks others feel about the disorder

EXPECTED OUTCOME

Child openly discusses feelings and concerns about the condition, therapies, and perceived reactions of others

■ **PATIENT GOAL 3:** Will cope with actual or perceived changes caused by illness

NURSING INTERVENTIONS/*RATIONALES*

Acknowledge feelings; facilitate sharing feelings with family members, other health professionals

Clarify misconceptions child may have acquired

Help child to identify positive aspects of situation *to facilitate coping*

EXPECTED OUTCOME

Child discusses the disorder and feelings regarding limitations it imposes

■ **PATIENT GOAL 4:** Will cope with disorder and its effects

NURSING INTERVENTIONS/*RATIONALES*

Help child assess own strengths and assets; emphasize strengths

Identify coping behaviors *so that they can be reinforced*

Support positive coping mechanisms and extinguish negative ones

The Child with Chronic Illness or Disability—cont'd

Help child set realistic goals *to facilitate coping*

Encourage as much independence as condition allows

Introduce child to other children who have adjusted well to this or a similar disorder

Suggest involvement with special groups and facilities for children with similar problems

EXPECTED OUTCOMES

Child realistically identifies own assets and strengths

Child verbalizes positive suggestions for adjusting to the disability

Child becomes involved with special group activities

■ **PATIENT GOAL 5:** Will exhibit improved self-esteem and self-concept

NURSING INTERVENTIONS/*RATIONALES*

Encourage an appealing physical appearance: good body hygiene; clean, straight teeth; good grooming; stylish hair and clothing; makeup for teenage girls

Assist with improving appearance and grooming

Point out positive aspects of child's coping, appearance, and capabilities

Promote constructive thinking in child; encourage child to maximize strengths

Reinforce positive behaviors

Help child to determine and engage in activities that foster self-esteem

   Promote independence *since this is an important part of self-esteem*

EXPECTED OUTCOMES

Child demonstrates a positive appearance and good body image (specify)

Child appears clean, well-groomed, and attractively dressed

Child exhibits behaviors that indicate elevated self-esteem (specify)

■ **PATIENT GOAL 6:** Will exhibit appropriate sense of control

NURSING INTERVENTIONS/*RATIONALES*

Channel need for control and feeling of effectiveness in appropriate directions

Encourage child to monitor own care as appropriate

Provide opportunities for child to make choices and participate in care when appropriate *to ensure sense of control*

Assess child for vocational planning (when appropriate)

EXPECTED OUTCOME

Child becomes actively involved in own care and management

■ **PATIENT GOAL 7:** Will be prepared for discharge

NURSING INTERVENTIONS/*RATIONALES*

Begin early in hospitalization to discuss "going home"

Help child develop independence and self-help capabilities

Encourage visits from friends *to help child assess the impact of any change in appearance or behavior that might interfere with the return to former environments*

EXPECTED OUTCOMES

Child verbalizes and otherwise demonstrates interest in going home

(See also:

   Nursing Care Plan: The Child in the Hospital, 268.)

   Nursing Care Plan: The Family of the Child Who Is Ill or Hospitalized, p. 282.)

   Nursing Care Plan: The Child Who Is Terminally Ill or Dying, p. 296.)

Unit 4

NURSING CARE PLAN

The Child Who Is Terminally Ill or Dying

Terminal illness—A condition wherein a life is near or approaching its end
Grief—Physical, emotional, and spiritual responses to bereavement, separation, or loss

Grief reaction—Complex of somatic and psychologic symptoms associated with some extreme sorrow or loss
Anticipatory grief—Grieving before an actual loss

ASSESSMENT

Perform a physical assessment.
Obtain a health history of the terminal illness and therapies.
Assess child's conception of self, a process that occurs in the following five stages, as the child acquires information about own situation.*
  Stage 1—Disease is a serious illness
        New identity of "sick" child
  Stage 2—Discovery of the relationship of medication and recovery
        Learns the taboos of disease and death
  Stage 3—Marked by an understanding of the purposes and implications of special procedures
        Sense of well-being begins to fade and perceives self as different from other children
  Stage 4—Illness is viewed as a permanent condition
        Sense of always being sick and never getting better
  Stage 5—Realization that there is only a finite number of medications
        Awareness (directly or indirectly) of the fatal prognosis
Assess child's understanding of and reactions to death (Table 4-4).
Observe for physical signs of approaching death:
  Loss of sensation and movement in the lower extremities, progressing toward the upper body
  Sensation of heat, although body feels cool

Loss of senses:
  Tactile sensation decreases
  Sensitive to light
  Hearing is last sense to fail
Confusion, loss of consciousness, slurred speech
Muscle weakness
Loss of bowel and bladder control
Decreased appetite/thirst
Difficulty swallowing
Change in respiratory pattern
  Cheyne-Stokes respirations (waxing and waning of depth of breathing with regular periods of apnea)
  "Death rattle" (noisy chest sounds from accumulation of pulmonary and pharyngeal secretions)
Weak, slow pulse; decreased blood pressure
Assess family's response to impending death.
Observe for manifestations of the normal grief reaction in family members (Box 4-6).
Assess family's support systems, coping mechanisms, and available resources.
Assess own ability to provide effective care for children who are dying:
  Be aware of own feelings.
  Identify own coping strategies.
  Explore ethical issues.
  Recognize signs of *burnout,* a state of physical, emotional, and mental exhaustion.
(See assessment of specific disorder.)

NURSING DIAGNOSIS: Altered growth and development related to terminal illness and/or impending death

■ **PATIENT GOAL 1:** Will receive adequate support during terminal phase

NURSING INTERVENTIONS/*RATIONALES*

Encourage family to remain near child as much as possible *to provide support through their presence*
Encourage child to talk about feelings; help family as they encourage child to express feelings
Provide safe, acceptable outlets for aggression
Answer questions honestly while maintaining a positive, hopeful approach
Explain all procedures and therapies, especially the physical effects child will experience
Help child distinguish between consequences of therapies and manifestations of disease process
Structure hospital environment to allow for maximum self-control and independence within the limitations imposed by child's developmental level and physical condition
Respect child's need for privacy without neglecting child
Provide for presence of customary support systems

EXPECTED OUTCOMES

Child expresses feelings freely
Child demonstrates an understanding of symptoms
Child feels supported by family and caregivers
Child is free to exert self-control and independence as desired and appropriate for age

■ **PATIENT GOAL 2:** Will exhibit minimal or no evidence of physical discomfort

NURSING INTERVENTIONS/*RATIONALES*

Appreciate that pain control is an essential component of physical and emotional care during terminal stage
Provide pain relief around the clock *to prevent recurrence of pain*
Encourage family to provide comfort measures child prefers (e.g., rocking, stroking)
Avoid excessive noise or light *that may irritate child*
Place all commodities within easy reach *to increase child's control and lessen need for excessive movement*
Use gentle, minimal, physical manipulation
Experiment with using heat or cold on painful areas (use cautiously *because of easy skin breakdown*)
Use atraumatic procedures whenever possible (e.g., noninvasive temperature monitoring) *to minimize discomfort*

*Bluebond-Langner M: Worlds of dying children and their well siblings, *Death Stud* 13:1-16, 1989.

Unit 4

The Child Who Is Terminally Ill or Dying—cont'd

TABLE 4-4 Children's Understanding of and Reactions to Death

Concepts of Death	Reactions to Death	Interventions
Infants and Toddlers		
Death has least significance to children under 6 months.	They may continue to act as though the dead person is alive.	Help parents deal with their feelings, allowing them more emotional reserve to meet the needs of their children.
After parent-child attachment and the development of trust is established, a loss, even temporary, of the significant person is profound.	As children grow older, they will be increasingly able and willing to let go of the dead person.	Encourage parents to remain as near to child as possible; but also be sensitive to parents' needs.
Prolonged separation during the first several years is thought to be more significant in terms of future physical, social, and emotional growth than at any subsequent age.	Ritualism is important; a change in lifestyle could be anxiety producing.	Maintain as normal an environment as possible to retain ritualism.
Toddlers are egocentric and can only think about events in terms of their own frame of reference—living.	This age-group reacts more to the pain and discomfort of a serious illness than to the probable fatal prognosis.	If a parent has died, encourage having consistent caregiver for child.
Their egocentricity and vague separation of fact and fantasy make it impossible for them to comprehend absence of life.		Promote primary nursing.
Instead of understanding death, this age-group is affected more by any change in lifestyle.		
Preschool Children		
Believe their thoughts are sufficient to cause death, and as a consequence feel the burden of guilt, shame, and punishment.	If they become seriously ill, they conceive of the illness as a punishment for their thoughts or actions.	Help parents deal with their feelings, allowing them more emotional reserve to meet the needs of their children.
Their egocentricity implies a tremendous sense of self-power and omnipotence.	May feel guilty and responsible for the death of a sibling.	Help parents to understand behavioral reactions of their children.
Usually have some connotation of the meaning of death.	Greatest fear concerning death is separation from parents.	Encourage parents to remain near the child as much as possible, to minimize the child's great fear of separation from parents.
Death is seen as a departure, a kind of sleep.	May engage in activities that seem strange or abnormal to adults.	If a parent has died, encourage having a consistent caregiver for child.
May recognize the fact of physical death but do not separate it from living abilities.	Because they have fewer defense mechanisms to deal with loss, young children may react to a less significant loss with more outward grief than the loss of a very significant person.	Promote primary nursing.
Death is seen as temporary and gradual; life and death can change places with one another.	The loss can be so deep, painful, and threatening that the child must deny it for the present to survive its overwhelming impact.	
No understanding of the universality and inevitability of death.	Behavior reactions such as giggling, joking, attracting attention, or regressing to earlier developmental skills indicate the need to distance themselves from tremendous loss.	

Continued

Unit 4

The Child Who Is Terminally Ill or Dying—cont'd

TABLE 4-4   Children's Understanding of and Reactions to Death—cont'd

Concepts of Death	Reactions to Death	Interventions
School-Age Children Still associate misdeeds or bad thoughts with causing death and feel intense guilt and responsibility for the event. Because of their higher cognitive abilities, they respond well to logical explanations and comprehend the figurative meaning of words. Have a deeper understanding of death in a concrete sense. Particularly fear the mutilation and punishment they associate with death. Personify death as a devil, monster, or bogeyman. May have naturalistic/physiologic explanations of death. By 9 or 10 years of age children have an adult concept of death, realizing that it is inevitable, universal, and irreversible.	Because of their increased ability to comprehend, they may have more fears, for example: The reason for the illness Communicability of the disease to themselves or others Consequences of the disease The process of dying and death itself Their fear of the unknown is greater than the known. The realization of impending death is a tremendous threat to their sense of security and ego strength. Likely to exhibit fear through verbal uncooperativeness rather than actual physical aggression. Very interested in postdeath services. May be inquisitive about what happens to the body.	Help parents deal with their feelings, allowing them more emotional reserve to meet the needs of their children. Encourage parents to remain near child as much as possible; but also be sensitive to parents' needs. Because of children's fear of the unknown, anticipatory preparation is very important. Since the developmental task of this age is industry, helping children maintain control over their bodies and increasing their understanding allows them to achieve independence, self-worth, and self-esteem and avoids a sense of inferiority. Encourage children to talk about their feelings and provide outlets for aggression. Encourage parents to honestly answer questions about dying rather than avoiding them or fabricating euphemisms. Encourage parents to share their moments of sorrow with their children. Provide preparation for postdeath services.
Adolescents Have a mature understanding of death. Still very much influenced by remnants of magical thinking and are subject to guilt and shame. Likely to see deviations from accepted behavior as reasons for their illness.	Straddle transition from childhood to adulthood. Have the most difficulty in coping with death. Least likely to accept cessation of life, particularly if it is their own. Concern is for the present much more than for the past or the future. May consider themselves alienated from their peers and unable to communicate with their parents for emotional support, feeling alone in their struggle. Adolescents' orientation to the present compels them to worry about physical changes even more than the prognosis. Because of their idealistic view of the world, they may criticize funeral rites as barbaric, money making, and unnecessary.	Help parents deal with their feelings, allowing them more emotional reserve to meet the needs of their children. Avoid alliances with either parent or child. Structure hospital admission to allow for maximum self-control and independence. Answer adolescents' questions honestly, treating them as mature individuals and respecting their need for privacy, solitude, and personal expression of emotions. Help parents understand their child's reactions to death/dying, especially that their concern for present crises, such as loss of hair, may be much greater than for future ones, including possible death.

Unit 4

The Child Who Is Terminally Ill or Dying—cont'd

Change position frequently; if difficult for child, coordinate with pain relief from analgesics *to make moving easier and less distressing*

Avoid pressure on bony prominences or painful sites (e.g., with water bed, flotation mattress); ensure good body aligment *to prevent skin breakdown*

Keep fresh air circulating in room (e.g., open window, use small fan)

Use pillows or other supports to prop child in comfortable position

Carry child (if possible) to other areas for diversion if desired

Place absorbent pads under hips *because child may be incontinent*

Help child to toilet if desired

Limit care to essentials:

May need to forego usual hygienic measures such as bath or clothing change, but provide comfort measures (e.g., mouth care, wiping forehead, gentle back rub)

*Administer anticholinergic drugs (atropine or scopolamine) *to reduce secretions* (lessens "death rattle," *which can be distressing to family*)

EXPECTED OUTCOME
Child exhibits minimal or no evidence of physical discomfort

■ **PATIENT GOAL 3:** Will receive adequate emotional support at time of dying

NURSING INTERVENTIONS/*RATIONALES*
Preserve child's physical closeness with family members (e.g., parent may want to rock child in chair or lie next to child in bed)

Teach family about supportive interventions

Talk to child even though child may not appear to be awake

Position self and others where child can easily see face (e.g., sitting at head of bed)

Speak to child in clear, distinct voice; avoid whispering

Avoid conversation about child in child's presence *to reduce anxiety/fear*

Offer calm reassurance and orient child to surroundings when awake

Phrase questions for "yes" or "no" answers *to conserve energy*

Avoid repeated measurements of vital signs, *which only disturb child*

Play favorite music *(may soothe child)*

EXPECTED OUTCOME
Child appears calm and relaxed

*Dependent nursing action.

Continued

BOX 4-6

Symptomatology of Normal Grief

Sensations of Somatic Distress

Feelings of tightness in the throat

Choking, with shortness of breath

Marked tendency to sighing

Empty feeling in the abdomen

Lack of muscular power

Intense subjective distress described as tension or mental pain

Preoccupation with Image of the Deceased

Hears, sees, or imagines that the dead person is present

Slight sense of unreality

Feeling of emotional distance from others

May believe that he or she is approaching insanity

Feelings of Guilt

Searches for evidence of failure in preventing the death

Accuses self of negligence or exaggerates minor omissions

Feelings of Hostility

Loss of warmth toward others

Tendency to irritability and anger

Wishes to not be bothered by friends or relatives

Loss of Usual Patterns of Conduct

Restlessness, inability to sit still, aimless moving about

Continual searching for something to do or what he or she thinks should be done

Lack of capacity to initiate and maintain organized patterns of activity

Modified from Lindemann E: Symptomatology and management of acute grief, *Am J Psychiatry* 101:141-143, 1944.

The Child Who Is Terminally Ill or Dying—cont'd

NURSING DIAGNOSIS: Altered nutrition: less than body requirements related to loss of appetite, disinterest in food

■ **PATIENT GOAL 1:** Will receive optimum nutrition

NURSING INTERVENTIONS/*RATIONALES*

Offer any food and fluids child desires
Provide small meals and snacks several times a day
Avoid excessive encouragement to eat or drink
Avoid foods with strong odors *because they may cause nausea*
Provide pleasant environment for eating
Serve foods that require the least energy to eat (soups, shakes)
Feed slowly *to conserve energy*
*Administer antiemetic as prescribed if nausea/vomiting is a problem
Provide mouth care before and after eating; lubricate lips with petrolatum *to prevent cracking and promote comfort*

EXPECTED OUTCOME

Child consumes some nutrients and fluids

NURSING DIAGNOSIS: Fear/anxiety related to diagnosis, tests, and therapies and prognosis

■ **PATIENT GOAL 1:** Will experience reduction of anxiety

NURSING INTERVENTIONS/*RATIONALES*

Explain all procedures and other aspects of care to child *to reduce anxiety and fear*
Remain with child or provide for constant attendance
Determine what child has been told about prognosis *so this information can be reinforced*
Determine what family wishes child to know about prognosis
Emphasize importance of honesty
Encourage child to express feelings
Answer child's questions openly and honestly while maintaining a hopeful approach
Involve parents in child's care
Remain nonjudgmental regarding child's behavior

EXPECTED OUTCOME

Child discusses fears without evidence of stress

NURSING DIAGNOSIS: Anticipatory grieving related to potential loss of a child

■ **PATIENT (FAMILY) GOAL 1:** Will receive adequate support

NURSING INTERVENTIONS/*RATIONALES*

Discuss the grieving process with family *so that family better understands normalcy of feelings*
Provide opportunities for family to express emotions
Help parents deal with their feelings, *allowing them more emotional reserve to meet the needs of their children*
Encourage parents to remain as near to child as possible; but also be sensitive to parents' needs
Provide information regarding child's status and anticipated reactions *to decrease anxiety/fear*
Help parents to understand behavioral reactions of their child, especially that child's concerns for present crisis, such as loss of hair, may be much greater than for future crises, including possible death
Facilitate family's assistance with child's care
Provide comfort measures for child and family
Encourage family to address own health care needs
Provide as much privacy as possible
Assist family in assessing their need for referral services (e.g., hospice services, specific organizations for grieving families)
Encourage parents to honestly answer child's questions about dying rather than avoiding questions or using euphemisms
Encourage parents to share their moments of sorrow with child
Discuss with parents appropriate involvement of siblings
Identify religious and cultural beliefs related to death (e.g., prayer, rites, rituals)
Provide preparation for postdeath services
Discuss with family their preferences for care if death is imminent
Arrange for appropriate spiritual care in accordance with family's beliefs and/or affiliations
Maintain contact with family
Provide support for families who choose home care/hospice for their child
(See Guidelines box and Box 4-7.)

EXPECTED OUTCOMES

Family expresses fears, concerns, and any special desires for child who is terminally ill
Family demonstrates an understanding of child's needs (specify)
Family members avail themselves of services as desired
(See also:
  Nursing Care Plan: The Child in the Hospital, p. 268.)
  Nursing Care Plan: The Family of the Child Who Is Ill or Hospitalized, p. 282.)

*Dependent nursing action.

The Child Who Is Terminally Ill or Dying—cont'd

■ **PATIENT GOAL 2:** Will exhibit no evidence of loneliness

NURSING INTERVENTIONS/*RATIONALES*

Offer calm reassurance to child

Reassure child of the love of others

Continue to set some limits for child *to provide a sense of security*

Spend time with child when not directly involved in care

Reinforce to child that what is happening is not child's fault *to decrease feelings of guilt*

Involve child in routine activities as tolerated

Maintain a "normal" atmosphere

Talk to child even though child may not appear to be awake:

Situate self and others where easily visible to child

Speak to child in clear, distinct voice; avoid whispering

Avoid conversation about child's condition in presence of child *to decrease anxiety/fear*

Play favorite music or read stories to child

Orient child to surroundings when awake

Phrase questions for "yes" or "no" answers when possible *to conserve child's energy*

Instruct/encourage parents in above interventions

EXPECTED OUTCOME

Child exhibits no evidence of loneliness

NURSING DIAGNOSIS: Anticipatory grieving related to imminent death of a child

---

■ **PATIENT (FAMILY) GOAL 1:** Will receive adequate support

NURSING INTERVENTIONS/*RATIONALES*

Be available to family

Inform family of what to expect at time of death

Convey an attitude of caring for both child and family

Encourage at least one family member to stay with child

Help family to provide care of child, as they desire, without forcing involvement

*Administer medications or other agents as prescribed *to reduce unpleasant manifestations:*

Oxygen *for respiratory distress*

Anticonvulsants *for seizures*

Anticholinergic drugs *to reduce secretions ("death rattle")*

Analgesics *for pain* (Community Focus box)

Stool softeners/laxatives *for constipation*

Antiemetics *for nausea/vomiting*

Help and encourage family members to express feelings appropriately

Encourage family members to meet their own physical needs

Provide privacy

Provide for physical comfort of family

Provide emotional support and comfort to family

Encourage family to talk to child

Involve family and other children in decision-making whenever possible, especially regarding alternatives for terminal care (hospital, home, hospice)

Support and assist family in giving explanations to other family members regarding child's status

Maintain nonjudgmental attitude toward behavior of family members

EXPECTED OUTCOMES

Family members discuss their feelings

Family members are actively involved in child's care

■ **PATIENT (FAMILY) GOAL 2:** Will receive adequate support for home care/hospice

NURSING INTERVENTIONS/*RATIONALES*

Teach family physical care of child

Provide family with means for contacting health professionals at any time (e.g., telephone numbers)

Maintain daily contact with family (e.g., telephone call, home visit)

Refer to community agencies as appropriate *for ongoing support*

Reassure family that they can readmit child to the hospital at any time

Help plan with family what to do and what to expect when the child dies

EXPECTED OUTCOMES

Family demonstrates ability to provide care for child

Family is in contact with appropriate support groups as desired

---

*Dependent nursing action.

Continued

Unit 4

The Child Who Is Terminally Ill or Dying—cont'd

GUIDELINES

Supporting Grieving Families*

General

Stay with the family; sit quietly if they prefer not to talk; cry with them if desired.

Accept the family's grief reactions; avoid judgmental statements (e.g., "You should be feeling better by now").

Avoid offering rationalizations for the child's death (e.g., "You should be glad your child isn't suffering anymore").

Avoid artificial consolation (e.g., "I know how you feel" or "You are still young enough to have another baby").

Deal openly with feelings such as guilt, anger, and loss of self-esteem.

Focus on feelings by using a feeling word in the statement (e.g., "You're still feeling all the pain of losing a child").

Refer the family to an appropriate self-help group or for professional help if needed.

At the Time of Death

Reassure the family that everything possible is being done for the child, if they wish lifesaving interventions.

Do everything possible to ensure the child's comfort, especially relief from pain.

Provide the child and family the opportunity to review special experiences or memories in their lives.

Express personal feelings of loss and/or frustrations (e.g., "We will miss him so much" or "We tried everything; we feel so sorry that we couldn't save him").

Provide information that the family requests, and be honest.

Respect the emotional needs of family members, such as siblings, who may need brief respites from the dying child.

Make every effort to arrange for family members, especially parents, to be with the child at the moment of death, if they wish to be present.

Encourage family members to talk to the child, even if he or she appears comatose.

Allow the family to stay with the dead child for as long as they wish and to rock, hold, or bathe the child.

Provide practical help when possible, such as collecting the child's belongings.

Help the family identify and contact a relative, friend, or other support person.

Respect religious and cultural beliefs, such as special rites or rituals.

Arrange for spiritual support, such as clergy; provide spiritual support as requested by child or family.

After the Death

Attend the funeral, visitation, or memorial service if there was a special closeness with the family.

Initiate and maintain contact (e.g., sending cards, telephoning, inviting them back to the unit, or making a home visit).

Refer to the dead child by name; discuss shared memories with the family.

Discourage the use of drugs or alcohol as a method of escaping grief.

Encourage all family members to communicate their feelings rather than remain silent to avoid upsetting another member.

Emphasize that grieving is a painful process that often takes *years* to resolve.

*The term *family* refers to all significant persons involved in the child's life, such as the parents, siblings, grandparents, and other close relatives or friends.

Unit 4

The Child Who Is Terminally Ill or Dying—cont'd

BOX 4-7

Strategies for Intervention with Survivors of Sudden Childhood Death

Arrival of the Family

Meet the family immediately and escort them to a private area.

A health care worker with bereavement training should remain with the family.

Provide information about the extent of illness or injury and treatment efforts.

If the health care worker must leave the family, or the family requests privacy, return in 15 minutes, so that the family does not feel forgotten.

Provide tissues, telephone, coffee, and a Bible or other religious objects as desired.

Pronouncement of Death

When available, the family's own physician should inform them of the child's death.

Alternatively, the physician or nurse should introduce themselves and establish calm, reassuring eye contact with the parents.

Honest, clear communication that avoids misinterpretation is essential.

Nonverbal communication such as hugging, touching, or remaining with the family in silence may be most empathetic.

Acknowledge the family's guilt, attempt to alleviate it, and deal openly and nonjudgmentally with anger.

Provide information, answer questions, and offer reassurance that everything possible was done for the child.

Viewing the Body

Offer the parents the opportunity to see the body; repeat the offer later if they decline.

Before viewing, inform the parents of bodily changes they should expect (tubes, injuries, cold skin).

A single staff member should accompany the family but remain inconspicuous.

Offer the opportunity to hold the child.

Allow the family as much time as they need.

Offer parents the opportunity for siblings to view the body.

Formal Concluding Process

Discuss and answer questions concerning autopsy and funeral arrangements; obtain signatures on the body release and autopsy forms.

Provide anticipatory guidance regarding symptoms of grief response and their normalcy.

Provide written materials about grief symptoms.

Escort the family to the exit or to their car if necessary.

Provide a follow-up phone call in 24 to 48 hours to answer questions and provide support.

Provide referral for community health nursing visit.

Provide referrals to local support and resource groups (e.g., bereavement groups, bereavement counselors, SIDS groups, Parents of Murdered Children, and Mothers Against Drunk Driving).

Modified from Back K: Sudden, unexpected pediatric death: caring for the parents, *Pediatr Nurs* 17(6):571-574, 1991.

COMMUNITY FOCUS

Pain Control/Terminal Sedation and the "Double Effect"

When children are dying, one of the essential goals is to provide comfort. Often meeting this goal requires the use of large doses of opioids to control pain. In some situations, opioids provide insufficient analgesia and sedatives, such as barbiturates, are used to provide deep or unconscious sedation. Since the level of sedation generally hastens a person's death by depressing respirations, this use of "terminal sedation" is sometimes viewed as a method of euthanasia or assisted suicide. In these situations, the family deals with the difficult decision of relieving suffering but possibly shortening life. Their choice is often influenced by the community's—both consumers' and professionals'—beliefs and attitudes about "mercy killing."

The principles involved in ethical decision-making provide a useful framework for understanding the legitimacy for administering large doses of opioids or sedatives to relieve pain in the dying. The principle of "double effect"

draws a distinction between the intended effects of a person's action and the unintentional but recognized effects of that action. Justification for the use of terminal sedation requires that the practitioner intend only to relieve the child's suffering but not cause death.* Since death is inevitable, it is not possible to determine if the cause was the disease or the drug.

Nurses need to understand that medication to control pain is essential and that the ethical principle of double effect can justify this practice. It is difficult enough for a family to face the loss of their child without also having to face the cynicism of the uninformed public or professional. Since it is usually the nurse who administers the final dose of medication, it is often a concern that this dose killed the child. Again the principle of double effect provides reassurance that the medication was given only to relieve pain and that the timing of death can never be predicted.

*Truog D and others: Barbiturates in the care of the terminally ill, *N Engl J Med* 327(23):1678-1682, 1992.

Unit 4

NURSING CARE OF COMMON PROBLEMS OF ILL AND HOSPITALIZED CHILDREN

Children are admitted to the hospital for a variety of health problems. Some experiences are the same for all children (e.g., admission); others are shared by a number of children in their unique circumstances. The following are some of the common problems that are experienced frequently but not universally by children in the hospital.

NURSING CARE PLAN

The Child Undergoing Surgery

ASSESSMENT

Perform a physical assessment. (See Unit 1.)
Assess the child's understanding of the impending surgery and postoperative expectations.

Assess child for evidence of infection.
Review results of laboratory tests for abnormal findings.

PREOPERATIVE CARE

> **NURSING DIAGNOSIS:** Risk for injury related to surgical procedure, anesthesia

- **PATIENT GOAL 1:** Will receive fully informed consent and sign appropriate documents

NURSING INTERVENTIONS/*RATIONALES*

Inquire whether parents have any questions about procedure *to determine their level of understanding and to provide for additional information from nurse or other professional*
Check chart for signed informed consent form or obtain informed consent
   Contact physician to determine if parents have been informed of procedure *because informed consent is physician's responsibility*
   Obtain and/or witness signature if not obtained earlier

EXPECTED OUTCOMES

Family receives fully informed consent
Family signs appropriate documents

- **PATIENT GOAL 2:** Will receive proper hygiene measures

NURSING INTERVENTIONS/*RATIONALES*

Bathe child, groom hair
Provide mouth care *to promote comfort while NPO*
Cleanse operative site according to prescribed method, if ordered, *to minimize risk of infection*

EXPECTED OUTCOME

Child is cleansed and prepared appropriately (specify)

- **PATIENT GOAL 3:** Will receive proper preparation

NURSING INTERVENTIONS/*RATIONALES*

Carry out special procedure as prescribed (e.g., colonic enemas)
*Administer antibiotics as ordered, observing for known side effects
Order and/or assist with special tests such as radiographs
Consult with practitioner for appropriate change in schedule or route of administration of any medication child ordinarily receives
Attire child appropriately (e.g., special operating room gown)
   Allow child to wear underwear or pajama bottoms, if possible, *to provide privacy*
   Label personal articles and clothing
Remove any makeup and/or nail polish *to observe for cyanosis*
Remove jewelry and/or prosthetic devices (e.g., mouth retainers) *because they may be lost or interfere with anesthesia/surgery*
Check for loose teeth
   Inform anesthesiologist if loose teeth are detected *to prevent aspiration of teeth during anesthesia*

EXPECTED OUTCOME

Child is prepared appropriately (specify)

- **PATIENT GOAL 4:** Will experience no complications

NURSING INTERVENTIONS/*RATIONALES*

Maintain child NPO (nothing by mouth) as ordered *to prevent aspiration during anesthesia* (See Practice Alert, p. 307.)
Be sure child is well hydrated before NPO begins, especially infants, *who are more at risk for dehydration*
Take and record vital signs
   Report any deviations from admission readings, especially elevated temperature, *which may indicate infection*
Have child void before preoperative medication is administered *to prevent bladder distention or incontinence during anesthesia*
   Record time of last voiding if unable to void
Be certain allergies are clearly indicated on chart *to decrease risk of adverse reaction*
Check laboratory values for any sign of systemic abnormality such as infection (increased white blood cells), anemia (decreased hemoglobin and/or hematocrit), or bleeding tendencies (reduced platelets or prolonged bleeding or clotting time)
Keep small infants warm during transport and waiting time

EXPECTED OUTCOMES

Child is preoperatively NPO for designated time
Child voids
Pertinent information about child is visible

*Dependent nursing action.

Unit 4

The Child Undergoing Surgery—cont'd

■ **PATIENT GOAL 5:** Will experience no injury

NURSING INTERVENTIONS/*RATIONALES*

Check that identification band is securely fastened
Check identification band with surgical personnel *to ensure correct identification*
Fasten siderails of bed or crib *to prevent falls*
Use restraints during transport by stretcher (or other conveyance) *to prevent falls*
Do not leave child unattended

EXPECTED OUTCOMES

Child is safe from immediate harm
Child is clearly and correctly identified

NURSING DIAGNOSIS: Anxiety/fear related to separation from support system, unfamiliar environment, knowledge deficit

---

■ **PATIENT GOAL 1:** Will demonstrate optimum sense of security

NURSING INTERVENTIONS/*RATIONALES*

Institute preoperative teaching *to reduce anxiety/fear*
Orient child to strange surroundings
Explain where parents will be while child is in operating room
Have someone stay with child *to provide increased sense of security*

EXPECTED OUTCOME

Child demonstrates minimum insecurity or anxiety

■ **PATIENT (FAMILY) GOAL 2:** Will demonstrate understanding of surgery and postoperative care

NURSING INTERVENTIONS/*RATIONALES*

Prepare for postoperative procedures as indicated (e.g., nasogastric tube, IV fluids, NPO, dressing changes, wound drains if necessary)
Explain reason for surgery; if special operative procedure is to be performed, explain basic principles and briefly outline care needed *to reinforce information given by practitioner*
Explain all preoperative procedures (e.g., blood work, any other laboratory test)
In emergency situation, explain most essential components of surgery (e.g., where child will be before and after surgery, anesthesia, dressing)
Accept behavioral reactions of parents and child *because these can be highly variable*

EXPECTED OUTCOMES

Child and family demonstrate an understanding of forthcoming events (specify methods of learning and evaluation)
*Family's behavioral reactions are accepted and supported

■ **PATIENT GOAL 3:** Will exhibit signs of optimum relaxation, sedation, and support before arriving in operating room

NURSING INTERVENTIONS/*RATIONALES*

†Administer preoperative sedation (preferably oral), if ordered, *to promote relaxation and sleep*
Place unfamiliar equipment out of child's view *to decrease anxiety/fear*

Place child in quiet room with minimum distraction *to promote relaxation and encourage sleep*
Do not leave child unattended
Explain what is happening, unless child is asleep
Encourage parents to stay with child as long as permitted and according to their wishes
Permit parents to hold child until child falls asleep, if desired
Encourage parents to accompany child as far as possible, preferably through induction of anesthesia
Allow significant objects to accompany child (e.g., a favorite toy) *to provide comfort and sense of security*

EXPECTED OUTCOMES

Child falls asleep or lies quietly
Child is not left alone

NURSING DIAGNOSIS: Altered family processes related to a surgical procedure

---

■ **PATIENT (FAMILY) GOAL 1:** Will receive adequate support and reassurance

NURSING INTERVENTIONS/*RATIONALES*

Reinforce and clarify information given by practitioner
Explain associated diagnostic tests and procedures (e.g., x-ray examinations)
Explain child's schedule:
    When child will receive premedication
    Time child will leave for surgery
    Where parents can wait for child to return
    Room to which child will return
    Postprocedural care and routines
Explore family's feelings regarding the procedure and its implications *to assess need for further intervention*
Include parents in preparation of child
Be available to family *to provide support and reassurance as needed*
(See also Nursing Care Plan: The Family of the Child Who Is Ill or Hospitalized, p. 282.)

EXPECTED OUTCOMES

Family demonstrates an understanding of procedure (specify demonstration) and related information (specify)
Family complies with directives (specify)

POSTOPERATIVE CARE

NURSING DIAGNOSIS: Risk for injury related to surgical procedure, anesthesia

---

■ **NURSE GOAL 1:** Receive child on return from surgery

NURSING INTERVENTIONS/*RATIONALES*

Place child in bed (unless transported in own bed or crib) using techniques appropriate to type of surgery *to prevent injury*
Hang IV apparatus and connect any needed equipment (e.g., suction apparatus, traction)
Place child in position of comfort and safety in accordance with surgeon's orders
Perform stat (immediate) activities

*Nursing outcome.
†Dependent nursing action.

Continued

The Child Undergoing Surgery—cont'd

EXPECTED OUTCOME

Child is transferred to bed without injury and with minimum
stress

■ **PATIENT GOAL 2:** Will exhibit signs of wound healing
without evidence of wound infection

NURSING INTERVENTIONS/*RATIONALES*

Use proper handwashing techniques and other universal pre-
cautions, especially if wound drainage is present
Employ careful wound care *to minimize risk of infection*
  Keep wound clean and dressings intact
  Apply dressings *that promote moist wound healing*
    (i.e., hydrocolloid dressings such as Duoderm)
  Change dressings if indicated, whenever soiled; carefully
    dispose of soiled dressings
  Carry out special wound care as prescribed (e.g., irrigation,
    drain care)
  Cleanse with prescribed preparation (if ordered)
  *Apply antibacterial solutions and/or ointments as ordered
    to prevent infection
  Report any unusual appearance or drainage *for early
    detection of infection*
Place diapers below abdominal dressing if appropriate *to
  prevent contamination*
When child begins oral feedings, provide nutritious diet as
  ordered *to promote wound healing*

EXPECTED OUTCOME

Child exhibits no evidence of wound infection

■ **PATIENT GOAL 3:** Will exhibit no evidence of complications

NURSING INTERVENTIONS/*RATIONALES*

Ambulate as prescribed *to decrease complications associated
  with immobility*
Maintain child NPO until fully awake *to prevent aspiration*
Encourage to void when awake
  Offer bedpan
  Boys may be allowed to stand at bedside
Notify practitioner if child is unable to void *to ensure appro-
  priate intervention*
Maintain abdominal decompression, chest tubes, or other
  equipment, if prescribed
Provide diet as prescribed; advance as appropriate

EXPECTED OUTCOME

Child exhibits no evidence of complications

NURSING DIAGNOSIS: Anxiety/fear related to
surgery, unfamiliar environment, separation from
support systems, discomfort

■ **PATIENT GOAL 1:** Will experience reduced anxiety

NURSING INTERVENTIONS/*RATIONALES*

Maintain calm, reassuring manner
Encourage expression of feelings *to facilitate coping*

Explain procedures and other activities before initiating
Answer questions and explain purposes of activities
Keep informed of progress
Remain with child as much as possible
Give encouragement and positive feedback for cooperation
  in care
Encourage parental presence as soon as permitted *to decrease
  stress of separation*
If emergency procedure, review child's memory of previous
  events *so that misconceptions can be clarified*

EXPECTED OUTCOMES

Child rests quietly and calmly
Child discusses procedures and activities without evidence of
  anxiety

NURSING DIAGNOSIS: Pain related to surgical
incision

■ **PATIENT GOAL 1:** Will experience either no pain or a
reduction of pain to level acceptable to child

NURSING INTERVENTIONS/*RATIONALES*

*Administer analgesics prescribed for pain around the clock
Do not wait until child experiences severe pain to intervene
  in order to prevent pain from occurring
Avoid palpating operative area unless necessary
Insert rectal tube, if indicated, *to relieve gas*
Encourage to void, if appropriate, *to prevent bladder distention*
Administer mouth care *to provide comfort*
Lubricate nostril *to decrease irritation* from nasogastric tube
  if present
Allow child position of comfort if not contraindicated
Perform nursing activities and procedures (e.g., dressing
  change, deep breathing, ambulation) after analgesia
*Administer antiemetics as ordered *for nausea and vomiting*
  and laxatives *to prevent constipation*
Monitor effectiveness of analgesics

EXPECTED OUTCOME

Child rests quietly and exhibits minimal or no evidence of
  pain (specify)

NURSING DIAGNOSIS: Risk for fluid volume deficit
related to NPO status before and/or after surgery, loss
of appetite, vomiting

■ **PATIENT GOAL 1:** Will receive adequate hydration

NURSING INTERVENTIONS/*RATIONALES*

Monitor IV infusion at prescribed rate *to ensure adequate
  hydration*
  Attach pediatric IV apparatus if not done in operating room
Offer fluids as soon as ordered or child tolerates
  Start with small sips of water or ice chips and advance as
    tolerated
Encourage to drink
  Tempt with favorite fluids, ice chips, or flavored ice pops

*Dependent nursing action.

The Child Undergoing Surgery—cont'd

EXPECTED OUTCOMES

Child exhibits no evidence of dehydration

Child takes and retains fluid when allowed (specify)

NURSING DIAGNOSIS: Risk for infection related to weakened condition, presence of infective organisms

■ **PATIENT GOAL 1:** Will maintain normal respiratory function

NURSING INTERVENTIONS/*RATIONALES*

Assess need for pain medication before respiratory therapy

Help to turn, deep breathe

Splint operative site with hand or pillow if possible before coughing (if coughing prescribed) *to minimize pain*

Assist with use of incentive spirometer or blow bottle

Perform percussion and vibration if indicated

Suction secretions if needed

Assess respirations, including breath sounds

EXPECTED OUTCOME

Lungs remain clear

NURSING DIAGNOSIS: Altered family processes related to situational crisis (emergency hospitalization of child), knowledge deficit

■ **PATIENT (FAMILY) GOAL 1:** Will receive adequate support and reassurance

NURSING INTERVENTIONS/*RATIONALES*

Explain all procedures *to reduce anxiety/fear*

Keep family informed of child's progress

Encourage expression of feelings *to facilitate coping*

Refer to public health nurse if indicated *for follow-up care*

Refer to appropriate agency or persons for specific help (e.g., social services, clergy)

(See also:

Nursing Care Plan: The Child in the Hospital, p. 268.)

Nursing Care Plan: The Family of the Child Who Is Ill or Hospitalized, p. 282.)

EXPECTED OUTCOMES

Family discusses child's condition and therapies comfortably

Family demonstrates an awareness of child's progress (specify method of evaluation)

Family members avail themselves of appropriate assistance

■ **PATIENT (FAMILY) GOAL 2:** Will demonstrate understanding of home care

NURSING INTERVENTIONS/*RATIONALES*

If dressing changes are required at home, teach parents sterile or aseptic procedures; provide written list of necessary equipment and instructions *for referral at home*

Instruct parents regarding administration of medications (if ordered), including possible side effects and untoward reactions, *to ensure adequate home care*

Instruct parents in care and management of special procedures (e.g., ostomy care, irrigations) *to ensure adequate home care*

EXPECTED OUTCOME

Family demonstrates an understanding of instructions (specify methods of learning and evaluation)

 PRACTICE ALERT

Current recommendations for the length of time children need to be NPO (nothing by mouth) before elective surgery in order to prevent pulmonary aspiration are as follows:*

Clear liquids	2 hours
Breast milk	4 hours
Infant formula	6 hours
Non-human milk	6 hours
Light meal (toast, clear liquids)	6 hours

*American Society of Anesthesiologists Task Force on Preoperative Fasting: Practice guidelines for preoperative fasting and the use of pharmacologic agents to reduce the risk of pulmonary aspiration: application to healthy patients undergoing elective procedures, *Anesthesiology* 90(3): 899, 1999.

NURSING CARE PLAN

The Child with Elevated Body Temperature

Set point—The temperature around which body temperature is regulated by a thermostat-like mechanism in the hypothalamus

Fever—An elevation in set point such that body temperature is regulated at a higher level; may be arbitrarily defined as temperature above 38° C (100.4° F)

Hyperthermia—A situation in which body temperature exceeds the set point, which usually results from the body or external conditions creating more heat than the body can eliminate, such as in heat stroke, aspirin toxicity, and hyperthyroidism

ASSESSMENT

Observe for clinical manifestations of fever:
Increase in body temperature above normal range
Flushed skin
Skin warm to touch

Glassy look to eyes
Increased respiratory rate
Tachycardia
Febrile seizures

NURSING DIAGNOSIS: Ineffective thermoregulation related to inflammatory process, elevated environmental temperature (fever)

- **PATIENT GOAL 1:** Will maintain temperature within normal limits

NURSING INTERVENTIONS/*RATIONALES*

*Administer antipyretic drug in appropriate dosage for child's weight (See p. 589.)
Use the following cooling measures, preferably 1 hour after administering antipyretic, *to lower the set point:*
Increase air circulation
Reduce environmental temperature
Place in lightweight clothing
Expose skin to air
Apply cool compress to skin (e.g., forehead)
Avoid chilling; if child shivers, apply more clothing or blankets *because shivering increases the body's metabolic rate*
Monitor temperature *to determine effectiveness of treatment*

EXPECTED OUTCOME

Body temperature remains within the acceptable limits (See inside front cover.)

NURSING DIAGNOSIS: Hyperthermia related to increased heat production

- **PATIENT GOAL 1:** Will maintain body temperature within normal limits

NURSING INTERVENTIONS/*RATIONALES*

Apply cooling blanket or mattress
Give tepid water bath of 20 to 30 minutes' duration (exact temperature range for tepid water bath has not been established; it is usually best to start with warm water and gradually add cooler water until a temperature is reached that is beneficial but does not cause chilling)
Apply cool, moist towels or washcloths; expose only one area of body at a time; change as needed; continue approximately 30 minutes
Avoid chilling
Never use isopropyl "rubbing" alcohol in bath or for sponging *because it may cause neurotoxic effects*
Monitor temperature *to prevent excessive body cooling*

EXPECTED OUTCOME

Temperature is reduced to acceptable limits (See inside front cover.)

---

*Dependent nursing action.

Unit 4

NURSING CARE PLAN

The Child with Fluid and Electrolyte Disturbance

Dehydration
  Isotonic (isosmotic, isonatremic)—Electrolyte and water deficits present in approximately balanced proportions
  Hypotonic (hyposmotic, hyponatremic)—Electrolyte deficit exceeds the water deficit

Hypertonic (hyperosmotic, hypernatremic)—Water loss in excess of electrolyte loss
Fluid excess
  Edema—Excess fluid in the interstitial spaces
  Water intoxification—Excessive intake of fluid

ASSESSMENT
Take a careful health history, especially regarding current health problem (e.g., length of illness, events that may have precipitated symptoms).
Perform a physical assessment.
Observe for manifestations of fluid and electrolyte disturbances (Table 4-5).
Perform specific assessments:
  Intake and output—Accurate measurements of fluid intake and output are vital to the assessment of dehydration. This includes oral and parenteral intake and losses from urine, stools, vomiting, fistulas, nasogastric suction, sweat, and wound drainage.
  Body weight—Measure regularly and at same time of day, usually each morning, to detect decreased or increased weight
  Urine—Assess frequency, volume, and color of urine
  Stools—Assess frequency, volume, and consistency of stools

  Vomitus—Assess for volume, frequency, and type of vomiting
  Sweating—Can be only estimated from frequency of clothing and linen changes
  Vital signs—Temperature (normal, elevated, or lowered depending on degree of dehydration), pulse, and blood pressure
  Skin—Assess for color, temperature, feel, turgor, and presence or absence of edema
  Mucous membranes—Assess for moisture, color, and presence and consistency of secretions; condition of tongue
  Fontanel (infants)—Sunken, soft, normal
  Behavior—Irritability, lethargy, comatose condition, characteristics of cry (infant), activity level, restlessness
  Sensory alterations—Presence of thirst
Assist with diagnostic procedures and tests (e.g., urinalysis, blood chemistry, complete blood count [CBC], blood gases).

NURSING DIAGNOSIS: Fluid volume deficit related to failure of regulatory mechanisms such as renal or hypothalamic

NURSING DIAGNOSIS: Fluid volume deficit related to active loss from renal, gastrointestinal (vomiting, diarrhea, nasogastric tube), or respiratory (hyperventilation) tracts; or from skin (diaphoresis, wounds)

■ **PATIENT GOAL 1:** Will have normal fluid volume

NURSING INTERVENTIONS/*RATIONALES*
Administer fluids as ordered
  Intravenous:
    *Administer fluid as prescribed
    Maintain desired drip rate
    *Add appropriate electrolytes as prescribed
    Maintain integrity of infusion site
  Oral:
    *Feed oral rehydration solutions as prescribed

EXPECTED OUTCOMES
Child receives sufficient fluids to replace losses
Child exhibits signs of adequate hydration (specify)

■ **PATIENT GOAL 2:** Will comply with therapeutic regimen

NURSING INTERVENTIONS/*RATIONALES*
Apply appropriate restraining methods where indicated *to maintain intravenous infusion*
Provide pacifier for infants who are NPO *to provide nonnutritive sucking*

EXPECTED OUTCOMES
Child does not interfere with fluid therapy
Infant engages in nonnutritive sucking

NURSING DIAGNOSIS: Risk for fluid volume deficit related to loss of appetite, NPO therapy, self-care deficit, immobility, altered sensorium

■ **PATIENT GOAL 1:** Will exhibit adequate hydration

NURSING INTERVENTIONS/*RATIONALES*
(See previous interventions.)
Employ play *for promoting fluid intake:*
  Make freezer pops using child's favorite juice
  Cut gelatin into fun shapes
  Make game of taking sip when turning page of book or in games such as "Simon says"
  Use small medicine cups; decorate the cups
  Color water with food coloring or Kool-Aid
  Have tea party; pour at small table
  Let child fill a syringe and squirt it into mouth or use it to fill small decorated cups
  Cut straws in half and place in small container (much easier for child to suck liquid)
  Decorate straw: cut out small design with two holes and pass straw through; place small sticker on straw
  Use a "crazy" straw
  Make a "progress poster"; give rewards for drinking a predetermined quantity

EXPECTED OUTCOMES
Child drinks a sufficient amount of fluid (specify type and amount)

Unit 4

Continued

The Child with Fluid and Electrolyte Disturbance—cont'd

Child exhibits evidence of adequate hydration (e.g., moist mucous membranes, good skin turgor, adequate urinary output for age)

> **NURSING DIAGNOSIS:** Fluid volume excess related to overhydration; failure of regulatory mechanisms

■ **PATIENT GOAL 1:** Will receive appropriate fluid intake

NURSING INTERVENTIONS/RATIONALES
Regulate fluid intake carefully
Monitor intravenous infusion
Prepare formula with correct amount of water
Employ strategies to prevent undesired intake:
 Review daily fluid restrictions with parents and child
 Suggest ways to divide total volume of fluid into small quantities to be spread over entire day

Keep mouth moist by other means, such as hard candy, ice chips, fine mist spray of cool water
Keep lips lubricated *to prevent cracking and promote comfort*

EXPECTED OUTCOME
Child exhibits no evidence of fluid gain

■ **PATIENT GOAL 2:** Will maintain appropriate fluid volume

NURSING INTERVENTIONS/RATIONALES
*Administer diuretic as prescribed, preferably early in day *to minimize night voiding*
Monitor progress *to ensure appropriate intervention*

EXPECTED OUTCOME
Child eliminates excess fluid

*Dependent nursing action.

TABLE 4-5   Significance of Clinical Observations Related to Fluid and Electrolyte Effects

Observation	Significant Variation	Possible Imbalance	Comments
Temperature	Elevated	Early water depletion Sodium excess	Elevated temperature will increase rate of water loss
	Lowered	Fluid volume deficit	Caused by reduced energy output Shock is outcome of severe fluid deficit
Pulse	Rapid, weak, thready, easily obliterated	Circulatory collapse may result from fluid deficit, hemorrhage, plasma-to-interstitial fluid shift	Pulse rate should include assessment of volume and quality, as well as rate Compare central with peripheral pulses
	Bounding, easily obliterated	Impending circulatory collapse Sodium deficit	Pulse may be influenced by activity or emotions
	Bounding, not easily obliterated	Fluid volume excess Interstitial fluid-to-plasma shift	
	Weak, irregular, rapid	Severe potassium deficit	
	Weak, irregular, slowing	Severe potassium excess	
	Increased	Sodium excess Magnesium deficit	
	Decreased	Magnesium excess	
Respiration	Slow, shallow	Respiratory alkalosis	Rapid respirations increase water loss
	Rapid, deep	Metabolic acidosis	Not a reliable sign of respiratory alkalosis in infants
	Dyspnea	Fluid volume excess, either general or pulmonary	
	Moist crackles	Fluid volume excess Pulmonary edema	
	Shallow	Potassium excess or deficit	
	Stridor	Severe calcium deficit	
Blood pressure	Increased	Fluid volume excess	Blood pressure not a reliable sign in young children
	Decreased	Sodium deficit Diminished vascular volume (loss of plasma-to-interstitial fluid shift) Severe potassium excess or deficit	Elasticity of blood vessels may keep blood pressure stable

Unit 4

The Child with Fluid and Electrolyte Disturbance—cont'd

TABLE 4-5   **Significance of Clinical Observations Related to Fluid and Electrolyte Effects—cont'd**

Observation	Significant Variation	Possible Imbalance	Comments
Skin			
Color	Pallor	Protein deficit	Environmental influences (such as a
		Fluid deficit	cool room or uncovered infant) and
		Fluid compartment shifts	fever may change skin color
	Flushed	Sodium excess	
Temperature	Cold, mottled extremities	Severe fluid volume deficit, even with fever	Caused by decreased peripheral blood flow
		Severe sodium depletion	
Feel	Dry	Fluid depletion	
		Sodium excess	
	Clammy, cold	Sodium deficit	
		Plasma-to-interstitial fluid shift	
		Hypotonic dehydration	
	Poor capillary filling	Fluid volume deficit	
Elasticity	Poor to very poor	Fluid depletion	Pinch of skin from abdomen or inner thigh is lifted and remains raised for several seconds
Pitting edema	Slight to severe	Fluid volume excess	Obese infants may appear normal; loss of foot creases may occur
		Plasma-to-interstitial fluid shift	
Mucous membranes	Dry	Fluid volume depletion	
	Longitudinal wrinkles on tongue		
	Sticky; rough, red, dry tongue	Sodium excess	
		Hypertonic dehydration	
Salivation and tearing	Absent	Fluid volume deficit	
Fontanels	Sunken	Fluid volume deficit	
	Bulging	Fluid volume excess	
Eyeballs	Sunken	Fluid volume deficit	
	Soft		
Sensory alterations	Tingling in fingers and toes	Calcium deficit	Sensory alterations unreliable in infants and young children who are unable to communicate symptoms
		Alkalosis	
	Abdominal cramps	Sodium deficit	
		Potassium excess	
	Muscle cramps	Calcium deficit	
		Potassium deficit	
	Lightheadedness	Respiratory alkalosis	
	Nausea	Calcium excess	
		Potassium excess	
		Potassium deficit	
	Thirst	Fluid deficit	May be difficult to assess in infants
		Sodium excess	May be masked by nausea
		Calcium excess	Any condition that reduces intravascular volume will stimulate thirst receptors
Neurologic signs	Hypotonia	Potassium deficit	
		Calcium excess	
	Flaccid paralysis	Severe potassium deficit	
		Severe potassium excess	
	Weakness	Metabolic acidosis	

Unit 4

Continued

The Child with Fluid and Electrolyte Disturbance—cont'd

TABLE 4-5 **Significance of Clinical Observations Related to Fluid and Electrolyte Effects—cont'd**

Observation	Significant Variation	Possible Imbalance	Comments
Neurologic signs—cont'd	Hypertonia 　Positive Chvostek 　　sign 　Tremors, cramps, 　　tetany 　Twitching	Calcium deficit Alkalosis with diminished calcium 　ionization Calcium deficit Magnesium deficit	Children may develop calcium deficit easily, since growing bones do not readily relinquish calcium to circulation
Behavior	Lethargy Irritability Comatose condition Lethargy with hyperirritability on stimulation Extreme restlessness	Fluid volume deficit overload Fluid volume deficit Hypotonic fluid deficit Profound acidosis of alkalosis Hypertonic fluid deficit Potassium excess	Behavioral changes are among first indications of dehydration as reported by parents
Weight	Loss 　Up to 5% (50 ml/kg) 　5%-9% (75 ml/kg) 　10% or higher 　　(100 ml/kg) Gain	Fluid deficit 　Mild 　Moderate 　Severe Protein or calorie deficiency Edema, general or pulmonary Ascites	Check for hepatomegaly; children sequester excess fluid in liver
Urine	Increased (polyuria) Diminished Oliguria Specific gravity 　Low (≤1.010) 　High (≥1.030) pH 　Acid 　Alkaline	Interstitial fluid-to-plasma shift Increased renal solute load Mild fluid deficit Moderate-to-severe fluid deficit Moderate-to-severe fluid deficit Plasma-to-interstitial fluid shift Sodium deficit Potassium excess Severe sodium excess Renal insufficiency Adequate hydration Fluid excess Renal disease Sodium deficit Fluid deficit Sodium excess Glycosuria Proteinuria Acidosis, metabolic or respiratory Alkalosis accompanied by severe 　potassium deficit Fluid deficit Alkalosis, metabolic or respiratory Hyperaldosteronism Acidosis accompanied by chronic 　renal infection and renal tubular 　dysfunction Diuretic therapy with carbonic 　anhydrase inhibitors	Normal range 　Infant: 2-3 ml/kg/hr 　Toddler/preschooler: 2 ml/kg/hr 　School-age child: 1-2 ml/kg/hr 　Adolescent: 0.5-1 ml/kg/hr (varies 　　with intake and other factors) Used to monitor hydration status in infants Fixed low reading occurs in renal disease

NURSING CARE PLAN

The Child with Special Nutritional Needs

The child with **special nutritional needs** has an imbalance between nutrient intake and nutrient expenditure or need.

(See specific nursing care plan for the child with disease-related nutritional alterations.)

ASSESSMENT

Take a dietary history. (See p. 94.)

Assess nutritional status. (See Clinical Assessment of Nutritional Status, p. 97.)

Review laboratory analyses of hemoglobin, hematocrit, albumin, creatinine, nitrogen, or any other specific nutrient measurement. (See p. 653.)

Observe child's eating behaviors.

NURSING DIAGNOSIS: Altered nutrition: less than body requirements related to fatigue, neuromuscular impairment, unconsciousness

■ **PATIENT GOAL 1:** Will consume adequate nourishment

NURSING INTERVENTIONS/*RATIONALES*

Provide feedings appropriate to age and capabilities

Feed child when he or she is well rested *so that child is more likely to eat*

*Administer appropriate diet by gavage, gastrostomy, or naso-gastric tubes as ordered

*Administer supplementary vitamins and minerals as ordered

EXPECTED OUTCOME

Child consumes an adequate amount with minimum effort (specify amount)

NURSING DIAGNOSIS: Altered nutrition: less than body requirements related to receiving nothing by mouth (NPO)

■ **PATIENT GOAL 1:** Will receive adequate nourishment and appropriate comfort measures

NURSING INTERVENTIONS/*RATIONALES*

*Administer intravenous fluids and/or total parenteral nutrition (TPN) as prescribed

Give pacifier *to provide nonnutritive sucking for infants*

Provide mouth care for children *to keep mouth clean and promote comfort:*

Brush teeth or use moist swabs or toothettes

Use emollient (petrolatum) on lips

Spray mouth with mist

EXPECTED OUTCOMES

Child receives sufficient nourishment

Infant engages in nonnutritive sucking

Child's mucous membranes remain moist and teeth are clean

NURSING DIAGNOSIS: Altered nutrition: less than body requirements related to loss of appetite, refusal to eat

■ **PATIENT GOAL 1:** Will receive adequate nourishment

NURSING INTERVENTIONS/*RATIONALES*

Take a dietary history (See p. 94.) and use information to make eating time as much like home as possible

Encourage parents or other family members to feed child or to be present at mealtimes

Have children eat at tables in groups; bring nonambulatory children to eating area in wheelchairs, beds, strollers, gurneys, or wagons

Use familiar eating utensils such as a favorite plate, cup, or bottle for small children

Make mealtimes pleasant; avoid any procedures immediately before or after eating; make sure child is rested and pain free

Have a nurse present at mealtimes to offer assistance, prevent disruptions, and praise children for their eating

Serve small, frequent meals rather than three large meals, or serve three meals and nutritious between-meal snacks

Bring in foods from home, especially if food preparation is very different from hospital's; consider cultural differences

Provide finger foods for young children

Involve children in food selection and preparation whenever possible

Serve small portions, and serve each course separately, such as soup first, followed by meat, potatoes, and vegetables, and ending with dessert; with young children, camouflage size of food by cutting meat thicker so less appears on plate or by folding a cheese slice in half; offer second helpings; ensure a variety of foods, textures, and colors

Provide food selections that are favorites of most children, such as peanut butter and jelly sandwiches, hot dogs, hamburgers, macaroni and cheese, pizza, spaghetti, tacos, fried chicken, corn on the cob, and fruit yogurt

Avoid foods that are highly seasoned, have strong odors, are served hot, or are all mixed together, unless typical of cultural practices

Provide fluid secretions that are favorites of most children, such as fruit punch, cola, ginger ale, sweetened tea, ice pops, sherbet, ice cream, milk and milkshakes, eggnog, pudding, gelatin, clear broth, or creamed soups

Offer nutritious snacks such as frozen yogurt or pudding, ice cream, oatmeal or peanut butter cookies, hot cocoa, cheese slices or "kisses," pieces of raw vegetables or fruit, and dried fruit or cereal

Make food service attractive and different, for example:

Serve a "picnic lunch" in a paper bag

Pack food in a Chinese-food container; decorate container

Put a "face" or a "flower" on a hamburger or sandwich using pieces of vegetables

Use a cookie cutter to shape a sandwich

Serve pudding, yogurt, or juice frozen as an ice pop

Make slurpies or snow cones by pouring flavored syrup on crushed ice

Add vegetable coloring to water or milk

Serve fluids through brightly colored or unusually shaped straws

*Dependent nursing action.

Continued

Unit 4

The Child with Special Nutritional Needs—cont'd

Make "bow tie" sandwiches by cutting them in triangles and placing two points together
Slice sandwiches into "fingers"
Grate mounds of cheese
Cut apples horizontally to make circles
Put a banana on a hot dog bun and spread with peanut butter
Break uncooked spaghetti into toothpick lengths and skewer cheese, cold meat, vegetables, or fruit chunks
Praise children for what they do eat
Do *not* punish children for not eating by removing their dessert or putting them to bed

EXPECTED OUTCOME

Child consumes an adequate amount of appropriate foods (specify type and amount)

NURSING DIAGNOSIS: Feeding deficit related to physical disability, mechanical restrictions, cognitive impairment

---

■ **PATIENT GOAL 1:** Will assist with self-feeding

NURSING INTERVENTIONS/*RATIONALES*

Assess child's self-feeding skills
Use self-help aids for feeding
Modify utensils *to facilitate self-help*

Place dishes and utensils within reach based on disability (specify)
   Place plate on child's chest (if unable to sit or turn)
   Employ a length of clean, clear plastic tubing for drinking (if straw is too short)
Serve easy-to-handle foods
Make meals as interesting and attractive as possible
Protect child and bed linens from possible spills with bib or towels

EXPECTED OUTCOME

Child assists with feeding as much as possible within limitations (specify amount of self-help)

■ **PATIENT GOAL 2:** Will be fed

NURSING INTERVENTIONS/*RATIONALES*

Allow child some autonomy in passive feeding
Include child in food selection and sequence of eating foods served (within limits of diet and sound nutrition)
Offer small bites, semisolid foods, and fluids through a straw for children lying in prone position *to prevent aspiration and to make eating/drinking easier*
Provide diet appropriate for age

EXPECTED OUTCOMES

Child participates in feeding activity according to ability
Child consumes a sufficient amount (specify)

NURSING CARE PLAN

The Child in Pain

The following is an operational definition that is useful in clinical practice: ***Pain is whatever the experiencing person says it is, existing whenever the person says it does.****

CHILD'S CONCEPT OF PAIN RELATED TO COGNITIVE DEVELOPMENT†

Age 2 to 7 years (preoperational thought):
Relates to pain primarily as physical, concrete experience
Thinks in terms of magical disappearance of pain
May view pain as punishment for wrongdoing
Tends to hold someone accountable for own pain and may strike out at that person

Age 7 to 10+ years (concrete operational thought):
Relates to pain physically (e.g., headache, stomachache)
Able to perceive psychologic pain, such as someone dying
Fears bodily harm and annihilation (body destruction and death)
May view pain as punishment for wrongdoing

Age 13 years and older (formal operational thought):
Able to give reason for pain (e.g., fell and hit nerve)
Perceives several types of psychologic pain
Has limited life experiences to cope with pain as adult might cope despite mature understanding of pain
Fears losing control during painful experience

ASSESSMENT

Use a variety of pain assessment strategies *because different strategies provide qualitative and quantitative information about pain;* one approach is

QUESTT:
Question the child
Use pain rating scales
Evaluate behavior
Secure parents' involvement
Take cause of pain into account
Take action

Question the child *because child's verbal statement and description of pain is most important factor in assessment.*
Have child locate pain by marking body part on a human figure drawing, or pointing to area with one finger on self, doll, stuffed animal, or "where Mommy or Daddy would put a bandage," *because children as young as toddler age, or even a child who has difficulty understanding pain scales, can usually locate pain on a drawing or on their body* (Fig. 4-1).
Be aware of reasons why children may deny or not tell the truth about pain (e.g., fear of receiving an injection if they admit to discomfort; belief that suffering is punishment for some misdeed; not appreciating degree of chronic pain; belief that nurses know when children have pain; lack of trust in telling a stranger [but readily admitting to parent that they are hurting]). Use a variety of words to describe pain (e.g., "ouch," "owie," "boo-boo," "feel funny," or "hurt") *because young child may not know what the word* **pain** *means and may need to describe pain using familiar language.* Use appropriate foreign language words (e.g., in Spanish, pain is "duele," "le le," "dolor," or "ai ai").

Use pain rating scales *because they provide subjective, quantitative measures of pain intensity* (Table 4-6).
Select a scale that is suitable to the child's age, abilities, and preference *because some scales are more appropriate for younger children than other scales* (e.g., scales using numbers require an understanding of numeric value, such as knowing that 5 is larger than 3).

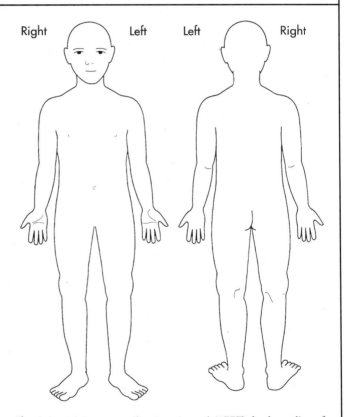

Right   Left   Left   Right

Fig. 4-1 Adolescent pediatric pain tool (APPT): body outlines for pain assessment. Instructions: "Color in the areas on these drawings to show where you have pain. Make the marks as big or as small as the place where the pain is." (From Savedra MC, Tesler MD, Holzemer WL, and Ward JA, School of Nursing, University of California-San Francisco; Copyright 1989, 1992.)

Continued

*McCaffery M, Pasero C: *Pain: a clinical manual,* ed 3, St Louis, 1999, Mosby.

†Hurley A, Whelan FG: Cognitive development and children's perception of pain, *Pediatr Nurs* 14(1):21-24, 1988.

Unit 4

TABLE 4-6 Pain Rating Scales for Children

Pain Scale/Description	Instructions	Recommended Age/Comments
FACES Pain Rating Scale* (Wong and Baker, 1988, 1999): Consists of six cartoon faces ranging from smiling face for "no pain" to tearful face for "worst pain"	**Original instructions:** Explain to child that each face is for a person who feels happy because there is no pain (hurt) or sad because there is some or a lot of pain. FACE 0 is very happy because there is no hurt. FACE 1 hurts just a little bit. FACE 2 hurts a little more. FACE 3 hurts even more. FACE 4 hurts a whole lot, but FACE 5 hurts as much as you can imagine, although you don't have to be crying to feel this bad. Ask child to choose face that best describes own pain. Record the number under chosen face on pain assessment record. **Brief word instructions:** Point to each face using the words to describe the pain intensity. Ask the child to choose face that best describes own pain and record the appropriate number.	For children as young as 3 years. Using original instructions without affect words, such as *happy* or *sad,* or brief words resulted in same pain rating, probably reflecting child's rating of pain intensity. For coding purposes, numbers 0, 2, 4, 6, 8, 10 can be substituted for 0-5 system to accommodate 0-10 system. The FACES provides three scales in one: facial expressions, numbers, and words.

0	1	2	3	4	5
No Hurt	Hurts Little Bit	Hurts Little More	Hurts Even More	Hurts Whole Lot	Hurts Worst

Oucher† (Beyer, Denyes, and Villar-ruel, 1992): Consists of six photographs of child's face representing "no hurt" to "biggest hurt you could ever have"; includes a vertical scale with numbers from 0-100; scales for black and Hispanic children have been developed (Villarruel and Denyes, 1991)	**Numeric Scale** Point to each section of scale to explain variations in pain intensity: "0 means no hurt." "This means little hurts" (pointing to lower part of scale, 1-29). "This means middle hurts" (pointing to middle part of scale, 30-69). "This means big hurts" (pointing to upper part of scale, 70-99). "100 means the biggest hurt you could ever have." Score is actual number stated by child. **Photographic Scale** Point to each photograph on Oucher and explain variations in pain intensity using following language: first picture from the bottom is "no hurt," second is "a little hurt," third is "a little more hurt," fourth is "even more hurt than that," fifth is "pretty much or a lot of hurt," and the sixth is the "biggest hurt you could ever have." Score pictures from 0-5, with the bottom picture scored as 0. **General** Practice using Oucher by recalling and rating previous pain experiences (e.g., falling off a bike). Child points to number or photograph that describes pain intensity associated with experience. Obtain current pain score from child by asking, "How much hurt do you have right now?"	For children 3-13 years. Use numeric scale if child can count to 100 by ones and identify larger of any two numbers, or by tens (Jordan-Marsh and others, 1994). Determine whether child has cognitive ability to use photographic scale; child should be able to seriate six geometric shapes from largest to smallest. Determine which ethnic version of Oucher to use. Allow the child to select a version of Oucher, or use version that most closely matches physical characteristics of child.

NOTE: Several variations of faces scales exist (Bieri and others, 1990; Kuttner and LePage, 1989; McGrath, de Veber, and Hearn, 1985).
**Wong-Baker FACES Pain Rating Scale Reference Manual* describing development and research of the scale is available from the Pain Resource Center, City of Hope National Medical Center, 1500 East Duarte Rd., Duarte, CA 91010; (626) 359-8111, ext. 3829; fax: (626) 301-8941; e-mail: mayday_pain@smtplink.coh.org; or Web site: www.mosby.com/WOW/. A compilation of many pain scales, including the FACES, is available free from Purdue Frederick Company, 100 Connecticut Ave., Norwalk, CT 06850-3950; (800) 733-1333 or (203) 853-0123, ext. 7378 or 7314; Web site: www.partnersagainstpain.com. The use of FACES with children is demonstrated in *Whaley and Wong's Pediatric Nursing Video Series,* "Pain Assessment and Management," narrated by Donna Wong, PhD, RN. Available from Mosby, 11830 Westline Industrial Dr., St. Louis, MO 63146; (800) 426-4545; fax: (800) 535-9935; Web site: www.mosby.com.
†Oucher is available for purchase from the Association for the Care of Children's Health, PO Box 25707, Alexandria, VA 22313; (703) 684-6179 or (800) 808-ACCH (2224); fax: (703) 684-1589; Web site: www.acch.org.

Unit 4

The Child in Pain—cont'd

TABLE 4-6 Pain Rating Scales for Children—cont'd

Pain Scale/Description	Instructions	Recommended Age/Comments
Poker Chip Tool‡ Uses four red poker chips placed horizontally in front of child (Hester and others, 1998)	Say to the child: "I want to talk with you about the hurt you may be having right now." Align the chips horizontally in front of the child on the bedside table, a clipboard, or other firm surface. Tell the child, "These are pieces of hurt." Beginning at the chip nearest the child's left side and ending at the one nearest the right side, point to the chips and say, "This [first chip] is a little bit of hurt and this [fourth chip] is the most hurt you could ever have." For a young child or for any child who may not fully comprehend the instructions, clarify by saying, "That means this [one] is just a little hurt, this [two] is a little more hurt, this [three] is more yet, and this [four] is the most hurt you could ever have." Do not give children an option for zero hurt. Research with the Poker Chip Tool has verified that children without pain will so indicate by responses such as "I don't have any." Ask the child, "How many pieces of hurt do you have right now?" After initial use of the Poker Chip Tool, some children internalize the concept "pieces of hurt." If a child gives a response such as "I have one right now," *before* you ask or before you lay out the poker chips, record the number of chips on the Pain Flow Sheet. Clarify the child's answer by words such as "Oh, you have a little hurt? Tell me about the hurt."	For children as young as 4 years.
Word-Graphic Rating Scale§ (Tesler and others, 1991): Uses descriptive words (may vary in other scales) to denote varying intensities of pain	Explain to child. "This is a line with words to describe how much pain you may have. This side of the line means no pain and over here the line means worst possible pain." (Point with your finger where "no pain" is, and run your finger along the line to "worst possible pain," as you say it.) "If you have no pain, you would mark like this." (Show example.) "If you have some pain, you would mark somewhere along the line, depending on how much pain you have." (Show example.) "The more pain you have, the closer to worst pain you would mark. The worst pain possible is marked like this." (Show example.) "Show me how much pain you have right now by marking with a straight, up-and-down line anywhere along the line to show how much pain you have right now." With a millimeter rule, measure from the "no pain" end to the mark and record this measurement as the pain score.	For children 4-17 years.

|———————————————————————————————————————|

No pain   Little pain   Medium pain   Large pain   Worst possible pain

‡Developed in 1975 by N.O. Hester, University of Colorado Health Sciences Center, School of Nursing, Denver, CO 80262. Also available in Spanish and French.

§Instructions for Word-Graphic Rating Scale from Acute Pain Management Guideline Panel: *Acute pain management in infants, children, and adolescents: operative and medical procedures: quick reference guide for clinicians,* ACHPR Pub No 92-0020, Rockville, MD, 1992, Agency for Health Care Policy and Research, Public Health Service, US Department of Health and Human Services. Word-Graphic Rating Scale is part of the Adolescent Pediatric Pain Tool and is available from Pediatric Pain Study, University of California, School of Nursing, Department of Family Health Care Nursing, San Francisco, CA 94143-0606; (415) 476-4040.

Continued

Unit 4

TABLE 4-6 Pain Rating Scales for Children—cont'd

Pain Scale/Description	Instructions	Recommended Age/Comments
Numeric Scale Uses straight line with end points identified as "no pain" and "worst pain" and sometimes "medium pain" in the middle; divisions along line are marked in units from 0 to 5 or 10 (high number may vary)	Explain to child that at one end of the line is a 0, which means that a person feels no pain (hurt). At the other end is usually a 5 or a 10, which means the person feels the worst pain imaginable. The numbers 1 to 5 or 10 are for a very little pain to a whole lot of pain. Ask child to choose a number that best describes own pain. 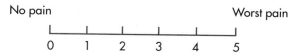	For children as young as 5 years, as long as they can count and have some concept of numbers and their values in relation to other numbers. Scale may be used horizontally or vertically. Number coding should be same as other scales used in a facility.
Visual Analogue Scale Defined as a vertical or horizontal line that is drawn to a certain length, such as 10 cm, and anchored by items that represent the extremes of the subjective phenomenon, such as pain, that is measured (Cline and others, 1992)	Ask child to place a mark on line that best describes amount of own pain. With a centimeter ruler, measure from the "no pain" end to the mark and record this measurement as the pain score.	For children as young as 4½ years, preferably at least 7 years. Vertical or horizontal scale may be used (Walco and Ilowite, 1991).
Color Tool Uses crayons or markers for child to construct own scale that is used with body outline (Eland and Banner, 1999)	Present eight crayons or markers to child in random order. Ask child to "pick a crayon with a color that reminds you of the most hurt (or pain) that you could possibly have"; once that crayon is selected, separate it from the others. Next, ask the child to select a crayon with a color that "reminds you of pain that is a little less than the pain we just talked about"; once the second crayon is selected, separate it from the group and place it with the first crayon selected. Ask the child to select a third crayon with a color "that reminds you of only a little pain"; separate this crayon and move it to the selected group. Finally, ask the child to select a crayon with a color that "reminds you of no hurt (or pain)" and separate that fourth color. Show the four crayons selected to the child and arrange them in order of "worst hurt (or pain)" to "no hurt (or pain)" and ask the child to show on the body outline "where the hurt is." If the child offers any verbal comments, note them.	Children as young as 4 years, provided they know their colors, are not color blind, and are able to construct the scale if in pain.

REFERENCES:

Beyer JE, Denyes, MJ, Villarruel AM: The creation, validation and continuing development of the Oucher: a measure of pain intensity in children, *J Pediatr Nurs* 7(5):335-346, 1992.

Bieri D and others: The FACES Pain Scale for the self-assessment of the severity of pain experienced by children: development, initial validation, and preliminary investigation for ratio scale properties, *Pain* 41(2):139-150, 1990.

Cline ME and others: Standardization of the visual analogue scale, *Nurs Res* 41(6):879-888, 1997.

Eland JA, Banner W: Analgesia, sedation, and neuromuscular blockade in pediatric critical care. In Hazinski MF, editor: *Manual of pediatric critical care*, St Louis, 1999, Mosby.

Hester NO and others: Putting pain measurement into clinical practice. In Finley GA, McGrath PJ, editors: *Measurement of pain in infants and children*, vol 10, Seattle, 1998, International Association for the Study of Pain Press.

Jordan-Marsh M and others: Alternative Oucher form testing gender ethnicity and age variations, *Res Nurs Health* 17:111-118, 1994.

Kuttner L, LePage T: Face scales for the assessment of pediatric pain: a critical review, *Can J Behav Sci* 21(2):198-209, 1989.

McGrath P, de Veber L, Hearn M: Multidimensional pain assessment in children. In Fields H, Dubner R, and Cervero F, editors: *Advances in pain research and therapy*, vol 9, New York, NY, 1985, Raven Press.

Tesler M and others: The Word-Graphic Rating Scale as a measure of children's and adolescents' pain intensity, *Res Nurs Health* 14:361-371, 1991.

Villarruel AM, Denyes MJ: Pain assessment in children: theoretical and empirical validity, *Adv Nurs Sci* 14(2):32-41, 1991.

Walco GA, Ilowite NT: Vertical versus horizontal visual analogue scales of pain intensity in children, *J Pain Symptom Manage* 6(3):200, 1991.

Wong D, Baker C: Pain in children: comparison of assessment scales, *Pediatr Nurs* 14(1):9-17, 1988.

Wong D, Baker C: Reference manual for the Wong-Baker FACES Pain Rating Scale, Tulsa, OK, 1999, Wong & Baker.

Unit 4

The Child in Pain—cont'd

ASSESSMENT—cont'd

Consider nurse preference in terms of convenience (e.g., ease of use and cost, availability).

Consider child preference in terms of ease of use.

Use same scale with child to avoid confusing child with different instructions.

Use pain assessment scale for pain only *because multiple uses of scale (e.g., as a general measure of the child's feelings) can cause child to lose interest in the scale.*

Teach child to use scale before pain is expected (e.g., preoperatively) *to facilitate its use when child is actually in pain.*

In introducing pain scale, explain that this is one way for children (and parents) to let nurse know if the child is hurting.

When analgesics are used, have child choose pain rating that is acceptable or satisfactory while active and at rest (may not be zero, because child may prefer fewer side effects to larger dose of analgesic) *since child's perception of comfort should guide interventions to meet the comfort/function goals.*

Consider using pain assessment scales for infants and young children (Tables 4-7 and 4-8) *because they provide a systematic and quantitative measure of pain.*

Evaluate behavior and physiologic changes when self report is not possible *because these changes are common indicators of pain in children and are especially valuable in assessing pain in nonverbal patients* (Box 4-8).

Facial expression is one of the most consistent indicators of acute pain in infants (Fig. 4-2).

Physiologic changes (e.g., increased heart rate, increased blood pressure, increased respirations, crying, sweating, decreased oxygen saturation, dilation of pupils, flushing or pallor, nausea, and muscle tension) are primarily seen in early onset of acute pain and subside with continuing or chronic pain, making them unreliable indicators of persistent acute or chronic pain.

Both behavioral and physiologic changes may indicate emotions other than pain (e.g., fear or anxiety); no single behavioral or physiologic change is an absolute indicator of pain, and absence of these changes does not mean absence of pain.

Observe for specific behaviors (e.g., pulling ears, rolling head from side to side, lying on side with legs flexed, limping, refusing to move a body part) that often indicate location of body pain.

Observe for improvement in behavior (e.g., less irritability, cessation of crying, sleeping, or playing) following administration of analgesics *because such behaviors provide excellent clues to pain existing before analgesic was given;* no change in behavior may mean that pain still exists and that analgesic was inadequate.

Be aware that children who are asleep may still have pain, *because children in pain may sleep from exhaustion, and opioids and adjuvant drugs may cause sedation without adequate analgesia.*

Use pain assessment record or adapt existing form to include pain assessment (e.g., fifth vital sign on vital sign sheet) to document effectiveness of interventions *because giving practitioners objective documentation of pain, rather than opinion, is more likely to lead to favorable change in analgesic orders* (Boxes 4-9 and 4-10).

Observe coping strategies child uses during painful procedure (e.g., talking, moaning, lying rigidly still, squeezing hand, and so on) *because children who undergo repeated painful procedures often develop effective coping strategies that can be encouraged in future experiences with pain.*

Secure parents' involvement *because they know their child best,* although they may not have seen their child in moderate to severe pain before.

Ask parents about child's behavior when in pain by taking a pain history (Box 4-11) before pain is expected *to recognize signs of existing pain early.*

Encourage parents to participate in assessing current pain by using the pain assessment record *because parents are the most consistent persons caring for the child and want to be involved in pain relief;* encourage their participation *to give them control and a sense of helping.*

Be aware that "proxy" pain ratings by parents often do not correlate well with the child's self-report *because only the person in pain knows amount of pain.*

Obtain information regarding ***current*** pain, such as duration, type, and location. Influencing factors may include: (1) precipitating events (those that cause or increase the pain), (2) relieving events (those that lessen the pain, such as medications), (3) temporal events (times when the pain is relieved or increased), (4) positional events (standing, sitting, lying down), and (5) associated events (meals, stress, coughing). Have parent or child describe pain in terms of interruption of daily activities.

Take cause of pain into account *because pathology or procedure may give clues to expected intensity and type of pain.*

Take action to meet the established comfort/function goals (child's acceptable pain level: one that permits function of expected activities) *because the only reason to assess pain is to be able to relieve it by using analgesic/adjuvant drugs and/or nonpharmacologic methods.* A pain rating above 3 on a 0 to 10 scale usually adversely affects function (e.g., activities of daily living, playing).

Nursing Care Plan text continued on p. 328.

 PRACTICE ALERT

A golden rule to follow in pain assessment is this: **Whatever is painful to an adult is painful to an infant or child, until proved otherwise.** Be aware that temperament affects coping style, and children with more positive moods may appear to be in less pain than they actually are. Children who use passive coping behaviors (offering no resistance, cooperating) may rate pain as more intense than children who use active coping behaviors (resisting, attacking). If children's behaviors appear to differ from their rating of pain, believe their pain rating, unless they appear to be in pain. In this case, assess possible reasons for denying pain.

Continued

Unit 4

The Child in Pain—cont'd

TABLE 4-7 CRIES Neonatal Postoperative Pain Scale*

	0	1	2
Crying	No	High pitched	Inconsolable
Requires O$_2$ for Sat >95%	No	<30%	>30%
Increased vital signs	Heart rate and blood pressure ≤ preoperative state	Heart rate and blood pressure increase <20% of preoperative state	Heart rate and blood pressure increase >20% of preoperative state
Expression	None	Grimace	Grimace/grunt
Sleepless	No	Wakes at frequent intervals	Constantly awake

Coding Tips for Using CRIES

Crying	The characteristic cry of pain is *high pitched.*
	If no cry, or cry that is not high pitched, **score 0.**
	If cry high pitched but infant is easily consoled, **score 1.**
	If cry is high pitched and infant is inconsolable, **score 2.**
Requires O$_2$ for Sat >95%	Look for *changes* in oxygenation. Infants experiencing pain manifest decreases in oxygenation as measured by Tco$_2$ or oxygen saturation. (Consider other causes of changes in oxygenation, such as atelectasis, pneumothorax, oversedation.)
	If no oxygen is required, **score 0.**
	If <30% O$_2$ is required, **score 1.**
	If >30% is required, **score 2.**
Increased vital signs	NOTE: Measure blood pressure (BP) last, because this may wake child, causing difficulty with other assessments.
	Use baseline preoperative parameters from a nonstressed period.
	Multiply baseline heart rate (HR) × 0.2, then add this to baseline HR to determine the HR that is 20% over baseline. Do likewise for BP. Use mean BP.
	If HR and BP are both unchanged or less than baseline, **score 0.**
	If HR or BP is increased but increase is <20% of baseline, **score 1.**
	If either one is increased >20% over baseline, **score 2.**
Expression	The facial expression most often associated with pain is a grimace. This may be characterized by lowered brow, eyes squeezed shut, deepened nasolabial furrow, open lips and mouth.
	If no grimace is present, **score 0.**
	If grimace alone is present, **score 1.**
	If grimace and noncry vocalization grunt is present, **score 2.**
Sleepless	This parameter is scored based on the infant's state during the hour preceding this recorded score.
	If the child has been continuously asleep, **score 0.**
	If the child has awakened at frequent intervals, **score 1.**
	If the child has been awake constantly, **score 2.**

Neonatal pain assessment tool developed at the University of Missouri-Columbia (Krechel SW, Bildner J: CRIES: a new neonatal postoperative pain measurement score: initial testing of validity and reliability, *Pediatr Anaesth* 5: 53-61, 1995). Copyright S. Krechel, MD and J. Bildner, RNC, CNS, 1995. Used with permission.

BP, Blood pressure; *HR,* heart rate.

*Ages of use: 32-60 weeks gestational age; a score of 4 or higher indicates need for pain management. *Scoring range:* 0 = no pain; 10 = worst pain.

The Child in Pain—cont'd

TABLE 4-8   FLACC Scale*

	0	1	2
Face	No particular expression or smile	Occasional grimace or frown, withdrawn, disinterested	Frequent to constant frown, clenched jaw, quivering chin
Legs	Normal position or relaxed	Uneasy, restless, tense	Kicking, or legs drawn up
Activity	Lying quietly, normal position, moves easily	Squirming, shifting back and forth, tense	Arched, rigid, or jerking
Cry	No cry (awake or asleep)	Moans or whimpers, occasional complaint	Crying steadily, screams or sobs, frequent complaints
Consolability	Content, relaxed	Reassured by occasional touching, hugging, or "talking to"; distractable	Difficult to console or comfort

*Ages of use: 2 months-7 years. *Scoring range:* 0 = no pain; 10 = worst pain.
From Merkel S, Voepel-Lewis T, Shayevitz J, Malviya S: The FLACC: a behavioral scale for scoring postoperative pain in young children, *Pediatr Nurs* 23(3):293-297, 1997. Used with permission of Jannetti Publications, Inc. and the University of Michigan Health System. Can be reproduced for clinical and research use.

BOX 4-8

Developmental Characteristics of Children's Responses to Pain

Young Infants

Generalized body response of rigidity or thrashing, possibly with local reflex withdrawal of stimulated area
Loud crying
Facial expression of pain (brows lowered and drawn together, eyes tightly closed, mouth open and squarish) (See Fig. 4-2.)
Demonstrates no association between approaching stimulus and subsequent pain

Older Infants

Localized body response with deliberate withdrawal of stimulated area
Loud crying
Facial expression of pain and/or anger (same facial characteristics as pain but eyes may be open)
Physical resistance, especially pushing the stimulus away *after* it is applied

Young Children

Loud crying, screaming
Verbal expressions of "Ow," "Ouch," or "It hurts"
Thrashing of arms and legs
Attempts to push stimulus away *before* it is applied

Uncooperative; need physical restraint
Request termination of procedure
Clings to parent, nurse, or other significant person
Requests emotional support, such as hugs or other forms of physical comfort
May become restless and irritable with continuing pain
All these behaviors may be seen in anticipation of actual painful procedure

School-Age Children

May display all behaviors of young child, especially *during* painful procedure, but less in anticipatory period
Stalling behavior, such as "Wait a minute" or "I'm not ready"
Muscular rigidity, such as clenched fists, white knuckles, gritted teeth, contracted limbs, body stiffness, closed eyes, wrinkled forehead

Adolescents

Less vocal protest
Less motor activity
More verbal expressions, such as "It hurts" or "You're hurting me"
Increased muscle tension and body control

Data from Craig KD and others: Developmental changes in infant pain expression during immunization injections, *Soc Sci Med* 19(12):1331:1337, 1984; and Katz E, Kellerman J, Siegel S: Behavioral distress in children with cancer undergoing medical procedures: developmental considerations, *J Consult Clin Psychol* 48(3):356-365, 1980.

Unit 4

The Child in Pain—cont'd

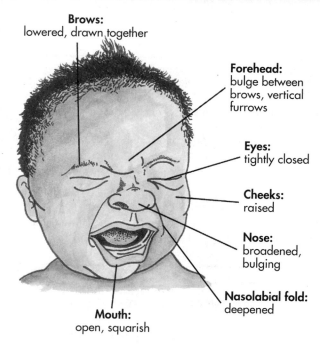

Brows:
lowered, drawn together

Forehead:
bulge between
brows, vertical
furrows

Eyes:
tightly closed

Cheeks:
raised

Nose:
broadened,
bulging

Nasolabial fold:
deepened

Mouth:
open, squarish

Fig. 4-2 Facial expression of physical distress is the most consistent behavioral indicator of pain in infants.

BOX 4-9

Pain Assessment Record

Directions for each column:

1. Record date and time of assessment and analgesic administration; assess analgesic effect _____ minutes later and then _____

2. Use a pain rating scale if child understands its use. Name of scale: _____

   Ratings: No pain = _____ Worst pain = _____ Comfort/function goals* _____

3. Record analgesic, dose, and route

4. Record possible indications or effects of pain, such as shallow breathing due to incisional pain, parental request for pain relief; record indications or effects of pain relief, such as "moves easily, playing"

5. Record any other side effects (e.g., nausea, itching)

6. Record LOS (see inset) R (respiratory function); record breaths per minute and/or other observations of respiratory status (e.g., depth of respiration, change in color of skin)

7. Signature or initials of person recording information

Level of Sedation (LOS) Scale†

S = Sleeping, easily aroused
   Requires no action
1 = Awake and alert
   Requires no action
2 = Occasionally drowsy, easy to arouse
   Requires no action
3 = Frequently drowsy, arousable, drifts off to sleep during conversation
   Notify practitioner and decrease dose
4 = Somnolent, minimal or no response to stimuli
   Notify practitioner and stop opioid

1 Date/time	2 Pain rating	3 Analgesic	4 Possible effects/indications of pain or relief of pain	5 Side effects	6 LOS/R	7 Signature

*Ask the child what pain rating would be acceptable in terms of usual function (e.g., activities of daily living, playing, attending school, and so on). From McCaffery M, Pasero C, editors: *Pain: a clinical manual,* ed 2, St Louis, 1999, Mosby.

†From Pasero C, McCaffery M: Providing epidural analgesia: how to maintain a delicate balance, *Nurs99* 29(8):34-39, 1999.

Unit 4

The Child in Pain—cont'd

BOX 4-10

Your Child's Pain Rating Scale

Please keep a record of how well your child's pain medicines are working. Rate your child's pain before and after pain medicine is given.

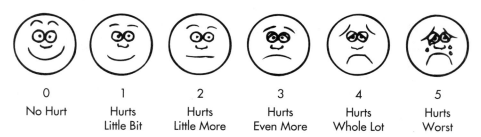

0	1	2	3	4	5
No Hurt	Hurts Little Bit	Hurts Little More	Hurts Even More	Hurts Whole Lot	Hurts Worst

Explain to your child that each face is for a person who has no hurt (pain) or some or a lot of hurt (pain). Point to each face and say the words under the face. Ask the child to pick the face that best describes how much hurt he (or she) has. Record the number of that face in the pain rating column. If your child's pain is above 2, or if you have other concerns with pain, let your nurse or physician know.

Date and time	Pain rating	Medicine I took	Side effects, such as drowsiness or upset stomach

Pain assessment record. Modified from Wong DL: Pain assessment in children. In Martin KS and others, editors: *Mosby's home health client teaching guides: Rx for teaching*, St Louis, 1997, Mosby. May be photocopied for clinical use.

The Child in Pain—cont'd

BOX 4-11

Pain Experience History

Child Form

Tell me what pain is.

Tell me about the hurt you have had before.

Do you tell others when you hurt? If yes, who?

What do you do for yourself when you are hurting?

What do you want others to do for you when you hurt?

What don't you want others to do for you when you hurt?

What helps the most to take your hurt away?

Is there anything special that you want me to know about you when you hurt? (If yes, have child describe.)

Parent Form

What word(s) does your child use in regard to pain?

Describe the pain experiences your child has had before.

Does your child tell you or others when he/she is hurting?

How do you know when your child is in pain?

How does your child usually react to pain?

What do you do for your child when he/she is hurting?

What does your child do for himself/herself when in pain?

What works best to decrease or take away your child's pain?

Is there anything special that you would like me to know about your child and his/her pain? (If yes, describe.)

Modified from Hester NO, Barcus CS: Assessment and management of pain in children, *Pediatr Nurs Update* 1:2-8, 1986.

The Child in Pain—cont'd

TRANSLATIONS OF FACES PAIN RATING SCALE*

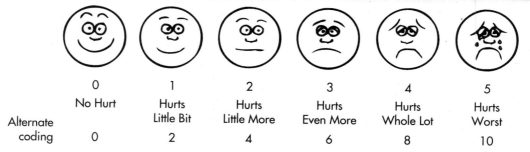

	0	1	2	3	4	5
	No Hurt	Hurts Little Bit	Hurts Little More	Hurts Even More	Hurts Whole Lot	Hurts Worst
Alternate coding	0	2	4	6	8	10

Original Instructions:

Explain to the person that each face is for a person who feels happy because he has no pain (hurt) or sad because he has some or a lot of pain. **Face 0** is very happy because he doesn't hurt at all. **Face 1** hurts just a little bit. **Face 2** hurts a little more. **Face 3** hurts even more. **Face 4** hurts a whole lot. **Face 5** hurts as much as you can imagine, although you don't have to be crying to feel this bad. Ask the person to choose the face that best describes how much hurt he has.

Rating scale is recommended for persons age 3 years and older.

Brief Word Instructions:

Point to each face using the words to describe the pain intensity. Ask the child to choose face that best describes own pain and record the appropriate number. NOTE: Use of these instructions is recommended.

Spanish

Expliquele a la persona que cada cara representa una persona que se siente feliz porque no tiene dolor o triste porque siente un poco o mucho dolor. **Cara 0** se siente muy feliz porque no tiene dolor. **Cara 1** tiene un poco de dolor. **Cara 2** tiene un poquito más de dolor. **Cara 3** tiene más dolor. **Cara 4** tiene mucho dolor. **Cara 5** tiene el dolor más fuerte que usted pueda imaginar, aunque usted no tiene que estar llorando para sentirse asi de mal. Pidale a la persona que escoja la cara que mejor describe su proprio dolor.

Esta escala se puede usar con personas de tres años de edad o más.

French

Expliquez á la personne que chaque visage représent un personne qui est heureux parce qu'elle n'a pas point du mal ou triste parce qu'il a un peu ou beaucoup du mal. **Visage 0** est trés heureux parce qu'elle n'a pas point du mal. **Visage 1** a un petit peu de mal. **Visage 2** a plus du mal. **Visage 3** a encore plus du mal. **Visage 4** a beaucoup du mal. **Visage 5** a autant mal que vous pouvez imaginer, bien que ces mauvais sentiments ne finissent pas nécessairement a vous faire pleurer. Demandez à la personne de choisir le visage qui convient le mieux avec ses sentiments.

Ces evaluations sont recommendés pour des personnes de trois ans et davantage.

Wong-Baker FACES Pain Rating Scale: Available at no charge from The Purdue Frederick Company, 100 Connecticut Ave., Norwalk, CT 06850-3590; (203) 853-0123, ext. 7378 or 7314. Spanish and Portuguese translations by Ellen Johnsen; French translation by Irene Sherman Liguori and Robert Marino; Italian translation by Madeline Mitchko and Ida DiPietropaolo; Romanian translation by Florin Nicolae; Bosnian translation by Dijana Groth; Vietnamese translation by Yen B. Isle; Chinese translation by Hung-Shen Lin; Japanese translation from *After the announcement of cancer,* Tokyo, 1993, Iwanami Shoten, Pub; German translation from Wong DL: *Pediatric quick reference,* Berlin, Wiesbaden, 1997, Ullstein Mosby.
*These three pages may be photocopied for clinical use. From Wong DL, Hess CS: *Wong and Whaley's Clinical manual of pediatric nursing,* ed 5.
Copyright © 2000, Mosby, St Louis.

Unit 4

The Child in Pain—cont'd

Italian

Spiegare a la persona che ogni facien è per una persona che si sente felice perchè non tiene dolore oppure triste perchè ha poco o molto dolore. **Faccia 0** è molto felice perchè non tiene dolore. **Faccia 1** tiene poco dolore. **Faccia 2** tiene un po più di dolore. **Faccia 3** tiene più dolore. **Faccia 4** tiene molto dolore. **Faccia 5** tiene molto dolore che non puoi immaginare però non devi piangere per tenere dolore. Domandi ala persona di scegliere quale faccia meglio descrive come si sente.

Grado scale è raccomandata a la persona di tre anni in sù.

Portuguese

Explique a pessoa que cada face representa uma pessoa que está feliz porque não têm dor, ou triste por ter um pouco ou muita dor. **Face 0** está muito feliz porque não têm nenhuma dor. **Face 1** tem apenas um pouco de dor. **Face 2** têm um pouco mais de dor. **Face 3** têm ainda mais dor. **Face 4** têm muita dor. **Face 5** têm uma dor máxima, apesar de que nem sempre provoca o choro. Peça a pessoa que escolhe a face que melhor descreve como ele se sente.

Esta escala é aplicável a pessoas de tres anos de idade ou mais.

Romanian

Explică persoanei că fiecare față este specifică diferitelor stări fizice; o persoană este ferioita pentru că nu are nici o durere ori tristă pentru că suferă puțin sau mai mult. **Fața 0** este foarte ferioită pentru că nu are absolut nici o durere. **Fața 1** are un pic de durere. **Fața 2** are ceva mai mult. **Fața 3** suferă și mai mult. **Fața 4** suferă foarte mult. **Fața 5** este greu de imaginat cât de mult suferă, căci nu trebuie neapărat să plângi, oricat de tare te-ar durea. Intreabă persoana să indice figura care-i desorie cel mai bine starea fizică.

Acest **grad de durere** este racomandat pentru persoanele de la 3 ani în sus.

Bosnian

Objasnite osobi da je svako lice namjenjeno za osobu koja se osjeća sretnom jer ne osjeća bol ili tužnom jer osjeća malo ili puno boli. Lice 0 je sretno jer ne osjeća nikakvu bol. Lice 1 osjeća samo malu bol. Lice 2 osjeća malo više boli. Lice 3 osjeća još veću bol. Lice 4 osjeća puno boli. Lice 5 osjeća onoliku bol koju je moguće zamisliti, što ne znači da osoba koja osjeća tu bol mora plakati. Upitajte osobu da izabere lice koje najbolje opisuju kako se osjeća. Skala procijene bola se preporučuje za osobe starosti 3 godine ili više.

Upirati prstom na svako lice objašnjavajući riječima intenzitet boli. Pitajte dijete da izabere lice koje najbolje opisuje njihovu bol i zabilježite odgovarajući broj.

German

Erläutern Sie dem Kind, daß jedes Gesicht zu einer Person gehört, die froh darüber ist, keine Schmerzen zu haben, oder die sehr traurig ist, weil sie mäßige bis starke Schmerzen hat. **Gesicht 0** ist sehr froh, weil es keine Schmerzen hat. **Gesicht 1** sagt, es tut ein bißchen weh. **Gesicht 2** hat ein bißchen mehr Schmerzen. **Gesicht 3** sagt, es tut noch mehr weh, und **Gesicht 4**, es tut ziemlich weh. **Gesicht 5** leidet unter so starken Schmerzen, wie Du Dir nur vorstellen kannst, auch wenn dabei nicht unbedingt Tränen fließen müssen. Bitten Sie das Kind, das Gesicht auszuwählen, das seinem Empfinden am besten entspricht. Empfohlen für Kinder ab 3 Jahren.

Vietnamese

Xin cắt nghĩa cho mỗi người, từng khuôn mặt của một người cảm thấy vui vẻ tại vì không có sự đau đớn hoặc, buồn vì có chút ít hay rất nhiều sự đau đớn. Cái **mặt** với **số 0** thì rất là vui tại vì mặt ấy không có sự đau đớn. **Mặt số 1** chỉ đau một chút thôi. **Mặt số 2** hơi đau hơn một chút nữa. **Mặt số 3** đau hơn chút nữa. **Mặt số 4** đau thật nhiều. **Mặt số 5** đau không thể tưởng tượng, mặc dù người ta không cần phải khóc mới cảm thấy được sự buồn khổ như thế.

Bạn hỏi từng người tự chọn khuôn mặt nào diễn tả được sự đau đớn của chính mình.

Continued

Unit 4

The Child in Pain—cont'd

Japanese

　3歳以上の患者に望ましい。それぞれの顔は、患者の痛み (pain, hurt) がないのでご機嫌な感じ、または、ある程度の痛み・沢山の痛みがあるので悲しい感じを表現していることを説明して下さい。0＝痛みがまったくないから、とても幸せな顔をしている、1＝ほんの少し痛い、2＝もう少し痛い、

3＝もっと痛い、4＝とっても痛い、5＝痛くて涙を流す必要はないけれども、これ以上の痛みは考えられないほど痛い。今、どのように感じているか最もよく表わしている顔を選ぶよう、患者に求めて下さい。

Chinese

　　解釋給人聽用每張臉譜來代表著一個人的感覺是因爲沒有疼痛〔傷痛〕而感快樂或是因爲些許疼痛或者是許多疼痛而感傷心。第零張臉是很快樂的因爲他一點也不覺得疼痛。第一張臉只痛一丁點兒。第二張臉又痛多了一些。第三張臉痛得更多

了。第四張臉是非常痛了。第五張臉是爲人們所能想像到的劇痛既使感到這樣難過，卻不一定哭出來。請這人選擇出最能代表他現在感覺的一張臉譜。此量表適用於三歲以上的人。

Continued from p. 319.

NURSING DIAGNOSIS: Pain related to (specify)

■ **PATIENT GOAL:** Will experience either no pain or a reduction of pain to level acceptable to child (equal to or less than comfort/function goal) when receiving analgesics

NURSING INTERVENTIONS/*RATIONALES*

Plan to administer prescribed analgesic before procedure *so that its peak effect coincides with painful event*

Plan preventive schedule of medication around the clock (ATC) or, if analgesic is ordered PRN, administer it at regular intervals when pain is continuous and predictable (e.g., postoperatively) *to maintain steady blood levels of analgesic*

Administer analgesia by least traumatic route whenever possible *to avoid causing additional pain;* avoid intramuscular or subcutaneous injections (Box 4-12).

Prepare child for administration of analgesia by using supportive statements (e.g., "This medicine I am putting in the IV will make you feel better in a few minutes")

Reinforce the effect of the analgesic by telling the child that he/she will begin to feel better in the appropriate amount of time, according to drug used; use a clock or timer to measure onset of relief with the child; reinforce the cause and effect of pain-analgesic *so the child becomes conditioned to expecting relief*

If an injection must be given, avoid saying, "I am going to give you an injection for pain" *since this is another pain in addition to the existing pain;* if the child refuses an injection, explain that the little hurt from the needle will take away the bigger hurt for a long time

Avoid statements such as, "This is enough medicine to take away anyone's pain," or "By now you shouldn't need so much pain medicine" *because they convey a judgmental and belittling attitude*

Give the child control whenever possible (e.g., using patient-controlled analgesia, choosing which arm for a venipuncture, taking bandages off, or holding the tape or other equipment)

*Administer prescribed analgesic; nonopioids, including acetaminophen (Tylenol, paracetamol) and nonsteroidal antiinflammatory drugs (NSAIDs), are suitable for mild to moderate pain (Table 4-9), opioids† are needed for moderate to severe pain (Table 4-10); a combination of the two analgesics (Box 4-14) attacks pain at the peripheral nervous system and at the central nervous system and provides increased analgesia without increased side effects.

Titrate (adjust) dosage for maximum pain relief with minimal side effects

Begin with recommended dosage for age and weight

Increase dosage and/or decrease interval between dosages if pain relief is inadequate

Nursing Care Plan text continued on p. 336.

PRACTICE ALERT

A frequent error in attempting to improve pain control is to change to another analgesic. If an opioid, such as morphine, hydromorphone, or fentanyl, is used, rarely is the problem one of drug choice. Rather, the problem is usually one of dosage. The correct intervention may be to increase the dose (if inadequate pain control) or decrease the dose (if side effects) before changing the analgesic. If a change to another analgesic is warranted because of adverse side effects or accumulation of active metabolites, the new drug should be at least equal in potency to the original analgesic.

---

*Dependent nursing action.

†The term *opioid* refers to natural or synthetic analgesics with morphine-like actions. It is preferred to the term *narcotic,* which in a legal context refers to any substance that causes psychologic dependence (such as cocaine, which is not an opioid). In older children and parents, the word "narcotic" also engenders fears of addiction that are unwarranted when opioids are used for pain control.

BOX 4-12

Routes and Methods of Analgesic Drug Administration

Oral

Preferred because of convenience, cost, and relatively steady blood levels

Higher dosages of oral form of opioids required for equivalent parenteral analgesia

Peak drug effect occurs after 1½ to 2 hours for most analgesics

Delay in onset is disadvantage when rapid control of severe pain or of fluctuating pain is desired

Sublingual/Buccal/Transmucosal

Tablet or liquid placed between cheek and gum (buccal) or under tongue (sublingual)

Highly desirable because more rapid onset than oral route

Less first-pass effect through liver than oral route, which normally reduces analgesia from oral opioids (unless sublingual/buccal form swallowed, which occurs often in children)

Few drugs commercially available in this form

Many drugs can be compounded into a sublingual troche or lozenge*

Fentanyl Oralet—Oral transmucosal fentanyl citrate in hard confection base on a plastic holder; used for preoperative or preprocedural sedation/analgesia

Actiq—Same formulation as Fentanyl Oralet; indicated only for management of breakthrough cancer pain in patients with malignancies who are already receiving and are tolerant to opioid therapy

Intravenous (IV) (Bolus)

Preferred for rapid control of severe pain

Provides most rapid onset of effect, usually in about 5 minutes

Advantage for acute pain, procedural pain, and breakthrough pain

Initial bolus dose is controversial; one recommendation is one-half IM dose

Needs to be repeated hourly for continuous pain control

Drugs with short half-life (morphine, fentanyl, hydromorphone) are preferred, to avoid toxic accumulation of drug

Intravenous (Continuous)

Preferred over bolus and IM for maintaining control of pain

Provides steady blood levels

Easy to titrate dosage

Amount of initial dose is controversial; one approach to calculating hourly infusion rate is to divide IM dose by drug's expected duration for IM route

Peak effect is delayed; for rapid pain relief, begin with initial IV bolus dose (See preceding section.)

Subcutaneous (SC) (Continuous)

Used when oral and IV routes not available

Provides equivalent blood levels to continuous IV infusion

Suggested initial bolus dose to equal 2-hour IV dose; total 24-hour dose usually equal to total IV or IM 24-hour dose

Patient-Controlled Analgesia (PCA)

Generally refers to self-administration of drugs, regardless of route

Typically uses programmable infusion pump (IV, epidural, or SC) that permits self-administration of boluses of medication at preset dose and time interval (*lockout interval* is time between doses)

PCA bolus administration may be combined with initial bolus and continuous (basal or background) infusion of opioid (Box 4-13)

Optimum lockout interval not known, but must be at least as long as time needed for onset of drug

Should effectively control pain during movement or procedures

Longer lockout requires larger dose

Family-Controlled Analgesia

One family member (usually a parent) or significant other is designated child's primary pain manager and has responsibility of pressing PCA button

Guidelines for selecting a primary pain manager for family-controlled analgesia:

Spends a significant amount of time with the patient

Is willing to assume responsibility of being primary pain manager

Is willing to accept and respect patient's reports of pain (if able to provide) as best indicator of how much pain the patient is experiencing; knows how to use and interpret a pain rating scale

Understands the purpose and goals of patient's pain management plan

Understands concept of maintaining a steady analgesic blood level

Recognizes signs of pain and side effects and adverse reactions to opioid

Nurse-Activated Dosing

Child's primary nurse is designated primary pain manager and is only person who presses PCA button during that nurse's shift

Guidelines for selecting primary pain manager for family-controlled analgesia apply to nurse-activated dosing

Data primarily from American Pain Society: *Principles of analgesic use in the treatment of acute pain or cancer pain,* ed 4, Glenview, IL, 1999, The Society; and McCaffery M, Pasero C: *Pain: a clinical manual,* ed 2, St Louis, 1999, Mosby.

*For further information about compounding drugs in troche or suppository form, contact: Technical Staff, Professional Compounding Centers of America (PCCA), PO Box 368, Sugar Land, TX 77487; (800) 331-2498; Web site: www.thecompounders.com.

Continued

Unit 4

BOX 4-12

Routes and Methods of Analgesic Drug Administration—cont'd

Nurse-Activated Dosing—cont'd

May be used in addition to a basal rate to treat break-through pain with bolus doses; patients are assessed q30 minutes for the need for a bolus dose

May be used without a basal rate as a means of maintaining analgesia with ATC bolus doses

BOX 4-13

Suggested Intravenous Patient Controlled Analgesia Opioid Infusion Orders

Drug	Basal Rate (µg/kg/hr)	Bolus Rate (µg/kg/dose)	Lockout Period (minutes)	Maximum Dose/hour (mg/kg)
Morphine	10-30	10-30	6-10	0.1-0.15
Hydromorphone	3-5	3-5	6-10	0.015-0.02
Fentanyl	0.5-1.0	0.5-1.0	6-10	0.002-0.004

From Yaster M, Krane EJ, Kaplan RF, et al: *Pediatric pain management and sedation handbook,* St Louis, 1997, Mosby, p. 100.

Intramuscular (IM)

NOT RECOMMENDED FOR PAIN CONTROL

Painful administration (hated by children)

Some drugs (e.g., meperidine) can cause tissue damage

Wide fluctuation in absorption of drug from muscle

Faster absorption from deltoid than from gluteal sites

Shorter duration and more expensive than oral drugs

Time consuming for staff

Intranasal

Midazolam (Versed) has been used as nasal spray

Although effective, route may be traumatic for children

Available commercially as Stadol NS (butorphanol); approved for those over 18 years of age; should not be used in patient receiving morphinelike drugs because butorphanol is partial antagonist

Intradermal

Used primarily for skin anesthesia (e.g., before lumbar puncture, bone marrow aspiration, arterial puncture, skin biopsy)

Local anesthetics (such as lidocaine) cause stinging, burning sensation

Duration of stinging may depend on type of "caine" used

To avoid stinging sensation associated with lidocaine:

Buffer the solution by adding 1 part sodium bicarbonate (1 mEq/ml) to 10 parts 1% or 2% lidocaine (Guidelines box)

Topical/Transdermal

EMLA (eutectic mixture of local anesthetics [lidocaine/prilocaine]) cream and anesthetic disc

Eliminates or reduces pain from most procedures involving skin puncture

Must be placed over puncture site and covered by occlusive dressing or applied as anesthetic disc for 1 hour or more before procedure (Guidelines box)

LAT (lidocaine/adrenaline/tetracaine) or *tetracaine/phenylephrine (tetraphen)*

Provides skin anesthesia about 15 minutes after application

Gel (preferable) or liquid placed on wounds for suturing (nonintact skin)

Cocaine should no longer be used because of the risk of systemic absorption and toxicity

Adrenalin must not be used on end arterioles (fingers, toes, tip of nose, penis, earlobes) because of vasoconstriction

Numby Stuff

Uses iontophoresis to transport lidocaine 2% and epinephrine 1:100,000 *(Iontocaine)* into the skin

A small battery-powered device delivers current via an electrode with Iontocaine and a ground electrode

Produces local dermal anesthesia in about 10 minutes to a depth of approximately 10 mm at maximum setting

May be frightening to young children when they see the device and feel the mild current

Child should be observed during iontophoresis

Transdermal fentanyl (Duragesic)

Available as "patch" for continuous cancer pain control

Safety and efficacy not established in children under 12 years

Not appropriate for initial relief of acute pain because of long interval to peak effect (from 12 to 24 hours); for rapid onset of pain relief, an immediate release opioid must be given

Orders for "rescue doses" of an immediate release opioid should be available for **breakthrough pain,** a flare of severe pain that "breaks through" the medication being administered at regular intervals for persistent pain

Has duration of up to 72 hours for prolonged pain relief

If respiratory depression occurs, several doses of naloxone may be needed

Vapocoolant

Use of spray coolant, such as Fluori-Methane, Frigiderm, or ethyl chloride; placed on the skin immediately before the needle puncture

Some children dislike the cold; spraying the coolant on a cotton ball then applying this to the skin may be less uncomfortable

Application of ice to the skin for 30 seconds has been found to be ineffective

The Child in Pain—cont'd

BOX 4-12

Routes and Methods of Analgesic Drug Administration—cont'd

Rectal

Alternative to oral or parenteral routes

Variable absorption rate

Generally disliked by children

Many drugs can be compounded into rectal suppositories*

Regional Nerve Block

Use of long-acting anesthetic (bupivacaine or ropivacaine) injected into nerves to block pain at site

Provides prolonged analgesia postoperatively, such as after inguinal herniorrhaphy

May be used to provide local anesthesia for surgery, such as dorsal penile nerve block for circumcision or for reduction of fractures

Inhalation

Use of anesthetics, such as nitrous oxide or halothane, to produce partial or complete analgesia for painful procedures

Occupational exposure to high levels of nitrous oxide may cause side effects

Epidural/Intrathecal

Involves catheter placed into epidural, caudal, or intrathecal space for continuous infusion or single or intermittent administration of opioid with or without a long-acting anesthetic (e.g., bupivacaine or ropivacaine)

Analgesia primarily from drug's direct effect on opioid receptors in spinal cord

Respiratory depression is rare but may have slow and delayed onset; can be prevented by checking level of sedation and respiratory rate and depth hourly for initial 24 hours and decreasing dose when excessive sedation is detected

Nausea, itching, and urinary retention are common dose-related side effects from the epidural opioid

Mild hypotension, urinary retention, and temporary motor and/or sensory deficits are common unwanted effects of epidural local anesthetic

*For further information about compounding drugs in troche or suppository form, contact: Technical Staff, Professional Compounding Centers of America (PCCA), PO Box 368, Sugar Land, TX 77487; (800) 331-2498; Web site: www.thecompounders.com.

Unit 4

The Child in Pain—cont'd

TABLE 4-9   Nonsteroidal Antiinflammatory Drugs (NSAIDs) Approved for Children*

Drug (Trade Name)	Dose	Comments
Acetaminophen (Tylenol and other brands)†	10-15 mg/kg/dose every 4-6 hours not to exceed 5 doses in 24 hours or 75 mg/kg/day, orally	Available in numerous preparations Nonprescription Higher dosage range may provide increased analgesia
Choline magnesium trisalicylate (Trilisate)	Children 37 kg or less: 50 mg/kg/day divided into 2 doses Children over 37 kg: 2250 mg/day divided into 2 doses	Available in suspension 500 mg/5 ml Prescription
Ibuprofen†		
Children's Motrin	Children 6 months: 5-10 mg/kg/dose every 6-8 hours not to exceed 40 mg/kg/day	Available in numerous preparations Nonprescription
Children's Advil	Children 6 months and older: 5-10 mg/kg/dose every 6-8 hours not to exceed 40 mg/kg/day	Available in suspension 100 mg/5 ml and drops 100 mg/2.5 ml Nonprescription
Naproxen (Naprosyn)	Children over 2 years: 10 mg/kg/day divided into 2 doses	Available in suspension 125 mg/5 ml and several different dosages for tablets Prescription
Tolmetin (Tolectin)	Children over 2 years: 20 mg/kg/day divided into 3 or 4 doses	Available in 200 mg, 400 mg, and 600 mg tablets Prescription

Taken from Olin BR and others: *Drug facts and comparisons,* ed 1998, St Louis, 1998, Facts and Comparisons.

NOTE: Newer formulations of NSAIDs, such as celecoxib (Celebrex), selectively inhibit one of the enzymes of cyclooxygenase (COX-2, which is responsible for pain transmission), but do not inhibit the other (COX-1). Inhibition of COX-1 decreases prostaglandin production, which is necessary for normal organ function. For example, prostaglandins help maintain gastric mucosal blood flow and barrier protection, regulate blood flow to the liver and kidneys, and facilitate platelet aggregation and clot formation. Theoretically, the COX-2 NSAIDs provide similar analgesic and antiinflammatory benefits with fewer side effects than the non-selective agents. Celebrex is approved for use in patients over 18 years of age.

*All NSAIDs in the table (except acetaminophen) have significant antiinflammatory, antipyretic, and analgesic actions. Acetaminophen has a weak antiinflammatory action, and its classification as an NSAID is controversial. Patients respond differently to various NSAIDs; therefore, changing from one drug to another may be necessary for maximum benefit.

Acetylsalicylic acid (aspirin) is also an NSAID but is not recommended for children because of its possible association with Reye syndrome. The NSAIDs in the table have no known association with Reye syndrome. However, caution should be exercised in prescribing any salicylate-containing drug (e.g., Trilisate) for children with known or suspected viral infection.

Side effects of ibuprofen, naproxen, and tolmetin include nausea, vomiting, diarrhea, constipation, gastric ulceration, bleeding, nephritis, and fluid retention. Acetaminophen and choline magnesium trisalicylate are well tolerated in the gastrointestinal tract and do not interfere with platelet function. NSAIDs (except acetaminophen) should not be given to patients with allergic reactions to salicylates. All the NSAIDs should be used cautiously in patients with renal impairment.

†For dosage recommendations for specific formulations of acetaminophen and ibuprofen, see pp. 589-590.

The Child in Pain—cont'd

TABLE 4-10 Dosage of Selected Opioids for Children

Drug	Approximate Equianalgesic Oral Dose	Approximate Equianalgesic Parenteral Dose	Recommended Starting Dose (Children Less Than 50-kg Body Weight)[a]	
			Oral	Parenteral[b]
Morphine[c]	30 mg every 3-4 hours (around-the-clock dosing)	10 mg every 3-4 hours	0.2-0.4 mg/kg every 3-4 hours 0.3-0.6 mg/kg time released every 12 hours	0.1-0.2 mg/kg IM every 3-4 hours 0.02-0.1 mg/kg IV bolus every 2 hours 0.015 mg/kg every 8 minutes PCA 0.01-0.02 mg/kg/hr IV infusion (neonates) 0.01-0.06 mg/kg/hr IV infusion (child)
Fentanyl (Sublimaze) (oral mucosal form—Fentanyl Oralet)[d]	1-1.5 mg	0.1 mg IV	5-15 µg/kg; maximum dose 400 µg	0.5-1.5 µg/kg IV bolus every ½ hour 1-2 µg/hr IV infusion
Codeine[c]	200 mg every 3-4 hours	130 mg every 3-4 hours	0.5-1 mg/kg every 3-4 hours	Not recommended
Hydromorphone[c] (Dilaudid)	7.5 mg every 3-4 hours	1.5 mg every 3-4 hours	0.06 mg/kg every 3-4 hours	0.015 mg/kg IV bolus every 2 hours
Hydrocodone (in Lorcet, Lortab, Vicodin, others)	30 mg every 3-4 hours	Not available	0.2 mg/kg every 3-4 hours[g]	Not available
Levorphanol (Levo-Dromoran)	4 mg every 6-8 hours	2 mg every 6-8 hours	0.04 mg/kg every 6-8 hours	0.02 mg/kg every 6-8 hours
Meperidine (Demerol)[f]	300 mg every 2-3 hours	100 mg every 3 hours	Not recommended	0.75 mg/kg every 2-3 hours
Methadone (Dolophine, others)	20 mg every 6-8 hours	10 mg every 6-8 hours	0.2 mg/kg every 6-8 hours	0.1 mg/kg every 6-8 hours
Oxycodone (Roxicodone, Oxycontin; also in Percocet, Percodan, Tylox, others)	20-30 mg every 3-4 hours	Not available	0.2 mg/kg every 3-4 hours[g]	Not available

Data from Acute Pain Management Guideline Panel: *Acute pain management: operative or medical procedures and trauma: clinical practice guideline,* AHCPR Pub No 92-0032, Rockville, MD, 1992, Agency for Health Care Policy and Research, Public Health Service, US Department of Health and Human Services; World Health Organization: *Cancer pain relief and palliative care in children,* Geneva, Switzerland, 1998, WHO; and Yaster M and others: *Pediatric pain management and sedation handbook,* St Louis, 1997, Mosby.

IV, Intravenous; *IM,* intramuscular; *PCA,* patient-controlled analgesia.

NOTE: Published tables vary in the suggested doses that are equianalgesic to morphine. Clinical response is the criterion that must be applied for each patient; titration to clinical response is necessary. Because there is not complete cross-tolerance among these drugs, it is usually necessary to use a lower than equianalgesic dose when changing drugs and to retitrate to response. Caution: Recommended doses do not apply to patients with renal or hepatic insufficiency or other conditions affecting drug metabolism and kinetics.

[a]Caution: Doses listed for patients with body weight less than 50 kg should not be used as initial starting doses in infants less than 6 months of age. For nonventilated infants under 6 months of age, the initial opioid dose should be about one fourth to one third of the dose recommended for older infants and children. For children with body weight greater than 50 kg, the usual adult dose should be used.

[b]IM injections should not be used.

[c]For morphine, hydromorphone, and oxymorphone, rectal administration is an alternate route for patients unable to take oral medications, but equianalgesic doses may differ from oral and parenteral doses because of pharmacokinetic differences.

[d]Fentanyl Oralet is indicated for use in a hospital setting only (1) as an anesthetic premedication in the operating room setting or (2) to induce conscious sedation before a diagnostic or therapeutic procedure in other monitored anesthesia care settings in hospital; is contraindicated in children who weigh less than 15 kg (33 lb).

[e]Caution: Codeine doses above 65 mg often are not appropriate because of diminishing incremental analgesia with increasing doses but continually increasing constipation and other side effects.

[f]Meperidine is not recommended for continuous pain control (e.g., postoperatively) because of risk of normeperidine toxicity. (See Practice Alert, p. 335.)

[g]Caution: Doses of aspirin and acetaminophen in combination with opioid/NSAID preparations must also be adjusted to patient's body weight.

Unit 4

The Child in Pain—cont'd

BOX 4-14

Selected Combination Opioid and Nonopioid Oral Analgesics—Nonaspirin Products*

Fioricet with Codeine	30 mg codeine 325 mg acetaminophen 50 mg butalbital 40 mg caffeine	Tylenol with Codeine No. 1	7.5 mg codeine 300 mg acetaminophen
		Tylenol with Codeine No. 2	15 mg codeine 300 mg acetaminophen
Hydrocet	5 mg hydrocodone 500 mg acetaminophen	Tylenol with Codeine No. 3	30 mg codeine 300 mg acetaminophen
Lorcet-HD	5 mg hydrocodone 500 mg acetaminophen	Tylenol with Codeine No. 4	60 mg codeine 300 mg acetaminophen
Lorcet Plus	7.5 mg hydrocodone 650 mg acetaminophen	Tylenol and Codeine Elixir (each 5 ml)	12 mg codeine 120 mg acetaminophen 7% alcohol
Lorcet 10/650	10 mg hydrocodone 650 mg acetaminophen	Tylox†	5 mg oxycodone HCl 500 mg acetaminophen
Lortab 2.5/500	2.5 mg hydrocodone 500 mg acetaminophen	Vicodin	5 mg hydrocodone 500 mg acetaminophen
Lortab 5/500	5 mg hydrocodone 500 mg acetaminophen	Vicodin ES	7.5 mg hydrocodone 750 mg acetaminophen
Lortab 10/500	10 mg hydrocodone 500 mg acetaminophen	Vicodin HP	10 mg hydrocodone 650 mg acetaminophen
Lortab Elixir (each 15 ml)	7.5 mg hydrocodone 500 mg acetaminophen		
Percocet-5†	5 mg oxycodone HCl 325 mg acetaminophen		

*Aspirin is not recommended for children because of its possible association with Reye syndrome. Analgesic compounds with aspirin include Darvon Compound, Darvon with A.S.A., Percodan, and Percodan-Demi. Darvon or Darvocet (propoxyphene) is not recommended; its analgesic effect is no greater than that from aspirin, acetaminophen, or other NSAIDs. Propoxyphene, an opioid, can depress respirations and its major metabolite is cardiotoxic and is a CNS stimulant that can produce seizures. (Dahl JL: Darvon, a drug with dubious distinction, *Cancer Pain Update* (48):3,6, Summer 1998.)

†All medications require a prescription, but these are classified as schedule II drugs (like morphine), and each filling requires a written prescription that includes the patient's name and address, the practitioner's DEA (Drug Enforcement Agency) number, and the date. The prescription must be filled within 5 days.

GUIDELINES

Using Buffered Lidocaine (BL)

Supplies: 8.4% sodium bicarbonate (1 mEq/ml), 1% to 2% lidocaine with or without epinephrine, syringe with removable needle, and a 30-gauge needle

Instructions:

Use 1 part sodium bicarbonate to 10 parts lidocaine (e.g., draw up 1 ml of lidocaine and 0.1 ml of sodium bicarbonate).

Change needle used to withdraw BL to 30-gauge needle for intradermal injection.

For venipuncture or port access, inject 0.1 ml or less BL intradermally directly over intended puncture site; anesthesia occurs almost immediately.

Suggested maximum dose of lidocaine for local anesthesia is 4.5 mg/kg.

If buffering lidocaine vial (e.g., 20 ml lidocaine with 2 ml sodium bicarbonate), solution may be used for 7 days if unrefrigerated or 14 days if refrigerated.

Using EMLA

Eutectic Mixture of Local Anesthetics-lidocaine 2.5% and prilocaine 2.5%)

Explain to child that EMLA is like a "magic cream that takes hurt away." Tap or lightly scratch site of procedure to show child that "skin is now awake."

Apply the "peel and stick" Anesthetic Disc or a thick layer (dollop) of EMLA cream over normal intact skin to anesthetize site (about one-half of a 5-gram tube; can use one-third of tube if puncture site is localized and superficial (e.g., intradermal injection or heel/finger puncture).

For venous access, apply to two sites; place enough cream on antecubital fossa to cover medial and lateral veins. Do not rub the cream.

If using the cream, place transparent adhesive dressing (e.g., Tegaderm) over EMLA. Make sure cream remains in a dollop or mound. A piece of plastic film (e.g., Saran Wrap) can be used, with tape to seal the edges. Use only as much adhesive as needed to prevent leakage.

To make the dressing less accessible, cover it loosely with a self-adhering Ace-type bandage (such as Coban) or an IV protector (such as IV House*). Label the dressing with "EMLA applied" and the date and time to distinguish it from other types of dressings. Instruct older children not to disturb the dressing. (Covering the dressing with an opaque material may reduce the attraction and discourage "fingering.") Supervise younger or cognitively-compromised children throughout the application time.

Leave EMLA on skin for at least 60 minutes for superficial puncture and 120 minutes for deep penetration (e.g., IM injection, biopsy). EMLA may be applied at home, and may need to be kept on longer in persons with dark and/or thicker skin. Anesthesia may last up to 4 hours after EMLA is removed.

Remove Disc or dressing before procedure and wipe cream from skin. For transparent dressing, grasp opposite sides, and while holding dressing *parallel* to skin, pull sides away from each other to stretch and loosen. An adhesive remover may be used.

Observe skin reaction (e.g., either blanched or reddened). If there is no obvious skin reaction, EMLA may not have penetrated adequately. Test skin sensitivity and reapply if needed.

Repeat tapping or lightly scratching on skin to show child that "skin is asleep" and that it cannot feel a needle.

After procedure, assess behavioral response. If child was upset, use pain scale (e.g., FACES) to help child distinguish between pain and fear. (See FACES Pain Rating Scale on p. 316.)

In the United States, EMLA is approved for use in infants born at 37 weeks of gestation and older.† It should not be used in those rare patients with congenital or idiopathic methemoglobinemia and in infants under the age of 12 months who are receiving treatment with methemoglobin-inducing agents such as sulfonamides, phenytoin (Dilantin), phenobarbital, and acetaminophen (Tylenol). Methemoglobin, a dysfunctional form of hemoglobin, reduces the blood's oxygen-carrying capacity, causing cyanosis and hypoxemia. The use of intravenous methylene blue promptly eliminates the methemoglobinemia.

NOTE: Although the package insert lists under "Warnings" that patients taking drugs associated with drug-induced methemoglobinemia, such as acetaminophen, are at greater risk for developing methemoglobinemia, there have been no reported cases of this complication occurring in children taking acetaminophen and using EMLA.

Follow the manufacturer's guidelines for MAXIMUM RECOMMENDED APPLICATION AREA TO INTACT SKIN FOR INFANTS AND CHILDREN

Age and Body Weight Requirements	Maximum Total Dose of EMLA	Maximum Application Area
1 to 3 months or <5 kg	1 g	10 cm² (1.25 × 1.25 in)
4 to 12 months and >5 kg	2 g	20 cm² (1.75 × 1.75 in)
1 to 6 years and >10 kg	10 g	100 cm² (4 × 4 in)
7 to 12 years and >20 kg	20 g	200 cm² (5.5 × 5.5 in)

NOTE: If a patient greater than 3 months old does not meet the minimum weight requirement, the maximum total dose of EMLA should be restricted to that which corresponds to the patient's weight.

*For more information, contact IV House, 7400 Foxmont Dr., Hazelwood, MO 63042-2198; (800) 530-0400; fax, (314) 831-3683; e-mail: ivhouse@icon-stl.net.

†See also the Community and Home Care Instruction on Applying EMLA, p. 615.

Meperidine (Demerol, Pethidine) is not recommended for chronic use (or for more than 48 hours at a time), such as for postoperative pain control, because of the accumulation of its metabolite, *normeperidine.* Normeperidine is a central nervous system stimulant that can produce anxiety, tremors, myoclonus, and generalized seizures. Normeperidine's half-life is 15 to 20 hours, compared with 3 hours for meperidine, and the central nervous system excitation is not reversed with naloxone.

Assess the child at least every 8 hours for early signs of toxicity, such as tremors in the outstretched hand, episodes of twitching or jerking, or increased agitation or excitability (may be upset easily). If normeperidine toxicity is suspected, discontinue the meperidine immediately, notify the practitioner, and request another opioid (e.g., morphine, oxycodone, hydromorphone [Dilaudid], or fentanyl) (Love, 1994). Do not administer naloxone. The pharmacist should complete an adverse drug reaction report to MedWatch.*

Love G: The dangers of normeperidine toxicity, *Am J Nurs* 94(6):14, 1994.

*The FDA Medical Products Reporting Program, Food and Drug Administration, 5600 Fishers Lane, Rockville, MD 20852-9787; (800) FDA-1088; fax, (800) FDA-0178; Web site, www.fda.gov/medwatch.

The Child in Pain—cont'd

Continued from p. 328.

If using parenteral route, change to oral route as soon as possible using equianalgesic (equal analgesic effect) dosages (See Tables 4-10 and 4-11.) *because of the first-pass effect (an oral opioid is rapidly absorbed from the gastrointestinal tract and enters the portal circulation, where it is partially metabolized before reaching the central circulation; therefore, oral dosages must be larger)*

Convert directly by giving next dose of analgesic orally in equivalent dosage without any parenteral form of the same drug, or

Convert gradually to oral form using the following steps:

Convert half the parenteral dose to an oral dose

Administer half the parenteral dose and the oral dose

Assess pain relief in 30 to 60 minutes

If pain relief is inadequate, increase the oral dose as needed

If sedation occurs, decrease the oral dose of opioid as needed, and request order for addition of nonopioid (e.g., acetaminophen) *to attack pain at peripheral nervous system and central nervous system*

When the parenteral and oral doses are effective, discontinue the parenteral dose and give twice the oral dose.

*Avoid combining opioids with so-called "potentiators," *because combining drugs such as promethazine (Phenergan) and chlorpromazine (Thorazine) add the additional risk of sedation and respiratory depression without increasing analgesia* (For drug alternatives to the Demerol, Phenergan, and Thorazine [DPT] mixture, see Box 4-16.)

Do not use placebos in the assessment or treatment of pain, *because deceptive use of placebos does not provide useful information about the presence or severity of pain, can cause side effects similar to those of opioids, can destroy child's and family's trust in the health care staff, and raises serious ethical and legal questions*

EXPECTED OUTCOMES

Child exhibits pain control (comfort level) that allows expected function/activities

Child accepts administration of analgesia with minimal distress

---

NURSING DIAGNOSIS: High risk for poisoning or injury related to sensitivity, excessive dose, decreased gastrointestinal motility

---

■ **PATIENT GOAL 1:** Will exhibit normal respiratory function

NURSING INTERVENTIONS/*RATIONALES*

Monitor rate and depth of respirations and level of sedation *because depression of these functions can lead to apnea*

Have emergency drugs and equipment in case of respiratory depression from opioids to begin therapy as soon as needed

If respirations or sedation are depressed:

Stop or reduce infusion by 25% when possible

Stimulate patient (shake gently, call by name, ask to breathe)

If patient cannot be aroused or is apneic:

*Administer naloxone (Narcan)†:

For children less than 40 kg: dilute 0.1 mg of naloxone in 10 ml of sterile saline to make 10 μg/ml solution and give 0.5 μg/kg

For children over 40 kg: dilute 0.4 mg ampule in 10 ml of sterile saline and give 0.5 ml

Administer bolus IV push every 2 minutes until effect is obtained

Closely monitor patient. Naloxone's duration of antagonist action may be shorter than that of opioid, requiring repeated doses of naloxone, and naloxone can precipitate withdrawal

*If respiratory depression is due to benzodiazepines (e.g., diazepam [Valium] or midazolam [Versed]), administer flumazenil (Romazicon). Pediatric dosing experience suggests 0.01 mg/kg (0.1 ml/kg) as loading dose; if inadequate or no response within 1 to 2 minutes, administer same dose and repeat as needed at 1-minute intervals for maximum dose of 1 mg (10 ml)

EXPECTED OUTCOME

Child's respirations and sedation level remain within acceptable limits (See inside front cover for normal variations.)

■ **PATIENT GOAL 2:** Child will not develop constipation and will receive treatment for other opioid-related side effects

NURSING INTERVENTIONS/*RATIONALES*

Decrease dose by 25% to determine if this dose decreases side effects while relieving pain

*Administer laxative (with or without stool softener) *to prevent constipation*

Stop or decrease medication if evidence of rash

*Administer antipruritic *for itching*

*Administer antiemetic for nausea and vomiting

Encourage child to lie quietly until nausea subsides *since movement increases nausea and vomiting*

Recognize signs of tolerance (e.g., decreasing pain relief, decreasing duration of pain relief)

Recognize signs of withdrawal following discontinuation of drug (physical dependence) (Box 4-15)

*Help treat tolerance and physical dependence appropriately *because these are involuntary, physiologic responses that occur from prolonged use of opioids*

Treat tolerance by increasing opioid dose

Suggested guidelines for preventing withdrawal syndrome in patients with physical dependence†:

Gradually reduce dose (similar to tapering of steroids):

Give one half of previous daily dose in every 6 hr doses for first 2 days

Then reduce dose by 25% every 2 days

Continue this schedule until total daily dose of 0.6 mg/kg/day of morphine (or equivalent) is reached

After 2 days on this dose, discontinue opioid

May also switch to oral methadone, using one fourth of equianalgesic dose as initial weaning dose and proceeding as described above

Never refer to child who is tolerant or physically dependent as addicted (Community Focus box)

EXPECTED OUTCOMES

Child has regular bowel movements

Child exhibits no evidence of rash or itching

Child receives appropriate treatment for tolerance or to prevent withdrawal if physically dependent

---

*Dependent nursing action.

†American Pain Society: *Principles of analgesic use in the treatment of acute pain and cancer pain,* ed 4, Glenview, IL, 1999, The Society.

Unit 4

The Child in Pain—cont'd

TABLE 4-11   Selected Analgesics (Equianalgesia)

Drug*	Equal to Oral Morphine (mg)	Equal to IM/IV Morphine (mg)
Hydromorphone (Dilaudid) 1 mg	4	1.3
Codeine 30 mg	4.5	1.5
Meperidine (Demerol) 50 mg	4.8	1.6
30 mg codeine + 300 mg acetaminophen (Tylenol No. 3)	7.2	2.4
Oxycodone 5 mg + 325 mg acetaminophen (Percocet)	7.2	2.4
Oxycodone 5 mg + 325 mg aspirin (Percodan)	7.2	2.4
Hydrocodone 5 mg + 500 mg acetaminophen (Vicodin, Lortab)	9	3
Oxycodone 5 mg + 500 mg acetaminophen (Tylox)	9	3
Dolophine (Methadone) 10 mg	15	7.5
Acetaminophen (Tylenol) 325 mg	2.7	0.9
Aspirin 325 mg	2.7	0.9
Acetaminophen (Tylenol Extra Strength) 500 mg	4	1.3
60 mg codeine + acetaminophen 300 mg (Tylenol No. 4)	11.7	3.9
Transdermal fentanyl patch (Duragesic) (based on 25 µg/hr patch applied every 3 days = 50 mg oral morphine every 24 hr or divided into 6 doses = 8.3 mg)	8.3	2.77

Courtesy of Betty R. Ferrell, PhD. FAAN, 1999. Used with permission.

*Oral medication with exception of fentanyl.

NOTE: When converting to oral oxycodone from oral morphine, an appropriate conservative estimate is 15 to 20 mg of oxycodone per 30 mg of morphine; however, when converting to oral morphine from oral oxycodone, an appropriate conservative estimate is 30 mg of morphine per 30 mg of oxycodone. (From McCaffery M, Pasero C: *Pain: a clinical manual,* ed 2, St Louis, 1999, Mosby, p. 198.)

BOX 4-15

Effects of Opioids

General Side Effects

Constipation (possibly severe)
Respiratory depression
Sedation
Nausea and vomiting
Agitation, euphoria
Mental clouding
Hallucinations
Orthostatic hypotension
Pruritus
Urticaria
Sweating
Miosis (may be sign of toxicity)
Anaphylaxis (rare)

Signs of Tolerance

Decreasing pain relief
Decreasing duration of pain relief

Signs of Withdrawal Syndrome in Patients with Physical Dependence

Initial signs:
  Lacrimation
  Rhinorrhea
  Yawning
  Sweating
Later signs:
  Restlessness
  Irritability
  Tremors
  Anorexia
  Dilated pupils
  Gooseflesh

The Child in Pain—cont'd

BOX 4-16

Suggested Medications for Conscious Sedation

Opioids*

Morphine sulfate, 0.05 to 0.10 mg/kg IV over 1 to 2 minutes given 5 minutes before procedure

Fentanyl, 1 to 2 µg/kg (0.001 to 0.002 mg/kg) IV 3 minutes before procedure

Fentanyl Oralet, 5 to 15 µg/kg, maximum to 400 µg, orally 20 to 40 minutes before procedure†

Hydromorphone (Dilaudid), 0.015-0.02 mg/kg IV over 1 to 2 minutes given 5 minutes before procedure.

Meperidine (if morphine sulfate or fentanyl is not available), 0.5 to 1.0 mg/kg IV over 1 to 2 minutes given 2 to 5 minutes before procedure or 1.5 mg/kg orally 45 to 60 minutes before procedure

Sedatives‡

Midazolam (Versed), 0.25 to 0.5 mg/kg (children 6 months to less than 6 years of age and less cooperative children may require a higher dose of up to 1 mg/kg), maximum to 20 mg, using oral preparation, 10 to 20 minutes, or 0.05 mg/kg IV 3 minutes before procedure

Diazepam (Valium), 0.2 to 0.3 mg/kg, maximum to 10 mg, orally 45 to 60 minutes before procedure

Pentobarbital (Nembutal), 1 to 3 mg/kg IV boluses to maximum of 100 mg until asleep

Chloral hydrate, 50 to 75 mg/kg, to maximum of 100 mg/kg or 2.5 g, orally or rectally 60 minutes before procedure

Modified from Zeltzer LK and others: Report of the subcommittee on the management of pain associated with procedures in children with cancer, *Pediatrics* 86(suppl):826-831, 1990; Coté CJ: Sedation for the pediatric patient, *Pediatr Clin North Am* 41(1):31-58, 1994; and Yaster M and others: *Pediatric pain management and sedation handbook,* St Louis, 1997, Mosby.

*Provide analgesia and sedation.

†Not recommended for children less than 15 kg. Lozenge should be sucked, not chewed and swallowed. If chewed, drug is less effective because part of it is metabolized by liver before entering bloodstream. Swallowing drug rapidly does not increase risk of respiratory depression during first 15 to 30 minutes, period of greatest risk for decreased respiration.

‡Provide sedation but no analgesia.

COMMUNITY FOCUS

Fear of Opioid Addiction

One of the reasons for the unfounded but prevalent fear of addiction to opioids used to relieve pain is a misunderstanding of physical dependence, tolerance, and addiction. Health professionals and the members of the community often confuse these terms, when in reality they are unrelated.

The American Society of Addiction Medicine defines these three terms as follows:

Physical dependence on an opioid is a physiologic state in which abrupt cessation of the opioid, or administration of an opioid antagonist, results in a withdrawal syndrome. Physical dependency on opioids is an expected occurrence in all individuals in the presence of continuous use of opioids for therapeutic or for nontherapeutic purposes. It does not, in and of itself, imply addiction.

Tolerance is a form of neuroadaptation to the effects of chronically administered opioids (or other medications). It is indicated by the need for increasing or more frequent doses of the medication to achieve the initial effects of the drug. Tolerance may occur both to the analgesic effects of opioids and to some of the unwanted side effects, such as respiratory depression, sedation, or nausea. The occurrence of tolerance is variable, but it does not, in and of itself, imply addiction.

Addiction, in the context of pain treatment with opioids, is characterized by a persistent pattern of dysfunctional opioid use that may involve any or all of the following:

- Adverse consequences associated with the use of opioids
- Loss of control over the use of opioids
- Preoccupation with obtaining opioids despite the presence of adequate analgesia

Unfortunately, individuals who have severe, unrelieved pain may become intensely focused on finding relief for their pain. Sometimes behaviors such as "clock watching" make patients appear to others to be preoccupied with obtaining opioids. However, this preoccupation focuses on finding relief from pain, not on using opioids for other reasons. This phenomenon has been termed "pseudoaddiction" and must not be confused with real addiction.

Nurses must educate older children, parents, and health professionals about the extremely low risk of real addiction (less than 1%) from the use of opioids to treat pain. Infants, young children, and comatose or terminally ill children simply cannot become addicted because they are incapable of a consistent pattern of drug-seeking behavior, such as stealing, drug-dealing, prostitution, and use of family income to obtain opioids for non-analgesic reasons.

From American Society of Addiction Medicine: *Public policy statement on the rights and responsibilities of physicians in the use of opioids for the treatment of pain,* April 16, 1997.

The Child in Pain—cont'd

■ **PATIENT GOAL 3:** Will feel less distress about the painful experience by using appropriate nonpharmacologic strategies

NURSING INTERVENTIONS/*RATIONALES*

Use nonpharmacologic interventions to supplement, not replace, pharmacologic interventions *because the major treatment of pain is with analgesics*

Assess the appropriateness of using nonpharmacologic interventions *because they are most useful for mild pain and when pain is reasonably well-controlled with analgesics;* used alone, they are not appropriate for moderate to severe pain

Employ nonpharmacologic strategies to help child manage pain *because techniques such as relaxation, rhythmic breathing, and distraction can make pain more tolerable*

Use strategy that is familiar to child or describe several strategies and let child select one (Guidelines box) *to facilitate child's learning and use of strategy*

Involve parent in selection of strategy *because parent knows child best*

Select appropriate person(s), usually parent, to assist child with strategy

Teach child to use specific nonpharmacologic strategies before pain occurs or before it becomes severe, *since these approaches appear to be most effective for mild pain*

Assist or have parent assist child with using strategy during actual pain, *because coaching may be needed to help child focus on required actions*

EXPECTED OUTCOMES

Child feels less distress about the painful experience

Child exhibits pain relief that allows child to perform expected activities

Child learns and implements effective coping strategies

Parent learns and supports use of nonpharmacologic interventions and effectively assists child in coping with pain

GUIDELINES

Nonpharmacologic Strategies for Pain Management

General Strategies

Use nonpharmacologic interventions to supplement, not replace, pharmacologic interventions and use for mild pain and pain that is reasonably well controlled with analgesics.

Form a trusting relationship with child and family.

Express concern regarding their reports of pain and intervene appropriately.

Take an active role in seeking effective pain management strategies.

Use general guidelines to prepare child for procedure.

Prepare child before potentially painful procedures but avoid "planting" the idea of pain. For example, instead of saying, "This is going to (or may) hurt," say, "Sometimes this feels like pushing, sticking, or pinching, and sometimes it doesn't bother people. Tell me what it feels like to you."

Use "nonpain" descriptors when possible (e.g., "It feels like heat" rather than "It's a burning pain"). This allows for variation in sensory perception, avoids suggesting pain, and gives child control in describing reactions.

Avoid evaluative statements or descriptions (e.g., "This is a terrible procedure" or "It really will hurt a lot").

Stay with child during a painful procedure.

Allow parents to stay with child if child and parent desire; encourage parent to talk softly to child and to remain near child's head.

Involve parents in learning specific nonpharmacologic strategies and in assisting child with their use.

Educate child about the pain, especially when explanation may lessen anxiety (e.g., that pain may occur after surgery and does not indicate something is wrong); reassure that child is not responsible for the pain.

For long-term pain control, give child a doll, which represents "the patient," and allow child to do everything to the doll that is done to the child; pain control can be emphasized through the doll by stating, "Dolly feels better after the medicine."

Teach procedures to child and family for later use.

Specific Strategies

Distraction

Involve parent and child in identifying strong distractors.

Involve child in play; use radio, tape recorder, CD player or computer game; have child sing or use rhythmic breathing.

Have child take a deep breath and blow it out until told to stop.*

Have child blow bubbles to "blow the hurt away."

Have child concentrate on yelling or saying "ouch" by focusing on "yelling as loud or soft as you feel it hurt: that way I know what's happening."

*French GM, Painter EC, Courty DL: Blowing away shot pain: a technique for pain management during immunization. *Pediatrics* 93(3):384-388, 1994.

Continued

Unit 4

The Child in Pain—cont'd

GUIDELINES

Nonpharmacologic Strategies for Pain Management—cont'd

Distraction—cont'd

Have child look through kaleidoscope (type with glitter suspended in fluid-filled tube) and encourage to concentrate by asking, "Do you see the different designs?"†

Use humor, such as watching cartoons, telling jokes or funny stories, or acting silly with child.

Have child read, play games, or visit with friends.

Relaxation

With an infant or young child:

Hold in a comfortable, well-supported position, such as vertically against the chest and shoulder.

Rock in a wide, rhythmic arc in a rocking chair or sway back and forth, rather than bouncing child.

Repeat one or two words softly, such as "Mommy's here."

With a slightly older child:

Ask child to take a deep breath and "go limp as a rag doll" while exhaling slowly; than ask child to yawn (demonstrate if needed).

Help child assume a comfortable position (e.g., pillow under neck and knees).

Begin progressive relaxation: starting with the toes, systematically instruct child to let each body part "go limp" or "feel heavy"; if child has difficulty with relaxing, instruct child to tense or tighten each body part and then relax it

Allow child to keep eyes open, since children may respond better if eyes are open rather than closed during relaxation

Guided Imagery

Have child identify some highly pleasurable real or imaginary experience.

Have child describe details of the event, including as many senses as possible (e.g., "feel the cool breezes," "see the beautiful colors," "hear the pleasant music").

Have child write down or tape record script.

Encourage child to concentrate only on the pleasurable event during the painful time; enhance the image by recalling specific details through reading the script or playing the tape.

Combine with relaxation and rhythmic breathing.

Positive Self-Talk

Teach child positive statements to say when in pain (e.g., "I will be feeling better soon," "When I go home, I will feel better, and we will eat ice cream").

Thought Stopping

Identify positive facts about the painful event (e.g., "It does not last long").

Identify reassuring information (e.g., "If I think about something else, it does not hurt as much").

Condense positive and reassuring facts into a set of brief statements, and have child memorize them (e.g., "Short procedure, good veins, little hurt, nice nurse, go home").

Have child repeat the memorized statements whenever thinking about or experiencing the painful event.

Cutaneous Stimulation

Includes simple rhythmic rubbing; use of pressure or electric vibrator; massage with hand lotion, powder, or menthol cream; application of heat or cold, such as vapocoolant spray on the site before giving injection or application of ice to the site opposite the painful area (e.g., if right knee hurts, place ice on left knee).

A more sophisticated method is **transcutaneous electrical nerve stimulation (TENS)** (use of controlled low-voltage electricity to the body via electrodes placed on the skin).

Another method is the use of **therapeutic electro membrane (TEM),** a high technology membrane electron reservoir fabricated from a non-woven, nonallergenic dressing that when placed in contact with the skin, releases the stored electrons in the form of microcurrent impulses.‡

Behavioral Contracting

Informal—May be used with children as young as 4 or 5 years of age:

Use stars or tokens as rewards.

Give uncooperative or procrastinating children (during a procedure) a limited time (measured by a visible timer) to complete the procedure.

Proceed as needed if child is unable to comply.

Reinforce cooperation with a reward if the procedure is accomplished within specified time.

Formal—Use written contract, which includes the following:

Realistic (seems possible) goal or desired behavior

Measurable behavior (e.g., agrees not to hit anyone during procedures)

Contract written, dated, and signed by all persons involved in any of the agreements

Identified rewards or consequences are reinforcing

Goals can be evaluated

Requires commitment and compromise from both parties (e.g., while timer is used, nurse will not nag or prod child to complete procedure)

---

†Vessey JA, Carlson KL, McGill J: Use of distraction with children during an acute pain experience. *Nurs Res* 43(6):369-372, 1994.

‡For more information contact Helio Medical Supplies, Inc., 2080A Walsh Avenue, Santa Clara, CA 95050; (888)-PAINTEM · (724-6836); e-mail: eileen@heliomed.com.

NURSING CARE PLAN

The Child at Risk for Infection

Infection is the invasion of the body by pathogenic microorganisms that reproduce and multiply, causing disease by local cellular injury, secretion of a toxin, or antigen-antibody reaction to the host.

The Centers for Disease Control and Prevention (CDC) and the Hospital Infection Control Practices Advisory Committee (HICPAC) revised the guidelines that were published in 1983. The revised guideline contains two levels of precautions:

Standard precautions synthesize the major features of universal (blood and body fluid) precautions (UP) (designed to reduce the risk of transmission of blood-borne pathogens) and body substance isolation (BSI) (designed to reduce the risk of transmission of pathogens from moist body substances). Standard precautions involve the use of *barrier protection,* such as gloves, goggles, gown, and/or mask, to prevent contamination from (1) blood; (2) all body fluids, secretions, and excretions *except sweat,* regardless of whether or not they contain visible blood; (3) nonintact skin; and (4) mucous membranes. Standard precautions are designed for the care of *all* patients to reduce the risk of transmission of microorganisms from both recognized and unrecognized sources of infection.

Transmission-based precautions are designed for patients documented or suspected to be infected or colonized with highly transmissible or epidemiologically important pathogens for which additional precautions beyond standard precautions are needed to interrupt transmission in hospitals. There are three types of transmission-based precautions: *airborne precautions, droplet precautions,* and *contact precautions.* They may be combined for diseases that have multiple routes of transmission (Box 4-17). When used either singu-

larly or in combination, they are to be used in addition to standard precautions.

Airborne precautions are designed to reduce the risk of airborne transmission of infectious agents. Special air handling and ventilation are required to prevent airborne transmission.

Droplet precautions are designed to reduce the risk of droplet transmission of infectious agents. Droplets are generated from the source person primarily during coughing, sneezing, or talking, and during the performance of certain procedures (e.g., suctioning and bronchoscopy).

Contact precautions are designed to reduce the risk of transmission of epidemiologically important microorganisms by direct or indirect contact. *Direct-contact transmission* involves skin-to-skin contact and physical transfer of microorganisms to a susceptible host from an infected or colonized person, such as occurs when personnel turn patients, bathe patients, or perform other patient care activities that require physical contact. Direct-contact transmission also can occur between two patients (e.g., by hand contact), with one serving as the source of infectious microorganisms and the other as a susceptible host. *Indirect-contact transmission* involves contact of a susceptible host with a contaminated intermediate object, usually inanimate, in the patient's environment.

PRACTICE ALERT

Handwashing is the most critical infection control practice.

ASSESSMENT

Take a careful health history, especially regarding evidence of contact with infective organisms, conditions that predispose the child to infection, medications that reduce the body's natural defenses (such as steroids and chemotherapeutic agents), and immunizations.

Observe for evidence of infection:
  Elevated temperature
  Swelling, tenderness, pain, and redness at site of infection

  Lethargy
    Loss of appetite
    Evidence of leukocytosis—Elevated WBC, appearance of pus
Monitor vital signs for early signs of infectious processes.
  Report any temperature elevation to practitioner.
Observe for signs of infection specific to child's illness.
Assist with diagnostic procedures and tests (e.g., collect specimens for culture, thoracentesis, or venipuncture).

NURSING DIAGNOSIS: Risk for infection related to impaired body defenses, presence of infective organisms

■ **PATIENT GOAL 1:** Will exhibit no evidence of infection

NURSING INTERVENTIONS/*RATIONALES*

Promote good health practices:
  Maintain adequate nutrition *to support body's natural defenses*
  Maintain good hygienic habits *to decrease exposure to infective organisms:*

Use good handwashing technique
Place child in room with noninfectious children; restrict visitors with active illnesses
Advise visitors (and hospital personnel) to practice good handwashing technique
Restrict contact with persons who have infections, including family, other children, friends, and members of staff
Use medical asepsis
Keep child dry and warm

EXPECTED OUTCOMES

Child and family apply good health practices
Child exhibits no evidence of infection

Continued

Unit 4

The Child at Risk for Infection—cont'd

■ **PATIENT (OTHERS) GOAL 2:** Will remain free from infection

NURSING INTERVENTIONS/*RATIONALES*
Implement standard precautions

Implement transmission-based precautions according to hospital policy

Instruct others (family, members of staff) in appropriate precautions

Teach affected children protective methods *to prevent spread of infection* (e.g., handwashing, handling genital area, care after using bedpan or toilet)

Try to keep infants and small children from placing hand and objects in contaminated areas

Superabsorbent disposable diapers with elastic legs contain urine and feces better than cloth diapers and *their use may reduce fecal contamination in the environment*

Assess home situation and implement protective measures as feasible in individual circumstances

*Administer antimicrobial medications if prescribed *to treat or prevent infection*

Support body's natural defenses (e.g., with good nutrition)

EXPECTED OUTCOME
Others remain free from infection

*Dependent nursing action.

BOX 4-17

Summary of Types of Precautions and Patients Requiring Them

Standard Precautions

Use standard precautions for the care of all patients

Airborne Precautions

In addition to standard precautions, use airborne precautions for patients known or suspected to have serious illnesses transmitted by airborne droplet nuclei. Examples of such illnesses include measles, varicella (including disseminated zoster), and tuberculosis

Droplet Precautions

In addition to standard precautions, use droplet precautions for patients known or suspected to have serious illnesses transmitted by large particle droplets. Examples of such illnesses include the following:

Invasive *Haemophilus influenzae* type b disease, including meningitis, pneumonia, epiglottitis, and sepsis

Invasive *Neisseria meningitidis* disease, including meningitis, pneumonia, and sepsis

Other serious bacterial respiratory infections spread by droplet transmission, including diphtheria (pharyngeal), mycoplasmal pneumonia, pertussis, pneumonic plague, streptococcal pharyngitis, pneumonia, or scarlet fever in infants and young children

Serious viral infections spread by droplet transmission, including adenovirus, influenza, mumps, parvovirus B19, rubella

Contact Precautions

In addition to standard precautions, use contact precautions for patients known or suspected to have serious illnesses easily transmitted by direct patient contact or by contact with items in the patient's environment. Examples of such illnesses include the following:

Gastrointestinal, respiratory, skin, or wound infections or colonization with multidrug-resistant bacteria judged by the infection control program to be of special clinical and epidemiologic significance based on current state, regional, or national recommendations

Enteric infections with a low infectious dose or prolonged environmental survival, including *Clostridium difficile.* For diapered or incontinent patients: enterohemorrhagic *Escherichia coli* O157:H7, *Shigella,* hepatitis A, or rotavirus

Respiratory syncytial virus, parainfluenza virus, or enteroviral infections in infants and young children

Skin infections that are highly contagious or that may occur on dry skin, including diphtheria (cutaneous); herpes simplex virus (neonatal or mucocutaneous); impetigo; major (noncontained) abscesses, cellulitis, or decubiti; pediculosis; scabies; staphylococcal furunculosis in infants and young children; and zoster (disseminated or in the immunocompromised host)

Viral/hemorrhagic conjunctivitis

Viral hemorrhagic infections (Ebola, Lassa, or Marburg)

Modified from Garner JS: Guideline for isolation precautions in hospitals, *Infect Control Hosp Epidemiol* 17(1):66, 1996.

NURSING CARE PLAN

Child and Family Compliance

Compliance is the extent to which the patient's or family's behavior coincides with the prescribed regimen (e.g., taking medications, following diets, executing other lifestyle changes).

FACTORS THAT ENHANCE COMPLIANCE

Individual/family factors:
  High self-esteem
  Positive body image
  High degree of autonomy
  Supportive and well-adjusted family
  Effective family communication
  Family expectation for successful completion of therapy

Care setting factors:
  Perceived satisfaction with care
  Positive interactions with practitioners
  Continuity of care
  Individualized care
  Minimum waiting time for appointments
  Convenient care setting

Treatment factors:
  Simple regimen
  Minimal disruption in usual lifestyle
  Short duration
  Inexpensive
  Visible benefits
  Tolerable side effects

ASSESSMENT

The most successful assessment of compliance combines at least two of the following methods:

Clinical judgment—The nurse judges family compliance. This method is subject to bias and inaccuracy unless the nurse carefully evaluates the criteria used in evaluation.

Self-reporting—The family is asked about their ability to carry out the prescribed treatments, although most people overestimate their compliance.

Direct observation—The nurse directly observes the patient or family perform the treatment. This method is difficult to employ outside the health care setting, and the family's awareness of being observed frequently affects their performance.

Monitoring appointments—The family's attendance at scheduled appointments is recorded, although this method only indirectly indicates compliance with the prescribed care.

Monitoring therapeutic response—The child's response in terms of benefit from treatment is monitored and, preferably, recorded on a graph or chart. Unfortunately, few treatments yield directly measurable results.

Pill counts—The nurse counts the number of pills remaining in the original container and compares the amount missing with the number of days the medication should have been taken. Although this is a simple method, families may forget to bring the container or may deliberately alter the number of pills to avoid detection. This method is also poorly suited to liquid medication, which is commonly prescribed in pediatrics.

Chemical assay—For certain drugs, such as digoxin, theophylline, and phenytoin, measurement of plasma drug levels provides information on the amount of drug recently ingested. However, this method is expensive, indicates only short-term compliance, and requires precise timing of the assay for accurate results.

NURSING DIAGNOSIS: Noncompliance related to (specify)

■ **PATIENT (FAMILY) GOAL 1:** Will exhibit compliance

NURSING INTERVENTIONS/*RATIONALES*

Encourage child and family to adhere to the prescribed treatment plan

Implement strategies to improve compliance (Box 4-18)

EXPECTED OUTCOMES

Child and family provide evidence of compliance (specify)

Child exhibits evidence of benefits from therapy (specify)

Unit 4

Continued

Child and Family Compliance—cont'd

BOX 4-18

Strategies to Improve Compliance

The best results occur when at least two strategies are employed. Ideally, such strategies are implemented before or concurrent with the initiation of therapy to avoid compliance problems.

Organizational strategies—Those interventions that are concerned with the care setting and the therapeutic plan:

Give specific appointments and names of health care professionals to be seen

Increase frequency of appointments

Designate a primary practitioner

Use mail and telephone reminders

Reduce waiting time for appointments

Reduce cost of treatment (e.g., generic brands of medications, free samples)

Reduce the treatment's disruption on the family's lifestyle

Use "cues" to minimize forgetfulness (e.g., pill dispensers, watches with alarms, charts to record completed therapy, reminders such as messages on the refrigerator or the bathroom mirror) and treatment schedules that incorporate the treatment plan into the daily routine (e.g., physical therapy after the evening bath)

Educational strategies—Those interventions that are concerned with instructing the family about the treatment plan:

Establish rapport; reduce anxiety and fear

Assess what the family knows and expects to learn, especially if they have concerns, and address their concerns before beginning teaching

Assess family's learning style; ask if they prefer having everything explained in detail or if they prefer knowing only the major facts

Use a variety of teaching materials (e.g., lecture, demonstration, video or slide presentation, written material)

Speak family's language, avoid jargon, and clarify all terms

Be specific when giving information; divide the information into small steps

Keep information short, simple, and concrete

Introduce most important information first

Use "verbal" headings to organize information, such as "There are two things you need to learn: how to give the medicine and what side effects to look for. First, how to give. . . . Second, what side effects . . ."

Stress how important the instructions are and the expected benefits; explain the detrimental effects of inadequate treatment, but avoid fear tactics

Evaluate the teaching by eliciting feedback to ensure that the family understands the information

Repeat information as needed

Reward the family for learning by giving verbal praise

Use "teachable moments"—times when family is most likely to accept new information (e.g., when a family member asks a question)

Behavioral strategies—Those interventions designed to modify behavior directly:

Involve significant others

Teach self-management skills (e.g., problem solving)

Provide positive reinforcement for accomplishment

Give verbal praise

Use concrete rewards (e.g., earning stars or tokens, a special privilege, gift)

Institute appropriate disciplinary techniques for non-compliance (e.g., time out for young children, withholding privileges for older children)

Implement behavioral contacting—a process in which the desired behavior is explicitly outlined in the form of a written contract

Essential components of a contract:

Goal or desired behavior is realistic and seems attainable

Behavior is measurable (e.g., agreeing to take the drug before leaving for school without reminding)

Contract is written and signed by all those involved in any of the agreements

Contract is dated and, if appropriate, has a date when specified goal should be reached (e.g., taking medication until the container is empty)

Reinforce with identified rewards or consequences

Goal is evaluated (e.g., counting the number of pills)

Use psychosocial services (e.g., counseling, psychotherapy, group therapy) when indicated

NURSING CARE OF THE NEWBORN

NURSING CARE PLAN

The Normal Newborn and Family

A **newborn** (neonate) is an infant, from birth to 4 weeks of age, born usually with a gestational age of 38 to 42 weeks.

ASSESSMENT

(See Newborn Assessment, p. 14.)
(See Assessment of Gestational Age, p. 22.)
Observe states of sleep and activity (Table 4-12).
Observe parental attachment behaviors:
  When the infant is brought to the parents, do they reach out for the child and call the child by name?
  Do the parents speak about the child in terms of identification (whom the infant looks like, what appears special about their child over other infants)?
  When parents are holding the infant, what kind of body contact is there? Do parents feel at ease in changing the infant's position? Are fingertips or whole hands used? Are there parts of the body they avoid touching or parts of the body they investigate and scrutinize?

When the infant is awake, what kinds of stimulation do the parents provide? Do they talk to the infant, to each other, or to no one? How do they look at the infant (direct visual contact, avoidance of eye contact or looking at other people or objects).
How comfortable do the parents appear in terms of caring for the infant? Do they express any concern regarding their ability, or disgust for certain activities, such as changing diapers?
What type of affection do they demonstrate to the newborn, such as smiling, stroking, kissing, or rocking?
If the infant is fussy, what kinds of comforting techniques do the parents use, such as rocking, swaddling, talking, or stroking?

NURSING DIAGNOSIS: Ineffective airway clearance related to excess mucus, improper positioning

■ **PATIENT GOAL 1:** Will maintain a patent airway

NURSING INTERVENTIONS/*RATIONALES*

Suction mouth and nasopharynx with bulb syringe as needed
  Compress bulb before insertion and suction pharynx, then nose, *to prevent aspiration of fluid*
  With mechanical suction, limit each suctioning attempt to 5 seconds with sufficient time between attempts *to allow reoxygenation*
Position infant on right side after feeding *to prevent aspiration*
Position infant on back during sleep
Perform as few procedures as possible on infant during first hour and have oxygen ready for use if respiratory distress should develop
Take vital signs according to institutional policy and more frequently, if necessary
  Observe for signs of respiratory distress and report any of the following immediately:
    Tachypnea
    Grunting, stridor
    Abnormal breath sounds
    Flaring alae nasi
    Cyanosis or pallor
Keep diapers, clothing, and blankets loose enough *to allow maximum lung (abdominal) expansion and to avoid overheating*
Clean nares of any crusted secretions during bath or when necessary
Check for patent nares

EXPECTED OUTCOMES

Airway remains patent
Breathing is regular and unlabored
Respiratory rate is within normal limits (See inside back cover for normal limits.)

NURSING DIAGNOSIS: Risk for altered body temperature related to immature temperature control, changes in environmental temperature

■ **PATIENT GOAL 1:** Will maintain stable body temperature

NURSING INTERVENTIONS/*RATIONALES*

Wrap infant snugly in a warmed blanket
Place infant in a preheated environment (under radiant warmer or next to mother)
Place infant on a padded, covered surface
Take infant's temperature on arrival at nursery or mother's room; proceed according to hospital policy regarding method and frequency of monitoring
Maintain room temperature between 24° and 25.5° C (75° to 78° F) and humidity about 40% to 50%
Give initial bath according to hospital policy
  Prevent chilling of infant during bath
  Postpone bath if there is any question regarding stabilization of body temperature
Dress infant in a shirt and diaper and swaddle in a blanket or cover with blanket
Provide infant with a head covering if heat loss is a problem *since large surface area of head favors heat loss*
Keep infant away from drafts, air conditioning vents, or fans
Place infant in a recessed cubicle with walls high enough *to shield from cross-ventilation*
Warm all objects used to examine or cover infant (e.g., place them under radiant warmer)
Uncover only one area of body for examination or procedures
Postpone circumcision until after temperature stabilizes, or use radiant warmer during procedure (Atraumatic Care box)
Be alert to signs of hypothermia or hyperthermia

EXPECTED OUTCOME

Infant's temperature remains at optimum level (36.5° to 37.5° C [97.7° to 99.5° F])

Continued

The Normal Newborn and Family—cont'd

TABLE 4-12 Implications for Parenting Relative to Infant's States of Sleep and Activity

Behavior	Duration	Implications for Parenting
Regular Sleep Closed eyes Regular breathing No movement except for sudden bodily jerks	4-5 hours/day, 10-20 minutes/ sleep cycle	External stimuli do not arouse infant Continue usual house noises Leave infant alone if sudden loud noise awakens infant and child cries
Irregular Sleep Closed eyes Irregular breathing Slight muscular twitching of body	12-15 hours/day, 20-45 minutes/ sleep cycle	External stimuli that did not arouse infant during regular sleep may minimally arouse child Periodic groaning or crying is usual; do not interpret as an indication of pain or discomfort
Drowsiness Eyes may be open Irregular breathing Active body movement	Variable	Most stimuli arouse infant Pick infant up during this time rather than leave in crib
Alert Inactivity Responds to environment by active body movement and by staring at close-range objects	2-3 hours/day	Satisfy infant's needs such as hunger Place infant in area of home where activity is continuous Place toys in crib or playpen Place objects within 17.5-20 cm (7-8 inches) of infant's view
Waking and Crying* May begin with whimpering and slight body movement Progresses to strong, angry crying, and uncoordinated thrashing of extremities	1-4 hours/day	Remove intense internal or external stimuli Stimuli that were effective during alert inactivity are usually ineffective Rock and swaddle to decrease crying

*Some classifications divide this fifth state into two states: alert with activity; and crying.

Unit 4

ATRAUMATIC CARE

Circumcision Anesthesia and Other Comfort Measures

Pharmacologic Interventions

Use of Topical Anesthetic Only

One hour before the procedure, administer acetaminophen (e.g., Tylenol) as ordered by the practitioner.

Place a thick layer of EMLA cream around the penis where the prepuce (foreskin) attaches to the glans. Avoid placing cream on the tip of the penis, where EMLA may come in contact with the urethral opening.

Cover the penis with a finger cot, a finger cut from a vinyl or latex glove, or a piece of plastic wrap and secure bottom of covering with tape. Avoid using Tegaderm or large amounts of tape on the skin, because removing the adhesive causes pain and can irritate the fragile skin.

If the infant urinates during the time EMLA is applied (1 to 2 hours), reapply the cream and covering.

Remove cream with clean cloth or tissue. Blanching or redness of skin is an expected reaction to application of EMLA under an occlusive dressing.

During procedure, allow infant to suck a pacifier coated with a mixture of sugar and water. To make an approximate 25% sucrose solution, add 1 teaspoon of table sugar to 4 teaspoons of sterile water. Use this solution to coat the pacifier, or administer 2 ml to the tongue 2 minutes before the procedure.*

Following procedure, apply A&D ointment on a 4 × 4 dressing before diapering infant. This prevents sticking of wound to dressing or diaper.

Administer acetaminophen as ordered by the practitioner 4 hours after the initial dose.

Use of Dorsal Penile Nerve Block (DPNB) or Ring Block*

One hour before the procedure, administer acetaminophen as ordered by the practitioner.

One to two hours before procedure, apply EMLA. For the DPNB, apply EMLA to the prepuce as described above and at the penile base. For the ring block, apply EMLA to the prepuce as described above and to the shaft of the penis. A topical anesthetic should be used in conjunction with the dorsal penile nerve block or ring block to avoid the pain of injecting the anesthetic.

Buffer the lidocaine with 8.4% sodium bicarbonate in a 10:1 ratio.

Use a 30-gauge needle to administer 0.8 ml of the buffered lidocaine; inject the anesthetic slowly. For the DPNB, 0.4 ml of the buffered lidocaine is infiltrated at the 2 o'clock and 10 o'clock positions at the penile base. For the ring block, 0.4 ml of buffered lidocaine is infiltrated subcutaneously on each side of the shaft of the penis below the prepuce.

For maximum anesthesia, wait 5 minutes following the injection of lidocaine. An alternative anesthesia is chloroprocaine, which is as effective as lidocaine after 3 minutes. Bupivacaine or ropivacaine provide a longer duration of anesthesia but may have a longer onset of action.

During the circumcision, allow infant to suck a pacifier coated with a mixture of sugar and water as previously described.

Apply A&D ointment to a 4 × 4 gauze and cover the wound before diapering infant. This prevents sticking of wound to dressing or diaper.

Administer acetaminophen as ordered by practitioner 4 hours after the initial dose.

Nonpharmacologic Interventions (to Accompany Pharmacologic Interventions)

If circumstraint board is used, pad with blankets and/or "lamb's wool." Preferably, use a circumcision chair.

Provide the parents, caregiver, or another staff member with the option to hold the infant during the procedure or to be present during the circumcision.

Prewarm any topical solutions to be used in sterile preparation of the surgical site by placing in a warm blanket or towel.

The infant's upper extremities should be swaddled or free from restraint. Lower extremities should be held or restrained using the circumstraint board for safety of the patient.

If the patient is not swaddled and is unclothed, perform the procedure under a radiant warmer to prevent hypothermia.

Shield infant's eyes from examination and radiant warmer lights.

Play infant relaxation music† before, during, and after procedure; allow parents or legal guardian the option to provide the music of their choice.

Following the procedure, remove restraints and swaddle. Immediately have the parent, other caregiver, or nursing staff hold the infant. Continue to have the infant suck on sucrose-coated pacifier.‡

*Note that these procedures differ among clinicians but represent current research findings. Data from "Standard of Practice, Infant Circumcisions," Boston City Hospital, Department of Nursing, Maternal-Child Health and Family-Centered Care, 1996, Boston, MA; Broadman LM and others: Post-circumcision analgesia: a prospective evaluation of subcutaneous ring block of the penis, *Anesthesiology* 67:339-402, 1987; Lander J and others: Comparison of ring block, dorsal penile nerve block and topical anesthesia for neonatal circumcision, *JAMA* 278:2157-2162, 1997; Marchette L and others: Pain reduction interventions during neonatal circumcision, *Nurs Res* 40(4):241-244, 1991; Mintz MR, Grillo R: Dorsal penile nerve block for circumcision, *Clin Pediatr* 28:590-591, 1989; Myron AV, Maguire DP: Pain perception in the neonate: implications for circumcision, *J Prof Nurs* 7:188-195, 1991; Spencer DM and others: Dorsal penile nerve block in neonatal circumcision: chloroprocaine versus lidocaine, *Am J Perinatol* 9(3):214-218, 1992; Williamson ML: Circumcision anesthesia: a study of nursing implications for dorsal penile nerve block, *Pediatr Nurs* 23:59-63, 1997; Yaster M and others: *Pediatric pain management and sedation handbook*, St Louis, 1997, Mosby.

†Suggested infant relaxation music: *Heartbeat Lullabies* by Terry Woodford. Available from Baby-Go-To-Sleep Center, Audio Therapy Innovations, Inc., PO Box 550, Colorado Springs, CO 80901; (800) 537-7748.

‡Circumcision information for parents is available from the American Academy of Pediatrics, 141 NW Point Blvd., PO Box 747, Elk Grove Village, IL 60009-0747; (800) 433-9016; Web site: www.aap.org.

Unit 4

The Normal Newborn and Family—cont'd

NURSING DIAGNOSIS: Risk for infection or inflammation related to deficient immunologic defenses, environmental factors, maternal disease

■ **PATIENT GOAL 1:** Will exhibit no evidence of infection

NURSING INTERVENTIONS/*RATIONALES*

Wash hands before and after caring for each infant
Wear gloves when in contact with body secretions
Use of cover gowns is controversial *because studies show they do not decrease infection rates but do increase costs*
Check that appropriate eye prophylaxis has been carried out
Check eyes daily for evidence of inflammation or discharge
Keep infant from potential sources of infection (e.g., persons with respiratory or skin infections, improperly prepared food sources, other unclean items)
Clean vulva in posterior direction *to prevent fecal contamination of vagina or urethra;* stress this to parents
While cleaning penis, do not retract foreskin; gently wipe away smegma
Maintain asepsis during circumcision
*If infant has been circumcised, cover area with a petrolatum jelly gauze dressing (except when Plastibell is used)
Check for voiding and bleeding after circumcision; disposable diaper may feel dry when wet, but crotch area will feel "clumpy" or "doughy" and heavy
Keep umbilical stump clean and dry
Place diapers below umbilical stump
Assess cord daily for odor, color, and drainage
*Apply antibacterial agent and/or alcohol to cord as ordered
*Administer hepatitis B vaccine (HBV) in vastus lateralis or deltoid muscle *because both sites afford maximum immune response*

EXPECTED OUTCOMES

Infant exhibits no evidence of infection or inflammation
Eyes remain clear with no evidence of irritation
Genital area is free of irritation
Cord appears dry, surrounding area free of infection
Infant receives HBV

NURSING DIAGNOSIS: Risk for trauma related to physical helplessness

■ **PATIENT GOAL 1:** Will be clearly and correctly identified

NURSING INTERVENTIONS/*RATIONALES*

Make certain infant is properly identified *for placement with correct mother*
Ensure that identification (ID) bands are properly and securely placed
Check infant's ID band often *to ensure infant identity is correct*
Discuss safety issues with parents, especially mother, *to prevent possible kidnapping*
Observe staff's ID badges and give infant only to properly identified personnel
Never leave infant alone in crib or room

EXPECTED OUTCOMES

Infant is clearly and correctly identified at all times
Parents observe safety practices
ID band remains in place

■ **PATIENT GOAL 2:** Will have no physical injury

NURSING INTERVENTIONS/*RATIONALES*

Avoid using rectal thermometer *because of risk of rectal perforation*
Never leave infant unsupervised on a raised surface without side barriers
Keep pointed or sharp objects away from infant
Always close diaper pins (if used) and place them away from infant's body
Keep own fingernails short and trimmed; avoid jewelry that can scratch infant
Employ appropriate methods of handling and transporting infant

EXPECTED OUTCOME

Infant remains free of physical injury

■ **PATIENT GOAL 3:** Will exhibit no evidence of bleeding

NURSING INTERVENTIONS/*RATIONALES*

*Administer vitamin K intramuscularly using vastus lateralis muscle as site of injection
Check circumcision site; assess for any oozing *that may indicate bleeding tendencies*

EXPECTED OUTCOME

Infant exhibits no evidence of bleeding

NURSING DIAGNOSIS: Altered nutrition: less than body requirements (risk) related to immaturity, parental knowledge deficit

■ **PATIENT GOAL 1:** Will receive optimum nutrition

NURSING INTERVENTIONS/*RATIONALES*

Assess strength of suck and coordination with swallowing *to identify possible problem affecting feeding*
Offer initial intake according to parent's preference, hospital policy, and practitioner's protocol
Prepare for demand feeding of breast-fed infants; night feedings determined by condition and preferences of mother
Offer bottle-fed infants 2 to 3 ounces of formula every 3 to 4 hours or on demand
Support and assist breast-feeding mothers during initial feedings and continue if necessary
Avoid routine water or supplemental feedings for breast-feeding infants because these may *decrease the desire to suck and cause nipple preference*
Encourage father or other support person to remain with mother to help her and infant with positioning, relaxation, and reinforcement
Encourage father or other support person to participate in bottle-feeding
Place infant on right side after feeding *to prevent aspiration*
Observe stool pattern

*Dependent nursing action.

Unit 4

The Normal Newborn and Family—cont'd

EXPECTED OUTCOMES

Infant demonstrates strong suck

Infant retains feedings

Infant receives an adequate amount of nutrients (specify amount and frequency of feedings)

Infant loses less than 10% of birth weight

> **NURSING DIAGNOSIS:** Altered family processes related to maturational crisis, birth of term infant, change in family unit

■ **PATIENT (FAMILY) GOAL 1:** Will exhibit parent-infant attachment behaviors

NURSING INTERVENTIONS/*RATIONALES*

As soon after delivery as possible, encourage parents to see and hold infant; place newborn close to face of parents *to establish visual contact*

Ideally, perform eye care after initial meeting of infant and parents, within 1 hour after birth *when infant is alert and most likely to visually relate to parent*

Identify for parents specific behaviors manifested by infant (e.g., alertness, ability to see, vigorous suck, rooting behavior, and attention to human voice)

Discuss with parents their expectations of fantasy child vs real child (if indicated)

Encourage parents to "talk out" their labor and delivery experience; identify any events that signify loss of control to either parent, especially mother

Identify behavioral steps in attachment process, and evaluate those aspects that could be considered positive and those that may represent inadequate or delayed parenting

Encourage family to room-in or to call for infant frequently if not rooming-in

Observe and assess reciprocity of cues between infant and parent *to identify behaviors that may need strengthening*

Assist parents in recognizing attention-nonattention cycles and in understanding their significance

Assess variables affecting development of attachment through observing infant and parent and interviewing each parent or other significant caregiver

EXPECTED OUTCOMES

Parents establish contact with infant immediately or soon after birth

Parents demonstrate attachment behaviors such as touching, eye contact, naming and calling infant by name, talking to infant, and participating in caregiving activities

Parents recognize attention-nonattention cycles

■ **PATIENT (SIBLING) GOAL 2:** Will demonstrate adjustment/attachment behaviors toward newborn

NURSING INTERVENTIONS/*RATIONALES*

Allow to visit and touch newborn when feasible

Explain physical differences in newborn, such as bald head, umbilical stump and clamp, and circumcision *to lessen any fear siblings might have*

Explain to siblings realistic expectations regarding newborn's abilities and needs

Requires complete care

Is not a playmate

Encourage siblings to participate in care at home *to make them feel part of the experience*

Encourage parents to spend individual time with other children at home *to reduce feelings of jealousy toward new sibling*

EXPECTED OUTCOME

Siblings express interest in newborn and have realistic expectations for their age

■ **PATIENT (FAMILY) GOAL 3:** Will be prepared for discharge and home care

NURSING INTERVENTIONS/*RATIONALES*

Discuss with parents correct preparation of formula:

Stress that proportions must not be altered to dilute or concentrate the formula

Discourage microwaving of bottles *to avoid burns*

Encourage use of support persons, such as lactation specialist or members of La Leche League, for assistance with breast-feeding

Instruct in other aspects of newborn care:

Bathing

Umbilical cord and circumcision care

Recognize states of activity for optimum interaction (See Table 4-12.)

Encourage participation in parenting classes, if offered

Discuss importance and proper use of federally approved car seat restraints

If infant is small, advise parents to use rolled blankets and towels in crotch area *to prevent slouch* and along sides *to minimize lateral movement,* but to never use padding underneath or behind infant *since it creates slackness in harness, leading to possible ejection from seat in a crash*

Refer to organizations that may rent car seat restraints

If parent-infant attachment is at risk, refer to appropriate agencies (social services, family and child services, at-risk programs)

EXPECTED OUTCOMES

Family demonstrates ability to provide care for infant

Family keeps appointments for follow-up care

Infant rides home in federally approved car seat restraint

Family members avail themselves of needed services

Unit 4

NURSING CARE PLAN

The High-Risk Newborn and Family

High-risk newborns are neonates who, regardless of gestational age or birth weight, have a greater than average chance of morbidity or mortality because of conditions or circumstances superimposed on the normal course of events associated with birth and the adjustment to extrauterine existence.

CLASSIFICATION ACCORDING TO SIZE
Low-birth-weight (LBW) infant—An infant whose birth weight is less than 2500 g, regardless of gestational age

Extremely low-birth-weight (ELBW) infant—An infant whose birth weight is less than 1000 g

Very-low-birth-weight (VLBW) infant—An infant whose birth weight is less than 1500 g

Moderately-low-birth-weight (MLBW)—An infant whose birth weight is 1501 to 2500 g

Appropriate-for-gestational-age (AGA) infant—An infant whose weight falls between the 10th and 90th percentiles on intrauterine growth curves

Small-for-date (SFD) or small-for-gestational-age (SGA) infant—An infant whose rate of intrauterine growth was slowed and whose birth weight falls below the 10th percentile on intrauterine growth curves

Intrauterine growth retardation (IUGR)—Found in infants whose intrauterine growth is retarded (sometimes used as a more descriptive term for the SGA infant)

Large-for-gestational-age (LGA) infant—An infant whose birth weight falls above the 90th percentile on intrauterine growth charts

CLASSIFICATION ACCORDING TO GESTATIONAL AGE
Premature (preterm) infant—An infant born before completion of 37 weeks of gestation, regardless of birth weight

Full-term infant—An infant born between the beginning of the 38th week and the completion of the 42nd week of gestation, regardless of birth weight

Postmature (postterm) infant—An infant born after 42 weeks of gestational age, regardless of birth weight

CLASSIFICATION ACCORDING TO MORTALITY
Live birth—Birth in which the neonate manifests any heartbeat, breathes, or displays voluntary movement, regardless of gestational age

Fetal death—Death of the fetus after 20 weeks of gestation and before delivery, with absence of any signs of life after birth

Neonatal death—Death that occurs in the first 27 days of life; early neonatal death occurs in the first week of life; late neonatal death occurs at 7 to 27 days

Perinatal mortality—Describes the total number of fetal and early neonatal deaths per 1000 live births

Postnatal death—Death that occurs at 28 days to 1 year

ASSESSMENT
See the following:
  Assessment of Gestational Age, p. 22
  Newborn Assessment, p. 14
  Guidelines for Physical Assessment
  Box 4-19
  Developmental Characteristics of Children's Responses to
    Pain, p. 321
Observe for clinical manifestations of prematurity:
  Very small, scrawny appearance
  Skin is red to pink with visible veins
  Fine, feathery hair; lanugo on back and face
  Little or no evidence of subcutaneous fat
  Head larger in relation to body
  Sucking pads prominent
  Lies in "relaxed attitude"
  Limbs extended
  Ear cartilages poorly developed
  Few fine wrinkles on palms and soles
  Clitoris prominent in female

  Scrotum underdeveloped, nonpendulous, with minimal
    rugae and undescended testes
  Lax, easily manipulated joints
  Absent, weak, or ineffectual grasping, sucking, swallowing,
    and gag reflexes
  Other neurologic signs are absent or diminished
  Unable to maintain body temperature
  Dilute urine
  Pliable thorax
  Periodic breathing, hypoventilation
  Frequent episodes of apnea
Observe for clinical manifestations of postmaturity:
  Absence of lanugo
  Little if any vernix caseosa, deep yellow or green in color
  Abundant or receding scalp hair
  Long fingernails
  Whiter skin than term newborns
  Skin frequently cracked, parchmentlike, and desquamating
  Wasted physical appearance, little subcutaneous tissue
  Long, thin appearance

Physical Assessment

General Assessment

Weigh daily, or more often if ordered, using electronic scale.

Measure length and head circumference periodically.

Describe general body shape and size, posture at rest, ease of breathing, presence and location of edema.

Describe any apparent deformities.

Describe any signs of distress: poor color, mouth open, head bobbing, grimace, furrowed brow.

Respiratory Assessment

Describe shape of chest (barrel, concave), symmetry, presence of incisions, chest tubes, or other deviations.

Describe use of accessory muscles: nasal flaring or substernal, intercostal, or subclavicular retractions.

Determine respiratory rate and regularity.

Auscultate and describe breath sounds: stridor, crackles, wheezing, wet diminished sounds, areas of absence of sound, grunting, diminished air entry, equality of breath sounds.

Determine whether suctioning is needed.

Describe cry (if not intubated).

Describe ambient oxygen and method of delivery; if intubated, describe size of tube, type of ventilator and settings, and method of securing tube.

Determine oxygen saturation by pulse oximetry, and partial pressure of oxygen and carbon dioxide by transcutaneous oxygen ($tcPo_2$) and transcutaneous carbon dioxide ($tcPco_2$).

Cardiovascular Assessment

Determine heart rate and rhythm.

Describe heart sounds, including any murmurs.

Determine the point of maximum intensity (PMI), the point at which the heartbeat sounds and palpates loudest (a change in the PMI may indicate a mediastinal shift).

Describe infant's color (variance may be of cardiac, respiratory, or hematopoietic origin): cyanosis, pallor, plethora, jaundice, mottling.

Assess color of nail beds, mucous membranes, lips.

Determine blood pressure. Indicate extremity used and cuff size; check each extremity at least once.

Describe peripheral pulses, capillary refill (<2 to 3 seconds), peripheral perfusion (mottling).

Describe monitors, their parameters, and whether alarms are in "on" position.

Gastrointestinal Assessment

Determine presence of abdominal distention: increase in circumference, shiny skin, evidence of abdominal wall erythema, visible peristalsis, visible loops of bowel, status of umbilicus.

Determine any signs of regurgitation and, if so, time related to feeding; character and amount of residual if gavage fed; if nasogastric tube in place, describe type of suction, drainage (color, consistency, pH, guaiac).

Describe amount, color, consistency, and odor of any emesis.

Palpate liver margin.

Describe amount, color, and consistency of stools; check for occult blood and/or reducing substances if ordered or indicated by appearance of stool.

Describe bowel sounds: presence or absence (must be present if feeding).

Genitourinary Assessment

Describe any abnormalities of genitalia.

Describe urine amount (as determined by weight), color, pH, labstick findings, and specific gravity (to screen for adequacy of hydration).

Check weight (the most accurate measure for assessment of hydration).

Neurologic-Musculoskeletal Assessment

Describe infant's movements: random, purposeful, jittery, twitching, spontaneous, elicited; level of activity with stimulation; evaluate based on gestational age.

Describe infant's position or attitude: flexed, extended.

Describe reflexes observed: Moro, sucking, Babinski, plantar, and other expected reflexes.

Determine level of response and consolability.

Determine changes in head circumference (if indicated); size and tension of fontanels, suture lines.

Determine pupillary responses in infant >32 weeks of gestation.

Temperature

Determine skin and axillary temperature.

Determine relationship to environmental temperature.

Skin Assessment

Describe any discoloration, reddened area, signs of irritation, blisters, abrasions, or denuded areas, especially where monitoring equipment, infusions, or other apparatus come in contact with skin; also check and note *any* skin preparation used (e.g., povidone-iodine tape).

Determine texture and turgor of skin: dry, smooth, flaky, peeling, etc.

Describe any rash, skin lesions, or birthmarks.

Determine whether intravenous infusion catheter or needle is in place, and observe for signs of infiltration.

Describe parenteral infusion lines: location, type (arterial, venous, peripheral, umbilical, central, peripheral central venous); type of infusion (medication, saline, dextrose, electrolyte, lipids, total parenteral nutrition); type of infusion pump and rate of flow; type of catheter or needle; and appearance of insertion site.

The High-Risk Newborn and Family—cont'd

BOX 4-19

Signs of Stress or Fatigue in Neonates

Autonomic Stress

Acrocyanosis
Deep, rapid respirations
Regular, rapid heart rate

Changes in State

Dull or sleep states
Crying or fussy
Glassy-eyed or strained alertness

Behavioral Changes

Unfocused and uncoordinated eyes
Limp arms and legs
Flaccid shoulders dropped back
Hiccups
Sneezes
Yawning
Straining while having a bowel movement

From Als H: Toward a synactive theory of development: promise for the assessment and support of infant and individuality, *Infant Ment Health J* 3:229-243, 1982.

The High-Risk Newborn and Family—cont'd

NURSING DIAGNOSIS: Ineffective breathing pattern related to pulmonary and neuromuscular immaturity, decreased energy, and fatigue

■ **PATIENT GOAL 1:** Will exhibit adequate oxygenation parameters (specify)

NURSING INTERVENTIONS/*RATIONALES*

Position for optimum air exchange

Place prone when feasible *since this position results in improved oxygenation, better-tolerated feedings, and more organized sleep-rest patterns*

Place supine with neck slightly extended and nose pointing to ceiling in "sniffing" position *to prevent any narrowing of airway*

Avoid neck hyperextension *because it reduces diameter of trachea*

Observe for deviations from desired functioning; recognize signs of distress: grunting, cyanosis, nasal flaring, apnea

Suction *to remove accumulated mucus from nasopharynx, trachea, and endotracheal tube*

Suction only as necessary based on assessment (e.g., auscultation of chest, evidence of decreased oxygenation, increased infant irritability)

Never suction routinely *because it may cause bronchospasm, bradycardia due to vagal nerve stimulation, hypoxia, and increased intracranial pressure (ICP), predisposing infant to intraventricular hemorrhage (IVH)*

Use proper suctioning technique *because improper suctioning can cause infection, airway damage, pneumothorax, and IVH*

Use two-person suction technique *because assistant can provide immediate hyperoxygenation before and after catheter insertion*

*Carry out percussion, vibration, and postural drainage only as prescribed *to facilitate drainage of secretions*

Avoid using Trendelenburg position *because it can contribute to increased ICP and reduced lung capacity from gravity pushing organs against diaphragm*

During diaper changes, raise infant slightly under hips; do not raise feet and legs

Use semiprone or side-lying position for infant with excessive mucus or while infant is being fed *to prevent aspiration*

Observe for signs of respiratory distress: nasal flaring, retractions, tachypnea, apnea, grunting, cyanosis, low oxygenation saturation (Sao_2)

†Carry out regimen prescribed for supplemental oxygen therapy (maintain ambient O_2 concentration at minimum Fio_2 level based on arterial blood gases, Sao_2, and transcutaneous oxygen [$tcpo_2$])

Maintain neutral thermal environment *to conserve utilization of O_2*

Closely monitor blood gas measurements ($tcpo_2$ and Sao_2 readings)

Apply and manage monitoring equipment correctly (e.g., cardiac or oxygen)

Demonstrate understanding of function of respiratory support apparatus

Mechanical ventilation apparatus

Insufflation bags with masks and/or endotracheal tube adaptor

Oxygen hoods/tents

Humidifier warmers

Observe and assess infant's response to ventilation and oxygenation therapy

EXPECTED OUTCOMES

Airway remains patent

Breathing provides adequate oxygenation and CO_2 removal

Respiratory rate and pattern is within appropriate limits for age and weight (specify)

Arterial blood gases and acid-base balance are within normal limits for gestational age

Tissue oxygenation is adequate

NURSING DIAGNOSIS: Ineffective thermoregulation related to immature temperature control and decreased subcutaneous body fat

■ **PATIENT GOAL 1:** Will maintain stable body temperature

NURSING INTERVENTIONS/*RATIONALES*

Place infant in incubator or radiant warmer, or clothe warmly and place in open crib *to maintain stable body temperature*

Monitor axillary temperature in unstable infants (use skin probe or air temperature control; check function of servocontrolled mechanism when used)

Regulate servocontrolled unit or air temperature control as needed *to maintain skin temperature within accepted range*

Use plastic heat shield as appropriate *to decrease heat and water losses*

Monitor for signs of hyperthermia: redness, flushing, diaphoresis (rarely)

Check temperature of infant in relation to ambient temperature and temperature of heating unit *to decrease radiant heat loss*

Avoid situations that might predispose infant to heat loss, such as exposure to cool air, drafts, bathing, cold scales, or cold mattress

Monitor serum glucose values *to ensure euglycemia*

EXPECTED OUTCOME

Infant's axillary temperature remains within normal range for postconceptual age (specify)

NURSING DIAGNOSIS: Risk for infection related to deficient immunologic defenses

■ **PATIENT GOAL 1:** Will exhibit no evidence of nosocomial infection

NURSING INTERVENTIONS/*RATIONALES*

Ensure that all caregivers wash hands before and after handling infant *to minimize exposure to infective organisms*

---

*Dependent nursing action.

Continued

The High-Risk Newborn and Family—cont'd

Ensure that all equipment in contact with infant is clean or sterile

Prevent personnel with upper respiratory tract or other communicable infections from coming into direct contact with infant

Isolate other infants with infections according to institutional policy

Instruct health care workers and parents in infection control procedures

*Administer antibiotics as ordered

Ensure strict asepsis and/or sterility with invasive procedures and equipment such as peripheral IV therapy, lumbar punctures, and arterial/venous catheter insertion

EXPECTED OUTCOME

Infant exhibits no evidence of nosocomial infection

NURSING DIAGNOSIS: Altered nutrition: less than body requirements (risk) related to inability to ingest nutrients because of immaturity and/or illness

---

■ **PATIENT GOAL 1:** Will receive adequate nourishment, with sufficient caloric intake to maintain positive nitrogen balance and exhibit appropriate weight gain

NURSING INTERVENTIONS/*RATIONALES*

*Maintain parenteral fluid or total parenteral nutrition therapy as ordered

Monitor for signs of intolerance to total parenteral therapy, especially to protein and glucose

Assess readiness to nipple feed, especially ability to coordinate swallowing and breathing

Nipple feed infant if strong sucking, swallowing, and gag reflexes are present (usually at gestational age of 34 to 35 weeks) *to minimize risk of aspiration*

Follow unit protocol for advancing volume and concentration of formula *to avoid feeding intolerance*

Use orogastric feeding if infant tires easily or has weak sucking, gag, or swallowing reflexes *because nipple feeding may result in weight loss*

Assist mother with expressing breast milk *to establish and maintain lactation until infant can breast-feed*

Assist mother with breast-feeding when feasible and desirable

EXPECTED OUTCOMES

Infant receives an adequate amount of calories and essential nutrients

Infant demonstrates a steady weight gain (approximately 20 to 30 g/day) once past acute phase of illness

---

NURSING DIAGNOSIS: Risk for fluid volume deficit or excess related to immature physiologic characteristics of preterm infant and/or immaturity or illness

---

■ **PATIENT GOAL 1:** Will exhibit adequate hydration status

NURSING INTERVENTIONS/*RATIONALES*

Monitor fluid and electrolytes closely with therapies that increase insensible water loss (IWL) (e.g., phototherapy, radiant warmer)

Implement strategies to minimize IWL, such as plastic covering and increased ambient humidity

Ensure adequate parenteral/oral fluid intake

Assess state of hydration (e.g., skin turgor, blood pressure, edema, weight, mucous membranes, urine specific gravity, electrolytes, fontanels)

Regulate parenteral fluids closely *to avoid dehydration, overhydration, or extravasation*

Avoid administering hypertonic fluids (e.g., undiluted medications, concentrated glucose infusions) *to prevent excess solute load on immature kidneys and fragile veins*

Monitor urinary output and laboratory values *for evidence of dehydration or overhydration* (adequate urinary output 1 to 2 ml/kg/hr)

Minimize use of adhesives *to preserve intact skin barrier*

EXPECTED OUTCOME

Infant exhibits evidence of fluid homeostasis

NURSING DIAGNOSIS: Risk for impaired skin integrity related to immature skin structure, immobility, decreased nutritional state, invasive procedures

---

■ **PATIENT GOAL 1:** Will maintain skin integrity

NURSING INTERVENTIONS/*RATIONALES*

(See Guidelines on neonatal skin care, p. 225.)

EXPECTED OUTCOME

Skin remains clean and intact with no evidence of irritation or injury

---

NURSING DIAGNOSIS: Risk for injury from variable cerebral blood flow, systemic hypertension or hypotension, and decreased cellular nutrients (glucose and oxygen) related to immature central nervous system and physiologic stress response

---

■ **PATIENT GOAL 1:** Will receive care to prevent injury and maintain appropriate systemic and cerebral blood flow, as well as adequate cerebral glucose and oxygen; will not exhibit evidence of intraventricular hemorrhage (unless preexisting condition)

NURSING INTERVENTIONS/*RATIONALES*

Decrease environmental stimulation *because stress responses, especially increased blood pressure, increase risk of elevated ICP*

Establish a routine that provides for undisturbed sleep-rest periods *to eliminate or minimize times of stress*

Use minimal handling, and handle or disturb infant only when absolutely necessary

Keep extra diapers under buttocks to facilitate changing soiled diapers; raise infant's hips, not feet and legs

Organize (cluster) care during normal waking hours as much as possible *to minimize sleep disruption and frequent intermittent noise*

Close and open drapes and dim lights *to allow for day/night schedule*

---

*Dependent nursing action.

Unit 4

The High-Risk Newborn and Family—cont'd

Cover incubator with cloth and place "do not disturb" sign nearby *to decrease light and alert others to infant's rest period*

Refrain from loud talking or laughing

Limit number of visitors and staff near infant at one time

Explain meaning of unfamiliar sounds to family

Keep equipment noise to minimum

Turn alarms as low as safely possible

Attend to alarms and telephones immediately

Place bedside equipment, such as ventilator or IV pump, away from head of bed

Turn outflow valve from ventilator away from infant's ear

Perform treatments requiring equipment at one time

Turn off bedside equipment such as suction and oxygen when it is not in use

Avoid loud, abrupt noises, such as throwing items in trash can, dropping items, placing items on top of incubator, closing doors and drawers, heavy traffic

Turn off any radios or televisions

May place soft earmuffs on infant

Assess and manage pain using pharmacologic and nonpharmacologic methods, *since pain increases blood pressure*

Recognize signs of physical stress and overstimulation *to institute appropriate interventions promptly*

Avoid hypertonic medications and solutions *because they increase cerebral blood flow*

Elevate head of bed or mattress between 15 and 20 degrees *to decrease ICP*

Maintain adequate oxygenation *because hypoxia increases cerebral blood flow and ICP* (See interventions under Nursing Diagnosis: Ineffective breathing pattern, p. 353.)

Avoid any sudden turning of head to side, *which restricts carotid artery blood flow and adequate oxygenation to brain*

EXPECTED OUTCOME

Infant exhibits no evidence of increased ICP or IVH

NURSING DIAGNOSIS: Pain related to procedures, diagnosis, treatment

■ **PATIENT GOAL 1:** Will experience either no pain or a reduction of pain

NURSING INTERVENTIONS/*RATIONALES*

Recognize that infants, regardless of gestational age, feel pain

Differentiate between clinical manifestations of pain and stress/fatigue

*Administer analgesics as prescribed, or advocate for more effective pain control

Use nonpharmacologic pain measures appropriate to infant's age and condition: repositioning, swaddling, containment, cuddling, rocking, music, reducing environmental stimulation, tactile comfort measures (stroking, patting), and nonnutritive sucking (pacifier)

Assess effectiveness of nonpharmacologic pain measures *because some measures (e.g., stroking) may increase premature infant's distress*

Encourage parents to provide comfort measures when possible

Convey an attitude of sensitivity and compassion for infant's discomfort

Discuss with family their concerns about infant's pain

Encourage family to speak with health practitioner about their concerns

EXPECTED OUTCOME

Infant exhibits no or minimal signs of pain

NURSING DIAGNOSIS: Altered growth and development related to preterm birth, unnatural NICU environment, separation from parents

■ **PATIENT GOAL 1:** Will attain normal growth and development potential

NURSING INTERVENTIONS/*RATIONALES*

Provide optimum nutrition *to ensure steady weight gain and brain growth*

Provide regular periods of undisturbed rest *to decrease unnecessary O_2 use and caloric expenditure*

Provide age-appropriate developmental intervention, including positioning

Recognize signs of overstimulation (e.g., flaccidity, yawning, staring, active averting, irritability, crying) *so that infant is allowed to rest*

Promote parent-infant interaction *since it is essential for normal growth and development*

Promote self-regulating behaviors (e.g., midline, flexed extremities; hands to mouth; and "nesting")

EXPECTED OUTCOMES

Infant exhibits a steady weight gain once past the acute phase of illness

Infant is exposed only to appropriate stimuli

Infant demonstrates quiet alert state interspersed with uninterrupted sleep periods of 50 to 60 minutes

---

NURSING DIAGNOSIS: Altered family processes related to situational/maturational crisis, knowledge deficit (birth of a preterm and/or ill infant), interruption of parental attachment process

■ **PATIENT (FAMILY) GOAL 1:** Will be informed of infant's progress

NURSING INTERVENTIONS/*RATIONALES*

Prioritize information *to help parents understand most important aspects of care, signs of improvement, or deterioration in infant's condition*

Encourage parents to ask questions about child's status

Answer questions; facilitate expression of concern regarding care and prognosis

Be honest; respond to questions with correct answers *to establish trust*

Encourage mother and father to visit and/or call unit often *so they stay informed of infant's progress*

Emphasize positive aspects of infant's status *to encourage sense of hope*

---

*Dependent nursing action.

Continued

The High-Risk Newborn and Family—cont'd

EXPECTED OUTCOME

Parents express feelings and concerns regarding infant and prognosis, and demonstrate understanding and involvement in care

■ **PATIENT (PARENT) GOAL 2:** Will exhibit positive attachment behaviors

NURSING INTERVENTIONS/*RATIONALES*

Encourage parents to visit as soon as possible *so that attachment process is initiated*

Encourage parents to:

Visit infant frequently

Touch, hold, and caress infant as appropriate for infant's physical condition

Become actively involved in infant's care

Bring clothing to dress infant as soon as condition permits

Reinforce parents' endeavors *to increase their self-confidence*

Be alert to signs of tension and stress in parents

Enable parents to spend time alone with infant

Help parents interpret infant's responses; comment regarding any positive response and signs of overstimulation or fatigue

Help parents by demonstrating infant care techniques and offer support

Identify resources (e.g., transportation, baby-sitting) *to enable parents to visit*

EXPECTED OUTCOMES

Parents visit infant soon after birth and at frequent intervals

Parents relate positively with infant (e.g., call infant by name, look at and touch infant)

Parents provide care for infant and demonstrate an attitude of comfort in relationships with infant

Parents identify signs of stress or fatigue in infant

■ **PATIENT (SIBLING) GOAL 3:** Will exhibit positive attachment behaviors

NURSING INTERVENTIONS/*RATIONALES*

Encourage siblings to visit infants when feasible

Explain environment, events, appearance of infant, and why infant cannot come home *to prepare them for visiting*

Provide photos of infant or other items if siblings are unable to visit

Encourage siblings to make pictures for infant or to bring other small items, such as a letter or drawing, to place in incubator or crib

EXPECTED OUTCOMES

Siblings visit infant in NICU or nursery

Siblings exhibit an understanding of explanations (specify)

Siblings receive infant-related items (specify)

■ **PATIENT (FAMILY) GOAL 4:** Will be prepared for home care

NURSING INTERVENTIONS/*RATIONALES*

Assess readiness of family (especially mother or other primary caregiver) to care for infant in home setting *to facilitate parents' transition to home with infant*

Teach necessary infant care techniques and observations

Encourage parent(s), when possible, to spend one or two nights in a hospital predischarge room with infant *to foster confidence in caring for infant at home*

Reinforce follow-up medical care

Refer to appropriate agencies or services *so that needed assistance is provided*

Encourage and facilitate involvement with parent support group or refer to appropriate support group(s) *for ongoing support*

Offer family opportunity to learn infant cardiopulmonary resuscitation and how to respond to choking incidents

EXPECTED OUTCOMES

Family demonstrates ability to provide care for infant

Family members state how and when to contact available services

Family members recognize importance of follow-up medical care

---

NURSING DIAGNOSIS: Anticipatory grieving related to unexpected birth of high-risk infant, grave prognosis, and/or death of infant

---

■ **PATIENT (FAMILY) GOAL 1:** Will acknowledge possibility of child's death and demonstrate healthy grieving behaviors

NURSING INTERVENTIONS/*RATIONALES*

Provide family with the opportunity to hold their infant before death and, if possible, to be present at the time of death

Support family's decision for terminating life support

Arrange for or perform appropriate baptism rite for infant

Provide family with the opportunity to see, touch, hold, bathe, caress, examine, and talk to their infant privately before and after death

Keep infant's body available for a few hours *to give family members who are hesitant an opportunity to see deceased infant if they change their minds;* rewarm as necessary

Provide photographs taken before and after infant's death for family to refer to at a later time *to make infant "real"*

Take photograph of infant being held or touched by an adult; avoid morgue-type photographs, *because they depersonalize child*

Dress infant in an appropriate dress or suit *to personalize child*

Provide other tangible remembrances of child's death (e.g., name tags, identification band, lock of hair, footprints, blanket)

Encourage family to name infant if they have not done so

Identify resources to assist with funeral arrangements *to facilitate parental grieving*

EXPECTED OUTCOME

Family discusses the reality of the death and conveys an attitude of realization

The High-Risk Newborn and Family—cont'd

■ **PATIENT (FAMILY) GOAL 2:** Will receive adequate emotional and physical support

NURSING INTERVENTIONS/*RATIONALES*

Be available to family *to provide support*

Provide appropriate religious support (e.g., clergy)

Discuss infant's illness and death with family

Talk with family openly and honestly about funeral arrangements

    Have information available regarding inexpensive services in the community

    Inform family of all options available *so that they can make informed decisions*

Provide opportunity for family to call the unit if they have any questions regarding infant's illness and death

May contact family after the death *to assess coping and status of grieving process*

Refer family to appropriate support group(s) *for ongoing support*

EXPECTED OUTCOMES

Family grieves for infant's death appropriately

Family demonstrates appropriate grieving behaviors (influenced by cultural, religious, and social factors) over infant's death

Unit 4

NURSING CARE PLAN

The Newborn with Hyperbilirubinemia

Hyperbilirubinemia is an excessive accumulation of bilirubin in the blood (Table 4-13).

ASSESSMENT

Obtain a maternal/fetal history:
Perform a newborn assessment. (See p. 14.)
Observe for manifestations of hyperbilirubinemia:
    Jaundice—Yellowish discoloration of skin:
        Bright yellow or orange—Unconjugated (indirect)
        Greenish, muddy yellow—Conjugated (direct)

Intensity of jaundice:
    Unrelated to degree of bilirubinemia
    Determined by serum bilirubin measurements
Assist with diagnostic procedures and tests (e.g., serum bilirubin levels, Coombs test [infants of Rh-negative mothers]).
Observe for evidence of dehydration (See Table 4-5, p. 310.) and hyperthermia.

TABLE 4-13   Comparison of Major Types of Unconjugated Hyperbilirubinemia*

	Physiologic Jaundice	Breast-Feeding–Associated Jaundice (Early Onset)	Breast Milk Jaundice (Late Onset)	Hemolytic Disease
Cause	Immature hepatic function plus increased bilirubin load from RBC hemolysis	Decreased milk intake related to fewer calories consumed by infant before mother's milk is well-established; enterohepatic shunting	Possible factors in breast milk that prevent bilirubin conjugation Less frequent stooling	Blood antigen incompatibility causes hemolysis of large numbers of RBCs Liver unable to conjugate and excrete excess bilirubin from hemolysis
Onset	After 24 hours (preterm infants, prolonged)	Second-fourth day	Fifth-seventh day	During first 24 hours (levels increase faster than 5 mg/dl/day)
Peak	72-90 hours	Third-fifth day	Tenth-fifteenth day	Variable
Duration	Declines on fifth-seventh day		May remain jaundiced for 3-12 weeks	
Therapy	Phototherapy if bilirubin levels increase significantly (rise in bilirubin greater than 5 mg/dl/day)†	Frequent (10-12 times/day) breast-feeding Phototherapy for bilirubin 17-22 mg/dl in healthy term infants†	Increase frequency of breast-feeding; use no supplementation such as glucose water; cessation of breast-feeding no longer recommended Temporary discontinuation of breast-feeding for up to 24 hours; if bilirubin levels decrease, breast-feeding can resume May include home phototherapy without discontinuing breast-feeding	*Postnatal*—Phototherapy; if severe, exchange transfusion *Prenatal*—Transfusion (fetus) Prevent sensitization (Rh incompatibility) of Rh-negative mother with RhoGAM

*Table depicts patterns of jaundice in term infants; patterns in preterm infants will vary according to factors such as gestational age, birth weight, and illness.
†Note that there is considerable controversy regarding the timing of initiation of phototherapy in healthy term infants with jaundice. (Maisels MJ: Jaundice. In Avery GB, Fletcher MA, MacDonald MG, editors: *Neonatology: pathophysiology and management of the newborn*, ed 4, Philadelphia, 1994, JB Lippincott.)

Unit 4

The Newborn with Hyperbilirubinemia—cont'd

NURSING DIAGNOSIS: Risk for injury from breakdown products of red blood cells in greater numbers than normal and functional immaturity of liver

■ **PATIENT GOAL 1:** Will receive appropriate therapy if needed to accelerate bilirubin excretion

NURSING INTERVENTIONS/RATIONALES

Initiate early feedings *to enhance excretion of bilirubin in the stool*

Assess skin for evidence of jaundice, *which indicates rising bilirubin levels*

Check bilirubin levels with transcutaneous bilirubinometry *to determine rising levels*

  Refer early discharged newborns for home visit *to check bilirubin levels*

Note time of initial jaundice *to distinguish physiologic jaundice (appears after 24 hours) from jaundice due to hemolytic disease or other causes (appears before 24 hours)*

Discuss signs of jaundice with the mother when infant is being discharged early *since clinical symptoms may not appear until infant is home*

Assess infant's overall status, especially factors that increase the risk of brain damage from hyperbilirubinemia (e.g., hypoxia, hypothermia, hypoglycemia, and metabolic acidosis)

Initiate phototherapy as prescribed *to decrease bilirubin levels*

EXPECTED OUTCOMES

Newborn begins feeding soon after birth
Newborn is exposed to prescribed light source

■ **PATIENT GOAL 2:** Will experience no complications from phototherapy

NURSING INTERVENTIONS/RATIONALES

Shield infant's eyes
  Make certain that lids are closed before applying shield *to prevent corneal irritation*
  Check eyes each shift for drainage or irritation
Place infant nude under light *for maximum skin exposure*
Change position frequently, especially during the first several hours of treatment, *to increase body surface exposure*
Monitor body temperature *to detect hypothermia or hyperthermia*
  Check axillary temperature
Chart duration of therapy, type of lights, distance of lights from infant, use of open or closed bassinet, and shielding of infant's eyes *to document correct use of phototherapy*
With increased stooling, cleanse skin frequently *to prevent perianal irritation*
Avoid use of oily applications on skin *to prevent tanning and burning*
Ensure adequate fluid intake *to prevent dehydration*

EXPECTED OUTCOME

Infant displays no evidence of eye irritation, dehydration, temperature instability, or skin breakdown

■ **PATIENT GOAL 3:** Will experience no complications from exchange transfusion (if therapy required)

NURSING INTERVENTIONS/RATIONALES

Give infant nothing by mouth before procedure (usually for 2 to 4 hours) *to prevent aspiration*

Check donor blood for correct blood group and Rh type *to prevent transfusion reaction*

Assist practitioner during procedure; ensure asepsis *to prevent infection*

Keep accurate records of amounts of blood infused and withdrawn *to maintain proper blood volume*

Maintain optimum body temperature of infant during procedure *to prevent hypothermia and cold stress or hyperthermia*

Observe for signs of exchange transfusion reaction (tachycardia or bradycardia, respiratory distress, dramatic change in blood pressure, temperature instability, and rash) *to initiate therapy promptly*

Have resuscitation equipment (e.g., supplemental oxygen, airway, manual resuscitation bag, endotracheal tube, and laryngoscope) at bedside *to be prepared for an emergency*

Check umbilical site for bleeding or infection

Monitor vital signs during and following transfusion *to detect complications such as cardiac dysrhythmias*

EXPECTED OUTCOMES

Infant exhibits no signs of adverse effects from exchange transfusion

Vital signs remain within normal limits (See inside back cover for normal variations.)

There is no evidence of infection or bleeding at infusion site

NURSING DIAGNOSIS: Altered family processes related to infant with potentially adverse physiologic response

■ **PATIENT (FAMILY) GOAL 1:** Will receive emotional support

NURSING INTERVENTIONS/RATIONALES

Discontinue phototherapy during family visits; remove infant's eye shields *to promote family interaction*

Emphasize benign nature of physiologic jaundice *to prevent undue parental concern and potential overprotection of child*

Assure family that skin will regain normal pigmentation

Advise breast-feeding mothers of possibility of prolonged jaundice

Emphasize benign nature of jaundice and benefits of human milk *to prevent early termination of breast-feeding*

EXPECTED OUTCOME

Family demonstrates an understanding of therapy and prognosis

■ **PATIENT (FAMILY) GOAL 2:** Will be prepared for home phototherapy (if prescribed)

Unit 4

Continued

The Newborn with Hyperbilirubinemia—cont'd

NURSING INTERVENTIONS/*RATIONALES*

Assess family's understanding of jaundice and proposed therapy *to ensure optimum results and safety*

Instruct family regarding:

Placement and care of lamp (See previous Patient Goal 2.)

Placement and care of fiberoptic biliblanket or bilibed (may be used alone or in conjunction with conventional phototherapy [above the baby]) *to maximize exposure and decrease bilirubin levels more rapidly*

Select correct size of biliblanket (preterm or term)

Expose as much skin as possible to fiberoptic light source

Cover biliblanket with an opaque cover when infant is being held

*Proper eye care:

Apply eye patches

Close lids before applying patches

Be certain patches fit snugly with no possibility of light leaks

Remove patches when light is discontinued (e.g., during feeding, bathing, and other caregiving activities) and at least once every 4 to 6 hours

*Proper positioning while under lamp:

Rotate to expose all areas of skin

Keep infant nude or dressed in mini-diaper

Providing increased fluid intake

Measuring axillary temperature

Keeping log of time spent under light, infant's color, feeding patterns, amount of feedings, diaper changes

Observing for signs of lethargy, change in sleeping pattern, any difficulty arousing infant, changes in stooling or voiding

Keeping diaper area clean and dry

Importance of bilirubin tests as prescribed

EXPECTED OUTCOME

Family demonstrates ability to provide home phototherapy for infant (specify learning and methods of demonstration)

*Not required for fiberoptic light source.

NURSING CARE PLAN

The Infant with Respiratory Distress Syndrome

Respiratory distress in the newborn period may be caused by surfactant deficiency, incomplete absorption of lung fluid (transient tachypnea of the newborn), meconium aspiration, viral or bacterial pneumonia, sepsis, mechanical obstruction, or hypothermia. This section pertains only to the type of respiratory distress caused by surfactant deficiency, or respiratory distress syndrome (RDS). RDS is an acute, severe lung disease that primarily affects preterm infants; it may be seen in 3% to 5% of term infants and in infants born of diabetic mothers.

ASSESSMENT

Perform a newborn physical and a clinical assessment of gestational age. (See p. 22.)

Perform a systematic assessment, with special emphasis on respiratory assessment. (See p. 378.)

Observe for manifestations of RDS:
Tachypnea (initially, then apnea)
Substernal and/or intercostal retractions
Inspiratory crackles
Expiratory grunt
Nasal flaring
Cyanosis
Labored breathing

As the disease progresses, observe for:
Flaccidity and inertness
Unresponsiveness
Frequent apneic episodes
Diminished breath sounds
Impaired thermoregulation
Respiratory failure

Severe disease associated with the following:
Shocklike state
Decreased cardiac output
Low systemic blood pressure

Assist with diagnostic procedures and tests (e.g., radiography, blood gas analysis).

NURSING DIAGNOSIS: Ineffective breathing pattern related to surfactant deficiency and alveolar instability

■ **PATIENT GOAL 1:** Will exhibit adequate oxygenation

NURSING INTERVENTIONS/*RATIONALES*

(See Nursing Diagnosis: Ineffective breathing related to pulmonary and neuromuscular immaturity, p. 353.)

Suction endotracheal tube (ET) as necessary before surfactant administration *to be certain airway is clear*

*Administer surfactant according to manufacturer's recommendations *to decrease alveolar surface tension*

Avoid suctioning for at least 2 hours after surfactant administration *to promote absorption into alveoli*

Observe for increased chest excursion after surfactant administration

Closely monitor blood gas measurements and pulse oximeter readings

Decrease ventilator settings, especially peak inspiratory pressure and oxygen, *to prevent hyperoxemia and overdistention of lungs*

Monitor patency of ET tube *to prevent blockage with mucus*

EXPECTED OUTCOME

(See Nursing Diagnosis: Ineffective breathing related to pulmonary and neuromuscular immaturity, p. 353.)

NURSING DIAGNOSIS: Risk for injury from increased intracranial pressure (ICP) related to immature central nervous system and physiologic stress response

■ **PATIENT GOAL 1:** Will exhibit normal ICP (unless increased ICP is related to infant's illness) and no evidence of intraventricular hemorrhage (IVH) (unless there is a preexisting condition)

NURSING INTERVENTIONS/*RATIONALES*

(See Nursing Interventions related to the prevention of increased ICP in Nursing Care Plan: The High-Risk Newborn and Family, p. 350.)

Maintain adequate oxygenation *because hypoxia increases cerebral blood flow and ICP* (See Nursing Interventions under Nursing Diagnosis: Ineffective breathing pattern on this page.)

EXPECTED OUTCOME

Infant exhibits no evidence of increased ICP or IVH

NURSING DIAGNOSIS: Altered family processes related to situational/maturational crisis, knowledge deficit (birth of a preterm and/or ill infant), interruption of parental attachment process

■ **PATIENT (FAMILY) GOAL 1:** Will be informed of infant's progress

NURSING INTERVENTIONS/*RATIONALES*

(See Nursing Diagnosis: Altered family processes, p. 355.)

Explain procedure of surfactant administration to parents *to increase their understanding and involvement in infant's care*

EXPECTED OUTCOMES

(See Nursing Diagnosis: Altered family processes, p. 355.)

(See also Nursing Care Plan: The High-Risk Newborn and Family, p. 350.)

*Dependent nursing action.

Unit 4

Neonatal Complications

TABLE 4-14	Metabolic Abnormalities in the Newborn	
	Hypoglycemia	**Hypocalcemia**
Definition	Blood glucose concentration significantly lower than that in the majority of infants of the same age and weight	Abnormally low levels of calcium in circulating blood
Types	Early transitional neonatal: large or normal-size infants who appear to suffer from hyper-insulinism Classic transient neonatal: infants who suffered intrauterine malnutrition that depleted glycogen and fat stores Secondary: a response to perinatal stresses that increase infant's metabolic needs relative to glycogen stores Recurrent, severe: caused by an enzymatic or metabolic-endocrine defect	Early onset: appears in first 24-48 hours, appears in preterm infants who experienced perinatal hypoxia; infants of diabetic mothers Late onset: cow's milk–induced hypocalcemia (neonatal tetany): apparent after first 7 days (high phosphorus/calcium ratio of cow's milk depresses parathyroid activity; reducing serum calcium levels); may be seen in infants with intestinal malabsorption, hypomagnesemia, or hypoparathyroidism
Clinical Manifestations	Vague, often indistinguishable from other conditions Cerebral signs: jitteriness, tremors, twitching, weak or high-pitched cry, lethargy, limpness, apathy, convulsions, and coma Other: cyanosis, apnea, irregular respirations, sweating, eye rolling, tachypnea, poor feeder Signs often transient but recurrent	Early onset: jitteriness, apnea, cyanotic episodes, high-pitched cry, abdominal distention Late onset: twitching, tremors, seizures
Laboratory Diagnosis	Plasma glucose concentrations less than 50 mg/dl (2.8 mMol/L)	Serum calcium less than 7 mg/dl (1.75 mMol/L) Ionized calcium less than 1.1 mMol/L
Treatment	Intravenous glucose administration Preventive: early feeding in normoglycemic infants	Early onset: increased milk feedings, administration of calcium supplements PO or IV Late onset: administration of calcium gluconate IV (slowly); vitamin D; oral calcium supplement
Nursing	(See Nursing Care Plan: The High-Risk Newborn and Family, p. 350.) Identify infants with hypoglycemia Reduce environmental factors that predispose infant to hypoglycemia (e.g., cold stress, perinatal asphyxia, respiratory distress) Use proper feeding techniques Administer intravenous glucose as prescribed	(See Nursing Care Plan: The High-Risk Newborn and Family, p. 350.) Identify infants with hypocalcemia Administer calcium as prescribed Observe for signs of acute hypercalcemia (e.g., vomiting, bradycardia) Manipulate environment to reduce stimuli that might precipitate a seizure or tremors (e.g., picking up infant suddenly, sudden jarring of crib)

Neonatal Complications—cont'd

TABLE 4-15	Respiratory Complications in the Newborn		
Description	**Specific Manifestations**	**Treatment**	**Nursing Considerations**
Respiratory Distress Syndrome (RDS) (See p. 361.)			
Meconium Aspiration Syndrome (MAS)			
Aspiration of amniotic fluid containing meconium into fetal or newborn trachea in utero or at first breath	Meconium stained at birth Tachypnea Hypoxia Depressed state Hypoventilation	Vigorous suction of hypopharynx at birth Intubation and suction of trachea Treat for respiratory distress Prevent hypoxia and acidosis	(See Nursing Care Plan: The Infant with Respiratory Distress Syndrome, p. 361.)
Apnea of Prematurity			
Lapse of spontaneous breathing for 20 seconds or longer, that may or may not be followed by bradycardia, color change, and oxygen desaturation	Persistent apneic spells	Observe for apnea Check for thermal stability Administer theophylline or caffeine Prevent hypoglycemia	Provide continuous electronic monitoring (respiratory and heart rate) Observe for presence and type of respirations Observe color Apply gentle tactile stimulation Suction nose and oropharynx if still apneic Apply artificial ventilation with bag-valve-mask and with sufficient pressure to see the chest rise like an easy shallow breath Assess for and manage any precipitating factors (e.g., temperature, reflux of stomach contents, abdominal distention, ambient oxygen) Observe for signs of theophylline toxicity: tachycardia (rate greater than 180 to 190 beats/min); and vomiting (later)
Pneumothorax			
Presence of extraneous air in pleural space as a result of alveolar rupture	Tachypnea or apnea Grunting, flaring nares Retractions Absent or diminished breath sounds Shift in point of maximum intensity of heart sounds Bradycardia/cyanosis Oxygen desaturation	Evacuate trapped air from pleural space through needle aspiration and/or chest tubes and closed drainage	Maintain close vigilance of infants with respiratory distress or those on assisted ventilation Provide appropriate care of chest drainage apparatus Keep emergency needle aspiration setup at bedside
Bronchopulmonary Dysplasia (BPD)			
Pathologic process related to alveolar damage from lung disease (respiratory distress syndrome), prolonged exposure to high oxygen concentrations, and use of positive-pressure ventilation	Retractions Elevated Pco_2 Barrel chest Inability to wean from mechanical ventilation Susceptibility to upper respiratory tract infections Frequent hospitalization for respiratory problems	Regulate fluids Support respiratory efforts Prevent and/or control respiratory infections Supplemental oxygen in hospital/home Medications: Diuretics Bronchodilators Corticosteroids (sometimes)	Provide opportunities for additional rest, fluids, and calories Provide small, frequent feedings to avoid overextending stomach, which interferes with respiration Observe for signs of overhydration or underhydration Assist with home oxygen therapy

Unit 4

Neonatal Complications—cont'd

TABLE 4-16   Cardiovascular Complications in the Newborn

Description	Clinical Manifestations	Therapeutic Management	Nursing Considerations
Patent Ductus Arteriosus (PDA)			
Failure of the fetal ductus arteriosis (artery connecting the aorta and pulmonary artery) to close within the first weeks of life	Decreased Po_2 Increased Pco_2 Apnea Bounding peripheral pulses Typical systolic or continuous murmur Respiratory insufficiency	Regulate fluids Provide respiratory support Administer indomethacin Perform ductal ligation Diuretics	(See Nursing Care Plan: The High-Risk Newborn and Family, p. 350.) Collect specimens as needed Assess renal function Monitor weight Assess respiratory status
Persistent Pulmomary Hypertension of the Newborn (PPHN)			
Severe pulmonary hypertension and large right-to-left shunt through foramen ovale and ductus arteriosus	Hypoxia Marked cyanosis Tachypnea with grunting and retractions Decreased peripheral pulses Acidosis	Regulate fluids Give supplemental oxygen Give assisted ventilation Administer vasodilators (sometimes) Monitor pH Prevent acidosis Inhaled nitric oxide ECMO	(See Nursing Care Plan: The High-Risk Newborn and Family, p. 350; and Nursing Care Plan: Respiratory Distress Syndrome, p. 361.) Reduce stress to infant, especially noxious stimuli that cause crying and struggling Decrease physical manipulation and disturbance
Anemia of Prematurity			
Loss of blood from hemorrhage in organs (during delivery), blood diseases Contributing: delayed erythropoiesis, poor iron stores (fetal), and repetitive blood specimen collection	Pallor Tachypnea Apnea Tachycardia Diminished activity Poor feeder	Administer iron-fortified formula and/or supplemental iron Transfuse with packed RBCs for severe anemia Administer recombinant human erythropoietin as prescribed Minimize blood withdrawal	Monitor amount of blood drawn for tests Administer iron as prescribed
Polycythemia/Hyperviscosity Syndrome			
Venous hematocrit 65% or greater owing to twin-to-twin or mother-to-fetus transfusion or increased RBC production	High incidence of: Cardiovascular symptoms (cyanosis, apnea) Seizures Hyperbilirubinemia Gastrointestinal abnormalities Hypoglycemia	Correct metabolic imbalances Implement partial exchange transfusion Provide appropriate therapy for associated problems	(See Nursing Care Plan: The High-Risk Newborn and Family, p. 350; and Nursing Care Plan: The Newborn With Hyperbilirubinemia, p. 358.)
Hemorrhagic Disease of the Newborn			
Bleeding disorder resulting from transient deficiency of vitamin K–dependent blood factors	Oozing blood from umbilicus or circumcision Bloody or black stools Hematuria Ecchymoses Epistaxis	Administer prophylactic vitamin K	Administer vitamin K (intramuscular)
Retinopathy of Prematurity (ROP)			
Replacement of retina by fibrous tissue and blood vessels	Progressive vascular growth of retina Eventual blindness	Arrest proliferation process—cryotherapy or laser surgery Administer prophylactic vitamin E (sometimes) Use supplemental oxygen judiciously and monitor carefully Early screening in infants <1500 grams at birth and/or gestational age <28 weeks	(See Nursing Care Plan: The High-Risk Newborn and Family, p. 350.) Monitor oxygen concentration

Neonatal Complications—cont'd

TABLE 4-17   Cerebral Complications in the Newborn

Description	Clinical Manifestations	Therapeutic Management	Nursing Considerations
Germinal Matrix/Intraventricular Hemorrhage (GM/IVH)			

Hemorrhage into and around ventricles caused by ruptured vessels as a result of an event that increases cerebral blood flow to area	Apnea
	Bradycardia
	Cyanosis
	Hypotonia
	Tense, bulging anterior fontanel (term)
	Widely separated sutures
	Drop in hematocrit
	Neurologic signs:
	   Twitching
	   Stupor
	   Apnea
	   Seizures
	Evident on ultrasonography, magnetic resonance imaging, and/or tomography
		Prevention: minimize cerebral blood flow fluctuations in first 24-72 hours of life
		Monitor closely for pneumothorax, shock, acidosis, hypo- or hyperglycemia
		Avoid rapid volume expansion
		Ventricular taps (drainage)
		Monitor for and correct metabolic acidosis, respiratory compromise
		Supportive care:
		   Provide ventilatory support
		   Maintain oxygenation
		   Regulate fluid and electrolytes, acid-base balance
		   Suppress or prevent seizures
			(See Nursing Care Plan: The High-Risk Newborn and Family, p. 350.)
			Prevent increased cerebral blood pressure
			Minimal handling protocol
			Elevate head
			Minimize crying
			Avoid pressure-producing procedures (e.g., pain, overstimulation, unnecessary suctioning)
			Support family

Hypoxic-Ischemic Encephalopathy			
Resultant cellular damage (neurologic) from hypoxic-ischemic injury	Variable from mild to severe Seizures Abnormal muscle tone (usually hypotonia) Disturbance of sucking and swallowing Apneic episodes Stupor or coma	Provide supportive care Provide adequate ventilation Maintain cerebral perfusion Prevent hypoxia Treat seizures	(See Nursing Care Plan: The High-Risk Newborn and Family, p. 350.) Observe for signs that indicate cerebral hypoxia Monitor ventilatory and intravenous therapy and nutrition Observe for and manage seizures Support family Provide guidelines for family management of permanent neurologic damage
Intracranial Hemorrhage			
Hemorrhage caused by ruptured vessels in the following areas resulting from trauma: Subdural Subarachnoid	Same as for GM/IVH Manifestations depend on size and location of bleeding	Same as for GM/IVH	Same as for GM/IVH

Continued

Unit 4

Neonatal Complications—cont'd

TABLE 4-17   Cerebral Complications in the Newborn—cont'd

Description	Clinical Manifestations	Therapeutic Management	Nursing Considerations

Neonatal Seizures	Subtle seizures:
	  Signs may appear alone or in combination
	  Clonic horizontal eye deviation
	  Repetitive blinking or fluttering of eyelids, staring
	  Twitching
	  Drooling
	  Sucking or other oral-buccal-lingual movements
	  Arm movements resembling rowing or swimming
	  Leg movements described as pedaling or bicycling
	  Apnea (common)
	
	Tonic seizures:
	  Usually manifest as extensions of all four limbs, similar to decerebrate rigidity
	  Upper limbs are maintained in stiffly flexed position resembling decorticate rigidity
	  Appear more frequently in preterm infants
	  Commonly associated with intraventricular hemorrhage
	Clonic seizures:
	  Rhythmic jerking movements, about 1 to 3 per second
	  May migrate randomly from one part of the body to another
	  Simultaneous involvement of separate areas
	  Seizure movements may start at different times and at different rates
	Myoclonic seizures:
	  Single or multiple flexion jerks of limbs
	  Often indicate a metabolic etiology
		Correct metabolic derangements
		Supportive care:
		  Respiratory
		  Cardiovascular
		Suppress seizure activity with anticonvulsants
		Treat underlying cause
			Recognize that a seizure is occurring
			Observe and record seizure accurately (See p. 474.)
			Administer oxygen, anticonvulsants, and other therapies as prescribed
			Observe response to therapy
			Interpret infant's behavior to family
			Support family
			(See Nursing Care Plan: The High-Risk Newborn and Family, p. 350.)

Neonatal Jitteriness or Tremulousness

Involuntary trembling, quivering, or jitteriness	Repetitive shaking of an extremity or extremities
	Observed with crying; may occur with changes in sleeping state or may be elicited with stimulation
	Relatively common in newborn
	Mild jitteriness may be considered normal during first 4 days of life
	Can be distinguished from seizures by several characteristics:
	  Not accompanied by ocular movement as are seizures
	  Dominant movement in jitteriness is tremor
	  Seizure movement is clonic jerking that cannot be stopped by flexion of affected limb
	  Jitteriness is highly sensitive to stimulation; seizures are not
		No therapy required
		Evaluate if symptoms persist beyond the fourth day of life
			Distinguish between tremors and seizures
			Simple test to rule out pathology in neonatal tremors in full term, stable newborns is to stimulate sucking: Place pacifier or examiner's gloved finger in mouth of infant, who is lying supine with both hands free; test indicates tremor if activity stops instantly with sucking and returns after finger or pacifier is removed

Unit 4

Neonatal Complications—cont'd

TABLE 4-18   Infection in the Newborn

Description	Clinical Manifestations	Therapeutic Management	Nursing Considerations

Sepsis, Septicemia
Generalized bacterial infection in the bloodstream
	General Signs
	Infant generally "not doing well"
	Poor temperature control: hypothermia (common), hyperthermia (rare)
	Poor feeding, feeding intolerance
	
	Circulatory System
	Pallor, cyanosis, or mottling
	Cold, clammy skin
	Hypotension
	Edema
	Abnormal heartbeat: bradycardia, tachycardia
	
	Respiratory System
	Irregular respirations, apnea, or tachypnea
	Cyanosis
	Grunting
	Dyspnea
	Retractions
	Oxygen desaturation
	
	Central Nervous System
	Diminished activity: lethargy, hyporeflexia, coma
	Increased activity: irritability, tremors, seizures
	Full fontanel
	Increased or decreased tone
	Abnormal eye movements
	
	Gastrointestinal System
	Poor feeding
	Vomiting, increased stomach residual after feeding
	Diarrhea or decreased stool
	Occult blood in stool
	Abdominal distention
	Hepatomegaly
	
	Hematopoietic System
	Jaundice
	Pallor
	Purpura, petechiae, ecchymoses
	Splenomegaly
	Bleeding
		Aggressive administration of antibiotics
		Immunotherapy
		Transfusion with polymorphonuclear leukocytes, if indicated
		Supportive therapy:
		  Oxygen
		  Fluid, electrolyte, and acid-base management
		Blood transfusions, if indicated
		Electronic monitoring of vital signs
		Neutral thermal environment
			(See Nursing Care Plan: The High-Risk Newborn and Family, p. 350.)
			Administer antibiotics and other medications as prescribed
			Collect needed specimens for laboratory examination
			Anticipate potential problems such as dehydration or hypoxia
			Be alert for evidence of extensions of infection (e.g., meningitis) and superimposed infections (e.g., candidiasis)
			Prevent spread of infection to other infants (See Nursing Care Plan: The Child at Risk for Infection, p. 341)
			Include blood pressure with routine vital signs (to detect shock)
			Observe for signs of septic shock (See p. 442.)

Unit 4

Continued

Neonatal Complications—cont'd

| TABLE 4-18 | Infection in the Newborn—cont'd | | |

Description	Clinical Manifestations	Therapeutic Management	Nursing Considerations
Necrotizing Enterocolitis (NEC)			
Acute inflammation of the bowel characterized by ischemic necrosis of the gastrointestinal tract mucosa that may lead to perforation and peritonitis	***Nonspecific Clinical Signs*** Lethargy Poor feeding Hypotension Vomiting Apnea Decreased urine output Unstable temperature Jaundice ***Specific Signs*** Distended (often shiny) abdomen Blood in the stools or gastric contents Gastric retention Localized abdominal wall erythema or induration Bilious vomitus	Discontinuation of all oral feedings Intravenous fluids and electrolytes Abdominal decompression via nasogastric suction Intravenous antibiotics Correction of fluid and electrolyte imbalance Surgical intervention when indicated Monitor for and correct metabolic acidosis and hypoglycemia Provide minimal enteral feedings as prescribed	(See Nursing Care Plan: The High-Risk Newborn and Family, p. 350.) Administer antibiotics as prescribed Monitor intravenous fluids and feedings Monitor vital signs and blood pressure (changes may indicate impending sepsis or shock) Check abdomen for distention frequently; measure girth Listen for presence of bowel sounds Assist with diagnostic procedures Prevent pressure on abdomen (loose or no diapering, position on side or back) Advance to oral feedings as prescribed Prevent spread of infection
Bullous Impetigo (Impetigo Neonatorum)			
Superficial skin infection most often caused by *Staphylococcus aureus*	Eruption of bullous vesicular lesions on previously untraumatized skin	Warm saline compresses followed by gentle cleansing and application of topical antibiotic several times a day	Prevent spread of infection Assess persons who have come in contact with infant (to determine possible source of infection) Observe other infants in nursery (to detect signs of infection) (See Nursing Care Plan: The Normal Newborn and Family, p. 345.)

Neonatal Complications—cont'd

TABLE 4-19   Neonatal Complications Associated with Maternal Conditions

Description	Clinical Manifestations	Therapeutic Management	Nursing Considerations
Infant of the Diabetic Mother (IDM)			
Characterized by hypoglycemia associated with increased insulin activity	Large for gestational age Very plump and full-faced Plethora Respiratory distress Listlessness and lethargy Hypoglycemia that appears shortly after birth	Careful observation of mother and fetus during gestation Frequent blood glucose determination Early feeding of breast milk or formula, if tolerated IV glucose infusion for critically ill infants	(See Nursing Care Plan: The Normal Newborn and Family, p. 345.) Provide feedings as indicated Observe for central nervous system signs (e.g., hyperirritability, tremors, and jitteriness) Observe for signs of hypoglycemia (See p. 485.), hyperbilirubinemia (See p. 358.), respiratory distress (See p. 361.), and polycythemia (See p. 364.)
Drug-Exposed Infant			
Passive addiction to a drug that mother has habitually taken during pregnancy	Variable, but include: Irritability Tremors Shrill cry Hypertonicity of muscles Frantic sucking of hands Poor feeding Hyperactivity Poor regulation of sleep-wake states Sweating Tachypnea (>60/min) Frequent sneezing Frequent yawning Vomiting Temperature instability Diarrhea Convulsions	Parenteral and/or oral administration of phenobarbital, diazepam, methadone, or chlorpromazine Supplemental parenteral fluids as indicated Decrease environmental stimuli	(See Nursing Care Plan: The Normal Newborn and Family, p. 345.) Provide adequate nutrition and hydration Reduce external stimuli that might trigger hyperactivity and irritability Reduce infant's ability to self-stimulate by wrapping snugly, holding infant tightly, and arranging nursing activities to reduce amount of disturbance Measure weight frequently, monitor intake and output, and administer supplemental parenteral fluids (to prevent malnutrition, dehydration, and electrolyte imbalance) Protect hyperactive infants from skin abrasions Monitor activity level and its relationship to other activities Recognize infant's predisposition to disorders (e.g., acquired immunodeficiency syndrome [AIDS], hepatitis B)

Unit 4

Continued

Neonatal Complications—cont'd

TABLE 4-19 Neonatal Complications Associated with Maternal Conditions—cont'd

Description	Clinical Manifestations	Therapeutic Management	Nursing Considerations
Infant Exposed to Cocaine			
Altered physiology and behavioral changes due to central nervous system stimulation and peripheral sympathomimetic effects	Decreased birth weight, length, and occipitofrontal circumference Neurologic signs: 　Seizures 　Jitteriness 　Tremors 　Irritability 　Poor interaction with others 　Intolerance to comforting 　　(e.g., cuddling) 　Abnormal sleep patterns 　Muscular rigidity 　Lethargic 　Poor suck, feeding 　Unconsolable, excessive, or 　　weak cry Possible teratogenic effects Necrotizing enterocolitis	Treatment, based on individualized assessment, may range from comfort measures to stimulation	Use patience with feedings Position infant to avoid eye-to-eye contact; gradually assume face-to-face position as tolerated Provide comfort measures as indicated (e.g., swaddling, vertical rocking, using a pacifier, infant massage) Assist family in the attachment process (See Nursing Care Plan: The Normal Newborn and Family, p. 345.) Assist family in understanding poor interactive abilities (e.g., gaze aversion, arching back, lack of responsiveness to cuddling) Refer to early intervention programs

TABLE 4-20 Infections Acquired from Mother Before, During, or After Birth*

Fetal or Newborn Effects	Comments and Nursing Considerations†
Human Immunodeficiency Virus (HIV)	
No significant difference between infected and uninfected infants at birth in most cases Possible manifestations include generalized lymphadenopathy, splenomegaly, hepatomegaly, failure to thrive, progressive developmental delays, recurrent infections (see below), chronic diarrhea, oral candidiasis, hepatitis, cardiomyopathy, and parotitis (American Academy of Pediatrics, 1997) ***Pneumocystis carinii pneumonia (PCP)*** is the most common opportunistic infection and may occur as early as 4-6 weeks after birth; more commonly it is seen between 3 and 6 months after birth in congenitally or perinatally acquired HIV Other infections that may be seen in the neonatal period include candida esophagitis, disseminated cytomegalovirus, and chronic or disseminated herpes (HSV)	Transmitted transplacentally, at birth, in breast milk, or in contaminated blood products (rare) Average age at diagnosis is 18 months Mandatory HIV testing of mother/newborn not recommended, but testing is recommended and encouraged following parental education (American Academy of Pediatrics, 1997); 90% of children infected with HIV have acquired it from the mother Risk of infection for infant born to HIV-seropositive mother is 13% to 39% (American Academy of Pediatrics, 1997) Treatment: oral zidovudine 2 mg/kg in newborn of HIV-seropositive mother (whether treated or not) at 8-12 hours of age and thereafter up to 6 weeks If the mother's HIV status is unknown, and she is in a high-risk category, breast-feeding should be discouraged Cesarean delivery in HIV-seropositive mother is now recommended.

*This table is not an exhaustive representation of all perinatally transmitted infections. For further information regarding specific diseases or treatment not listed here, the reader is referred to American Academy of Pediatrics, Committee on Infectious Diseases: *1997 Red book report of the Committee on Infectious Diseases,* ed 24, Elk Grove Village, IL, 1997, The Academy.
†Isolation precautions depend on institutional policy. (See Infection Control, p. 341.)

Unit 4

Neonatal Complications—cont'd

TABLE 4-20   Infections Acquired from Mother Before, During, or After Birth*—cont'd

Fetal or Newborn Effects	Comments and Nursing Considerations†
Chickenpox (Varicella-Zoster Virus)	
First or early second trimester exposure—congenital varicella syndrome: limb dysplasia, microcephaly, cortical atrophy, chorioretinitis, cataracts, cutaneous scars, other anomalies, auditory nerve palsy, mental retardation Severe varicella may occur in newborn if mother develops varicella 5 days before or up to 2 days after delivery	Transmitted: first or early second trimester (congenital varicella syndrome); intrapartum (infection) Treatment: exposed infants—varicella-zoster immune globulin (VZIG) to infants born to mothers with onset of disease within 5 days before or 2 days after delivery (7 days before and 7 days after in United Kingdom); oral acyclovir (if infected) Isolation precautions 21 days after birth (if hospitalized) or 28 days if infant received VZIG; no isolation for varicella syndrome
Chlamydia Infection (*Chlamydia Trachomatis*)	
Conjunctivitis, pneumonia	Transmitted: last trimester or intrapartum; most common sexually transmitted disease in the United States Treatment: antibiotics (oral erythromycin or sulfonamide for 14 days) Silver nitrate, erythromycin, and tetracycline given for ophthalmia neonatorum does not protect against or prevent chlamydia
Group B Beta Hemolytic Streptococcus (GBS)	
May be asymptomatic at birth Early onset: first few days of life; mild to severe bacteremia (See Sepsis, p. 367.) and respiratory distress; high mortality rate when affected. Late onset: after 7 days—usually meningitis but may have septicemia as well; moderate incidence of neurologic damage from meningitis	Transmission: transplacental (ascending) and/or during birth GBS colonizes maternal reproductive, rectal and urinary tract, yet is asymptomatic Colonizes fetal/neonatal GI tract and spreads; severity of neonatal illness and colonization proportional to maternal colonization Implicated as a factor in early onset preterm labor Intrapartum screening protocols for GBS colonization in mother; treatment with antibiotics prior to delivery decreases fetal transmission. Risk factors for maternal screening include: preterm labor or rupture of membranes <35-37 weeks gestation, prolonged rupture of membranes >18 hours, maternal intrapartum fever, previous birth of newborn with GBS, chorioamnionitis Neonatal: monitor closely for respiratory distress, especially in first 24 hours of life, if feeding difficulties, or if apnea. If suspect GBS, obtain CBC with differential, blood cultures and/or diagnostic lab as ordered Parenteral antibiotics (penicillin) are effective against GBS Severe early onset GBS causes respiratory distress, septic shock, and persistent fetal circulation (See PPHN, p. 364.) often requiring inhaled nitric oxide or ECMO and pharmacologic support of blood pressure and cardiac function
Enterovirus (Coxsackie Virus Group A and B, Echovirus Enterovirus)	
Signs of septicemia, including poor feeding, vomiting, diarrhea, fever; cardiac enlargement, arrhythmias, congestive heart failure; lethargy, seizures, meningeal involvement	Transmitted by fecal-oral or respiratory route from mother/father to newborn in peripartum period

Unit 4

Continued

Neonatal Complications—cont'd

TABLE 4-20   Infections Acquired from Mother Before, During, or After Birth*—cont'd

Fetal or Newborn Effects	Comments and Nursing Considerations†
Cytomegalovirus (CMV) May be asymptomatic at birth; if acquired perinatally, no clinical illness usually seen Growth retardation (small for gestational age) Microcephaly, cerebral calcifications, chorioretinitis Jaundice, hepatosplenomegaly Petechial or purpuric rash Neurologic sequelae: seizure disorders, sensorimotor deafness, mental retardation, hearing loss	Transmitted: throughout pregnancy or during delivery; via CMV positive breast milk Affected individuals excrete virus in urine, saliva, and other body secretions Virus detected in urine or tissue by electron microscopy Pregnant women or immunocompromised person should avoid close contact with known cases Treatment: antiviral agent ganciclovir; however, current data for treatment of infants are inconclusive; CMV-IVIG may also be used Standard precautions; isolation not required; strict hand-washing
Parvovirus B19 (Erythema Infectiosum, Fifth Disease) Fetal hydrops and death from anemia and heart failure, early exposure Anemia from later exposure No teratogenic effects established Ordinarily, low risk of ill effect to fetus after first half of pregnancy	Transmitted: transplacentally First or early second trimester infection produces most serious effects Pregnant health care workers should not care for patients who might be highly contagious (e.g., aplastic crisis) Routine exclusion of pregnant women from workplace where disease is occurring is not recommended Intrauterine blood transfusion may be effective in some cases of fetal hydrops
Gonococcal Disease (*Neisseria Gonorrhoeae*) Ophthalmitis Neonatal gonococcal arthritis, septicemia, meningitis Scalp abscess (from infected fetal monitoring site)	Transmitted: last trimester or intrapartum Apply prophylactic medication to eyes at time of birth Obtain cultures as required Treatment: tetracycline or third-generation cephalosporin Concomitant infection with *Chlamydia trachomatis* is common
Hepatitis B Virus (HBV) May be asymptomatic Chronic hepatitis and death as a result of liver disease; 90% risk of chronic liver disease if infected in perinatal period	Transmitted: transplacentally, contaminated (HBsAg positive) maternal secretions during delivery Treatment: hepatitis B immune globulin and HB vaccine to all infants of HBsAG-positive mothers Breast-feeding considered safe if newborn has received HBIG and HB vaccine Prevention: universal immunization of all infants with HBV vaccine and routine screening of pregnant women

*This table is not an exhaustive representation of all perinatally transmitted infections. For further information regarding specific diseases or treatment not listed here, the reader is referred to American Academy of Pediatrics, Committee on Infectious Diseases: *1997 Red book report of the Committee on Infectious Diseases,* ed 24, Elk Grove Village, IL, 1997, The Academy.
†Isolation precautions depend on institutional policy. (See Infection Control, p. 341.)

Unit 4

Neonatal Complications—cont'd

TABLE 4-20 Infections Acquired from Mother Before, During, or After Birth*—cont'd	
Fetal or Newborn Effects	**Comments and Nursing Considerations†**
Herpes, Neonatal (Herpes Simplex Virus)	
Cutaneous lesions: vesicles at 6 to 10 days of age; may have no lesions	History of primary genital infection in mother/partner in 33% to 50% of cases
Disseminated disease resembles sepsis	Transmitted: intrapartum, either ascending and/or direct contact, especially primary infection
Ocular conjunctivitis, keratitis, chorioretinitis	
Associated with preterm births	May be transmitted from mother/father with nongenital lesions in postpartum or in nursery from infected infant
Initial symptoms may occur at birth or as late as 4-6 weeks of age	Cesarean section sometimes a preventive measure for mothers with active genital lesions if membranes ruptured less than 4-6 hours before delivery
Early nonspecific signs: fever, lethargy, poor feeding, irritability, vomiting	Vaginal delivery of infants of mothers with recurrent infection thought to be at lower risk
May include hyperbilirubinemia, seizures, flaccid or spastic paralysis, apneic episodes, respiratory distress, lethargy, or coma (CNS encephalopathy)	Suggest infants room-in with mother in private room until discharge as health permits
	Treatment: Acyclovir p.o. for 14-21 days; ophthalmic drug if eyes affected
Listeriosis (*Listeria*)	
Early onset: pneumonia, septicemia, granulomatosis infantisepticum (rare)	Transmitted: transplacentally or by aspiration of secretions at birth
Late onset (after first week): meningitis, septicemia	Treatment: parenteral ampicillin and gentamicin
Transplacental: stillbirth or preterm delivery	Standard precautions
	If infection detected antenatally, maternal antibiotic therapy may prevent fetal/perinatal illness
Lyme Disease (*Borrelia Burgdorferi*)	
Stillbirth	Transmitted: transplacentally
Congenital defects reported: congenital heart disease, syndactyly, cortical blindness	Immediate treatment of affected pregnant women with appropriate antibiotic
Prematurity	Advise pregnant women to avoid tick exposure in endemic areas
Rash	
Rubella, Congenital (Rubella Virus)	
Eye defects: cataracts (unilateral or bilateral), glaucoma, retinopathy	Transmitted: first trimester; early second trimester
CNS signs: microcephaly, seizures, severe mental retardation	Pregnant women should avoid contact with infected persons, including infants with congenital rubella syndrome
Congenital heart defects: patent ductus arteriosus, pulmonary artery stenosis	Emphasize vaccination of all unimmunized postpubertal males and females, susceptible adolescents, and adult females of childbearing age
Auditory: high incidence of delayed hearing loss	
Intrauterine growth retardation	Caution women against pregnancy for at least 3 months after vaccination
Thrombocytopenia, hepatomegaly, purple skin lesions, "blueberry muffin" appearance	Contact isolation for infant with congenital rubella; such infants may shed virus in secretions up to 1 year of age
Mild form may have no clinical manifestation	Breast-feeding not contraindicated
Syphilis, Congenital (*Treponema Pallidum*)	
Stillbirth, hydrops fetalis prematurity	Transmitted: transplacentally, at any time or at birth
Asymptomatic in some cases in first few weeks	Most severe form of syphilis
Hemolytic anemia, hepatomegaly, thrombocytopenia, lymphadenopathy	Treatment: parenteral penicillin and close follow-up for possible retreatment up to 1 year of age
After 2 years—CNS, bones, teeth, joints, eyes and skin, rhinitis	Standard precautions; contact isolation until newborn has received antibiotic treatment for at least 24 hours

Continued

Unit 4

Neonatal Complications—cont'd

TABLE 4-20 Infections Acquired from Mother Before, During, or After Birth*—cont'd

Fetal or Newborn Effects	Comments and Nursing Considerations†
Toxoplasmosis (*Toxoplasma Gondii*)	
Asymptomatic infants in 70% to 90% of cases	Transmitted: throughout pregnancy
Hydrocephaly, cerebral calcifications, chorioretinitis (classic triad)	Predominant host for organism is cats
Microcephaly, seizures, mental retardation, deafness	May be transmitted through cat feces or by eating poorly cooked or raw infected meat
Encephalitis, myocarditis, hepatosplenomegaly, anemia, diarrhea, vomiting, purpura, maculopapular rash, hepatomegaly, splenomegaly, jaundice, thrombocytopenia	Caution pregnant women to avoid contact with cat feces (e.g., emptying cat litter boxes) or to wear gloves if contact is unavoidable
	Treatment: pyrimethamine sulfadiazine
	Standard precautions in newborns

*This table is not an exhaustive representation of all perinatally transmitted infections. For further information regarding specific diseases or treatment not listed here, the reader is referred to American Academy of Pediatrics, Committee on Infectious Diseases: *1997 Red book report of the Committee on Infectious Diseases,* ed 24, Elk Grove Village, IL, 1997, The Academy.

†Isolation precautions depend on institutional policy. (See Infection Control, p. 341.)

TABLE 4-21 Congenital Effects of Maternal Ingestion of Alcohol and Smoking

Fetal or Newborn Effects	Comments and Nursing Considerations
Alcohol (Fetal Alcohol Syndrome [FAS])	
Often asymptomatic and difficult to detect except by maternal history	Exact quantity of alcohol needed to produce teratogenic effects in fetus is not known
Other manifestations may include:	Women with histories of heavy drinking should be counseled regarding risks to fetus
Facial features: hypoplastic maxilla, micrognathia, hypoplastic philtrum, short palpebral fissures	Provide mother with resources for treatment to decrease or eliminate alcoholic intake
Neurologic: mental retardation, motor retardation, microcephaly, hypotonia, hearing disorders, seizures	
Growth: prenatal growth retardation, persistent postnatal growth lag	
Behavior: irritability (infant), hyperactivity (child)	
Congenital heart defects	
Maternal Tobacco Smoking	
Fetal growth retardation	Women should be counseled regarding risks to fetus
Increased perinatal deaths, including sudden infant death syndrome (SIDS)	Provide with resources to help eliminate smoking
Increased spontaneous abortions	
Preterm delivery	
Postnatal: growth and intellectual and emotional developmental deficits	

Neonatal Complications—cont'd

TABLE 4-22   Common Autosomal Aberrations

Syndrome	Chromosome Abnormality and Nomenclature	Average Incidence (Live Birth)*	Major Clinical Manifestations
Cri-du-chat	Deletion of short arm of No. 5 chromosome—46,XY,5p–	1:50,000	Distinctive weak, high-pitched, mewlike cry resembling the cry of a cat; small head; hypertelorism; failure to thrive; severe mental retardation—profound with age
Trisomy 13 (Patau)	Trisomy of No. 13 chromosome—47,XY,+13	1:4000-15,000	Cleft lip and palate (frequently bilateral); ear malformations; microphthalmia; polydactyly; eye defects; cardiac defects; mental retardation; early death
Trisomy 18 (Edward)	Trisomy of No. 18 chromosome—47,XY,+18	1:3500-8000	Deformed and low-set ears; micrognathia; rockerbottom feet; overlapping (index over third) fingers; prominent occiput; hypertelorism; cardiac defects; mental retardation; failure to thrive; early death
Trisomy 21 (Down)	Trisomy of No. 21 chromosome—47,XY,+21 (trisomy); 46,XY,+(14;21) (translocation); 46,XY/47,XY,+21 (mosaic)	1:700†	Brachycephaly with flat occiput; inner epicanthal folds; small ears, nose, and mouth with protruding tongue; muscular hypotonia; broad, short hands with stubby fingers and transverse palmar crease; broad, stubby feet with wide space between big and second toes; cardiac defects; mental retardation; variable life expectancy

*Data from Nora JJ, Fraser FC: *Medical genetics: principles and practice,* ed 3, Philadelphia, 1989, Lea & Febiger.
†Risk related to maternal age: age 30 years = 1:900; age 35 years = 1:300; age 40 years = 1:100; age 45 years = 1:30.

TABLE 4-23   Infants with Inborn Errors of Metabolism (IEM)

Description	Clinical Manifestations	Therapeutic Management	Nursing Considerations
Congenital Hypothyroidism			
Thyroid deficiency; if untreated, results in abnormal physical and mental development	May be detected in utero by ultrasound evaluation on inadequate skeletal growth. Preterm infants often experience a transient hypothyroxinemia which usually requires no treatment since the condition corrects itself with increasing maturity. Preterm infants, however, require screening to differentiate the transient state from those requiring treatment. ***At Birth*** Wide range, from no symptoms or subtle to the following: Gestation ≥42 weeks Birth weight ≥4 kg (8.8 lb) Widened posterior and anterior fontanels	Lifelong replacement therapy with thyroid hormone preparation Regular monitoring of thyroxine (T_4) and thyroid-stimulating hormone (TSH) levels	Ensure that screening is done on all neonates Treatment may be initiated prior to neonatal screen results with suggestive symptoms of condition Observe for signs of inadequate treatment (fatigue, sleepiness, decreased appetite, constipation) Observe for signs of overdose (rapid pulse, dyspnea, irritability, insomnia, fever, sweating, weight loss) Make certain family understands the therapeutic measures prescribed and how to recognize possible complications Provide guidelines for family (e.g., explanations of disorder, need for lifelong treatment, and compliance with therapeutic regimen)

Continued

Unit 4

Neonatal Complications—cont'd

TABLE 4-23 Infants with Inborn Errors of Metabolism (IEM)—cont'd

Description	Clinical Manifestations	Therapeutic Management	Nursing Considerations
Congenital Hypothyroidism—cont'd			
	At Birth—cont'd		(See Nursing Care Plan: The Child with Chronic Illness or Disability, p. 287.)
	Hypothermia, 95° F or less		(See also Nursing Care Plan: Child and Family Compliance, p. 343.)
	Peripheral cyanosis		
	Respiratory distress		
	Edema		
	Prolonged physiologic jaundice		
	Abdominal distention		
	Vomiting		
	Hoarse cry		
	Delayed passage of meconium		
	Feeding difficulties		
	Hypoactivity		
	Lethargy, hypotonia		
	Before 3 Months of Age		
	Umbilical hernia		
	Mottled and dry skin		
	Constipation		
	Large tongue		
	Cold to touch		
	Excessive sleepiness		
	Eyelid edema		
	Long, coarse hair		
	Anemia		
	Hypotension, bradycardia		
	Narrow pulse pressure		
	Enlarged lingual thyroid		
	Asymmetric goiter		
	Hypoglycemia		
	Difficulty feeding related to lethargy		
	Minimal crying		
	Elongated nasal bridge		
	Older Child		
	Short stature		
	Infantile proportions persist; length of trunk long relative to legs		
	Decreased metabolic rate; weight gain, often leading to obesity		
	Infantile facial features of myxedema		
	Short forehead		
	Wide, puffy eyes; wrinkled eyelids		
	Broad, short, upturned nose		
	Hair often dry, brittle, or lusterless, extending far down onto forehead		
	Sensorineural hearing loss		
	Dentition delayed and usually defective		
	Decreased cognitive attention (ADHD)		
	Intellectual deficit of varying degrees		
	Impaired motor skills		

TABLE 4-23   Infants with Inborn Errors of Metabolism (IEM)—cont'd

Description	Clinical Manifestations	Therapeutic Management	Nursing Considerations
Phenylketonuria (PKU)			
Genetic disease, inherited as an autosomal-recessive trait, caused by absence of the enzyme phenylalanine hydroxylase that is necessary for metabolism of essential amino acid phenylalanine into the amino acid tyrosine	Phenylpyruvic acid in urine (musty odor) and sweat Increased phenylalanine blood levels Decreased tyrosine Decreased melanin (fair skin, blond hair, blue eyes) Decreased plasma levels of catecholamines Decreased levels of serotonin Central nervous system damage: mental retardation, hyperactivity, seizures Growth retardation Osteopenia Decreased bone mineral density	Routine PKU screening of all neonates; repeat screening in 2 weeks if initial screen was before 24 hours of age Lifelong low-phenylalanine diet, especially before and during pregnancy Frequent monitoring of phenylalanine blood levels (maintain serum levels between 2.0-8.0 mg/dl) Initiate diet before 3 weeks of age for optimal growth and intelligence	Refer to qualified nutritionist Provide low-phenylalanine diet Explain or clarify information about the disorder Teach family how to provide lifelong low-phenylalanine diet Give practical suggestions for food preparation and selection Explain reasons for frequent monitoring of phenylalanine levels Provide emotional support to help family and child adjust to difficult diet and common sequelae of condition (intellectual impairment, especially speech and learning and behavior problems) Help parents identify hidden sources of phenylalanine such as sweetener Aspartame Refer for genetic counseling and follow-up care (See Nursing Care Plan: The Child with Chronic Illness or Disability, p. 287.) (See also Nursing Care Plan: Child and Family Compliance, p. 343.)
Galactosemia			

Inborn error of carbohydrate metabolism, inherited as autosomal-recessive trait, in which absent hepatic enzymes prevent the conversion of galactose to glucose; the subsequent accumulation of galactose is toxic to the brain, liver, ovaries, and kidneys
Three subtypes of the condition exist with GALT (galactose-1-phosphate uridyl transferase) being the most severe form (classic galactosemia)
	Appear normal at birth
	After ingesting milk, signs appear (e.g., vomiting, weight loss, drowsiness, diarrhea)
	Weight loss
	Sepsis, especially *E. coli* septicemia
	Jaundice
	Seizures
	Cirrhosis
	Enlarged spleen
	Cataracts
	Cerebral damage
	Dehydration
	Long Term
	  Speech and language disorders
	  Cognitive delay
	  Growth retardation
	  Gross and fine motor impediments
	  Gonadal dysfunction (females)
		Elimination of all milk and galactose-containing foods, including breast milk, from the diet	Newborn screening
			Initiate feedings with a soy-based formula such as Isomil or Prosobec; may also use a protein hydrolysate formula such as Nutramigen or Progestimil
			Help family identify hidden sources of galactose (or lactose) such as certain medications (sulfonamides, doxycycline, cleocin, erythromycin; consult with pharmacist for others)
			Provide prescribed diet
			Teach family about the disorder
			Teach family how to eliminate all milk and galactose-containing foods from the diet
			Provide emotional support to help family and child adjust to diet and common sequelae of condition (developmental delay, speech problems, and growth retardation)
			(See Nursing Care Plan: The Child with Chronic Illness or Disability, p. 287.)
			(See also Nursing Care Plan: Child and Family Compliance, p. 343.)

NURSING CARE OF THE CHILD WITH RESPIRATORY DYSFUNCTION

Respiratory dysfunction is an interference with the ability of the pulmonary system to exchange oxygen and carbon dioxide adequately.

NURSING CARE PLAN

The Child with Respiratory Dysfunction

ASSESSMENT

Obtain histories:

Family history of allergies, genetic disorders

Patient history of previous respiratory dysfunction; recent evidence of exposure to infection, allergens or other irritants, trauma

Perform a physical assessment of the chest and lungs. (See p. 50.)

Observe respirations for:

Rate—Rapid (tachypnea), normal, or slow for the particular child

Depth—Normal depth, too shallow (hypopnea), too deep (hyperpnea); usually estimated from the amplitude of thoracic and abdominal excursion

Ease—Effortless, labored (dyspnea), orthopnea, associated with intercostal and/or substernal retractions (inspiratory "sinking in" of soft tissues in relation to the cartilaginous and bony thorax), pulsus paradoxus (blood pressure falls with inspiration and rises with expiration), flaring nares, head bobbing (head of sleeping child with suboccipital area supported on parent's forearm bobs forward in synchrony with each inspiration), grunting, or wheezing

Labored breathing—Continuous, intermittent, becoming steadily worsening, sudden onset, at rest or on exertion, associated with wheezing, grunting, or associated with pain

Rhythm—Variation in rate and depth of respirations

Observe for:

Evidence of infection—Elevated temperature, enlarged cervical lymph nodes, inflamed mucous membranes, and purulent discharges from the nose, ears, or lungs (sputum)

Cough—Characteristics of the cough (if present): under what circumstances the cough is heard (e.g., night only, on arising); the nature of the cough (paroxysmal with or without wheeze, "croupy" or "brassy"); frequency of cough; associated with swallowing or other activity; character of the cough (moist or dry); productivity

Wheeze—Expiratory or inspiratory, high-pitched or musical, prolonged, slowly progressive or sudden, associated with labored breathing

Cyanosis—Note distribution (peripheral, perioral, facial, trunk as well as face), degree, duration, associated with activity

Chest pain—May be a complaint of older children. Note location and circumstances: localized or generalized, referred to base of neck or abdomen, dull or sharp, deep or superficial, associated with rapid, shallow respirations or grunting

Sputum—Supervised older children may provide sputum sample; young children may need bulb suction to provide a sample; note volume, color, viscosity, and odor

Bad breath—May be associated with some respiratory infections

---

NURSING DIAGNOSIS: Ineffective airway clearance related to mechanical obstruction, inflammation, increased secretions, discomfort, perceptual and cognitive impairment, pain

■ **PATIENT GOAL 1:** Will maintain patent airway

NURSING INTERVENTIONS/*RATIONALES*

Aspirate (suction) secretions from airway as needed, limiting each suction attempt to 5 seconds with sufficient time between attempts *to allow reoxygenation*

Position supine with head in "sniffing" position with neck slightly extended and nose pointed to ceiling

Avoid neck hyperextension

Position *to prevent aspiration of secretions:*

Semiprone position

Side-lying position

Assist child in expectorating sputum by coughing; use bulb suction in infants

*Provide nebulization with appropriate solution and equipment as prescribed

Observe child closely after aerosol therapy *to prevent aspiration because large volumes of sputum may be thinned suddenly* (in cystic fibrosis)

*Administer expectorants if prescribed

*Perform chest physiotherapy if prescribed

Give nothing by mouth to prevent aspiration of fluids (e.g., child with severe tachypnea)

Use pain control measures (See Nursing Care Plan: The Child in Pain, p. 315.)

Have emergency equipment available

EXPECTED OUTCOMES

Airway remains clear

Child breathes easily; respirations are within normal limits (See inside front cover.)

---

*Dependent nursing action.

The Child with Respiratory Dysfunction—cont'd

■ **PATIENT GOAL 2:** Will expectorate secretions adequately

NURSING INTERVENTIONS/*RATIONALES*

Ensure adequate fluid intake *to liquefy secretions*
Provide humidified atmosphere *to prevent crusting of nasal secretions and drying of mucous membranes*
Explain importance of expectoration to child and family
Assist child in coughing effectively; provide tissues
Remove accumulated mucus; suction if needed
Perform percussion, vibration, and postural drainage *to facilitate drainage of secretions*

EXPECTED OUTCOME

Older child expectorates secretions without undue stress and fatigue

> **NURSING DIAGNOSIS:** Ineffective breathing pattern related to inflammatory process, pain, neurologic or musculoskeletal impairment

■ **PATIENT GOAL 1:** Will exhibit normal respiratory function

NURSING INTERVENTIONS/*RATIONALES*

Position for maximum ventilatory efficiency (i.e., open airway and provide for maximum lung expansion):
  Allow position of comfort (e.g., tripod position of child with epiglottitis; see p. 382) or use high Fowler position
  Avoid constricting clothing or bedding
  Use pillows and padding *to maintain open airway* (e.g., in infant, child with hypotonia)
Promote rest and sleep
*Place in tent or hood (infant) if prescribed *to provide increased humidity and supplemental oxygen*
Implement measures to reduce anxiety and apprehension (See Patient Goal 3.)
Organize activities to allow for minimal expenditure of energy and adequate rest and sleep
Encourage relaxation techniques (See pp. 339-340.)
Teach child and family measures to ease respiratory efforts:
  Use cool mist humidifier in child's room
  Warm mist provided by steam from running hot water in a closed bathroom may be helpful (spasmodic croup)

EXPECTED OUTCOMES

Child rests and sleeps quietly
Respirations are unlabored
Respirations remain within normal limits (See inside front cover for normal variations.)

■ **PATIENT GOAL 2:** Will receive optimum oxygen supply

NURSING INTERVENTIONS/*RATIONALES*

Position for maximum ventilatory efficiency (See Patient Goal 1.)
*Place in tent or hood with cool vapor, if prescribed
*Provide oxygen as prescribed and/or needed

EXPECTED OUTCOMES

Child breathes easily

Respirations remain within normal limits (See inside front cover for normal variations.)

■ **PATIENT GOAL 3:** Will experience reduction of fear and anxiety

NURSING INTERVENTIONS/*RATIONALES*

Explain unfamiliar procedures and equipment to the child
Remain with child during procedures
Use calm, reassuring manner *to reduce child's anxiety*
Provide constant attendance during acute phase of illness
Provide comfort measures child prefers (e.g., rocking, stroking)
Provide security devices such as familiar toy, blanket
Encourage parental attendance and, when possible, involvement in child's care
Do nothing to make the child more anxious than he or she already is
Maintain a relaxed manner
Establish rapport with child and parents
Instill confidence in both parents and child
Try to avoid any intrusive procedures
Be aware of child's rest/sleep cycle or pattern in planning nursing activities
Relieve pain (See Nursing Care Plan: The Child in Pain, p. 315.)
Provide diversional activities appropriate to child's age, condition, and capabilities
*Administer sedatives and/or analgesics as indicated if ordered *for restlessness and pain*
*Administer medications that promote breathing (e.g., bronchodilators, expectorants) as ordered

EXPECTED OUTCOMES

Child responds positively to comfort and pain reduction measures
Child remains calm and cooperative
Child exhibits no signs of distress
Parents remain with child and provide comfort
Child engages in quiet activities appropriate for age, interests, and condition

> **NURSING DIAGNOSIS:** Risk for suffocation related to airway obstruction (internal, external), inadequate oxygen

■ **PATIENT GOAL 1:** Will not suffocate

NURSING INTERVENTIONS/*RATIONALES*

Remove impediment to air exchange where possible (e.g., pillow over face, secretions, inadequate oxygen)
Avoid situations that predispose patient to airway obstruction or oxygen depletion
Have emergency equipment readily available
Be prepared to assist with tracheostomy and obtain parental permission for procedure
Implement appropriate emergency management of airway obstruction (See p. 648.) and/or CPR (See p. 642.)

EXPECTED OUTCOME

Child breathes easily

Unit 4

The Child with Respiratory Dysfunction—cont'd

NURSING DIAGNOSIS: Activity intolerance related to imbalance between oxygen supply and demand

■ **PATIENT GOAL 1:** Will maintain adequate energy levels

NURSING INTERVENTIONS/RATIONALES

Assess child's level of physical tolerance

Assist child in those activities of daily living that may be beyond tolerance

Provide diversional activities appropriate to child's age, condition, capabilities, and interest

Provide diversional play activities that promote rest and quiet but prevent boredom and withdrawal

Provide rest and sleep periods appropriate to age and condition

Instruct child to rest when feeling tired

Balance rest and activity when ambulatory

EXPECTED OUTCOMES

Child plays and rests quietly and engages in activities appropriate to age and capabilities (specify)

Child exhibits no evidence of increased respiratory distress

Child tolerates increasingly more activity

■ **PATIENT GOAL 2:** Will receive optimum rest

NURSING INTERVENTIONS/RATIONALES

Provide quiet environment

Organize activities *for maximum sleep time*

Schedule visiting to allow sufficient rest

Encourage parents to remain with child

*Administer sedatives and analgesics as indicated if ordered *for restlessness and pain*

Encourage frequent rest periods and regular sleep times

Follow child's usual routine for bedtime, nap time

Implement measures to ensure sleep, such as quiet, darkened room

EXPECTED OUTCOMES

Child remains calm, quiet and relaxed

Child gets a sufficient amount of rest (specify)

NURSING DIAGNOSIS: Pain related to inflammatory process, surgical incision

■ **PATIENT GOAL 1:** Will experience either no pain or a reduction of pain to level acceptable to child

**NURSING INTERVENTIONS/RATIONALES
AND EXPECTED OUTCOMES**

(See Nursing Care Plan: The Child in Pain, p. 315.)

NURSING DIAGNOSIS: Fear/anxiety related to hospitalization, difficulty breathing

■ **PATIENT GOAL 1:** Will experience reduction of fear and anxiety

**NURSING INTERVENTIONS/RATIONALES
AND EXPECTED OUTCOMES**

(See Patient Goal 3, p. 379.)

NURSING DIAGNOSIS: Altered family processes related to illness and/or hospitalization of a child

■ **PATIENT (FAMILY) GOAL 1:** Will experience reduction of anxiety

NURSING INTERVENTIONS/RATIONALES

Recognize parental concern and need for information and support

Explain therapy and child's behavior

Provide support as needed

Encourage family to become involved in child's care

EXPECTED OUTCOMES

Parents ask appropriate questions, discuss child's condition and care calmly, and become involved positively in child's care

(See also:

Nursing Care Plan: The Family of the Child Who Is Ill or Hospitalized, p. 282.)

Nursing Care Plan: The Child in the Hospital, p. 268.)

*Dependent nursing action.

Unit 4

NURSING CARE PLAN

The Child with Acute Respiratory Infection

Acute respiratory infection is an inflammatory process caused by viral, bacterial, atypical (mycoplasma), or aspiration of foreign substances, which involves any or all parts of the respiratory tract.

  Upper respiratory tract (upper airway)—Consists of the nose and pharynx

Croup syndromes—Consists of the epiglottis, larynx, and trachea (the structurally stable, nonreactive portion of the airway)

  Lower respiratory tract—Consists of the bronchi and bronchioles (which constitute the reactive portion of the airway because of their smooth muscle content and ability to constrict) and the alveoli

ASSESSMENT

(See assessment of respiratory function, p. 378.)

(See also physical assessment of chest and lungs, p. 50.)

Assist with diagnostic procedures and tests (e.g., radiography, throat culture, thoracentesis, venipuncture for blood analysis).

Observe for general clinical manifestations of acute respiratory tract infection (Box 4-20.)

Identify factors affecting type of illness and response to acute respiratory infection (e.g., age and size of child, ability to resist infection, contact with infected children, coexisting disorders affecting respiratory tract).

Assess respiratory status:

  Monitor respirations for rate, depth, pattern, presence of retractions, and flaring nares.

Auscultate lungs:

  Evaluate breath sounds (type and location).

  Detect presence of crackles or wheezes.

  Detect areas of consolidation.

  Evaluate effectiveness of chest physiotherapy.

Observe for presence or absence of retractions, nasal flaring.

Observe color of skin and mucous membranes for pallor and cyanosis.

Observe for presence of hoarseness, stridor, and cough.

Monitor heart rate and regularity.

Observe behavior:

  Restlessness

  Irritability

  Apprehension

Observe for signs of the following:

  Chest pain

  Abdominal pain

  Dyspnea

Observe for clinical manifestations of respiratory infection (specific):

I. Upper respiratory tract infections

Nasopharyngitis—Viral infection, *acute rhinitis* or *coryza*, equivalent of the "common cold" in adults

Edema and vasodilation of mucosa

Younger child

  Fever

  Irritability, restlessness

  Sneezing

  Vomiting and/or diarrhea, sometimes

  Decreased appetite

Older child

  Low-grade fever

  Dryness and irritation of nose and throat

  Sneezing, chilly sensation

  Muscular aches

  Cough, sometimes

Pharyngitis—Throat (including the tonsils) is principal anatomic site of pharyngitis (sore throat).

Younger child

  Fever

  General malaise

  Anorexia

  Moderate sore throat

  Headache

  Mild to moderate hyperemia

Older child

  Fever (may reach 40° C)

  Headache

  Anorexia

  Dysphagia

  Abdominal pain

  Vomiting

  Mild to fiery red, edematous pharynx

    Hyperemia of tonsils and pharynx; may extend to soft palate and uvula

    Often abundant follicular exudate that spreads and coalesces to form pseudomembrane on tonsils

    Cervical glands enlarged and tender

Influenza ("Flu")—Caused by three antigenically distinct orthomyxoviruses: types A and B, which cause epidemic disease; and type C, which is epidemiologically unimportant

May be subclinical, mild, moderate, or severe

Overt illness:

  Dry throat and nasal mucosa

  Dry cough

  Tendency toward hoarseness

  Sudden onset of fever and chills

  Flushed face

  Photophobia

  Myalgia

  Hyperesthesia

  Prostration (sometimes)

  Subglottal croup common (especially in infants)

II. Croup syndromes

Croup is a general term applied to a symptom complex characterized by hoarseness, a resonant cough described as "barking" (croupy), varying degrees of inspiratory stridor, and varying degrees of respiratory distress resulting from swelling or obstruction in the region of the larynx.

Acute laryngitis—Infection is usually viral; primary clinical manifestation is hoarseness; common illness of older children and adolescents.

May be accompanied by other upper respiratory symptoms: coryza, sore throat, nasal congestion

May be accompanied by systemic manifestations: fever, headache, myalgia, malaise

Symptoms vary with the infecting virus

Acute laryngotracheobronchitis (LTB)—Viral infection; most common of the croup syndromes; usually occurs in children less than 5 years of age

Continued

Unit 4

The Child with Acute Respiratory Infection—cont'd

ASSESSMENT—cont'd

Onset is slowly progressive:
  URI
  Inspiratory stridor
  Brassy cough
  Hoarseness
  Dyspnea
  Suprasternal retractions
  Restlessness
  Irritability
  Low-grade fever
  Nontoxic appearance
  May progress to hypoxia and respiratory failure

Acute spasmodic laryngitis (spasmodic croup)—Viral infection with allergic and psychogenic factors in some cases; distinct from laryngitis and LTB by characteristic paroxysmal attacks of laryngeal obstruction that occur chiefly at night; usually occurs in children age 1 to 3 years.

Onset is sudden; at night:
  URI
  Croupy cough
  Stridor
  Hoarseness
  Dyspnea
  Restlessness
  Child appears anxious, frightened
  Symptoms waken child
  Symptoms disappear during day
  Tends to recur

Acute epiglottitis (supraglottitis)—Bacterial (usually *H. influenzae*) infection; serious obstructive inflammatory process that requires immediate attention; occurs principally in children between 3 and 7 years of age, but can occur from infancy to adulthood.

Onset is abrupt; rapidly progressive:
  Sore throat
  Drooling
  Absence of spontaneous cough
  Agitation
  Throat is red, inflamed with distinctive large, cherry-red, edematous epiglottitis (Practice Alert)
  High fever
  Toxic appearance
  Rapid pulse and respirations
  Stridor aggravated when supine
  Child will sit upright, leaning forward, with chin thrust out, mouth open and tongue protruding; tripod position
  Thick, muffled voice
  Croaking, "froglike" sound on inspiration
  Anxious and frightened expression
  Suprasternal and substernal retractions may be visible
  Child seldom struggles to breathe (breathing slowly and quietly provides better air exchange)
  Sallow color of mild hypoxia to frank cyanosis

Acute tracheitis—Bacterial (usually *S. aureus*) infection of the mucosa of the upper trachea; is a distinct entity with features of both croup and epiglottitis; may cause airway obstruction severe enough to cause respiratory arrest; occurs in children ages 1 month to 6 years.

Onset is moderately progressive:
  Follows previous URI
  Begins with signs and symptoms similar to LTB

  Croupy cough
  Stridor unaffected by position
  Copious purulent secretions—may be severe enough to cause respiratory arrest
  Toxic appearance
  High fever
  No response to LTB therapy

III. Lower respiratory tract infections

Asthmatic bronchitis—Exaggerated response of bronchi to infection; most commonly caused by viruses but may be any variety of URI pathogens; bronchospasm, exudation, and edema of bronchi are similar to asthma in older children; occurs in late infancy and early childhood.
  Previous URI
  Wheezing
  Productive cough
  (See also Assessment of bronchial asthma, p. 392.)

Viral-induced bronchitis—Inflammation of large airways (trachea and bronchi); usually occurs in association with viral URI but other agents (e.g., bacteria, fungi, allergic disorders, airborne irritants) can trigger symptoms; seldom occurs as an isolated entity in childhood; affects children in first 4 years of life.
  Persistent dry, hacking cough (worse at night), becoming productive in 2 to 3 days
  Tachypnea
  Low-grade fever

Respiratory syncytial virus (RSV)/bronchiolitis—Acute viral infection with maximum effect at the bronchiolar level; usually affects children 2 to 12 months; rare after age 2 years
  Begins as simple URI with serous nasal discharge
  May be accompanied by mild fever
  Gradually develops increasing respiratory distress
  Dyspnea
  Paroxysmal, nonproductive cough
  Tachypnea with flaring nares and retractions
  Emphysema
  Child may be wheezing

IV. Pneumonias

Pneumonia, inflammation of the pulmonary parenchyma, is common throughout childhood but occurs more frequently in infancy and early childhood. Clinically, pneumonia may occur either as a primary disease or as a complication of some other illness. Morphologically, pneumonias are recognized as the following types:

  Lobar pneumonia—All or a large segment of one or more pulmonary lobes is involved. When both lungs are affected, it is known as bilateral or "double" pneumonia.

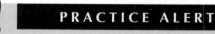

! PRACTICE ALERT !

Epiglottitis

Avoid throat examination or culture in suspected epiglottitis because this can precipitate further or complete obstruction.

The Child with Acute Respiratory Infection—cont'd

Bronchopneumonia—Begins in the terminal bronchioles, which become clogged with mucopurulent exudate to form consolidated patches in nearby lobules; also called *lobular pneumonia.*

Interstitial pneumonia—The inflammatory process is more or less confined within the alveolar walls (interstitium) and the peribronchial and interlobular tissues.

Pneumonitis is a localized acute inflammation of the lung without the toxemia associated with lobar pneumonia.

The pneumonias are more often classified according to the etiologic agent: viral, atypical (mycoplasma), bacterial, or aspiration of foreign substances. Pneumonia may be caused less often by histomycosis, coccidioidomycosis, and other fungi.

Viral pneumonia—Occurs more frequently than bacterial pneumonia; seen in children of all age-groups; often associated with viral URIs, and RSV accounts for the largest percentage.

May be acute or insidious

Symptoms variable:

Mild—Low-grade fever, slight cough, malaise

Severe—High fever, severe cough, prostration

Cough usually unproductive early in disease

A few wheezes or crackles heard on auscultation

Atypical pneumonia—Etiologic agent is mycoplasma; occurs principally in the fall and winter months; more prevalent where there are crowded living conditions.

May be sudden or insidious

General systemic symptoms:

Fever

Chills (older children)

Headache

Malaise

Anorexia

Myalgia

Followed by:

Rhinitis

Sore throat

Dry, hacking cough

Nonproductive early, then seromucoid sputum, to mucopurulent or blood streaked

Fine crepitant crackles over various lung areas

Bacterial pneumonia—Includes pneumococcal, staphylococcal, and streptococcal pneumonias; clinical manifestations differ from other types of pneumonia; individual microorganisms produce a distinct clinical picture.

Onset abrupt:

Usually preceded by viral infection

Toxic, acutely ill appearance

Fever

Malaise

Rapid, shallow respirations

Cough

Chest pain often exaggerated by deep breathing

Pain may be referred to abdomen

Chills

Meningismus

V. Pulmonary tuberculosis (TB)

Caused by *Mycobacterium tuberculosis;* other factors that influence development of TB include the following: heredity (resistance to the infection may be genetically transmitted); sex (morbidity and mortality higher in adolescent girls); age (lower resistance in infants, higher incidence during adolescence); stress (emotional or physical); nutritional state; and intercurrent infection (especially human immunodeficiency virus [HIV], measles, and pertussis).

Extremely variable

May be asymptomatic or produce a broad range of symptoms:

Fever

Malaise

Anorexia

Weight loss

Cough may or may not be present (progresses slowly over weeks to months)

Aching pain and tightness in the chest

Hemoptysis (rare)

With progression

Respiratory rate increases

Poor expansion of lung on the affected side

Diminished breath sounds and crackles

Dullness to percussion

Fever persists

Generalized symptoms are manifested

Child develops pallor, anemia, weakness, and weight loss

VI. Aspiration of foreign substances

Inflammation of lung tissue can occur as the result of irritation from foreign material (e.g., vomitus, small objects, oral secretions, or inhalation of smoke) and aspiration of food. Young children are especially prone to aspiration of foreign substances, and weak and debilitated children are subject to aspiration of food, vomitus, or secretions.

Foreign body (FB) aspiration—Clinical manifestations and changes produced depend on the degree and location of obstruction and type of FB:

Choking

Gagging

Sternal retractions

Wheezing

Cough

Inability to speak or breathe (larynx)

Decreased airway entry, dyspnea (bronchi)

Signs of acute distress requiring immediate and quick action:

Cannot speak

Becomes cyanotic

Collapses

Aspiration pneumonia—May result from aspiration of fluids, food, vomitus, nasopharyngeal secretions, amniotic fluid and debris (during birth process), hydrocarbons, lipids, and talcum powder. Aspiration of fluid or food substances is a particular hazard in children who have difficulty with swallowing; who are unable to swallow because of paralysis, weaknesses, debility, congenital anomalies, or absent cough reflex; or who are force fed, especially while crying or breathing rapidly. Irritated mucous membranes become a site for secondary bacterial infection.

Inhalation injury—Results from inhalation of smoke (noxious substances are primarily products of incomplete combustion) or other noxious gases

Local injury (smoke)

Suspected with a history of flames in a closed space whether burns are present or not

Unit 4

Continued

The Child with Acute Respiratory Infection—cont'd

ASSESSMENT—cont'd

Sooty material around nose, in sputum
Singed nasal hairs
Mucosal burns of nose, lips, mouth, throat
Hoarse voice
Cough
Inspiratory and expiratory stridor
Signs of respiratory distress (See p. 401.)
Systemic injury
    Gases that are nontoxic to the airways (e.g., carbon monoxide [CO] and hydrogen cyanide) can cause injury and death by interfering with or inhibiting cellular respiration

Mild CO poisoning:
    Headache
    Visual disturbances
    Irritability
    Nausea
Severe CO poisoning:
    Confusion
    Hallucinations
    Ataxia
    Coma
    Pallor
    Cyanosis
    May be bright, cherry-red lips and skin

NURSING DIAGNOSIS: Ineffective breathing pattern related to inflammatory process

■ **PATIENT GOAL 1:** Will exhibit normal respiratory function

NURSING INTERVENTIONS/*RATIONALES*

Position for maximum ventilation (i.e., open airway and allow maximum lung expansion)
Allow position of comfort (e.g., tripod position of child with epiglottitis, or maintain head elevation of at least 30 degrees)
Check child's position frequently to ensure child does not slide down *to avoid compressing the diaphragm*
Avoid constricting clothing or bedding
Use pillows and padding to maintain open airway (e.g., in infant or child with hypotonia)
*Provide increased humidity and supplemental oxygen by placing child in small tent or hood (infant) or administer via nasal cannula or mask (preferred methods for children older than infancy because of safety issues)
Promote rest and sleep by scheduling appropriate activity and rest periods
Encourage relaxation techniques
Teach child and family measures to ease respiratory efforts (e.g., appropriate positioning)
For most respiratory illnesses use cool-mist humidifier in child's room
    For spasmodic croup, create warm mist by running hot water in a closed bathroom (warm mist may be helpful because of its relaxing effect, but mostly because child is being held upright in the shower)

EXPECTED OUTCOMES

Respirations remain within normal limits (See inside back cover for normal variations.)
Respirations are unlabored
Child rests and sleeps quietly

■ **PATIENT GOAL 2:** Will receive optimum oxygen supply

NURSING INTERVENTIONS/*RATIONALES*

Position for maximum ventilatory efficiency (See Goal 1.)
Use pulse oximetry to monitor oxygen saturation
Place in cool, humidified environment, using appropriate oxygen delivery system
*Provide oxygen as prescribed and/or needed

EXPECTED OUTCOMES

Child breathes easily

Respirations remain within normal limits (See inside back cover for normal variations.)
Oxygen saturation is ≥95%

NURSING DIAGNOSIS: Fear/anxiety related to difficulty breathing, unfamiliar procedures, and possibly environment (hospital)

■ **PATIENT GOAL 1:** Will experience reduction of fear/anxiety

NURSING INTERVENTIONS/*RATIONALES*

Explain unfamiliar procedures and equipment to child in developmentally appropriate terms
Establish rapport with child and parents
Remain with child and parent during procedures
Use calm, reassuring manner
Provide frequent attendance during acute phase of illness
Provide comfort measures child prefers (e.g., rocking, stroking, music)
Provide attachment objects (e.g., familiar toy, blanket)
Encourage family-centered care with increased parental attendance and, when possible, involvement
Do nothing to make child more anxious or fearful
Instill confidence in both parents and child
Try to avoid any intrusive or painful procedures
Be aware of child's rest/sleep cycle or pattern in planning nursing activities
Assess and implement appropriate pain management therapy (i.e., sedatives and/or analgesics) (See Nursing Care Plan: The Child in Pain, p. 315.)
Provide diversional activities appropriate to child's cognitive ability and condition
*Administer medications that promote improved ventilation (e.g., bronchodilators, expectorants) as prescribed

EXPECTED OUTCOMES

Child exhibits no signs of respiratory distress or physical discomfort
Parents remain with child and provide comfort
Child engages in quiet activities appropriate for age, interest, condition, and cognitive level

---

NURSING DIAGNOSIS: Ineffective airway clearance related to mechanical obstruction, inflammation, increased secretions, pain

---

*Dependent nursing action.

Unit 4

The Child with Acute Respiratory Infection—cont'd

BOX 4-20

Signs and Symptoms Associated with Respiratory Infections in Infants and Small Children

Fever

May be absent in newborn infants

Greatest at ages 6 months to 3 years

Temperature may reach 39.5° to 40.5° C (103° to 105° F), even with mild infections

Often appears as first sign of infection

May be listless and irritable, or somewhat euphoric and temporarily more active than normal; some children talk with unaccustomed rapidity

Tendency to develop high temperatures with infection in certain families

May precipitate febrile seizures

Febrile seizures uncommon after 3 or 4 years of age

Meningismus

Meningeal signs without infection of the meninges

Occurs with abrupt onset of fever

Accompanied by:

Headache

Pain and stiffness in the back and neck

Presence of Kernig and Brudzinski signs

Subsides as temperature drops

Anorexia

Common with most childhood illnesses

Frequently the initial evidence of illness

Almost invariably accompanies acute infections in small children

Persists to a greater or lesser degree throughout febrile stage of illness; often extends into convalescence

Vomiting

Small children vomit readily with illness

A clue to the onset of infection

May precede other signs by several hours

Usually short-lived, but may persist during the illness

Diarrhea

Usually mild, transient diarrhea, but may become severe

Often accompanies respiratory infections, especially viral ones

Is frequent cause of dehydration

Abdominal Pain

Common complaint

Sometimes indistinguishable from pain of appendicitis

Mesenteric lymphadenitis may be a cause

Muscle spasms from vomiting may be a factor, especially in nervous, tense children

Nasal Blockage

Small nasal passages of infants easily blocked by mucosal swelling and exudation

Can interfere with respiration and feeding in infants

May contribute to the development of otitis media and sinusitis

Nasal Discharge

Frequently accompanies respiratory infections

May be thin and watery (rhinorrhea) or thick and purulent, depending on the type and/or stage of infection

Associated with itching

May irritate upper lip and skin surrounding the nose

Cough

Common feature of respiratory disease

May be evident only during the acute phase

May persist several months after a disease runs its course

Respiratory Sounds

Sounds associated with respiratory disease:

Cough

Hoarseness

Grunting

Stridor

Wheezing

Auscultation:

Wheezing

Crackles

Absence of sound

Sore Throat

Frequent complaint of older children

Younger children (unable to describe symptoms) may not complain, even when highly inflamed

Often, child will refuse to take oral fluids or solids

Elastic nature of the tissues in young children may cause less pressure on nerve endings

Unit 4

The Child with Acute Respiratory Infection—cont'd

■ **PATIENT GOAL 1:** Will maintain patent airway

NURSING INTERVENTIONS/*RATIONALES*

Position child in proper body alignment *to allow better lung expansion and improved gas exchange, as well as to prevent aspiration of secretions (prone, semiprone, side-lying; for infants not at risk for aspiration, use supine or side-lying position for sleeping)*

Suction secretions from airway as needed
    Limit each suction attempt to 5 seconds with sufficient time between attempts *to allow reoxygenation*

Position supine with head in "sniffing" position (neck slightly extended and nose pointed to ceiling)
    Avoid neck hyperextension

Assist child in expectorating sputum
    Administer expectorants if prescribed
    Perform chest physiotherapy

Give nothing by mouth *to prevent aspiration of fluids* (e.g., in child with severe tachypnea)

*Administer appropriate pain management

Have emergency equipment available *to avoid delay in treatment if needed*

Avoid throat examination and culture with suspected epiglottitis *because it could cause airway obstruction*

Assist child in splinting any incisional/injured area *to maximize effects of coughing and chest physiotherapy*

EXPECTED OUTCOMES

Airways remain clear

Child breathes easily; respirations are within normal limits (See inside front cover.)

■ **PATIENT GOAL 2:** Will expectorate secretions adequately

NURSING INTERVENTIONS/*RATIONALES*

Ensure adequate fluid intake *to liquefy secretions*

Provide humidified atmosphere *to prevent crusting of nasal secretions and drying of mucous membranes*

Explain importance of expectoration to child and family

Assist child in coughing effectively; provide tissues

Remove accumulated mucus; suction if needed

*Administer pain medications as indicated before attempting to clear airway

Provide nebulization with appropriate solution and equipment as prescribed

Assist with splinting *so child will experience minimal discomfort*

*Perform percussion, vibration, and postural drainage *to facilitate drainage of secretions*

EXPECTED OUTCOME

Older child expectorates secretions without undue stress and fatigue; younger child able to have a productive cough

NURSING DIAGNOSIS: Risk for infection related to presence of infective organisms

■ **PATIENT GOAL 1:** Will exhibit no signs of secondary infection

NURSING INTERVENTIONS/*RATIONALES*

Maintain aseptic environment, using sterile suction catheters and good handwashing

Isolate child as indicated *to prevent nosocomial spread of infection*

Administer antibiotics as prescribed *to prevent or treat infection*

Provide nutritious diet according to child's preferences and ability to consume nourishment *to support body's natural defenses*

Encourage good chest physiotherapy

Teach child and/or family to recognize symptoms early

EXPECTED OUTCOME

Child exhibits evidence of diminishing symptoms of infection

■ **PATIENT GOAL 2:** Will not spread infection to others

NURSING INTERVENTIONS/*RATIONALES*

Use standard precautions (See Nursing Care Plan: The Child at Risk for Infection, p. 341.)

Instruct others (parents, members of staff) in appropriate precautions

Teach affected children protective methods to prevent spread of infection (e.g., handwashing, disposal of soiled tissues)

Limit the number of visitors/family members and screen for any recent illness in visitors

Try to keep infants and small children from placing hands and objects in contaminated areas

Assess home situation and implement protective measures as feasible in individual circumstances

*Administer antimicrobial medications if prescribed

EXPECTED OUTCOME

Others remain free from infection

NURSING DIAGNOSIS: Activity intolerance related to inflammatory process, imbalance between oxygen supply and demand

■ **PATIENT GOAL 1:** Will maintain adequate energy levels

NURSING INTERVENTIONS/*RATIONALES*

Assess child's level of physical tolerance

Assist child in those activities of daily living that may be beyond tolerance

Provide diversional activities appropriate to child's age, condition, capabilities, and interests

Provide diversional play activities that promote rest and quiet but prevent boredom and withdrawal

Provide rest and sleep periods appropriate to age and condition

Instruct child to rest when feeling tired

Balance rest and activity when ambulatory

EXPECTED OUTCOMES

Child plays and rests quietly and engages in activities appropriate to age and capabilities (specify)

Child exhibits no evidence of increased respiratory distress

Child tolerates increasingly more activity

*Dependent nursing action.

The Child with Acute Respiratory Infection—cont'd

■ **PATIENT GOAL 2:** Will receive optimum rest

NURSING INTERVENTIONS/*RATIONALES*

Provide quiet environment

Organize activities for maximum sleep time

Do not perform nonessential treatments or procedures *to maximize rest*

Schedule visiting to allow for sufficient rest

Encourage parents to remain with child

Schedule treatments or other activities around the needs of the child *so that fatigue will be minimized*

*Administer sedatives and analgesics as indicated if ordered *for restlessness and pain*

Encourage frequent rest periods and regular sleep times

Follow child's usual routine for bedtime and nap time

Implement measures to ensure sleep, such as quiet, darkened room

EXPECTED OUTCOMES

Child remains calm, quiet, and relaxed

Child rests a sufficient amount (specify)

NURSING DIAGNOSIS: Pain related to inflammatory process, surgical incision

---

■ **PATIENT GOAL 1:** Will experience either no pain or a reduction of pain/discomfort to level acceptable to child

NURSING INTERVENTIONS/*RATIONALES*

Use local measures (gargles, troches, warmth or cold) to reduce throat pain

Apply heat or cold as appropriate to affected area

Administer analgesic as prescribed (See Nursing Care Plan: The Child in Pain, p. 315.)

Assess response to pain control measures (See Pain Assessment Record, p. 323.)

Encourage diversional activities appropriate to age, condition, and capabilities

EXPECTED OUTCOME

Child has either no pain or an acceptable level of pain

NURSING DIAGNOSIS: Altered family processes related to illness and/or hospitalization of a child

---

■ **PATIENT (FAMILY) GOAL 1:** Will experience reduction of anxiety and increased ability to cope

NURSING INTERVENTIONS/*RATIONALES*

Recognize parental concerns and need for information and support

Explore family's feelings and "problems" surrounding hospitalization and the child's illness

Explain therapy and child's behavior

Provide support as needed

Encourage family-centered care and encourage family to become involved in the child's care

EXPECTED OUTCOMES

Parents ask appropriate questions, discuss child's condition and care calmly, and become involved positively in the child's care

(See also:

Nursing Care Plan: The Family of the Child Who Is Ill or Hospitalized, p. 282.)

Nursing Care Plan: The Child in the Hospital, p. 268.)

*Dependent nursing action.

NURSING CARE PLAN

The Child with a Tonsillectomy

Tonsillectomy is the surgical removal of the palatine tonsils with or without removal of the adenoids (adenoidectomy)

ASSESSMENT

Preoperative

(See Nursing Care Plan: The Child Undergoing Surgery, p. 304.)

Perform routine physical assessment.

Note any evidence of bleeding tendencies.

Note any evidence of infection.

Examine laboratory results for bleeding and clotting times; report any abnormalities.

Note presence of any loose teeth.

Postoperative

(See Nursing Care Plan: The Child Undergoing Surgery, p. 304.)

Assess for evidence of hemorrhage:

  More than usual frequency of swallowing (note frequency when child is sleeping)

  Frequent clearing of throat

Bleeding in throat (insert tongue depressor carefully, using good light source)

Vomiting of bright red (fresh) blood (blood-tinged mucus expected; may be small amounts of dark red or brown [old] blood)

Increased pulse

Decreased blood pressure (late sign)

Pallor

Restlessness (may be difficult to differentiate from general discomfort of surgery)

Assess for evidence of respiratory distress:

  Stridor

  Restlessness

  Agitation

  Increased respiratory rate

  Progressive cyanosis

NURSING DIAGNOSIS: Risk for injury from hemorrhage related to raw, denuded surfaces of tonsil sockets

■ **PATIENT GOAL 1:** Will exhibit no evidence of bleeding

NURSING INTERVENTIONS/*RATIONALES*

Discourage child from coughing frequently or clearing the throat

Avoid use of gargles or vigorous toothbrushing

Avoid foods that are irritating (e.g., high-acid fruit juices, dry toast, raw vegetables) or highly seasoned

Encourage cool liquids or semisoft foods

Avoid placing hard objects in mouth (e.g., straws, toys)

Assess child for evidence of bleeding/hemorrhage (See Assessment above.)

Notify practitioner immediately if continuous bleeding is suspected *since surgery may be required to ligate the bleeding vessel*

Have suction equipment at the bedside; when suctioning is necessary, suction carefully *to avoid trauma to the operative site*

Explain to parents that any sign of bleeding requires immediate medical attention *because hemorrhage may occur 5 to 10 days after surgery as a result of tissue sloughing from the healing process*

EXPECTED OUTCOMES

Child does not aggravate the operative site

There is no evidence of bleeding or hemorrhage

If bleeding occurs, it is quickly assessed and appropriate interventions are implemented

---

NURSING DIAGNOSIS: Pain related to surgical site

■ **PATIENT GOAL 1:** Will have either no pain or a reduction of pain to level acceptable to child

NURSING INTERVENTIONS/*RATIONALES*

*Administer analgesics as prescribed

  Regularly scheduled pain medication is recommended for first 24 hours

*Administer mild sedation as prescribed *for irritability and to lessen crying, which may irritate operative site, thus increasing chance of bleeding*

*Administer medications by route appropriate to child's condition (e.g., rectal or parenteral) *to avoid painful swallowing;* liquid form may also be appropriate for older children *because of throat pain*

*Administer local anesthetics such as tetracaine lollipops or give child ice pops

*Administer antiemetic (transdermal form may be available) *to prevent vomiting*

Avoid offering irritating liquids and solid foods *to avoid irritating the operative site*

Apply an ice collar as tolerated (many children prefer not to have this)

Use nonpharmacologic pain reduction techniques (See p. 339.)

(See Nursing Care Plan: The Child in Pain, p. 315.)

EXPECTED OUTCOMES

Child exhibits absence of or minimum evidence of pain

Child accepts administration of medications with minimum distress

Child rests comfortably

---

*Dependent nursing action.

The Child with a Tonsillectomy—cont'd

■ **PATIENT GOAL 2:** Will exhibit no evidence of increased irritation to operative site

NURSING INTERVENTIONS/*RATIONALES*

Offer diet as tolerated and indicated:
  Cool, liquid diet (usually for first 24 hours) (e.g., water, crushed ice, flavored ice pops, diluted fruit juice)
  Soft diet (usually started 48 to 72 hours) (e.g., gelatin, cooked fruits, sherbet, soup, mashed potatoes)
  Advance to regular diet as tolerated
Avoid fluids with a red or brown color *to distinguish fresh or old blood from the ingested liquids* (not universally accepted)
Avoid substances that irritate denuded areas (e.g., citrus juices, rough foods, highly seasoned foods, carbonated beverages)
Avoid placing hard objects in mouth (e.g., straws, toys)

EXPECTED OUTCOME

Child exhibits minimum acceptable level of discomfort

NURSING DIAGNOSIS: Impaired swallowing related to inflammation and pain

---

■ **PATIENT GOAL 1:** Will receive adequate fluids and nourishment

NURSING INTERVENTIONS/*RATIONALES*

Maintain intravenous fluids, as prescribed, until liquids are tolerated
Offer appropriate diet as tolerated (See previous interventions.)
Provide pain relief (See p. 388.) *so that child is better able to swallow*
Position for optimum swallowing (e.g., high Fowler position, sitting)
Explain to child and family the importance of drinking and eating *because this promotes healing by increasing blood supply to tissues and provides necessary fluids and nourishment*

EXPECTED OUTCOME

Child consumes an adequate amount of fluids and nourishment

■ **PATIENT GOAL 2:** Will not aspirate secretions

NURSING INTERVENTIONS/*RATIONALES*

Assist child to expectorate mucus and drainage without coughing or clearing the throat
Have suction equipment at bedside
Position child on side or stomach while sleeping *to minimize risk of aspiration*

EXPECTED OUTCOME

Child disposes of mucus and drainage appropriately

NURSING DIAGNOSIS: Risk for fluid volume deficit related to nothing by mouth before surgery, reluctance to swallow

---

■ **PATIENT GOAL 1:** Will exhibit adequate hydration

NURSING INTERVENTIONS/*RATIONALES*

Administer fluids as ordered:
  Intravenous
    *Administer fluids as prescribed
    Maintain desired drip rate
    *Add appropriate electrolytes as prescribed
    Maintain integrity of infusion site
  Oral
    Determine and then provide child's fluid preferences
    Employ play for promoting fluid intake (See p. 309.)
Relieve pain *because child is more likely to ingest fluids if pain is controlled* (See also Nursing Diagnosis: Pain related to surgical site, p. 388.)
Maintain and record intake and output
Assess for evidence of hydration
Provide oral hygiene *to encourage interest in taking fluids*

EXPECTED OUTCOMES

Child drinks a sufficient amount of fluids (specify type and amount)
Child exhibits evidence of adequate hydration (e.g., moist mucous membranes, good skin turgor, adequate urinary output for age)
Child receives intravenous fluids as ordered

NURSING DIAGNOSIS: Anxiety/fear related to unfamiliar event, discomfort

---

■ **PATIENT GOAL 1:** Will exhibit absence of or minimum anxiety/fear

NURSING INTERVENTIONS/*RATIONALES*

Explain source of discomfort
(See Nursing Care Plan: The Child in the Hospital, p. 268.)
(See also Nursing Care Plan: The Child Undergoing Surgery, p. 304.)
Anticipate needs
Keep child and bed free from any blood-tinged excretions *since this is often frightening to children*
Reassure child regarding any blood-tinged drainage
Keep emesis basin within easy reach

EXPECTED OUTCOMES

Child rests quietly and readily attends to verbal and nonverbal communication
Child communicates needs and wants in a calm manner

NURSING DIAGNOSIS: Altered family processes related to a child hospitalized for surgery

---

■ **PATIENT (FAMILY) GOAL 1:** Will receive adequate support

**NURSING INTERVENTIONS/*RATIONALES*
AND EXPECTED OUTCOMES**

(See the following:
  Nursing Care Plan: The Family of the Child Who Is Ill or Hospitalized, p. 282.)
  Nursing Care Plan: The Child in the Hospital, p. 268.)
  Nursing Care Plan: The Child Undergoing Surgery, p. 304.)

*Dependent nursing action.

Unit 4

NURSING CARE PLAN

The Child with Acute Otitis Media

Otitis media—An inflammation of the middle ear without reference to etiology or pathogenesis

Acute otitis media (AOM)—A rapid and short onset of signs and symptoms lasting approximately 3 weeks

Otitis media with effusion (OME)—An inflammation of the middle ear in which a collection of fluid is present in the middle ear space

Chronic otitis media with effusion—A middle ear effusion that persists beyond 3 months

ASSESSMENT

Observe for evidence of AOM:

Follows an URI

Otalgia (earache)

Fever

Purulent discharge may or may not be present

Infant or very young child

Crying

Fussy, restless, irritable

Tendency to rub, hold, or pull affected ear

Rolls head side to side

Difficulty comforting child

Loss of appetite

Older child

Crying and/or verbalizes feelings of discomfort

Irritability

Lethargy

Loss of appetite

Otoscopic examination of AOM reveals an intact membrane that appears bright red and bulging, with no visible bony landmarks or light reflex; OME findings may include a slightly injected, dull gray membrane, obscured landmarks, and a visible fluid level or meniscus behind the eardrum if air is present above the fluid.

Observe for evidence of chronic otitis media:

Hearing loss

Difficulty communicating

Feelings of fullness, tinnitus, and/or vertigo may be present

---

NURSING DIAGNOSIS: Pain related to pressure caused by inflammatory process

■ **PATIENT GOAL 1:** Will experience either no pain or a reduction of pain/discomfort to level acceptable to child

NURSING INTERVENTIONS/*RATIONALES*

*Administer analgesics/antipyretics *to reduce pain and fever*

Position for comfort according to needs of individual child

Select local comfort measures according to child's level of cooperation and provision of maximum relief

Apply external heat (with heating pad on low setting, wrapped in a towel) over the ear with child lying on the affected side *to promote comfort*

Apply an ice bag over affected ear *to reduce edema and pressure*

Avoid chewing by offering liquid or soft foods

Position with affected ear in dependent position; have child lie on affected side

(See also Nursing Care Plan: The Child in Pain, p. 315.)

EXPECTED OUTCOME

Child sleeps and rests quietly and exhibits no signs of discomfort.

NURSING DIAGNOSIS: Risk for infection/injury related to inadequate treatment/presence of infective organisms

■ **PATIENT GOAL 1:** Will not experience recurrence of infection

NURSING INTERVENTIONS/*RATIONALES*

Emphasize the importance of following instructions, especially regarding administration of antibiotics:

Maintain regularity of administration

Complete the course of therapy

Explain that although the symptoms usually subside within 24 to 48 hours, the infection is not completely gone until all the prescribed antibiotic is taken

Stress importance of follow-up care.

(See also Community and Home Care Instructions, p. 598.)

Use preventive practices:

Hold or sit infant upright for feedings

Encourage gentle nose blowing during upper respiratory infection, rather than forceful noseblowing, *because of the risk of transferring organisms from the eustachian tube to the middle ear*

Use blowing games (e.g., have older child blow up balloons) or chew sugarless gum *to promote aeration of middle ear during an UPI*

Eliminate tobacco smoke and known or potential allergens from child's environment

EXPECTED OUTCOMES

Child remains free of infection

Family complies with directives (specify)

■ **PATIENT GOAL 2:** Will not experience complications from illness or treatment modalities

NURSING INTERVENTIONS/*RATIONALES*

(See previous patient goal.)

Cleanse external canal of draining ear with sterile cotton swabs or pledgets soaked in normal saline or hydrogen peroxide

When there is profuse drainage, cleanse exudate from ear and surrounding skin and apply moisture barriers such as petrolatum jelly *to prevent excoriation*

When ear wicks or lightly rolled sterile gauze packs have been placed in ear after surgery:

Keep loose enough to allow drainage to flow out of ear *because infection may be transferred to mastoid process*

Avoid getting wicks wet during baths and shampoos

*Dependent nursing action.

Unit 4

The Child with Acute Otitis Media—cont'd

Explain use of ear plugs, if recommended by practitioner when myringotomy tubes are in place *to prevent contaminated water from entering the middle ear during swimming or bathing*

Notify practitioner if grommet (usually tiny, white, spool-shaped plastic tube) falls out of ear canal

Explain to family that this is normal; no immediate intervention needed

Explain to family potential complications of OM that can occur with inadequate treatment:

Conductive hearing loss

Perforated, scarred eardrum

Mastoiditis (inflammation of mastoid air cell system)

Cholesteatoma (cystlike lesion that can invade and destroy surrounding auditory structures)

Intracranial infections, such as meningitis

Explain prevention of ear discomfort during airplane travel:

*Nasal mucosa-shrinking spray or oral decongestant may be prescribed if child has URI

Bottle- or breastfeed, offer pacifier, or offer chewing gum (older child) during descent

EXPECTED OUTCOMES

Child recovers from infection and/or surgery without complications

Child remains comfortable during airplane travel

NURSING DIAGNOSIS: Altered family processes related to illness and/or hospitalization of child, temporary hearing loss

---

■ **PATIENT (FAMILY) GOAL 1:** Will receive adequate support

NURSING INTERVENTIONS/*RATIONALES*

Prepare family for surgical procedure (myringotomy), if appropriate

(See also Nursing Care Plan: The Family of the Child Who Is Ill or Hospitalized, p. 282.)

EXPECTED OUTCOME

Family demonstrates an understanding of procedure

■ **PATIENT (FAMILY) GOAL 2:** Will demonstrate positive coping behaviors toward child (specify)

NURSING INTERVENTIONS/*RATIONALES*

Explain that temporary hearing loss is common with OM *since family may be unaware of this*

Counsel parents about possible behavioral changes with hearing loss, including lack of awareness of environmental sounds

Caution parents that child is not ignoring them or misbehaving; child may be unaware of being spoken to

Speak louder, closer, and facing child

Use patience when communicating with child

Encourage further evaluation if hearing loss persists beyond the acute stage of illness

(See also Nursing Care Plan: The Child with Impaired Hearing, p. 522.)

EXPECTED OUTCOMES

Family will demonstrate positive coping behaviors toward child (specify)

Family will seek appropriate health care for child

---

*Dependent or independent nursing action.

NURSING CARE PLAN

The Child with Asthma

Asthma is a reversible obstructive process characterized by an increased responsiveness and inflammation of the airways, especially the lower airway.

Status asthmaticus is an acute, severe, and prolonged asthma attack in which respiratory distress continues despite vigorous therapeutic measures, especially the administration of sympathomimetics.

ASSESSMENT

Perform a physical assessment. (See p. 28.)

(See also assessment of chest and lungs, p. 50.)

(See also assessment of respirations, p. 378.)

Obtain a family history, especially regarding presence of atopy in family members.

Obtain a health history, including any evidence of atopy (e.g., eczema, rhinitis); evidence of possible precipitating factor(s); previous episodes of shortness of breath, wheezing, and coughing; and any complaints of itching at the front of neck or upper part of back.

Observe for manifestations of bronchial asthma:

Cough

Hacking, paroxysmal, irritative, and nonproductive

Becomes rattling and productive of frothy, clear, gelatinous sputum

Respiratory-related signs

Shortness of breath

Prolonged expiratory phase

Audible wheeze

Often appears pale

May have a malar flush and red ears

Lips deep, dark, red color

May progress to cyanosis of nail beds, circumoral

Restlessness

Apprehension

Anxious facial expression

Sweating may be prominent as the attack progresses

During infancy retractions may occur; clinical symptoms of asthma may be less obvious

Older children may sit upright with shoulders in a hunched-over position, hands on the bed or chair, and arms braced

Speaks with panting and short or broken phrases

Chest

Hyperresonance on percussion

Coarse, loud breath sounds

Wheezes throughout the lung fields

Prolonged expiration

Crackles

Generalized inspiratory and expiratory wheezing; increasingly high pitched

With repeated episodes:

Barrel chest

Elevated shoulders

Use of accessory muscles of respiration

Facial appearance—Flattened malar bones, circles beneath the eyes, narrow nose, prominent upper teeth

Observe for manifestations of severe respiratory distress and impending respiratory failure:

Profuse sweating

Child sits upright; refuses to lie down

Suddenly becomes agitated

Suddenly becomes quiet when previously agitated

Assist with diagnostic procedures and tests (e.g., blood gases, electrolytes, pH; oximetry; urine specific gravity; radiography; pulmonary function tests).

Assess environment for presence of possible allergenic factors.

NURSING DIAGNOSIS: Risk for suffocation related to interaction between individual and allergen(s)

■ **PATIENT GOAL 1:** Will experience no asthmatic episode

NURSING INTERVENTIONS/*RATIONALES*

Teach child and family how to avoid conditions or circumstances that precipitate asthmatic episode

Assist parents in eliminating allergens or other stimuli that trigger exacerbations (See Guidelines box, p. 394, for complete listing.)

Meal planning to eliminate allergenic foods

Removal of pets

Modification of environment:"allergy-proof" home (Guidelines box), especially no smoking in home

Avoid extremes of environmental temperature

When child is exposed to cold air, recommend breathing through nose (not mouth) and wearing a mask or scarf, or cupping hand over nose and mouth, *to create a reservoir of warm air to breathe*

Assist parents in obtaining and/or installing device to control environment (e.g., dehumidifier, air conditioner, electronic air filter)

Teach child and family to recognize early signs and symptoms *so that an impending episode can be controlled before it becomes distressful*

Teach child and family correct use of bronchodilators and antiinflammatory drugs (e.g., corticosteroids, cromolyn sodium), their adverse effects, and the dangers of overuse or underuse of drugs

Teach child how equipment works

Teach child correct use of inhalers, nebulizers, and peak expiratory flow meters (PEFMs) (See Guidelines boxes, p. 397.)

Teach child and family prophylactic treatment when appropriate (e.g., prevent exercise-induced bronchospasm by using medication before exercise)

Explain to child and family possible benefits of hyposensitization therapy when allergen(s) can be defined and cannot be avoided (e.g., pollen, mold) or controlled satisfactorily by drugs

*Administer hyposensitization therapy if prescribed

EXPECTED OUTCOMES

Family makes every effort to remove or avoid possible allergens or precipitating events

Child/family are able to detect signs of an impending episode early and implement appropriate actions

Child/family are able to administer medications and use inhalers and other equipment

*Dependent nursing action.

Unit 4

The Child with Asthma—cont'd

■ **PATIENT GOAL 2:** Will experience optimum health

NURSING INTERVENTIONS/*RATIONALES*

Encourage sound health practices *to support body's natural defenses:*
  Balanced, nutritious diet
  Adequate rest
  Good hygiene
  Appropriate exercise
  Follow-up care
Prevent respiratory infection, *since it can trigger an attack or aggravate the asthmatic state:*
  Avoid exposure to infection
  Take meticulous care of equipment *to avoid bacterial and/or fungal growth*
  Use good handwashing

EXPECTED OUTCOMES

Child and parents practice sound health practices
Child exhibits no evidence of infection

NURSING DIAGNOSIS: Ineffective airway clearance related to allergenic response and inflammation in the bronchial tree

---

■ **PATIENT GOAL 1:** Will exhibit evidence of improved ventilatory capacity

NURSING INTERVENTIONS/*RATIONALES*

Instruct and/or supervise breathing exercises and controlled breathing *to promote proper diaphragmatic breathing, side expansion, and improved chest wall mobility*
Use play techniques for breathing exercises with young children (e.g., blow a pinwheel or blow cotton balls on table) *to extend expiratory time and increase expiratory pressure*
Teach correct use of prescribed medications
Teach correct use of PEFM, nebulizer, and metered-dose inhaler (MDI) if indicated
Teach family to perform percussion and postural drainage and to encourage coughing if indicated
Encourage physical exercise
  Recommend activities requiring short bursts of energy (e.g., baseball, sprints, skiing) *since they may be better tolerated than activities requiring endurance* (e.g., soccer, distance running)
  Recommend swimming *because child breathes air saturated with moisture, and exhaling underwater prolongs expiration and increases end-expiratory pressure*
  Restrict physical activity only when child's condition makes it necessary
Encourage child not to smoke
Assist child and family in selecting activities appropriate to child's capabilities and preferences
Encourage good posture *for maximum lung expansion*

EXPECTED OUTCOMES

Child breathes easily and without dyspnea

Child exhibits improved ventilatory capacity (specify)
Child engages in activities according to abilities and interests (specify)

NURSING DIAGNOSIS: Activity intolerance related to imbalance between oxygen supply and demand

---

■ **PATIENT GOAL 1:** Will receive optimum rest

NURSING INTERVENTIONS/*RATIONALES*

Encourage activities appropriate to child's condition and capabilities (specify)
Provide ample opportunities for sleep, rest, and quiet activities to conserve oxygen supply

EXPECTED OUTCOMES

Child engages in appropriate activities (specify)
Child appears rested

NURSING DIAGNOSIS: Altered family processes related to having a child with a chronic illness

---

■ **PATIENT (FAMILY) GOAL 1:** Will exhibit positive adaptation to the condition

NURSING INTERVENTIONS/*RATIONALES*

Foster positive family relationships
Reinforce positive coping mechanisms of child and family
Use every opportunity to increase parents' and child's understanding of the disease and its therapies *since adequate knowledge is related to family's timely use of preventive and emergency interventions*
Reinforce the need for responding to early signs of impending asthma episode using prescribed medications as needed *to decrease potential for a severe exacerbation*
Intervene appropriately if there is evidence of maladaptation
  Be alert to signs of parental rejection or overprotection
  Be alert to signs that child is depressed and make appropriate referral for psychologic support *since depressed children, especially adolescents, may not comply with therapies as a means of passive suicide*
Teach child and family how to give respiratory treatments *to eliminate any confusion regarding medications or inhalers/nebulizers*
Encourage family to contact school personnel (e.g., nurse, teachers, coaches, principal) to develop a consistent plan of care for school setting
Refer family to appropriate support groups and community agencies

EXPECTED OUTCOMES

Family copes with symptoms and effects of the disease and provides a normal environment for the child
(See also Nursing Care Plan: The Child with Chronic Illness or Disability, p. 287.)

Continued

Unit 4

The Child with Asthma—cont'd

GUIDELINES

Allergy-Proofing the Home

Keep humidity between 30% and 50%; use dehumidifier and/or air conditioner if available; keep air conditioners clean and free of mold; do not use vaporizers or humidifiers.

Encase pillows in zippered, allergen-impermeable covers; or wash pillows in hot water (at least 54.4° C [130° F]) every week.

Encase mattress and box springs in zippered, allergen-impermeable covers.

Use foam rubber mattress and pillows or Dacron pillows and synthetic blankets.

Wash bed linens every 7 to 10 days in hot water (at least 54.4° C).

Encase polyester comforters in allergen-impermeable covers or wash in hot water (at least 54.4° C) every week; if possible, use cotton blankets instead of comforters.

Do not use a canopy above the bed; children should not sleep on a bottom bunk bed.

Store nothing under the bed; keep clothing in a closet with the door shut.

Use washable window shades; avoid heavy curtains; if curtains are used, launder them frequently.

Remove all carpeting, if possible; if not possible, vacuum carpet once or twice a week while the child wears a mask; have child remain out of the room while vacuuming and for 30 minutes after vacuuming.

If possible, use a central vacuum cleaner with a collecting bag outside of the home; or use cleaner filters (e.g., high-efficiency particulate air [HEPA] filters).

Have air and heating ducts cleaned annually; change or clean filters monthly; cover heating vents with filter material (e.g., cheesecloth) to prevent circulation of dust, especially when heat is turned on in the fall.

Remove unnecessary furniture, rugs, stuffed or real animals, toys, books, upholstered furniture, plants, aquariums, and wall hangings from child's room.

Use wipeable furniture (wood, plastic, vinyl, or leather) in place of upholstered furniture; avoid rattan or wicker furniture.

Cover walls with washable paint or wallpaper.

Limit child's exposure to animals (e.g., rabbits, gerbils, hamsters) at school; teach child to stay away from zoos, petting farms, and neighbor's pets.

Change child's clothes after playing outdoors; wash child's hair nightly if child has been outside and pollen count is high.

Keep child indoors while lawn is being mowed, bushes/trees are being trimmed, or when pollen count is high.

Keep windows and doors closed during pollen season; use air conditioner if possible or go to places that are air conditioned, such as libraries and shopping malls, when the weather is hot.

Wet-mop bare floors weekly; wet-dust and clean child's room weekly; child should not be present during cleaning activities.

Wash showers and shower curtains with bleach or Lysol at least once a month.

Limit or avoid child's exposure to tobacco and wood smoke; do not allow cigarette smoking in the house or car; select daycare centers, play areas, and shopping malls that are smoke-free.

Avoid odors, dust, or sprays (e.g., perfumes, talcum powder, room deoderizers, chalk dust at school, fresh paint, and cleaning solutions).

Do not use the cellar (basement) as a play area if it is damp; use a dehumidifier in a damp basement.

Cover all food, including pet food, and put food away in cabinets.

Store garbage in closed containers.

Use pesticide sprays, roach bait traps, and boric acid powder to kill cockroaches; if living in an apartment or adjacent housing, encourage neighbors to work together to get rid of cockroaches.

Repair leaking or dripping faucets; seal cracks and crevices in cabinets and pantry areas.

The Child with Asthma—cont'd

STATUS ASTHMATICUS (SPECIAL NEEDS)

> **NURSING DIAGNOSIS:** Risk for suffocation related to bronchospasm, mucus secretions, edema

■ **PATIENT GOAL 1:** Will experience cessation of bronchospasm

NURSING INTERVENTIONS/*RATIONALES*

Establish IV infusion *for administration of medication and hydration*

*Administer aerosolized bronchodilators and either oral or IV corticosteroids with or without epinephrine as prescribed *to relieve bronchospasm*

Interview parents to determine medications given before admission to avoid possible overdose

Carefully monitor IV aminophylline infusion or oral theophylline *for maximum efficacy and minimum side effects*

Closely monitor vital signs before, during, and after administration for maximum efficacy and minimum side effects

Have emergency equipment and medications readily available *to prevent delay in treatment*

EXPECTED OUTCOMES

Child breathes more easily
Child does not suffocate

■ **PATIENT GOAL 2:** Will exhibit normal respiratory function

NURSING INTERVENTIONS/*RATIONALES*

Administer humidified oxygen by tent, face mask, or cannula *to maintain satisfactory oxygenation*

Closely monitor oxygen saturations and blood gases via pulse oximetry *to detect early or impending hypoxia*

Closely monitor percentage of oxygen delivered *since high levels may depress respirations*

Position for optimum lung expansion
Use high Fowler position
Provide overbed table with pillow on which to lean if more comfortable for child

Implement measures to reduce fear/anxiety *to decrease respiratory efforts and oxygen consumption*
Encourage relaxation techniques *to decrease anxiety and promote lung expansion*

Administer sedatives and tranquilizing agents, if prescribed, with extreme caution and not when agitation is caused by anoxia, *since these drugs can depress respirations and mask signs of anoxia*

Organize activities to allow for rest, sleep, and minimum expenditure of energy

EXPECTED OUTCOMES

Child's respirations are unlabored and within normal limits (See inside front cover.)
Child rests and sleeps comfortably
Child does not experience decreased oxygen saturations

■ **PATIENT GOAL 3:** Will successfully expel bronchial secretions

NURSING INTERVENTIONS/*RATIONALES*

Provide adequate hydration, oral or IV, *to liquefy secretions for easier removal*

Maintain NPO, if necessary, *to prevent aspiration of fluids and food*

Provide humidified atmosphere *to prevent drying of mucous membranes*

Encourage child to cough effectively
Provide tissues
Explain need to remove secretions

Suction, using correct technique, only when necessary

Do not use chest physiotherapy (CPT) during an acute episode, *since it will only agitate an already-anxious, dyspneic child and aggravate the episode*

Position, if necessary, *to prevent aspiration of secretions*
Semiprone
Side-lying

EXPECTED OUTCOMES

Secretions are adequately and easily expelled
Child coughs effectively
Child does not aspirate secretions, food, or fluids

> **NURSING DIAGNOSIS:** Risk for fluid volume deficit related to difficulty taking fluids, insensible fluid losses from hyperventilation, and diaphoresis

■ **PATIENT GOAL 1:** Will exhibit adequate hydration

NURSING INTERVENTIONS/*RATIONALES*

Maintain IV infusion at appropriate rate *since fluid therapy will enhance liquefaction of secretions* (IVs are usually run two-thirds to three-quarters maintenance [unless dehydration present] in order to minimize the risk of pulmonary edema because of high inspiratory pressures)

Encourage oral fluids
Offer fluids when acute respiratory distress subsides *to decrease risk of aspiration*
Avoid cold liquids *since they can trigger reflex bronchospasm*
Give fluids (and food) in small, frequent feedings *to avoid abdominal distention that might interfere with diaphragmatic excursion*
Use play techniques appropriate to child's age *to encourage fluid intake* (See p. 309.)

Measure intake and output

Correct dehydration slowly *since overhydration can increase the accumulation of interstitial pulmonary fluid and lead to increased airway obstruction*

EXPECTED OUTCOME

Child exhibits adequate hydration

> **NURSING DIAGNOSIS:** Risk for injury (respiratory acidosis, electrolyte imbalance) related to hypoventilation, dehydration

■ **PATIENT GOAL 1:** Will not experience acidosis

NURSING INTERVENTIONS/*RATIONALES*

Closely monitor blood pH *since pH less than 7.25 impairs systemic, pulmonary, and coronary blood flow, and normal pH enhances effect of bronchodilators*

*Administer sodium bicarbonate as ordered *to prevent or correct acidosis*

Maintain IV infusion *for administration of emergency medications and to prevent dehydration*

*Dependent nursing action.

Continued

The Child with Asthma—cont'd

Prevent vomiting and subsequent dehydration; initially, child will experience alkalosis, but vomiting that becomes severe or uncontrolled can lead to acidosis

Implement measures to improve ventilation *because hypoventilation may cause an accumulation of carbon dioxide, which will decrease pH*

EXPECTED OUTCOME

Child exhibits no evidence of respiratory acidosis

■ **PATIENT GOAL 2:** Will exhibit normal serum electrolytes

NURSING INTERVENTIONS/*RATIONALES*

Closely monitor serum electrolytes *since dehydration, as well as medications, can alter normal serum electrolytes*

Maintain IV infusion at appropriate rate

Prevent dehydration and vomiting *since they cause electrolyte imbalances*

EXPECTED OUTCOME

Child exhibits normal serum electrolytes

NURSING DIAGNOSIS: Altered family processes related to emergency hospitalization of child

---

■ **PATIENT (FAMILY) GOAL 1:** Will experience reduction of anxiety

NURSING INTERVENTIONS/*RATIONALES*

Keep parents informed of child's condition

Encourage expression of feelings, especially about the severity of condition and prognosis

Allow parents to be with child as much as possible by encouraging family-centered care concepts

Point out any evidence of improvement *to encourage positive coping behaviors*

When possible, schedule treatments and care to child's routines

Reduce sensory stimuli by maintaining quiet, relaxed environment

EXPECTED OUTCOMES

Family verbalizes concerns and spends time with child

Family exhibits no signs of distress

(See also:
  Nursing Care Plan: The Family of the Child Who Is Ill or Hospitalized, p. 282.)
  Nursing Care Plan: The Child in the Hospital, p. 268.)

The Child with Asthma—cont'd

GUIDELINES

Use of a Peak Expiratory Flow Meter (PEFM)

1. Before each use, make sure the sliding marker or arrow on the PEFM is at the bottom of the numbered scale.
2. Stand up straight.
3. Remove gum or any food from the mouth.
4. Close your lips tightly around the mouthpiece. Be sure to keep your tongue away from the mouthpiece.
5. Blow out as hard and as quickly as you can, a "fast, hard puff."
6. Note the number by the marker on the numbered scale.
7. Repeat entire routine three times; but wait at least 30 seconds between each routine.
8. Record the *highest* of the three readings, not the average.
9. Measure your peak expiratory flow rate (PEFR) close to the same time and same way each day (e.g., morning and evening; or before and/or 15 minutes after taking medication).
10. Keep a chart of your PEFRs.

GUIDELINES

Use of a Metered-Dose Inhaler (MDI)*

Steps for Checking How Much Medicine Is in the Canister

1. If the canister is new, it is full.
2. If the canister has been used repeatedly, it might be empty. (Check product label to see how many inhalations should be in each canister.)
3. To check how much medicine is left in the canister, put the canister (not the mouthpiece) in a cup of water. Do not use this method with MDIs that contain hydrofluoroalkanes or dry powder.
   a. If the canister sinks to the bottom, it is full.
   b. If the canister floats sideways on the surface, it is empty.

Steps for Using the Inhaler

1. Remove the cap and hold inhaler upright.
2. Shake the inhaler.
3. Tilt the head back slightly and breathe out slowly.
4. With the inhaler in an upright position, insert the mouthpiece:
   a. About 3 to 4 cm from the mouth *or*
   b. Into an aerochamber *or*
   c. Into the mouth, forming an airtight seal between the lips and the mouthpiece
5. At the end of a normal expiration, depress the top of the inhaler canister firmly to release the medication (into either the aerochamber or the mouth) and breathe in slowly (about 3 to 5 seconds). Relax the pressure on the top of the canister.
6. Hold the breath for at least 5 to 10 seconds to allow the aerosol medication to reach deeply into the lungs.
7. Remove the inhaler and breathe out slowly through the nose.
8. Wait 1 minute between puffs (if an additional one is needed).
9. To determine if child is using the inhaler properly, have child use the device in front of a mirror. If vapor does not appear on the mirror, the inhaler is being used correctly.

Modified from National Heart, Lung, and Blood Institute, National Institutes of Health: *Guidelines for the diagnosis and management of asthma,* Pub No 91-3042, Bethesda, MD, Aug 1991.

*NOTE: Inhaled dry powder such as Pulmicort requires a different inhalation technique. To use a dry powder inhaler, the base of the device is turned until a click is heard. It is important to close the mouth tightly around the mouthpiece of the inhaler and inhale rapidly.

Unit 4

NURSING CARE PLAN

The Child with Cystic Fibrosis

Cystic fibrosis is a genetic multisystem disorder that primarily affects the exocrine (mucus-producing) glands.

ASSESSMENT

Perform a physical assessment. (See p. 28.)

Take health and family histories.

Observe for any of the following clinical manifestations of cystic fibrosis:

Meconium ileus (newborn)

Abdominal distention

Vomiting

Failure to pass stools

Rapid development of dehydration

Gastrointestinal

Large, bulky, loose, frothy, extremely foul-smelling stools

Voracious appetite (early in disease)

Loss of appetite (later in disease)

Weight loss

Marked tissue wasting

Failure to grow

Distended abdomen

Abdominal cramps

Foul-smelling flatus

Thin extremities

Sallow skin

Evidence of deficiency of fat-soluble vitamins (i.e., A, D, E, K)

Anemia

Pulmonary

Initial manifestations:

Wheezy respirations

Dry, nonproductive cough

Eventually:

Increased dyspnea

Paroxysmal cough

Evidence of obstructive emphysema and patchy areas of atelectasis

Progressive involvement:

Overinflated, barrel-shaped chest

Cyanosis

Clubbing of fingers and toes

Repeated episodes of bronchitis and bronchopneumonia

Assist with diagnostic procedures that include:

Chest radiography for evidence of generalized obstructive emphysema, atelectasis, bronchopneumonia

Sweat chloride concentrations (greater than 60 mEq/L is diagnostic)

Pancreatic enzyme measurements from stool specimens

Fat-absorption tests of stool specimens

Pulmonary function tests

NURSING DIAGNOSIS: Ineffective airway clearance related to secretion of thick, tenacious mucus

- **PATIENT GOAL 1:** Will expectorate mucus

NURSING INTERVENTIONS/RATIONALES

Assist child to expectorate sputum *to promote airway clearance*

*Provide nebulization with appropriate solution and equipment as prescribed

Suction if needed *to clear secretions*

Perform chest physiotherapy *to loosen secretions*

Teach child how to use Flutter Clearance Device† *to facilitate removal of mucus*

Teach child how to use ThAIRapy vest‡ which provides high-frequency chest wall oscillation *to help loosen secretions*

Encourage child to force expiration ("huffing") with the glottis partially closed *to help move secretions from the small airways to large airways where they can be expectorated*

Observe child closely after aerosol therapy and chest physiotherapy *to prevent aspiration because large volumes of sputum may be thinned suddenly*

*Administer DNase (recombinant human deoxyribonuclease) as prescribed *to decrease viscosity of mucus*

Encourage physical exercise *to stimulate mucus secretion*

EXPECTED OUTCOMES

Child will expectorate mucus

Child will engage in physical exercise appropriate to child's condition

---

NURSING DIAGNOSIS: Impaired gas exchange related to airway obstruction

- **PATIENT GOAL 1:** Will demonstrate signs of adequate gas exchange

NURSING INTERVENTIONS/RATIONALES

Maintain patent airway

Position *for maximum ventilatory efficiency* such as high Fowler position or sitting, leaning forward

Promote expectoration of mucus secretions

Monitor vital signs, arterial blood gases, and pulse oximetry readings *to detect/prevent hypoxemia*

*Administer supplemental oxygen as prescribed/needed

Closely monitor child, *since oxygen-induced carbon dioxide narcosis is a hazard of oxygen therapy in the child with chronic pulmonary disease*

Encourage physical exercise appropriate to child's condition *because it is often effective in clearing accumulated lung secretions and in increasing the capacity to endure exercise before experiencing dyspnea*

EXPECTED OUTCOMES

Respiratory rate is regular and within normal limits (See inside front cover.)

Blood gases/oxygen saturation values are within normal limits

Tissue oxygenation is adequate

Child engages in physical exercise appropriate to child's condition

---

*Dependent nursing action.

†Manufactured by Scandipharm, Inc., 22 Inverness Center Parkway, Birmingham, AL 35342; (205) 991-8085 or (800) 950-8085; Web site, www.scandipharm.com.

‡For information about the ThAIRapy vest, contact American Biosystems, 20 Yorkton Ct., St. Paul, MN 55117; (800) 426-4224.

The Child with Cystic Fibrosis—cont'd

NURSING DIAGNOSIS: Ineffective breathing pattern related to tracheobronchial obstruction

- **PATIENT GOAL 1:** Will exhibit normal respiratory function

NURSING INTERVENTIONS/*RATIONALES*

Allow position of comfort

Promote rest

Maintain patent airway

Encourage deep breathing by use of spirometry or developmentally appropriate games

Encourage child to engage in appropriate exercise

Implement measures to reduce anxiety and apprehension

Organize activities *to allow for minimum expenditure of energy*

EXPECTED OUTCOMES

Child rests and sleeps quietly

Respirations are unlabored

Respirations remain within normal limits (See inside front cover.)

NURSING DIAGNOSIS: Altered nutrition: less than body requirements related to inability to digest nutrients, loss of appetite (advanced disease)

- **PATIENT GOAL 1:** Will exhibit signs of adequate digestion

NURSING INTERVENTIONS/*RATIONALES*

*Administer pancreatic enzymes with meals and snacks as prescribed *since replacement of enzymes is necessary for digestion to occur in the child with pancreatic insufficiency*

Teach child and family proper administration of pancreatic enzymes:

Take with meals or snacks

Capsules can be swallowed whole or opened and sprinkled on food but not crushed or chewed

Observe frequency and nature of stools *because fewer, less fatty and less foul-smelling stools indicate adequate enzyme replacement*

Monitor child's physical growth (height, weight) *because appropriate growth correlates to adequate digestion of nutrients*

EXPECTED OUTCOMES

Child will receive appropriate amount of pancreatic enzyme medication

Child will not have more than two or three stools per day

Child will have an appropriate increase in height and weight

- **PATIENT GOAL 2:** Will receive adequate nourishment

NURSING INTERVENTIONS/*RATIONALES*

Provide well-balanced, high-calorie, high-protein diet with any modifications that may be prescribed *because impaired intestinal absorption places child at risk for malnutrition*

Implement measures to encourage adequate nourishment, especially when appetite is diminished because of infection and/or progressive lung involvement (See Nursing Care Plan: The Child with Special Nutritional Needs, p. 313.)

Provide adequate salt, especially when sweating (e.g., due to fever, hot weather, physical exertion) *since abnormally high sodium and chloride concentrations in the sweat predispose child to rapid loss of these electrolytes*

Salt supplementation through food or liquids (e.g., a sports drink such as Gatorade) may be necessary during periods of salt depletion

Identify sodium content of formula infant receives and of liquids the older child drinks

Caution child and family about not restricting salt intake

*Administer water-miscible multivitamin preparations, as prescribed *because impaired digestion and absorption of fat decreases the uptake of fat-soluble vitamins (i.e., A, D, E, K)*

*Administer iron preparations, as prescribed, *because impaired digestion can cause iron-deficiency anemia*

*Administer supplemental tube feedings or total parenteral nutrition, when prescribed, for the child experiencing failure to thrive despite adequate nutritional support

EXPECTED OUTCOMES

Child eats a well-balanced diet and exhibits a satisfactory weight gain

Child receives adequate electrolytes, especially sodium

Child does not experience vitamin deficiency, anemia, or malnutrition

NURSING DIAGNOSIS: Altered growth and development related to inadequate digestion of nutrients

- **PATIENT GOAL 1:** Will receive adequate nourishment for growth

NURSING INTERVENTIONS/*RATIONALES*

(See previous Patient Goal 2.)

Monitor child for steady growth by charting on height and weight growth chart *since failure to take in adequate nutrients can lead to impaired growth*

EXPECTED OUTCOME

Child exhibits normal growth

- **PATIENT GOAL 2:** Will attain maximum expected developmental potential

**NURSING INTERVENTIONS/*RATIONALES*
AND EXPECTED OUTCOMES**

(See Nursing Care Plan: The Child with Chronic Illness or Disability, p. 287.)

*Dependent nursing action.

Continued

Unit 4

The Child with Cystic Fibrosis—cont'd

NURSING DIAGNOSIS: Risk for infection related to impaired body defenses, presence of mucus as medium for growth of organisms

■ **PATIENT GOAL 1:** Will exhibit no evidence of infection

NURSING INTERVENTIONS/*RATIONALES***
Instruct family and child (if old enough) in administration of prophylactic antibiotics, if prescribed
Instruct family to have child immunized yearly against influenza and pneumococcus
Teach child/family about importance of good handwashing, especially before handling respiratory equipment

EXPECTED OUTCOME
Child is free of infection

NURSING DIAGNOSIS: Altered family processes related to situational crises

■ **PATIENT (FAMILY) GOAL 1:** Will receive adequate support

NURSING INTERVENTIONS/*RATIONALES***
Refer to appropriate support groups and agencies
(See Nursing Care Plan: The Family of the Child Who Is Ill or Hospitalized, p. 282.)

(See also Nursing Care Plan: The Child with Chronic Illness or Disability, p. 287.)

EXPECTED OUTCOMES
Family demonstrates the ability to cope with child's illness (specify behaviors)
Family contacts and becomes involved with appropriate agencies

NURSING DIAGNOSIS: Impaired social interaction related to frequent hospitalizations, confinement to home, fatigue

(See Nursing Diagnosis: Impaired social interaction, p. 293.)

NURSING DIAGNOSIS: Anticipatory grieving related to perceived potential loss of child

(See Nursing Diagnosis: Anticipatory grieving, p. 495.)
(See also:
   Nursing Care Plan: The Child with Chronic Illness or Disability, p. 287.)
   Nursing Care Plan: The Child in the Hospital, p. 268.)
   Nursing Care Plan: The Family of the Child Who Is Ill or Hospitalized, p. 282.)

NURSING CARE PLAN

The Child with Respiratory Failure

Respiratory insufficiency:
1. Increased work of breathing but with gas exchange function near normal (ventilatory insufficiency)
2. Inability to maintain normal blood gas tensions and development of hypoxemia and acidosis secondary to carbon dioxide retention

Respiratory failure—Inability of the respiratory apparatus to maintain adequate oxygenation of the blood, with or without carbon dioxide retention

Respiratory arrest—Cessation of respiration

Apnea—Absence of airflow (breathing)
Central—Absence of airflow and respiratory effort
Obstructive—Absence of airflow but presence of respiratory effort
Mixed—Absence of airflow and respiratory effort (central apnea), followed by resumption of respiratory effort without airflow (obstructive apnea)
Normal apnea—Short periods of central apnea (≤15 seconds) can be normal at any age
Pathologic apnea—Respiratory pause that is prolonged (≥20 seconds) or associated with cyanosis, marked pallor or hypotonia, or bradycardia

ASSESSMENT

(See Nursing Care Plan: The Child with Respiratory Dysfunction, p. 378.)

Be alert to the possibility of respiratory failure in children with predisposing conditions:

Obstructive lung disease—Increased resistance to airflow in either upper or lower respiratory tract
Restrictive lung disease—Impaired lung expansion resulting from loss of lung volume, decreased distensibility, or chest wall disturbance
Primary inefficient gas transfer—Insufficient alveolar ventilation for carbon dioxide removal or impaired oxygenation of pulmonary capillary blood as a result of dysfunction of the respiratory control mechanism or a diffusion defect

Observe for manifestations of respiratory failure:
Cardinal signs:
Restlessness
Tachypnea
Tachycardia
Diaphoresis
Early but less obvious signs:
Mood changes, such as euphoria or depression
Headache

Altered depth and pattern of respirations
Hypertension
Exertional dyspnea
Anorexia
Increased cardiac output and renal output
Central nervous system symptoms (decreased efficiency, impaired judgment, anxiety, confusion, restlessness, irritability, and depressed level of consciousness)
Flaring nares
Chest wall retractions
Expiratory grunt
Wheezing and/or prolonged expiration
Signs of more severe hypoxia:
Hypotension or hypertension
Dimness of vision
Somnolence
Stupor
Coma
Dyspnea
Depressed respirations
Bradycardia
Cyanosis, peripheral or central
Assist with diagnostic procedures and tests (e.g., blood gases and pH, oximetry, radiography, pulmonary function).

NURSING DIAGNOSIS: Impaired gas exchange related to altered oxygen supply, altered pulmonary blood flow, alveolar-capillary membrane changes

■ **PATIENT GOAL 1:** Will exhibit signs of improved ventilatory capacity and gas exchange

NURSING INTERVENTIONS/*RATIONALES*
Position for optimum lung expansion:
Elevate head, unless contraindicated
Frequently check positioning *because if child "slides down," the abdomen compresses the diaphragm, causing decreased lung expansion*
Maintain proper body alignment
Maintain open airway
Avoid neck hyperextension; use "sniffing" position
Encourage child to expectorate secretions
Suction secretions, using correct technique, when necessary
*Administer supplemental oxygen (nasal prongs, mist tent, incubator, hood, or mechanical ventilator) as prescribed/ needed

Maintain child NPO, if necessary, *to prevent aspiration*
Provide ongoing assessment:
Visual observation of skin color *to estimate arterial oxygen saturation*
Observation of respiratory effort or distress
Observation of diaphragmatic movement, lung expansion, and use of accessory muscles
Auscultation of breath sounds
Closely monitor blood gas measurements and pulse oximeter and transcutaneous oxygen readings *to detect changes in oxygenation*
Have emergency equipment and medications readily available *to prevent delay in treatment*
Anticipate possible need for intubation, tracheostomy, and mechanical ventilation
Organize activities to allow for periods of rest and sleep *to decrease oxygen consumption*
Implement measures that reduce fear and anxiety *to decrease respiratory efforts and oxygen consumption*

EXPECTED OUTCOME
Child exhibits improved ventilatory capacity and gas exchange (specify)

*Dependent nursing action.

Continued

The Child with Respiratory Failure—cont'd

NURSING DIAGNOSIS: Risk for suffocation related to mechanical or functional obstruction to airflow

- **PATIENT GOAL 1:** Will continue or resume breathing

NURSING INTERVENTIONS/*RATIONALES*

Implement appropriate emergency management of airway obstruction (See p. 648.) and/or Cardiopulmonary Resuscitation (See p. 643.)

EXPECTED OUTCOMES

Child resumes breathing
Child's airway remains open

NURSING DIAGNOSIS: Altered family processes related to situational crisis (seriously ill child)

- **PATIENT (FAMILY) GOAL 1:** Will receive adequate support

NURSING INTERVENTIONS/*RATIONALES*

Keep family informed of child's progress
Explain procedures and therapies
Reinforce information regarding child's condition
Encourage expression of feelings, especially about the severity of condition and prognosis
Arrange for presence of family support systems, if possible (e.g., friends, clergy)

EXPECTED OUTCOMES

Family exhibits evidence of understanding and coping (specify)
(See also:
   Nursing Care Plan: The Family of the Child Who Is Ill or Hospitalized, p. 282.)
   Nursing Care Plan: The Child in the Hospital, p. 268.)

COMMUNITY FOCUS

Importance of Cardiopulmonary Certification in the Schools

Today many children with respiratory disorders and special needs, such as those with tracheostomies, are mainstreamed into regular classrooms. Some of these children have health conditions that could result in the necessity to perform emergency care (i.e., cardiopulmonary resuscitation [CPR]). However, a survey of educators and classroom aides who had medically fragile children in their classrooms revealed that only 40% of these individuals had current CPR certification.* Sixty-eight percent of these individuals also stated that they did not feel adequately prepared to deal with potential emergency situations involving medically fragile children. As medical technology advances, the number of children who could require CPR in the schools will increase, as will the need for interdisciplinary collaboration between members of the health care team and those in the educational system. School nurses can work with teachers, classroom aides, and various community groups to facilitate this collaboration. For example, school nurses can use their contacts in the community to inform community groups of the need for CPR training and first aid classes in the schools. In addition, school nurses can provide in-service classes on emergency procedures, develop contingency plans and protocols to be used in emergency situations, and inform teachers and aides of community sites where they can receive CPR training.

*Krier JJ: Involvement of educational staff in the health care of medically fragile children, *Pediatr Nurs* 19(3):251-254, 1993.

Unit 4

NURSING CARE OF THE CHILD WITH GASTROINTESTINAL DYSFUNCTION

The gastrointestinal tract consists of the alimentary canal (mouth, esophagus, stomach, intestines, colon, and rectum), liver, pancreas, and gallbladder.

NURSING CARE PLAN

The Child with Gastrointestinal Dysfunction

ASSESSMENT

Take a careful health history, including history of present illness.

Observe for manifestations of gastrointestinal dysfunction:

Failure to thrive—Deceleration from established growth pattern, or consistently below the 5th percentile for height and weight on standard growth charts; sometimes accompanied by developmental delays

Spitting up or regurgitation—Passive transfer of gastric contents into the esophagus or mouth

Vomiting—Forceful ejection of gastric contents; involves a complex process under central nervous system control that causes salivation, pallor, sweating, and tachycardia; usually accompanied by nausea

    Projectile vomiting—Vomiting accompanied by vigorous peristaltic waves and typically associated with pyloric stenosis or pylorospasm

Nausea—Unpleasant sensation vaguely referred to the throat or abdomen with an inclination to vomit

Constipation—Passage of firm or hard stools or infrequent passage of stools with associated symptoms such as difficulty expelling the stools, blood-streaked stools, and abdominal discomfort

Encopresis—Overflow of incontinent stool causing soiling; often due to fecal retention or impaction

Diarrhea—Increase in the number of stools with an increased water content as a result of alterations of water and electrolyte transport by the GI tract; may be acute or chronic

Hypoactive, hyperactive, or absent bowel sounds—Evidence of intestinal motility problems that may be caused by inflammation or obstruction

Abdominal distention—Protuberant contour of the abdomen that may be caused by delayed gastric emptying, accumulation of gas or stool, inflammation, or obstruction

Abdominal pain—Pain associated with the abdomen that may be localized or diffuse, acute or chronic; often caused by inflammation, obstruction, or hemorrhage

Gastrointestinal bleeding—May be from an upper or lower GI source and may be acute or chronic

    Hematemesis—Vomiting of bright red blood or denatured blood that results from bleeding in the upper GI tract or from swallowed blood from the nose or oropharynx

Hematochezia—Passage of bright red blood per rectum, usually indicating lower GI tract bleeding

Melena—Passage of dark-colored, "tarry" stools due to denatured blood, suggesting upper GI tract bleeding or bleeding from the right colon

Jaundice—Yellow coloration of the skin and sclerae associated with liver dysfunction

Dysphagia—Difficulty swallowing caused by abnormalities in the neuromuscular function of the pharynx or upper esophageal sphincter or by disorders of the esophagus

Dysfunctional swallowing—Impaired swallowing due to central nervous system defects or structural defects of the oral cavity, pharynx, or esophagus; can cause feeding problems or aspiration

Fever—Common manifestation of illness in children with GI disorders; usually associated with dehydration, infection, or inflammation

Observe the manifestations of possible mechanical/paralytic intestinal obstruction:

Colicky abdominal pain—Results from peristalsis attempting to overcome the obstruction

Abdominal distention—Result of accumulation of gas and fluid above the level of the obstruction

Vomiting—Often the earliest sign of a high obstruction; a later sign of lower obstruction (may be bilious or feculent)

Constipation and obstipation—Early signs of low obstructions; later signs of higher obstructions

Dehydration—Results from losses of large quantities of fluid and electrolytes into the intestine

Rigid and boardlike abdomen—Results from increased distention

Bowel sounds—Gradually diminish and cease

Respiratory distress—Occurs as the diaphragm is pushed up into the pleural cavity

Shock—Plasma volume diminishes as fluids and electrolytes are lost from the bloodstream into the intestinal lumen

Sepsis—Caused by bacterial proliferation with invasion into the circulation

Assist with diagnostic procedures (e.g., upper/lower GI series, fiberoptic endoscopy, esophagoscopy, sigmoidoscopy, colonoscopy, manometry, radiography, mucosal biopsy).

Collect specimens for stool examination, blood analyses (e.g., RBC, WBC, enzyme studies).

Continued

Unit 4

The Child with Gastrointestinal Dysfunction—cont'd

NURSING DIAGNOSIS: Impaired swallowing related to pain, neuromuscular impairment, presence of mechanical devices (e.g., ET tube), long-term, nonoral feedings

■ **PATIENT GOAL 1:** Will swallow without aspiration

NURSING INTERVENTIONS/*RATIONALES*
Elevate head of bed to prevent aspiration
Assess neurologic function before attempting feeding *to prevent aspiration*
Stroke anterior aspect of throat (external) in distal to proximal direction *to encourage swallowing*
Relieve pain, if present, *to encourage swallowing*
Use strategies *to overcome feeding resistance* (Box 4-21)

EXPECTED OUTCOME
Child swallows without aspiration

■ **PATIENT GOAL 2:** Will receive adequate fluids and nourishment by alternative means

NURSING INTERVENTIONS/*RATIONALES*
Feed child by enteral means *to provide nourishment*
  Nasogastric tube (continuous or intermittent) (See p. 252.)
  Gastrostomy (See p. 253.)
*Feed child by parenteral means *to provide nourishment*
  Total parenteral nutrition (See p. 251.)
Monitor intake, output, and weight *to assess adequacy of nourishment*

EXPECTED OUTCOMES
Child consumes sufficient calories and nutrients
Child demonstrates satisfactory weight gain

NURSING DIAGNOSIS: Risk for fluid volume deficit related to active losses in stools or vomitus

■ **PATIENT GOAL 1:** Will have normal fluid volume

NURSING INTERVENTIONS/*RATIONALES*
*Administer IV fluids as ordered *to prevent dehydration*
*Administer oral rehydration solutions as ordered *to prevent dehydration*
Modify diet as appropriate *to decrease losses and promote hydration*
Monitor intake, output, and weight *to assess hydration*
Encourage fluid intake as appropriate *to promote hydration*
Use play *to encourage fluid intake* (See p. 309.)

EXPECTED OUTCOMES
Child receives sufficient fluids to replace losses
Child exhibits signs of adequate hydration (specify)

NURSING DIAGNOSIS: Diarrhea related to dietary indiscretions, food sensitivity, helminths, microorganisms

■ **PATIENT GOAL 1:** Will exhibit adequate hydration

**NURSING INTERVENTIONS/*RATIONALES*
AND EXPECTED OUTCOMES**
(See previous patient goal.)

■ **PATIENT GOAL 2:** Will experience reduction in excessive intestinal losses

NURSING INTERVENTIONS/*RATIONALES*
Modify diet as appropriate *to decrease losses*
Avoid foods known to be irritating or known to cause an allergic response *to decrease losses*
*Administer antimicrobials as ordered *to treat infection*
(See also Nursing Care Plan for specific condition.)

EXPECTED OUTCOME
Child exhibits normal bowel elimination

NURSING DIAGNOSIS: Constipation related to immobility, neuromuscular impairment, medications

■ **PATIENT GOAL 1:** Will experience adequate bowel elimination

NURSING INTERVENTIONS/*RATIONALES*
Modify diet as appropriate *to prevent constipation*
  High-fiber diet (Box 4-22)
  Increased fluid intake
Establish regular time for elimination (e.g., after a meal) *to encourage defecation*
Provide privacy for toileting appropriate to child's age and development *to promote relaxation for defecation*
Increase child's physical activity, if appropriate, *to help prevent constipation*
Teach child and family about bowel function, interventions, and need for persistence *in preventing constipation*
*Administer mineral oil (give carefully *to avoid risk of aspiration*) or stool softeners as prescribed *to prevent constipation*
*Administer enemas and/or suppositories as prescribed *for evacuation*

EXPECTED OUTCOMES
Child exhibits normal bowel elimination
(See also:
  Specific gastrointestinal disorder for appropriate interventions.)
  Nursing Care Plan: The Child in the Hospital, p. 268.)
  Nursing Care Plan: The Family of the Child Who Is Ill or Hospitalized, p. 282.)

*Dependent nursing action.

Unit 4

The Child with Gastrointestinal Dysfunction—cont'd

BOX 4-21

Components of a Care Plan to Overcome Feeding Resistance

Simulate normal feeding interactions:
 Hold and cuddle infant in "en face" feeding position.
 Engage in eye contact with infant.
 Engage in verbal interaction with infant.
Provide tactile stimulation:
 Begin with torso and progress to head and neck.
 Apply firm, consistent pressure.
 Use palm or hand or textured object (e.g., wash cloth).
 Gradually move toward mouth, cheeks, and lips.
 Stroke oral area from cheeks to lips.
 Pace according to child's tolerance.
Overcome oral hypersensitivity (sensitivity to intraoral stimulation).
 Provide oral stimulation as above.
 When external oral stimulation is tolerated, attempt massage of gums and tongue (use finger or soft rubber item).
 Massage gums from center and move toward molar region, working gradually from anterior to posterior.

Withdraw stimulus and close child's mouth if child gags.
Encourage oral exploration:
 Assist child in mouthing hands, fingers, toes, or soft rubber toys.
 Play oral games, e.g., blowing a kiss, kissing an object (toy animal).
Provide oral feedings:
 Introduce small volumes (even 3 to 5 ml) as early as possible.
 Offer feedings consistently (water, formula).
 Avoid force feeding.
Provide feeding stimulation during tube feedings:
 Hold child in feeding position.
 Provide oral stimulation during bolus feedings.
 Give oral feedings before tube feedings.
 Give bolus feedings in response to hunger when possible rather than on predetermined schedule.
Provide nonnutritive sucking to encourage use of oral musculature.

Data from Orr MJ, Allen SS: Optimal oral experiences for infants on long-term total parenteral nutrition, *Nutr Clin Pract* 9:288-295, 1986.

BOX 4-22

High-Fiber Foods

Bread, Grains

Whole-grain bread or rolls
Whole-grain cereals
Bran
Pancakes, waffles, and muffins with fruit or bran
Unrefined (brown) rice

Vegetables

Raw vegetables, especially broccoli, cabbage, carrots, cauliflower, celery, lettuce, and spinach
Cooked vegetables, such as those listed above, and asparagus, beans, brussels sprouts, corn, potatoes, rhubarb, squash, string beans, and turnips

Fruits

Raw fruits, especially those with skins or seeds, other than ripe banana or avocado
Raisins, prunes, or other dried fruits

Miscellaneous

Nuts, seeds, legumes (beans), popcorn
High-fiber snack bars

Unit 4

NURSING CARE PLAN

The Child with Appendicitis

Appendicitis is an inflammation of the vermiform appendix (blind sac at the end of the cecum).

ASSESSMENT

Take a careful history of illness.
Observe for clinical manifestations of appendicitis (Community Focus box):
　Right lower quadrant abdominal pain
　Fever
　Rigid abdomen
　Decreased or absent bowel sounds
　Vomiting (commonly follows onset of pain)
　Constipation or diarrhea may be present
　Anorexia
　Tachycardia, rapid, shallow breathing
　Pallor
　Lethargy
　Irritability
　Stooped posture

Observe for signs of peritonitis:
　Fever
　Sudden relief from pain (after perforation)
　Subsequent increase in pain, which is usually diffuse and accompanied by rigid guarding of the abdomen
　Progressive abdominal distention
　Tachycardia
　Rapid, shallow breathing
　Pallor
　Chills
　Irritability
Assist with diagnostic procedures (e.g., white blood count, abdominal radiography).

PREOPERATIVE CARE

> **NURSING DIAGNOSIS:** Pain related to inflamed appendix

■ **PATIENT GOAL 1:** Will experience either no pain or a reduction of pain to level acceptable to child

NURSING INTERVENTIONS/*RATIONALES*
(See Nursing Care Plan: The Child in Pain, p. 315.)
Allow position of comfort (usually with legs flexed) *because it may vary among children*
Provide small pillow *for splinting of abdomen*
*Administer analgesia *to provide pain relief*

EXPECTED OUTCOME
Child rests quietly, reports and/or exhibits no evidence of discomfort

> **NURSING DIAGNOSIS:** Risk for fluid volume deficit related to decreased intake and losses secondary to loss of appetite, vomiting

■ **PATIENT GOAL 1:** Will receive fluids for adequate hydration

NURSING INTERVENTIONS/*RATIONALES*
Maintain NPO *to minimize losses through vomiting and to minimize abdominal distention*
Maintain integrity of infusion site *for IV fluids and electrolytes*
*Administer IV fluids and electrolytes as prescribed
Monitor intake and output *to assess hydration*

EXPECTED OUTCOMES
Child receives sufficient fluids to replace losses
Child exhibits signs of adequate hydration (specify)

> **NURSING DIAGNOSIS:** Risk for infection related to possibility of rupture

■ **PATIENT GOAL 1:** Will experience minimized risk of infection

NURSING INTERVENTIONS/*RATIONALES*
Closely monitor vital signs, especially for increased heart rate and temperature and rapid, shallow breathing, *to detect ruptured appendix*
Observe for other signs of peritonitis (e.g., sudden relief of pain [sometimes] at time of perforation, followed by increased, diffuse pain and rigid guarding of the abdomen, abdominal distention, bloating, belching [from accumulation of air], pallor, chills, and irritability) *for appropriate treatment to be initiated*
Avoid administering laxatives or enemas *because these measures stimulate bowel motility and increase risk of perforation*
Monitor WBC count *as indicator of infection*

COMMUNITY FOCUS

Acute Appendicitis

Abdominal pain is a common complaint among school-age children and one that school nurses, teachers, and coaches hear frequently. In some instances, however, abdominal pain may indicate acute appendicitis. School nurses and nurse practitioners in school-based clinics should become very familiar with the "typical" pattern of symptoms in acute appendicitis and how to assess and evaluate an acute abdomen. School nurses also need to impress on teachers and coaches the importance of early referral to the health suite for further assessment. Early referral to the health suite and an alert school nurse or nurse practitioner may mean the difference between an uncomplicated appendectomy and a delayed diagnosis of a perforated appendix with peritonitis.

*Dependent nursing action.

The Child with Appendicitis—cont'd

EXPECTED OUTCOMES

Child remains free of symptoms of peritonitis

Signs of peritonitis are recognized early (specify)

POSTOPERATIVE CARE

(See Postoperative Care in Nursing Care Plan: The Child Undergoing Surgery, p. 305.)

RUPTURED APPENDIX

NURSING DIAGNOSIS: Risk for infection related to presence of infective organisms in abdomen

- **PATIENT GOAL 1:** Will experience minimized risk of spread of infection

NURSING INTERVENTIONS/*RATIONALES*

Provide wound care and dressing changes as prescribed *to prevent infection*

Monitor vital signs and WBC count *to assess presence of infection*

*Administer antibiotics as prescribed

EXPECTED OUTCOME

Child demonstrates resolution of peritonitis as evidenced by lack of fever, clean wound, normal WBC

NURSING DIAGNOSIS: Risk for injury related to absence of bowel motility

- **PATIENT GOAL 1:** Will not experience abdominal distention, vomiting

NURSING INTERVENTIONS/*RATIONALES*

Maintain NPO in early postoperative period *to prevent abdominal distention and vomiting*

Maintain NG tube decompression *until bowel motility returns*

Assess abdomen for distention, tenderness, presence of bowel sounds *to assess presence of peristalsis*

Monitor passage of flatus and stool *as indicator of bowel motility*

EXPECTED OUTCOME

Child does not exhibit signs of discomfort; abdomen remains soft and nondistended; child does not vomit

NURSING DIAGNOSIS: Altered family processes related to illness and hospitalization of child

- **PATIENT (FAMILY) GOAL 1:** Will receive adequate support

NURSING INTERVENTIONS/*RATIONALES*

Encourage expression of feelings and concerns *to enhance coping*

Encourage child to discuss hospital admission and treatments *in order to clarify misconceptions*

(See also:

Nursing Care Plan: The Child in the Hospital, p. 268.)

Nursing Care Plan: The Family of the Child Who Is Ill or Hospitalized, p. 282.)

EXPECTED OUTCOMES

Child and family express feelings and concerns

Child and family demonstrate understanding of hospitalization and treatments

*Dependent nursing action.

Unit 4

NURSING CARE PLAN

The Child with Acute Diarrhea (Gastroenteritis)

Acute diarrhea (gastroenteritis) is an inflammation of the stomach and intestines caused by various bacteria, viral, and parasitic pathogens.

(See Table 4-24, Infectious Causes of Acute Diarrhea.)

ASSESSMENT

Obtain a careful history of illness including the following:
  Possible ingestion of contaminated food or water
  Possible infection elsewhere (e.g., respiratory or urinary tract infection)
Perform a routine physical assessment.
Observe for manifestations of acute gastroenteritis (Table 4-24).
Assess state of dehydration (Table 4-25).

Record fecal output—Number, volume, characteristics
Observe and record presence of associated signs—Tenesmus, cramping, vomiting
Assist with diagnostic procedures (e.g., collect specimens as needed; stools for pH, blood, sugar, frequency; urine for pH, specific gravity, frequency; CBC, serum electrolytes, creatine, BUN).
Detect source of infection (e.g., examine other members of household and refer for treatment where indicated).

NURSING DIAGNOSIS: Fluid volume deficit related to excessive GI losses in stool or emesis

- **PATIENT GOAL 1:** Will exhibit signs of rehydration and maintain adequate hydration

NURSING INTERVENTIONS/*RATIONALES*

*Administer oral rehydration solutions (ORS) *for both rehydration and replacement of stool losses*
  Give ORS frequently in small amounts, especially if child is vomiting, *because vomiting, unless severe, is not a contraindication to using ORS*
*Administer and monitor IV fluids as prescribed *for severe dehydration and vomiting*
*Administer antimicrobial agents as prescribed *to treat specific pathogens causing excessive GI losses*
After rehydration, offer child regular diet as tolerated *because studies show that early reintroduction of normal diet is beneficial in reducing number of stools and weight loss and in shortening duration of illness*
Alternate ORS with a low-sodium fluid such as water, breast milk, lactose-free formula, or half-strength lactose-containing formula *for maintenance fluid therapy*
Maintain strict record of intake and output (urine, stool, and emesis) *to evaluate effectiveness of interventions*
Monitor urine specific gravity every 8 hours or as indicated *to assess hydration*
Weigh child daily *to assess for dehydration*
Assess vital signs, skin turgor, mucous membranes, and mental status every 4 hours or as indicated *to assess hydration*
Discourage intake of clear fluids such as fruit juices, carbonated soft drinks, and gelatin *because these fluids usually are high in carbohydrates, low in electrolytes, and have a high osmolality*
Instruct family in providing appropriate therapy, monitoring intake and output, and assessing for signs of dehydration *to ensure optimum results and improve compliance with the therapeutic regimen*

EXPECTED OUTCOME

Child exhibits signs of adequate hydration (specify)

NURSING DIAGNOSIS: Altered nutrition: less than body requirements related to diarrheal losses, inadequate intake

- **PATIENT GOAL 1:** Will consume nourishment adequate to maintain appropriate weight for age

NURSING INTERVENTIONS/*RATIONALES*

After rehydration, instruct breast-feeding mother to continue feeding breast milk *because this tends to reduce severity and duration of illness*
Avoid giving BRAT diet (bananas, rice, apples, and toast or tea) *because this diet is low in energy and protein, too high in carbohydrates, and low in electrolytes*
Observe and record response to feedings *to assess feeding tolerance*
Instruct family in providing appropriate diet *to gain compliance with therapeutic regimen*
Explore concerns and priorities of family members *to improve compliance with therapeutic regimen*

EXPECTED OUTCOME

Child takes prescribed nourishment and exhibits a satisfactory weight gain

---

NURSING DIAGNOSIS: Risk for infection related to microorganisms invading GI tract

- **PATIENT (OTHERS) GOAL 1:** Will not exhibit signs of gastrointestinal infection

NURSING INTERVENTIONS/*RATIONALES*

Implement standard precautions or other hospital infection-control practices, including appropriate disposal of stool and laundry and appropriate handling of specimens *to reduce risk of spreading infection*
Maintain careful handwashing *to reduce risk of spreading infection*
Apply diaper snugly *to reduce likelihood of fecal spread*
Use superabsorbent disposable diapers *to contain feces and decrease chance of diaper dermatitis*
Attempt to keep infants and small children from placing hands and objects in contaminated areas
Teach children, when possible, protective measures such as handwashing after using toilet *to prevent spread of infection*
Instruct family members and visitors in isolation practices, especially handwashing, *to reduce risk of spreading infection*

EXPECTED OUTCOME

Infection does not spread to others

*Dependent nursing action.

Unit 4

The Child with Acute Diarrhea (Gastroenteritis)—cont'd

TABLE 4-24 Infectious Causes of Acute Diarrhea

Organism	Pathology	Characteristics	Comments
VIRAL AGENTS			
Rotavirus Incubation period: 1-3 days	Invasion of epithelium of small bowel mucosa Severely distorted mucosal architecture with atrophic mucosa and severe inflammatory changes Decreased absorption of salt and water	Abrupt onset Fever (38° C or above) lasting approximately 48 hours Nausea/vomiting Abdominal pain Associated upper respiratory tract infection Diarrhea may persist for more than a week	Incidence higher in cool weather (80% in winter) Affects all age-groups; 6- to 24-month-old infants more vulnerable Usually mild and self-limited Important cause of nosocomial infections in hospitals and gastroenteritis in children attending daycare centers
Norwalk-like organisms Incubation period: 1-3 days	Mechanism of effect unknown Blunting of villi and inflammatory changes in lamina propria (small bowel and colon) Reduced enzymes	Fever Loss of appetite Nausea/vomiting Abdominal pain Diarrhea Malaise	Sources of infection: drinking water, recreation water, food (including shellfish) Affects all ages Self-limited (2-3 days)
BACTERIAL AGENTS			
Pathogenic *Escherichia coli* Incubation period: highly variable; depends on strain	Usually caused by enterotoxin production (small bowel) Reduced absorption and increased secretion of fluids and electrolytes	Onset gradual or abrupt Variable clinical manifestations Most—green, watery diarrhea with blood and mucus; becomes explosive Vomiting may be present from onset Abdominal distention Diarrhea Fever, appears toxic	Incidence higher in summer Usually interpersonal transmission but may transmit via inanimate objects A cause of nursery epidemics With symptomatic treatment only, may continue for weeks Full breast-feeding has a protective effect Symptoms generally subside in 3-7 days Relapse rate approximately 20%
Salmonella groups (nontyphoidal)—gram-negative, non-encapsulated, non-sporulating Incubation period: 6-72 hours for gastroenteritis (usually less than 24); 3-60 days for enteric fever (usually 7-14)	Penetration of lamina propria Local inflammation—no extensive destruction Stimulation of intestinal fluid excretion Systemic invasion of other sites	Rapid onset Variable symptoms—mild to severe Nausea, vomiting, and colicky abdominal pain followed by diarrhea, occasionally with blood and mucus Fever Hyperactive peristalsis and mild abdominal tenderness Symptoms usually subside within 5 days May have headache and cerebral manifestations (e.g., drowsiness, confusion, meningismus, or seizures) Infants may be afebrile and nontoxic May result in life-threatening septicemia and meningitis	Two thirds of patients are younger than 20 years of age; highest incidence in children younger than age 5 years, especially infants Highest incidence occurs from July through October, lowest from January through April Transmission primarily via contaminated food and drink—most from animal sources, including fowl, mammals, reptiles, and insects Most common sources are poultry and eggs In children—pets (e.g., dogs, cats, hamsters, and especially pet turtles) Communicable as long as organisms are excreted

Unit 4

Continued

TABLE 4-24   Infectious Causes of Acute Diarrhea—cont'd

Organism	Pathology	Characteristics	Comments
BACTERIAL AGENTS—cont'd			
Salmonella typhi	Rapid invasion of blood-stream from minor sites of inflammation Marked inflammation and necrosis of intestinal mucosa and lymphatics	Variable in infants Older children—irregular fever, headache, malaise, lethargy Diarrhea occurs in 50% at early stage Cough is common In a few days fever rises and is consistent; fatigue, cough, abdominal pain, anorexia, and weight loss develop; diarrhea begins	Decreased incidence in last decade Acute symptoms may persist for a week or more Transmitted by contaminated food or water (primary), infected animals (e.g., pet turtles)
Shigella groups—gram-negative, nonmotile anaerobic bacilli Incubation period: 1-7 days, usually 2-4	Enterotoxin Stimulates loss of fluids and electrolytes Invasion of epithelium with superficial mucosal ulcerations *S. dysenteriae* forms exotoxin	Onset variable but usually abrupt Fever and cramping abdominal pain initially Fever—may reach 40.5° C Convulsions in approximately 10%—usually associated with fever Patient appears sick Headache, nuchal rigidity, delirium Watery diarrhea with mucus and pus starts approximately 12-48 hours after onset Stools preceded by abdominal cramps; tenesmus and straining follow Symptoms usually subside in 5-10 days	Approximately 60% of cases in children younger than age 9 years, with more than one third between ages 1 and 4 years Peak incidence in late summer Transmitted directly or indirectly from infected persons Communicable for 1-4 weeks Self-limited disease Treat with antibiotics Severe dehydration and collapse can occur Acute symptoms may persist for a week or more
Yersinia enterocolitica Incubation period: dose-dependent; 1-3 weeks	Oxidase−, urease+, nonlactase-fermenting, gram− rods	Diarrhea—may be bloody Fever (>38.7° C) Abdominal pain in right lower quadrant (RLQ) Vomiting, diarrhea	Seen more commonly in winter Majority in first 3 years of life Transmitted by food and pets Can resemble appendicitis May be relapsing and last for weeks
Campylobacter jejuni Incubation period: 1-7 days or longer	Precise mechanism unclear Jejunum, ileum, and colon involvement Extensive ulceration with hemorrhagic ileitis Broadening and flattening of mucosa	Fever Abdominal pain—often severe, cramping, periumbilical Watery, profuse, foul-smelling diarrhea with blood Vomiting	Person-to-person transmission May be transmitted by pets (e.g., cat, dog, hamster) Food (especially chicken) and waterborne transmission Relapse possible Most patients recover spontaneously Antibiotics may speed recovery Peak incidence in summer
Vibrio cholerae (cholera) groups Incubation period: usually 2-3 days; range from few hours to 5 days	Enterotoxin causes increased secretion of chloride and possibly bicarbonate Intestinal mucosa congested with enlarged lymph follicles Intact mucosal surface	Sudden onset of profuse, watery diarrhea without cramping, tenesmus, or anal irritation, although children may complain of cramping Stools are intermittent at first, then almost continuous Stools are bloody with mucus	Rare in infants younger than 1 year old Mortality high in both treated and untreated infants and small children Transmitted via contaminated food and water Attack confers immunity

The Child with Acute Diarrhea (Gastroenteritis)—cont'd

TABLE 4-24 Infectious Causes of Acute Diarrhea—cont'd

Organism	Pathology	Characteristics	Comments
BACTERIAL AGENTS—cont'd			
Clostridium difficile	Toxin stimulates colonic secretion by damaging epithelium	Diarrhea with blood in stools	May cause pseudomembranous colitis Follows antibiotic therapy
FOOD POISONING			

Staphylococcus
  Incubation period:
  4-6 hours
	Produce heat-stable enterotoxin	Nausea, vomiting
		Severe abdominal cramps
		Profuse diarrhea
		Shock may occur in severe cases
		May be a mild fever
			Transferred via contaminated food—inadequately cooked or refrigerated (e.g., custards, mayonnaise, cream-filled or cream-topped desserts)
			Self-limited; improvement apparent within 24 hours
			Excellent prognosis

Clostridium perfringens
  Incubation period:
  8-24 hours,
  usually 8-12
	Produces heat-resistant and heat-sensitive toxins	Moderate to severe crampy, midepigastric pain	Self-limited illness
			Transmission by commercial food products, most often meat and poultry

Clostridium botulinum
  Incubation period:
  12-26 hours
  (range, 6 hours
  to 8 days)
	Highly potent neurotoxin	Nausea, vomiting
		Diarrhea
		Central nervous system (CNS) symptoms with curare-like effect
		Dry mouth, dysphagia
			Transmitted by contaminated food products
			Variable severity—mild symptoms to rapidly fatal within a few hours
			Antitoxin administration

TABLE 4-25 Clinical Manifestations of Dehydration

	Isotonic (Loss of Water and Salt)	Hypotonic (Loss of Salt in Excess of Water)	Hypertonic (Loss of Water in Excess of Salt)
Skin			
Color	Gray	Gray	Gray
Temperature	Cold	Cold	Cold or hot
Turgor	Poor	Very poor	Fair
Feel	Dry	Clammy	Thickened, doughy
Mucous membranes	Dry	Slightly moist	Parched
Tearing and salivation	Absent	Absent	Absent
Eyeball	Sunken and soft	Sunken	Sunken
Fontanel	Sunken	Sunken	Sunken
Body temperature	Subnormal or elevated	Subnormal or elevated	Subnormal or elevated
Pulse	Rapid	Very rapid	Moderately rapid
Respirations	Rapid	Rapid	Rapid
Behavior	Irritable to lethargic	Lethargic to comatose; convulsions	Marked lethargy with extreme hyperirritability on stimulation

Unit 4

The Child with Acute Diarrhea (Gastroenteritis)—cont'd

NURSING DIAGNOSIS: Impaired skin integrity related to irritation caused by frequent, loose stools

- **PATIENT GOAL 1:** Skin will remain intact

NURSING INTERVENTIONS/*RATIONALES*

Change diaper frequently *to keep skin clean and dry*

Cleanse buttocks gently with bland, nonalkaline soap and water or immerse child in a bath for gentle cleansing *because diarrheal stools are highly irritating to skin*

Apply ointment such as zinc oxide *to protect skin from irritation* (type of ointment may vary for each child and may require a trial period)

Expose slightly reddened intact skin to air whenever possible *to promote healing;* apply protective ointment to very irritated or excoriated skin *to facilitate healing*

Avoid using commercial baby wipes containing alcohol on excoriated skin *because they will cause stinging*

Observe buttocks and perineum for infection, such as *Candida, so that appropriate therapy can be initiated*

*Apply appropriate antifungal medication *to treat fungal infection of skin*

EXPECTED OUTCOME

Child has no evidence of skin breakdown

NURSING DIAGNOSIS: Anxiety/fear related to separation from parents, unfamiliar environment, distressing procedures

- **PATIENT GOAL 1:** Will exhibit signs of comfort

NURSING INTERVENTIONS/*RATIONALES*

Provide mouth care and pacifier for infants *to provide comfort*

Encourage family visitation and participation in care as much as the family is able, *to prevent stress associated with separation*

Touch, hold, and talk to child as much as possible *to provide comfort and relieve stress*

Provide sensory stimulation and diversion appropriate for child's developmental level and condition *to promote optimum growth and development*

EXPECTED OUTCOMES

Child exhibits minimal signs of physical or emotional distress

Family participates in child's care as much as possible

NURSING DIAGNOSIS: Altered family processes related to situational crisis, knowledge deficit

- **PATIENT (FAMILY) GOAL 1:** Family will understand about child's illness and its treatment and will be able to provide care

NURSING INTERVENTIONS/*RATIONALES*

Provide information to family about child's illness and therapeutic measures *to encourage compliance with therapeutic regimen, especially at home*

Assist family in providing comfort and support to child

Permit family members to participate in child's care as much as they desire, *to meet needs of both child and family*

Instruct family regarding precautions *to prevent spread of infection*

Arrange for posthospitalization health care *for continued assessment and treatment*

Refer family to a community health care agency *for supervision of home care as needed*

EXPECTED OUTCOME

Family demonstrates ability to care for child, especially at home

*Dependent nursing action.

NURSING CARE PLAN

The Child with Inflammatory Bowel Disease

Ulcerative colitis is a chronic inflammatory process involving the mucosa and submucosa of the colon and rectum.
Crohn disease is a chronic inflammatory process that may involve any part of the GI tract but most commonly affects the terminal ileum. The disease characteristically involves all layers of the bowel wall (transmural).

ASSESSMENT
(See Assessment of gastrointestinal dysfunction, p. 403.)
Observe for manifestations of inflammatory bowel disease (IBD) (Table 4-26).
Assist with diagnostic procedures and tests (e.g., rectosigmoid-oscopy, barium enema, stool examination, biopsy, and blood studies).
Assess parent-child relationships:
   Explore attitudes and feelings of child and parents.
   Elicit clues to possible parent-child disharmony, school problems, and other sources of stress.

Continued

TABLE 4-26   Comparison of Inflammatory Bowel Diseases: Ulcerative Colitis and Crohn Disease

Characteristics	Ulcerative Colitis	Crohn Disease
Intestinal bleedings	Common, mild to severe	Uncommon, mild to severe
Diarrhea	Often severe	Mild to severe
Abdominal pain	Less frequent	Common
Anorexia	Mild to moderate	May be severe
Weight loss	Mild to moderate	May be severe
Growth retardation	Usually mild	May be severe
Anal and perianal lesions	Rare	Common
Fistulas and strictures	Rare	Common

Unit 4

The Child with Inflammatory Bowel Disease—cont'd

NURSING DIAGNOSIS: Altered nutrition: less than body requirements related to chronic inflammatory process, diarrheal losses, loss of appetite, malabsorption, increased nutritional requirements

■ **PATIENT GOAL 1:** Will exhibit signs of reduced GI tract inflammation

NURSING INTERVENTIONS/*RATIONALES*

*Administer corticosteroids as prescribed *to reduce or eliminate inflammation*

Provide instructions for tapering medication *to eliminate untoward effects*

*Administer sulfasalazine as prescribed *to control inflammatory process*

*Administer folic acid supplements as prescribed *because sulfasalazine interferes with absorption and utilization of folic acid*

Stress importance of continued drug therapy *to prevent exacerbation of inflammatory process*

EXPECTED OUTCOME

Child will exhibit signs of reduced GI tract inflammation (specify)

■ **PATIENT GOAL 2:** Will consume sufficient nourishment for growth and development

NURSING INTERVENTIONS/*RATIONALES*

Provide well-balanced, high-protein, high-calorie diet *for maximum nutritional benefit*

Recommend low fiber diet if fiber foods produce symptoms

*Provide multivitamin, iron, and folic acid supplements as prescribed *to minimize deficiencies*

*Provide fish oil preparation as prescribed *for its antiinflammatory action and possible increased absorption of nutrients*

Include child and family in meal planning (e.g., favorite foods) *to increase child's intake*

Encourage small, frequent meals and snacks rather than three large meals a day *to increase child's daily food intake*

Serve meals and snacks around medication schedule when symptoms are controlled

Avoid foods that are known to aggravate condition

Relieve discomfort of mouth sores, if present, *so that child does not avoid eating because of mouth discomfort*

*Provide special enteral formulas (either by mouth or nasogastric infusion) or total parenteral nutrition, as prescribed, *to improve child's nutritional status*

Provide appropriate home care instructions (See p. 618.) *for maximum benefit without complications*

(See also Nursing Care Plan: The Child with Special Nutritional Needs, p. 313.)

EXPECTED OUTCOME

Child consumes sufficient nourishment (specify)

NURSING DIAGNOSIS: Altered family processes related to child's illness

■ **PATIENT (FAMILY) GOAL 1:** Will be prepared for temporary or permanent colostomy or ileostomy

NURSING INTERVENTIONS/*RATIONALES*

Explain procedure and relationship to disease process *to facilitate understanding*

Consult with enterostomal therapist, if available, *for teaching*

Teach ostomy care (See p. 626.)

Refer to appropriate agency and/or support group *for ongoing support*

EXPECTED OUTCOMES

Child and family demonstrate an understanding of procedures, surgery, and enterostomy care

(See also:

Nursing Care Plan: The Family of the Child Who Is Ill or Hospitalized, p. 282.)

Nursing Care Plan: The Child in the Hospital, p. 268.)

Nursing Care Plan: The Child with Chronic Illness or Disability, p. 287.)

*Dependent nursing action.

NURSING CARE PLAN

The Child with Peptic Ulcer Disease

Peptic ulcer is an erosion of the mucosal, submucosal, and sometimes muscular layer of the stomach, pylorus, or duodenum.

ASSESSMENT

Perform a routine physical assessment.

Assess for use of medications (aspirin, nonsteroidal antiinflammatory drugs, steroids), alcohol, or smoking.

Observe for manifestations of peptic ulcer disease (PUD):

Neonates (usually gastric and secondary)
Perforation may occur
Often massive hemorrhage
The same as seen in stress ulcers

Infants to 2-year-old children (gastric or duodenal, primary or secondary)
Poor eating, vomiting, melena, irritability, hematemesis
Vague discomfort
Usually bleed rather than perforate

2- to 6-year old children (gastric or duodenal)
Vomiting, generalized or epigastric pain, melena, hematemesis

Wake at night or early morning crying with pain
Perforation more likely in secondary ulcers

6- to 9-year-old children (usually duodenal and primary)
Pain—Burning or tenderness in epigastrium related to fasting state, melena, hematemesis, vomiting
May be related to emotional stress

Over 9 years (usually duodenal)
Vomiting, epigastric pain, melena, hematemesis
More typical of adult type

Take a careful health history, especially regarding pattern of pain.

Assist with diagnostic procedures and tests (e.g., radiography, barium swallow, endoscopy, blood studies, stool examination for occult blood, gastric acid measurement [occasionally]).

Observe for signs of hemorrhage.

> **NURSING DIAGNOSIS:** Pain related to ulceration

■ **PATIENT GOAL 1:** Will experience either no pain or a reduction of pain to level acceptable to child

NURSING INTERVENTIONS/*RATIONALES*

Implement nonpharmacologic pain management (See p. 339.)

*Implement measures to promote healing of inflamed mucosa (See Nursing Interventions/*Rationales* that follow)

Avoid administering aspirin or nonsteroidal antiinflammatory drugs if an analgesic/antipyretic is needed for other reasons *because these increase mucosal ulceration*

EXPECTED OUTCOMES

Child exhibits either no evidence of pain or a reduction of pain to level acceptable to child
(See also Nursing Care Plan: The Child in Pain, p. 315.)

> **NURSING DIAGNOSIS:** Risk for injury related to secretion of gastric juices and interference with protective mechanisms

■ **PATIENT GOAL 1:** Will exhibit signs of healing of inflamed mucosa

NURSING INTERVENTIONS/*RATIONALES*

*Administer antacids 1 and 3 hours after each meal and at bedtime as ordered *to protect mucosa and neutralize acid*

*Administer other mucosal protective agents (such as sucralfate and bismuth-containing preparations) as prescribed

*Administer histamine (H_2) receptor antagonists or other antisecretory agents as prescribed *to suppress gastric acid production*

*Administer antibiotics as prescribed *because* Helicobacter pylori *can be associated with ulcers*

Implement strategies to improve compliance with medication regimen (See Nursing Care Plan: Child and Family Compliance, p. 343.)

Teach child and family about the disease process and rationale for drug therapy *to increase compliance*

Explain to child and family that dietary modifications are not necessary

Explain to older child that smoking and alcohol contribute to ulcer formation

EXPECTED OUTCOMES

Child and family comply with medication regimen
Child exhibits signs of healing of inflamed mucosa

---

*Dependent nursing action.

Continued

Unit 4

The Child with Peptic Ulcer Disease—cont'd

■ **PATIENT GOAL 2:** Will experience reduction of stress

NURSING INTERVENTIONS/*RATIONALES*

Explore feelings and attitudes *for clues to stress-provoking situations*

Help child and family to recognize and avoid stress-producing situations *since stress may have precipitated or may aggravate the condition*

Refer for psychologic counseling, if appropriate, *to help child cope more constructively with stress*

EXPECTED OUTCOMES

Child discusses feelings and concerns
Family seeks counseling if recommended

NURSING DIAGNOSIS: Altered family processes related to a child with an illness

■ **PATIENT (FAMILY) GOAL 1:** Will receive adequate support

**NURSING INTERVENTIONS/*RATIONALES*
AND EXPECTED OUTCOMES**

(See Nursing Care Plan: The Family of the Child Who Is Ill or Hospitalized, p. 282.)

(See also Nursing Care Plan: The Child in the Hospital, p. 268.)

NURSING CARE PLAN

The Child with Acute Hepatitis

Hepatitis is an acute or chronic inflammation of the liver.
Hepatitis of viral etiology is caused by at least six types of virus:

Hepatitis A virus (HAV, previously designated *infectious hepatitis*)

Hepatitis B virus (HBV, previously designated *serum hepatitis*)

Hepatitis C virus (HCV, previously designated *parenterally transmitted non-A non-B hepatitis virus*)

Hepatitis D virus (HDV, occurs in children already infected with HBV)

Hepatitis E virus (enterically transmitted non-A non-B hepatitis virus)

Hepatitis G virus (HGV, blood-borne)

ASSESSMENT

Perform a routine physical assessment.

Take a careful health history, especially regarding:

Contact with persons known to have hepatitis

Questionable sanitation practices (e.g., drinking impure water)

Eating certain foods (e.g., raw shellfish taken from polluted water)

Previous blood transfusions

Ingestion of hepatotoxic drugs (e.g., salicylates, sulfonamides, antineoplastic agents, acetaminophen, anticonvulsants)

Parenteral administration of illicit drugs, or sexual contact with persons who use these drugs

Observe for manifestations of hepatitis (Table 4-27).

Assist with diagnostic procedures and tests (e.g., blood examination for presence of antibodies, and liver function tests).

> **NURSING DIAGNOSIS:** Risk for infection related to presence of hepatitis virus

■ **PATIENT (OTHERS) GOAL 1:** Will not contract infection

NURSING INTERVENTIONS/*RATIONALES*

Carry out standard precautions (See p. 346.) *to prevent spread of infection*

Use proper handwashing technique *to prevent spread of infection*

Apply diaper snugly *to reduce likelihood of fecal spread*

Use superabsorbent disposable diapers *to contain feces*

Attempt to keep infants and small children from placing hands and objects in contaminated areas

Explain to child and family the usual ways in which hepatitis A (fecal-oral route) and hepatitis B (parenteral route) are spread

Teach child and family infection control measures

Refer family to community health nurse, if appropriate, *for further assistance with infection control practices*

Refer child with a history of illicit drug use to an appropriate drug program for counseling

*Administer standard immune globulin (IG) as prescribed in situations of preexposure (such as travel to areas with prevalence of HAV) or within 2 weeks of exposure *to prevent hepatitis A*

*Administer hepatitis B immune globulin (HBIG) as prescribed *to prevent HBV within 72 hours of exposure* (e.g., following accidental needle puncture, newborn whose mother is HB$_s$Ag-positive)

*Administer hepatitis B immunization as prescribed for newborns, adolescents, and high-risk children

*Administer hepatitis A immunization as prescribed to high-risk children (See Immunizations, p. 190.)

EXPECTED OUTCOME

Infection does not spread to others

> **NURSING DIAGNOSIS:** Altered family processes related to situational crisis, knowledge deficit

■ **PATIENT (FAMILY) GOAL 1:** Will understand about child's illness and its treatment and will be able to provide care

NURSING INTERVENTIONS/*RATIONALES*

Provide support to family

Teach family about child's illness, treatment, and home care

Caution family against administering any medication without consent of practitioners *since liver may be unable to detoxify the drug sufficiently*

EXPECTED OUTCOMES

Family demonstrates the ability to provide home care for the child (specify learning and method of demonstration)

(See also:

Nursing Care Plan: The Child in the Hospital, p. 268.)

Nursing Care Plan: The Family of the Child Who Is Ill or Hospitalized, p. 282.)

©2000 Mosby, Inc. All rights reserved.

*Dependent nursing action.

Unit 4

TABLE 4-27 Comparison of Clinical Features of Hepatitis Types A, B, and C

Characteristics	Type A	Type B	Type C
Onset	Usually rapid, acute	More insidious	Usually insidious
Fever	Common and early	Less frequent	Less frequent
Anorexia	Common	Mild to moderate	Mild to moderate
Nausea and vomiting	Common	Sometimes present	Mild to moderate
Rash	Rare	Common	Sometimes present
Arthralgia	Rare	Common	Rare
Pruritus	Rare	Sometimes present	Sometimes present
Jaundice	Present (many cases anicteric)	Present	Present

NURSING CARE PLAN

The Child with Celiac Disease

Celiac disease is a malabsorption disease of the proximal small intestine that is characterized by abnormal mucosa with permanent intolerance to gluten.

ASSESSMENT

Perform a routine physical assessment.

Take a careful health history, especially regarding bowel habits related to intake.

Observe for manifestations of celiac disease (CD):
Diarrhea may be acute or insidious
Stools often watery, pale, foul smelling
Anorexia
Abdominal pain
Abdominal distention

Muscle wasting, especially in buttocks and extremities
Vomiting
Anemia
Constipation
Behavior changes common:
Irritability
Fretfulness
Assist with diagnostic procedures and tests (e.g., stool collection, intestinal biopsy, serum IgG, and IgA antibodies).

NURSING DIAGNOSIS: Altered nutrition less than body requirements related to malabsorption

■ **PATIENT GOAL 1:** Will exhibit signs of reduced irritation of intestinal mucosa

NURSING INTERVENTIONS/*RATIONALES*

Provide gluten-free diet *to promote healing of intestinal mucosa and prevent malabsorption*

Avoid lactose-containing milk products if child experiences lactose intolerance (which usually improves as intestinal mucosa heals)

*Administer corticosteroids, if prescribed, *to decrease severe bowel inflammation*

Monitor characteristics of stools *to assess for reduced bowel inflammation following gluten withdrawal*

EXPECTED OUTCOME

Child consumes specified diet and displays no evidence of bowel inflammation

■ **PATIENT GOAL 2:** Will consume adequate nourishment

NURSING INTERVENTIONS/*RATIONALES*

Provide prescribed diet

Arrange conference with dietitian *to help select foods compatible with diet and child's preferences*

*Administer supplemental water-miscible vitamins, folic acid, and iron as ordered *to treat specific nutritional deficiencies*

Monitor height and weight *to assess adequacy of nourishment*

EXPECTED OUTCOMES

Child consumes prescribed diet
Child exhibits appropriate growth

■ **PATIENT (FAMILY) GOAL 3:** Will be prepared for life-long dietary control of disease

NURSING INTERVENTIONS/*RATIONALES*

Assess child and family's understanding of the disorder and treatment *to ensure optimum results and safety*

Explain reason for eliminating gluten from diet, including long-range complications, *to encourage compliance*

Give written list of common food sources of wheat, rye, barley, and oats

Emphasize suitable substitutes, especially rice, corn, and millet

Stress importance of reading labels of prepared food *for hidden sources of gluten* (e.g., gluten is often added to foods as hydrolyzed vegetable protein)

Give instructions concerning vitamin and mineral supplements

Encourage child and family to express feelings and concerns while focusing on ways in which child can still feel normal

Encourage child and family to find new recipes using suitable ingredients *to decrease boredom with food restrictions*

Make referral to community health nurse or nutritionist *for continued dietary counseling and support*

Refer to organizations that provide support and guidance for children with celiac disease

EXPECTED OUTCOMES

Child and family demonstrate understanding of dietary restrictions (specify learning and method of demonstration)
Child and family comply with prescribed diet
Child and family utilize appropriate resources

*Dependent nursing action.

Unit 4

The Child with Celiac Disease—cont'd

NURSING DIAGNOSIS: Risk for injury related to celiac crisis

■ **PATIENT GOAL 1:** Will not experience complications from celiac crisis

NURSING INTERVENTIONS/*RATIONALES*

Monitor intravenous fluids closely *to prevent dehydration or overhydration*

Give mouth care during period when nothing is given by mouth *to promote comfort*

Observe child closely for signs of metabolic acidosis (e.g., weakness, irritability, decreasing level of consciousness, irregular heartbeat, poor muscular control) from intestinal fluid losses

Observe child closely for signs of dehydration

Monitor nasogastric suctioning and record drainage

Observe for signs of shock *so that treatment is initiated early*

*Administer steroids as ordered *to decrease inflammation;* when discontinued by decreasing doses, observe for return of signs suggestive of celiac disease

If hyperalimentation is required, observe all precautions to prevent infection *since this is a possible complication*

EXPECTED OUTCOMES

Child recovers from crisis uneventfully

Complications are recognized and appropriate care is instituted

NURSING DIAGNOSIS: Altered family processes related to a child with a chronic illness

■ **PATIENT (FAMILY) GOAL 1:** Family will receive adequate support

NURSING INTERVENTIONS/*RATIONALES*
AND EXPECTED OUTCOMES

Refer to appropriate support group(s) and agencies

(See also Nursing Care Plan: The Child with Chronic Illness or Disability, p. 287.)

*Dependent nursing action.

Unit 4

NURSING CARE PLAN

The Child with Hirschsprung Disease

Hirschsprung disease (congenital aganglionic megacolon) is a congenital anomaly that results in mechanical obstruction from inadequate motility of part of the intestine.

ASSESSMENT

Perform a routine physical assessment.

Take a careful health history, especially relative to bowel patterns.

Assess general hydration and nutritional status.

Monitor bowel elimination pattern.

Measure abdominal circumference.

Observe for manifestations of Hirschsprung disease:

Newborn period

Failure to pass meconium within 24-48 hours after birth

Reluctance to ingest fluids

Bile-stained vomitus

Abdominal distention

Intestinal obstruction

Infancy

Inadequate weight gain

Constipation

Abdominal distention

Episodes of diarrhea and vomiting

Ominous signs (often signify the presence of enterocolitis):

Bloody diarrhea

Fever

Severe lethargy

Childhood (symptoms more chronic)

Constipation

Ribbonlike, foul-smelling stools

Abdominal distention

Fecal masses may be palpable

Child usually has poor appetite and poor growth

Assist with diagnostic procedures and tests (e.g., radiography, rectal biopsy, and anorectal manometry).

PREOPERATIVE CARE

> **NURSING DIAGNOSIS:** Risk for injury related to decreased bowel motility

■ **PATIENT GOAL 1:** Will be prepared for surgical procedure

NURSING INTERVENTIONS/*RATIONALES*

*Administer saline enemas as prescribed *to empty bowel*

*Administer systemic antibiotics as prescribed *to reduce bacterial flora in bowel*

*Administer antibiotic colon irrigations as prescribed *to reduce bacterial flora in bowel*

*Administer fluid and electrolytes as prescribed *to stabilize child for surgery*

Measure and record abdominal circumference *since progressive distention is a serious sign*

Measure at largest diameter of abdomen (usually at level of umbilicus)

Mark point of measurement with pen *to ensure reliability*

Leave tape measure in place beneath child and take measurements at same time as vital signs *to avoid unnecessarily disturbing child*

In child with enterocolitis:

Closely monitor vital signs and blood pressure for signs of shock

Observe for symptoms of bowel perforation (e.g., fever, increasing abdominal distention, vomiting, increased tenderness, irritability, dyspnea, and cyanosis)

(See Preparation for procedures, p. 219.)

(See also Nursing Care Plan: The Child Undergoing Surgery, preoperative care, p. 304.)

Clarify any misconceptions about colostomy

Stress to child and family that the colostomy is temporary

EXPECTED OUTCOMES

Bowel is prepared for surgical procedure

Child and family demonstrate an understanding of the surgery and its implications

POSTOPERATIVE CARE

(See Nursing Care Plan: The Child Undergoing Surgery, postoperative care, p. 305.)

> **NURSING DIAGNOSIS:** Altered family processes related to situational crisis (hospitalized child)

■ **PATIENT (FAMILY) GOAL 1:** Will receive adequate support

NURSING INTERVENTIONS/*RATIONALES* AND EXPECTED OUTCOMES

(See Nursing Care Plan: The Family of the Child Who Is Ill or Hospitalized, p. 282.)

■ **PATIENT (FAMILY) GOAL 2:** Will be prepared for home care

NURSING INTERVENTIONS/*RATIONALES*

Encourage family and older child to assist with dressing changes during early postoperative period *to enhance teaching of colostomy care and promote acceptance of body change*

Teach colostomy care (See Community and Home Care Instructions: Caring for the Child with a Colostomy, p. 626.)

Enlist the aid of enterostomal therapist, if available

EXPECTED OUTCOMES

Child and family demonstrate the ability to provide ostomy care at home

(See also Nursing Care Plan: The Child in the Hospital, p. 268.)

*Dependent nursing action.

NURSING CARE PLAN

The Child with Intussusception

Intussusception is an invagination, or telescoping, of one portion of the intestine into another, resulting in obstruction beyond the defect.

ASSESSMENT

Perform a routine physical assessment.

Take a careful health history, especially regarding family's description of symptoms.

Observe stooling pattern and behavior preoperatively and postoperatively.

Observe child's behavior.

Observe for manifestations of intussusception:

  Sudden acute abdominal pain:

    Child screams and draws the knees onto the chest

    Child appears normal and comfortable during intervals between episodes of pain

  Vomiting

  Lethargy

  Passage of red currant jelly-like stools (stool mixed with blood and mucus)

Soft abdomen (early in disease)

  Tender, distended abdomen (later in disease)

  Palpable sausage-shaped mass in upper right quadrant

  Empty lower right quadrant (Dance sign)

  Eventual fever, prostration, and other signs of peritonitis

Observe for more chronic manifestations of intussusception:

  Diarrhea

  Anorexia

  Weight loss

  Occasional vomiting

  Periodic pain

  Pain without other symptoms (older child)

Assist with diagnostic procedures and tests (e.g., abdominal radiograph and barium enema).

PREOPERATIVE CARE

NURSING DIAGNOSIS: Pain related to invagination of bowel

■ **PATIENT GOAL 1:** Will experience either no pain or a reduction of pain to level acceptable to child

NURSING INTERVENTIONS/*RATIONALES*

(See Nursing Care Plan: The Child in Pain, p. 315.)

EXPECTED OUTCOME

Child exhibits signs of no pain or signs of minimum discomfort

■ **PATIENT (FAMILY) GOAL 2:** Will be prepared for surgical or nonsurgical correction

NURSING INTERVENTIONS/*RATIONALES*

Explain intussusception and nonsurgical hydrostatic reduction and/or surgery *to help prepare family and older child*

  Intussusception can be demonstrated by pushing the end of a finger on a rubber glove back into itself

  Hydrostatic reduction can then be simulated by filling the glove with water to push the "finger" out

  Discuss possibility of surgical correction if the nonsurgical procedure fails

Assess all stools, *since passage of a normal brown stool usually indicates reduction of intussusception*

Report to practitioner, *who may choose to alter diagnostic/therapeutic plan of care based on this information*

Explain risk of recurrence to family *so that prompt medical attention is sought*

(See Preparation for procedures, p. 219.)

(See also Nursing Care Plan: The Child Undergoing Surgery, p. 304.)

EXPECTED OUTCOME

Child and family demonstrate an understanding of the prescribed therapy

NURSING DIAGNOSIS: Altered family processes related to a child with a serious disorder

■ **PATIENT (FAMILY) GOAL 1:** Will receive adequate support

NURSING INTERVENTIONS/*RATIONALES* AND EXPECTED OUTCOMES

(See Nursing Care Plan: The Family of the Child Who Is Ill or Hospitalized, p. 282.)

(See also Nursing Care Plan: The Child in the Hospital, p. 268.)

POSTOPERATIVE CARE

(See Nursing Care Plan: The Child Undergoing Surgery, p. 305.)

Unit 4

NURSING CARE PLAN

The Child with Enterobiasis (Pinworms)

Enterobiasis is an intestinal infestation with the nematode *Enterobius vermicularis,* the common pinworm.

ASSESSMENT
Perform a routine physical assessment.
Observe for manifestations of pinworms:
  Intense perianal itching (principal symptom)
  Evidence of itching in young children includes the following:
    General irritability
    Restlessness
    Poor sleep
    Bed-wetting
    Distractibility
Short attention span
Perianal dermatitis and excoriation secondary to itching
If worms migrate, possible vaginal and urethral infection
Assist with diagnostic procedures and tests (e.g., collect stool for laboratory testing for ova and parasites; or collect tape test [a loop of transparent tape, sticky side out, is placed around the end of a tongue depressor, which is then pressed firmly against the child's perianal area on awakening before child has a bowel movement or bathes]).

NURSING DIAGNOSIS: Risk for injury related to presence of organisms (pinworms)

■ **PATIENT GOAL 1:** Will exhibit no evidence of pinworms

NURSING INTERVENTIONS/*RATIONALES*
*Teach family to administer antihelminthics as prescribed *to treat enterobiasis*
Remind of need to take a second dose of medication in 2 weeks, if prescribed, *to ensure total eradication of pinworms*

EXPECTED OUTCOME
Child exhibits no evidence of pinworms

NURSING DIAGNOSIS: Risk for infection related to presence of organisms (pinworms)

■ **PATIENT (OTHERS) GOAL 1:** Will not exhibit evidence of infection

NURSING INTERVENTIONS/*RATIONALES*
Teach child and family preventive measures:
  Handwashing after toileting and before eating *to reduce likelihood of spreading infection*
  Keep child's fingernails short *to minimize chance of ova collecting under nails*

Daily showering rather than tub bathing
Discourage child from biting nails, placing fingers in mouth, and scratching anal area
Dress child in one-piece outfit *to prevent access to anal area*
Dispose of diapers in a closed receptacle as soon as they are soiled

EXPECTED OUTCOME
Child and others remain free of infestation

NURSING DIAGNOSIS: Altered family processes related to a child with an infestation

■ **PATIENT (FAMILY) GOAL 1:** Will receive adequate support

NURSING INTERVENTIONS/*RATIONALES*
Help family comply with therapy
Help family and community cope with repeated infestations *since it is the most common helminthic infection in the United States*
Refer to appropriate public health agencies, especially regarding repeated infestations, *for follow-up care*

EXPECTED OUTCOMES
Family complies with therapy
Family contacts appropriate agency for follow-up care

*Dependent nursing action.

Unit 4

NURSING CARE PLAN

The Child with Giardiasis

Giardiasis is an inflammatory intestinal infestation with the protozoan *Giardia lamblia.*

ASSESSMENT

Perform a routine physical assessment.

Take a careful health history, especially relative to contact with water (e.g., mountain lakes, streams, and pools), possible contaminated food, and animals.

Observe for manifestations of giardiasis:

Infants and young children

Diarrhea

Vomiting

Anorexia

Failure to thrive

Children over 5 years of age

Abdominal cramps

Intermittent loose stools

Constipation

Stools may be malodorous, watery, pale, greasy

Most infections resolve spontaneously in 4 to 6 weeks.

Rarely, chronic form occurs:

Intermittent loose, foul-smelling stools

Possibility of:

Abdominal bloating

Flatulence

Sulfur-tasting belches

Epigastric pain

Vomiting

Headache

Weight loss

Assist with diagnostic procedures and tests (e.g., multiple stool specimens for identification of organisms and/or cysts, and CIE and ELISA tests).

NURSING DIAGNOSIS: Risk for injury related to presence of organisms *(Giardia)*

■ **PATIENT GOAL 1:** Will exhibit no evidence of infestation

NURSING INTERVENTIONS/*RATIONALES*

*Administer, or teach family to administer, antiprotozoal agents as prescribed *to eradicate* Giardia

EXPECTED OUTCOME

Child exhibits no evidence of infestation

NURSING DIAGNOSIS: Risk for infection related to presence of organisms *(Giardia)*

■ **PATIENT (OTHERS) GOAL 1:** Will not exhibit evidence of infection

NURSING INTERVENTIONS/*RATIONALES*

Always wash hands and fingernails with soap and water before eating and handling food and after toileting

Avoid placing fingers in mouth or biting nails

Discourage children from scratching bare anal area

Change diapers as soon as they are soiled and dispose in plastic bags in closed receptacle out of children's reach

Do not rinse diapers in toilet

Disinfect toilet seats and diaper-changing areas; use dilute household bleach (10% solution) or an antibacterial product such as Lysol and wipe clean with paper towels

Drink water that is specially treated, especially if camping

Wash all raw fruits and vegetables or food that has fallen on the floor or ground

Avoid foods grown in soil fertilized with human excreta

Teach children to defecate only in a toilet, not on the ground

Keep dogs and cats away from playgrounds or sandboxes

Avoid swimming in pools frequented by diapered children

Wear shoes outside

Educate day care staff regarding appropriate sanitation practices *since Giardia is prevalent among children in daycare centers.*

EXPECTED OUTCOME

Child and others do not become infected with organism

NURSING DIAGNOSIS: Altered family processes related to a child with an infestation

■ **PATIENT (FAMILY) GOAL 1:** Will receive adequate support

NURSING INTERVENTIONS/*RATIONALES*

Help family comply with therapy

Offer suggestions to decrease side effects of quinacrine and to increase its palatability:

Administer drug with or after meals

Crush tablets and mix with a strong flavoring (e.g., jam or syrup)

(See also Community and Home Care Instructions related to administration of medications, p. 597.)

EXPECTED OUTCOMES

Family complies with therapy

Child takes prescribed medication with minimum or no distress

OTHER COMMON INTESTINAL PARASITES

(See Table 4-28.)

---

*Dependent nursing action.

Continued

Unit 4

The Child with Giardiasis—cont'd

TABLE 4-28   Selected Intestinal Parasites

Clinical Manifestations	Comments
ASCARIASIS—*ASCARIS LUMBRICOIDES* (COMMON ROUNDWORM)	
Light infections: asymptomatic Heavy infections: anorexia, irritability, nervousness, enlarged abdomen, weight loss, fever, intestinal colic Severe infections: intestinal obstruction, appendicitis, perforation of intestine with peritonitis, obstructive jaundice, lung involvement—pneumonitis	Transferred to mouth by way of contaminated food, fingers, or toys Largest of the intestinal helminths Affects principally young children 1-4 years of age Prevalent in warm climates
HOOKWORM DISEASE—*NECATOR AMERICANUS*	
Light infections in well-nourished individuals: no problems Heavier infections: mild to severe anemia, malnutrition May be itching and burning ("ground itch") followed by erythema and a papular eruption in areas to which the organism migrates	Transmitted by discharging eggs on the soil; infection picked up from direct skin contact with contaminated soil Wearing shoes is recommended, although children playing in contaminated soil expose many skin surfaces
STRONGYLOIDIASIS—*STRONGYLOIDES STERCORALIS* (THREADWORM)	
Light infection: asymptomatic Heavy infection: respiratory signs and symptoms; abdominal pain, distention; nausea and vomiting; diarrhea—large, pale stools, often with mucus Threat to life in children with weakened immunologic defenses	Transmission is same as for hookworm except autoinfection common Older children and adults affected more often than young children Severe infections may lead to severe nutritional deficiency
VISCERAL LARVA MIGRANS—*TOXOCARA CANIS* (DOGS); INTESTINAL TOXOCARIASIS—*TOXOCARA CATI* (CATS)	
Symptoms depend on reactivity of infected individual May be asymptomatic except for eosinophilia Specific diagnosis difficult	Transmitted by contamination of hands from direct contact with dog, cat, or objects; or from ingestion of soil Dogs and cats should be kept away from areas where children play; sandboxes are especially important transmission areas Periodic deworming of diagnosed dogs and cats recommended Control of dog and cat population helpful Continued education and laws needed to prevent indiscriminate canine and feline defecation
TRICHURIASIS—*TRICHURIS TRICHIURA* (WHIPWORM)	
Light infections: asymptomatic Heavy infections: abdominal pain and distention, diarrhea	Transmitted from contaminated soil, vegetables, toys, and other objects Most frequent in warm, moist climates Occurs most often in undernourished children living in unsanitary conditions

NURSING CARE PLAN

The Child with Cleft Lip and/or Cleft Palate

Cleft lip (CL) is a malformation resulting from failure of the maxillary and median nasal processes to fuse during embryonic development.

Cleft palate (CP) is a midline fissure of the palate resulting from failure of the two sides to fuse during embryonic development.

ASSESSMENT

Perform a physical assessment:
   Inspect palate, both visually and by placing fingers directly on palate.

Observe feeding behaviors.
Observe infant-family interactions.

PREOPERATIVE CARE

> **NURSING DIAGNOSIS:** Altered nutrition: less than body requirements related to physical defect

■ **PATIENT GOAL 1:** Will consume adequate nourishment

NURSING INTERVENTIONS/*RATIONALES*

Administer diet appropriate for age (specify)
Assist mother with breast-feeding if this is mother's preference *because the newborn with either defect can breast-feed*
   Position and stabilize nipple well back in oral cavity *so that tongue action facilitates milk expression*
   Stimulate let-down reflex manually or with breast pump before nursing *since suction required to stimulate milk may initially be absent*
Modify feeding techniques to adjust to defect *since infant's ability to suck is reduced*
   Hold child in upright (sitting) position *to minimize risk of aspiration*
Use special feeding appliances *that compensate for infant's feeding difficulty*
   Try to nipple feed infant *to meet infant's need for sucking and to promote muscle development for speech*
   Position nipple between infant's tongue and existing palate *to facilitate compression of nipple*
   When using devices without nipples (e.g., Breck feeder, Asepto syringe), deposit formula on back of tongue *to facilitate swallowing* and adjust flow according to infant's swallowing *to prevent aspiration*
Bubble (burp) frequently *because of tendency to swallow excessive amounts of air*
Encourage parents to begin feeding infant as soon as possible *so that they become adept in feeding technique before discharge*
Monitor weight *to assess adequacy of nutritional intake*

EXPECTED OUTCOMES

Infant consumes an adequate amount of nutrients (specify amount)
Infant exhibits appropriate weight gain

> **NURSING DIAGNOSIS:** Risk for altered parenting related to infant with a highly visible physical defect

■ **PATIENT (FAMILY) GOAL 1:** Will demonstrate acceptance of infant

NURSING INTERVENTIONS/*RATIONALES*

Allow expression of feelings *to encourage family's coping*
Convey attitude of acceptance of infant and family *because parents are sensitive to affective attitudes of others*
Indicate by behavior that child is a valuable human being *to encourage acceptance of infant*
Describe results of surgical correction of defect
   Use photographs of satisfactory results *to encourage feeling of hope*
Arrange meeting with other parents who have experienced a similar situation and coped successfully

EXPECTED OUTCOMES

Family discusses feelings and concerns regarding child's defect, its repair, and future prospects
Family exhibits an attitude of acceptance of infant
(See also Nursing Care Plan: The Child Undergoing Surgery, Preoperative Care, p. 304.)

POSTOPERATIVE CARE

> **NURSING DIAGNOSIS:** Risk for trauma of the surgical site related to surgical procedure, dysfunctional swallowing

■ **PATIENT GOAL 1:** Will experience no trauma to operative site

NURSING INTERVENTIONS/*RATIONALES*

Position on back or side or in infant seat (CL) *to prevent trauma to operative site*
Maintain lip protective device (CL) *to protect the suture line*
Use nontraumatic feeding techniques *to minimize risk of trauma*
Restrain elbows only as necessary *to prevent access to operative site*
   Use jacket restraints on older infant *to prevent rolling onto abdomen and rubbing face on sheet*
Avoid placing objects in the mouth following CP repair (e.g., suction catheter, tongue depressor, straw, pacifier, small spoon) *to prevent trauma to operative site*
Prevent vigorous and sustained crying *that can cause tension on sutures*
Cleanse suture line gently after feeding and as necessary in manner ordered by surgeon (CL) *since inflammation or infection will interfere with healing and the cosmetic effect of surgical repair*
Teach cleansing and restraining procedures, especially when infant will be discharged before suture removal *to minimize complications after discharge*

Unit 4

Continued

The Child with Cleft Lip and/or Cleft Palate—cont'd

EXPECTED OUTCOME
Operative site remains undamaged

■ **PATIENT GOAL 2:** Will exhibit no evidence of aspiration

NURSING INTERVENTIONS/*RATIONALES*
Position *to allow for drainage of mucus* (partial side-lying position, semi-Fowler position) and *to prevent aspiration of formula*

EXPECTED OUTCOME
Child manages secretions and formula without aspiration

NURSING DIAGNOSIS: Altered nutrition: less than body requirements related to difficulty eating following surgical procedure

■ **PATIENT GOAL 1:** Will consume adequate nourishment

NURSING INTERVENTIONS/*RATIONALES*
Monitor IV fluids (if prescribed)
Administer diet appropriate for age and as prescribed for postoperative period (specify)
Involve family in determining best feeding methods *since family assumes feeding responsibility at home*
Modify feeding technique *to adjust to defect and surgical repair*
  Feed in sitting position *to minimize risk of aspiration*
  Use special appliances *that compensate for feeding difficulties without causing trauma to operative site*
  Bubble frequently *because of tendency to swallow large amounts of air*
  Assist with breast-feeding if method of choice
Teach feeding and suctioning techniques to family *to ensure optimum home care*

EXPECTED OUTCOMES
Infant consumes an adequate amount of nutrients (specify amounts)

Family demonstrates ability to carry out postoperative care
Infant exhibits appropriate weight gain

NURSING DIAGNOSIS Pain related to surgical procedure

■ **PATIENT GOAL 1:** Will experience optimum comfort level

NURSING INTERVENTIONS/*RATIONALES*
Assess behavior and vital signs for evidence of pain
*Administer analgesics and/or sedatives as ordered
Remove restraints periodically while supervised *to exercise arms, provide relief from restrictions, and to observe skin for signs of irritation*
Provide cuddling and tactile stimulation and other nonpharmacologic interventions as needed *for optimum comfort*
Involve parents in infant's care *to provide comfort and sense of security*

EXPECTED OUTCOME
Infant appears comfortable and rests quietly

NURSING DIAGNOSIS: Altered family processes related to child with a physical defect, hospitalization

■ **PATIENT (FAMILY) GOAL 1:** Will receive adequate support

**NURSING INTERVENTIONS/*RATIONALES*
AND EXPECTED OUTCOMES**
(See Nursing Care Plan: The Family of the Child Who Is Ill or Hospitalized, p. 282.)
Refer family to appropriate agencies and support groups
(See also Nursing Care Plan: The Child with Chronic Illness or Disability, p. 287.)

*Dependent nursing action.

NURSING CARE PLAN

The Infant with Hypertrophic Pyloric Stenosis

Hypertrophic pyloric stenosis is an obstruction at the pyloric sphincter by hypertrophy of the circular muscle of the pylorus.

ASSESSMENT

Perform a physical assessment.

Take a health history, especially regarding eating behaviors and vomiting patterns.

Observe for manifestations of hypertrophic pyloric stenosis:
   Projectile vomiting
      Usually occurs shortly after a feeding but may not occur for several hours
      May follow each feeding or appear intermittently
      Nonbilious vomitus; may be blood-tinged
   Infant hungry, avid nurser; eagerly accepts a second feeding after vomiting episode

No evidence of pain or discomfort except that of chronic hunger

Weight loss

Signs of dehydration

Distended upper abdomen

Readily palpable olive-shaped tumor in the epigastrium just to the right of the umbilicus

Visible gastric peristaltic waves that move from left to right across the epigastrium

Assist with diagnostic procedures and tests (e.g., upper GI series, ultrasound, and serum electrolytes).

NURSING DIAGNOSIS: Fluid volume deficit related to persistent vomiting

■ **PATIENT GOAL 1:** Will receive appropriate volume of fluids

NURSING INTERVENTIONS/*RATIONALES*

Maintain intravenous fluids as prescribed *to promote hydration and prevent dehydration*

Monitor laboratory data *to determine fluid and electrolyte imbalances*

Monitor intake, output, and urine specific gravity *to determine hydration status*

Monitor vital signs and daily weights *to assess hydration*

Assess skin turgor and mucous membranes *as indicators of adequate hydration*

EXPECTED OUTCOMES

Infant receives sufficient fluids to replace losses

Infant exhibits signs of adequate hydration as evidenced by normal vital signs and skin turgor, moist mucous membranes, and adequate urine output

NURSING DIAGNOSIS: Altered nutrition; less than body requirements related to persistent vomiting

■ **PATIENT GOAL 1:** Will consume adequate nourishment

NURSING INTERVENTIONS/*RATIONALES*

*Initiate postoperative feedings as prescribed

Begin with small feedings at frequent intervals *to prevent vomiting*

Observe and record infant's responses to feedings *to determine amount and frequency of subsequent feedings*

Reestablish breast-feeding or encourage family to feed infant *to prepare for discharge and continued nourishment*

EXPECTED OUTCOME

Infant consumes and retains a sufficient amount of nourishment

NURSING DIAGNOSIS: Altered family processes related to hospitalization of infant

(See the following:
   Nursing Care Plan: The Family of the Child Who Is Ill or Hospitalized, p. 282.)
   Nursing Care Plan: The Child Undergoing Surgery, p. 304.)
   Nursing Care Plan: The Child in Pain, p. 315.)

Unit 4

*Dependent nursing action.

NURSING CARE PLAN

The Infant with Esophageal Atresia and Tracheoesophageal Fistula

Esophageal atresia is a malformation caused by failure of the esophagus to develop a continuous passage; the esophagus may or may not form a connection with the trachea (tracheoesophageal fistula, TEF).

Type A (5% to 8%)—Blind pouch at each end of the esophagus, widely separated and with no communication to the trachea

Type B (rare)—Blind pouch at each end of the esophagus with fistula from trachea to upper esophageal segment

Type C (80% to 95%)—Proximal esophageal segment terminates in a blind pouch, and the distal segment is connected to the trachea or primary bronchus by a short fistula at or near the bifurcation

Type D (rare)—Both upper and lower esophageal segments connected to the trachea

Type E (less frequent than A or C)—Otherwise normal trachea and esophagus connected by a common fistula

ASSESSMENT

Perform newborn assessment. (See p. 14.)

Observe for manifestations of esophageal atresia and tracheoesophageal fistula:

Excessive salivation and drooling

Choking

Cyanosis

Apnea

Increased respiratory distress following feeding

Abdominal distention

Assist with diagnostic procedures (e.g., chest and abdomen radiography; catheter gently passed into the esophagus meets with resistance if the lumen is blocked).

Monitor frequently for signs of respiratory distress.

NURSING DIAGNOSIS: Ineffective airway clearance related to abnormal opening between esophagus and trachea or obstruction to swallowing

■ **PATIENT GOAL 1:** Will maintain patent airway

NURSING INTERVENTIONS/*RATIONALES*

Suction as necessary *to remove accumulated secretions from oropharynx*

Position supine with head elevated on an inclined plane (at least 30 degrees) *to decrease pressure against thoracic cavity and to minimize reflux of gastric secretions up distal esophagus and into trachea and bronchi*

*Administer oxygen as prescribed and monitor closely (pulse oximetry, blood gases) *to help relieve respiratory distress*

Do not use positive pressure (e.g., resuscitation bag/mask) *since it may introduce air into stomach and intestines, creating additional pressure in thoracic cavity*

Administer nothing by mouth *to prevent aspiration*

Maintain intermittent or continuous suction of esophageal segment, if ordered preoperatively, *to keep blind pouch empty of secretions*

Leave gastrostomy tube, if present, open to gravity drainage *so that air can escape, minimizing risk of regurgitation of gastric contents into trachea*

EXPECTED OUTCOMES

Airway remains patent

Infant does not aspirate secretions

Respirations remain within normal limits

NURSING DIAGNOSIS: Impaired (difficulty) swallowing related to mechanical obstruction

■ **PATIENT GOAL 1:** Will receive adequate nourishment

NURSING INTERVENTIONS/*RATIONALES*

*Administer gastrostomy feedings as prescribed *to provide nourishment until oral feedings are possible*

Progress to oral feedings as prescribed according to infant's condition and surgical correction

Observe closely *to make certain infant is able to swallow without choking*

Monitor intake, output, and weight *to assess adequacy of nutritional intake*

Give infant pacifier *to provide nonnutritive sucking*

Teach family appropriate feeding techniques *to prepare for discharge*

EXPECTED OUTCOME

Infant receives sufficient nourishment and exhibits a satisfactory weight gain

■ **PATIENT GOAL 2:** Patient will learn to take oral feedings (following complete repair)

NURSING INTERVENTIONS/*RATIONALES*

Introduce foods one at a time *to evaluate tolerance of food item*

Provide age-appropriate foods with various textures and flavors *to stimulate interest in eating*

Begin with pureed foods and progress to more solid foods as child shows readiness

Cut food in small, noncylindrical pieces *to prevent choking*

Avoid foods such as whole hot dogs or large pieces of meat *to decrease risk of choking*

Teach child to chew foods well *to decrease risk of choking*

Refer to speech or occupational therapist, if appropriate, *to facilitate learning*

EXPECTED OUTCOME

Child takes an adequate amount of nourishment and displays no evidence of feeding resistance, malnutrition, or dysphagia

---

NURSING DIAGNOSIS: Risk for injury related to surgical procedure

■ **PATIENT GOAL 1:** Will not experience trauma to surgical site

*Dependent nursing action.

The Infant with Esophageal Atresia and Tracheoesophageal Fistula—cont'd

NURSING INTERVENTIONS/*RATIONALES*

Suction only with catheter premeasured to a distance that does not reach to surgical site *to prevent trauma to mucosa*

EXPECTED OUTCOME

Child does not exhibit evidence of injury to surgical site

NURSING DIAGNOSIS: Anxiety related to difficulty swallowing, discomfort from surgery

■ **PATIENT GOAL 1:** Will experience a sense of security without discomfort

NURSING INTERVENTIONS/*RATIONALES*

Provide tactile stimulation (e.g., cuddling, rocking) *to facilitate optimum development and promote comfort*

Administer mouth care *to keep mouth clean and mucous membranes moist*

Offer pacifier frequently *to provide nonnutritive sucking*

*Administer analgesics as prescribed

Encourage parents to participate in child's care *to provide comfort and security*

EXPECTED OUTCOMES

Infant rests calmly, is alert when awake, and engages in non-nutritive sucking

Mouth remains clean and moist

Child experiences either no pain or minimal pain

NURSING DIAGNOSIS: Altered family processes related to child with a physical defect

■ **PATIENT (FAMILY) GOAL 1:** Will be prepared for home care of child

NURSING INTERVENTIONS/*RATIONALES*

Teach family skills and observations needed for home care:
Positioning *to prevent aspiration*
Signs of respiratory distress *to prevent delay in treatment*
Signs of complications (e.g., refusal to eat, dysphagia, increased coughing) *so practitioner can be notified*
Acquiring needed equipment and services
Care of gastrostomy and esophagostomy when infant has staged surgery, including techniques such as suctioning, feeding, care of operative site and/or ostomies, dressing changes, *to ensure appropriate care after discharge*

EXPECTED OUTCOMES

Family demonstrates ability to provide care to infant, an understanding of signs of complications, and appropriate actions

(See also:
Nursing Care Plan: The Family of the Child Who Is Ill or Hospitalized, p. 282.)
Nursing Care Plan: The High-Risk Newborn and Family, p. 350.)

*Dependent nursing action.

Unit 4

NURSING CARE PLAN

The Infant with an Anorectal Malformation

Anorectal malformation (imperforate anus) is a congenital malformation in which the rectum has no outside opening. (See Table 4-29 for classification of malformations.)

ASSESSMENT

Perform newborn assessment (See p. 14.) with special attention to perineal area.

Observe for passage of meconium. Note if meconium appears at an inappropriate orifice.

Observe for ribbonlike stools in older infant or young child who has history of difficult defecation or abdominal distention.

Assist with diagnostic procedures (e.g., endoscopy, radiography, ultrasound, IV pyelogram, voiding cystourethrogram).

NURSING DIAGNOSIS: Risk for injury related to inability to evacuate rectum, surgery

- **PATIENT GOAL 1:** Will not experience complications preoperatively and postoperatively

NURSING INTERVENTIONS/*RATIONALES*

Avoid taking rectal temperatures preoperatively and postoperatively *to prevent rectal trauma*

*Maintain nasogastric suction, if implemented, *for abdominal decompression*

Maintain scrupulous anal and perineal care *to prevent skin irritation and infection*

Observe stool patterns *to detect normal pattern or abnormality*

Position infant side-lying prone with hips elevated, or supine with legs suspended at a 90-degree angle, *to prevent pressure on perineal sutures*

EXPECTED OUTCOME

Child does not experience complications

NURSING DIAGNOSIS: Altered nutrition: less than body requirements related to inability to feed

- **PATIENT GOAL 1:** Will consume adequate nourishment

NURSING INTERVENTIONS/*RATIONALES*

*Monitor intravenous fluids as prescribed *to maintain hydration while NPO*

Offer nothing by mouth until peristalsis is established

Offer pacifier *to satisfy nonnutritive sucking needs until bowel elimination is achieved*

Provide formula or diet appropriate for age as soon as peristalsis is detected

EXPECTED OUTCOME

Child consumes a sufficient amount of nourishment when peristalsis resumes

---

NURSING DIAGNOSIS: Altered family processes related to the care of a child with a physical defect, hospitalization

- **PATIENT (FAMILY) GOAL 1:** Will be prepared for home care

NURSING INTERVENTIONS/*RATIONALES*

Teach care needed for home management:

Rectal dilation, if appropriate

Wound care

Colostomy care (See Community and Home Care Instructions, p. 626.)

Bowel habit training

Diet modification (e.g., fiber)

(See also Nursing Care Plan: The Family of the Child Who Is Ill or Hospitalized, p. 282.)

EXPECTED OUTCOME

Family demonstrates the ability to provide home care for the infant

*Dependent nursing action.

TABLE 4-29   Classification of Anorectal Malformations

Level	Male	Female
High	Anorectal agenesis	Anorectal agenesis
	With rectoprostatic-urethral fistula	With rectovaginal fistula
	Without fistula	Without fistula
	Rectal atresia	Rectal atresia
Intermediate	Recto-bulbar-urethral fistula	Rectovestibular fistula
		Rectovaginal fistula
	Agenesis without fistula	Agenesis without fistula
Low	Anocutaneous fistula	Anovestibular fistula
	Anal stenosis	Anocutaneous fistula
		Anal stenosis
		Cloaca
	Rare malformations	Rare malformations

From Stephens FD and others: *Pediatr Surg Int* 1:200, 1986.

Hernias and Abdominal Wall Defects

A **hernia** is a protrusion of a portion of an organ or organs through an abnormal opening (Table 4-30).

Omphalocele and **gastroschisis** are two of the more common forms of abdominal wall defects.

TABLE 4-30   Summary Outline of Hernias and Abdominal Wall Defects

Type	Manifestations/Diagnostic Evaluation	Management

DIAPHRAGMATIC
Through foramen of Bochdalek: protrusion of part of the abdominal organs through an opening in the diaphragm
	Symptoms—Mild to severe respiratory distress within a few hours after birth; tachypnea, cyanosis, dyspnea, and severe acidosis
	Breath sounds absent in affected area; bowel sounds may be present
	Vomiting, abdominal pain
	Rarely asymptomatic
	Diagnosis made by radiographic study
		Therapeutic:
		  In utero surgical repair of herniated diaphragm and ligation of fetal trachea (which is reopened before birth)
		  Supportive treatment of respiratory distress and correction of acidosis; possible use of extracorporeal membrane oxygenation
		  Prophylactic antibiotic administration
		  Surgical reduction of hernia and repair of defect
		Nursing:
		  Preoperative
		    Prevent crying
		    Maintain suction, oxygen, and intravenous fluids
		    Place in semi-Fowler position
		    Assist with diagnostic and preoperative procedures
		    Administer medications
		  Postoperative
		    Carry out routine postoperative care and observation
		    Use comfort measures
		    Support parents

HIATAL
Sliding: Protrusion of an abdominal structure (usually the stomach) through the esophageal hiatus
	Symptoms—Dysphagia, failure to thrive, vomiting, neck contortions, frequent unexplained respiratory problems, bleeding
	Diagnosis made by fluoroscopy
		Therapeutic:
		  Surgical repair of defect
		Nursing:
		  Be alert to significant signs
		  Carry out routine postoperative care

ABDOMINAL
Umbilical: Soft skin-covered protrusion of intestine and omentum through a weakness in the abdominal wall around the umbilicus
	Inspection and palpation of abdomen
	High incidence in black infants
	Spontaneous closure by age 3-4 years
		Therapeutic:
		  No treatment of small defects
		  Operative repair if persists
		  Strangulation requires immediate attention
		Nursing:
		  Discourage use of home remedies (e.g., belly bands, coins)
		  Reassure parents

Omphalocele: Protrusion of intraabdominal viscera into the base of the umbilical cord; the sac is covered with peritoneum without skin
Gastroschisis: Protrusion of intraabdominal contents through a defect in the abdominal wall lateral to the umbilical ring; there is never a peritoneal sac
	Obvious on inspection
	Observe for other malformations
		Therapeutic:
		  Surgical repair of defect
		  Preoperative
		    Large lesions—Gradual reduction of abdominal contents
		    Prophylactic antibiotic administration
		Nursing (preoperative):
		  Keep sac or viscera moist
		  Use overhead warming unit
		  Carry out routine care of intravenous line, nasogastric suction
		  Give nothing by mouth
		  Use comfort measures

Unit 4

NURSING CARE OF THE CHILD WITH CARDIOVASCULAR DYSFUNCTION

NURSING CARE PLAN

The Child with Cardiovascular Dysfunction

The **cardiovascular system** consists of the heart and blood vessels.

Cardiac dysfunction refers to dysfunction, congenital or acquired, of the heart or the blood vessels.

ASSESSMENT

Perform physical assessment with detailed examination of the heart. (See p. 56).

(See physiologic measurement of pulse and blood pressure, p. 36)

Assess general appearance, behavior, and function:

Inspection

Nutritional state—Failure to thrive, poor weight gain, poor feeding habits, fatigue during feeding, or sweating during feeding are associated with heart disease

Color—Cyanosis is a common feature of congenital heart disease, and pallor is associated with anemia, which frequently accompanies heart disease

Chest deformities—An enlarged heart sometimes distorts the chest configuration

Unusual pulsations—Visible pulsations are sometimes present

Respiratory excursion—The ease or difficulty of respirating (e.g., tachypnea, dyspnea, presence of expiratory grunt, shortness of breath, persistent cough) or frequent respiratory infections

Clubbing of fingers—Associated with some types of congenital heart disease

Behavior—Assuming knee-chest position or squatting is typical of some types of heart disease; exercise intolerance

Palpation and percussion

Chest—Helps discern heart size and other characteristics (such as thrills) associated with heart disease

Abdomen—Hepatomegaly and/or splenomegaly may be evident

Peripheral pulses—Rate, regularity, and amplitude (strength) may reveal discrepancies

Auscultation

Heart—Detect presence of heart murmurs

Heart rate and rhythm—Observe for discrepancies between apical and peripheral pulses

Character of heart sounds—Reveals deviations in heart sounds and intensity that help localize heart defects

Lungs—May reveal crackles, wheezes

Blood pressure—Deviations present in some cardiac conditions (e.g., discrepancies between upper and lower extremities)

Assist with diagnostic procedures and tests (e.g., electrocardiography, radiography, echocardiography, fluoroscopy, ultrasonography, angiography, blood analysis [blood count, hemoglobin, packed cell volume, blood gases], and cardiac catheterization). (See p. 433.)

Unit 4

NURSING CARE PLAN

The Child Who Undergoes Cardiac Catheterization

Cardiac catheterization is a diagnostic procedure in which a radiopaque catheter, introduced into heart chambers via large peripheral vessels, is observed by fluoroscopy or image intensification; pressure measurements and blood samples provide additional sources of information.

PREPROCEDURAL CARE

ASSESSMENT
Perform routine physical assessment, including the following:
  Accurate height (essential for correct catheter selection) and weight
  Previous allergic reactions (e.g., contrast agents, iodine)
  Signs and symptoms of infection
  Presence of diaper rash (femoral access may be needed)
  Assessment and marking of pedal pulses (dorsalis pedis, posterior tibial)
  Pulse oximetry (especially in child with cyanosis)

NURSING DIAGNOSIS: Anxiety and fear related to diagnostic procedure, unfamiliar environment

■ **PATIENT GOAL 1:** Will experience reduction of anxiety/fear

NURSING INTERVENTIONS/*RATIONALES*
(See Preparation for Procedures, p. 219.)
(See also Preoperative care, p. 304.)
*Administer sedation and analgesia as prescribed
Encourage family to provide support to child while waiting for procedure
Take to cardiac catheterization room
  Transport infant in bassinet, crib, or incubator with extra diapers, blanket, and pacifier
  Transport older child on gurney with comfort object (doll, toy, blanket)
  Distract child during procedure by playing tapes of favorite stories or songs; talk to child

EXPECTED OUTCOME
Child is transported to cardiac catheterization room with minimum distress to child and family

POSTPROCEDURAL CARE

ASSESSMENT
(See Postoperative Assessment, p. 305.)
(See also Assessment in following care plan.)

NURSING DIAGNOSIS: Risk for injury related to operative procedure, blood loss during catheterization, contrast medium

■ **PATIENT GOAL 1:** Will exhibit no evidence of complications

NURSING INTERVENTIONS/*RATIONALES*
Assess physiologic status *so that complications are detected early*
Vital signs, including heart rate counted for 1 full minute, *for evidence of arrhythmias or bradycardia*

Blood pressure, especially for hypotension, *which may indicate hemorrhage from cardiac perforation or bleeding at the site of initial catheterization*
Pulses, especially below the catheterization site, for equality and symmetry (pulse distal to the site may be weaker for the first few hours after catheterization but should gradually increase in strength)
Temperature and color of the affected extremity, *since coolness or blanching may indicate arterial obstruction*
General color and oxygenation by oximetry
Check dressing for evidence of bleeding or hematoma formation in the femoral or antecubital area
If bleeding occurs, apply direct continuous pressure 2.5 cm (1 inch) above the percutaneous site *to localize pressure over the vessel puncture*
Keep affected extremity as straight as possible, as prescribed, *to facilitate healing of cannulated vessel*
  Younger child can be held in parent's lap with correct position maintained
  Avoid hip flexion (when femoral site used) *to prevent bleeding*
Keep child relatively quiet *to decrease risk of bleeding*
Keep incision and dressing clean and dry *to prevent infection*
Provide warmth if child is chilled from exposure during procedure
Avoid either overheating or chilling
*Administer withheld digitalis and other medications, if ordered
Encourage early fluid intake *to prevent hypoglycemia and dehydration*
*Provide diet as prescribed; advance as tolerated

EXPECTED OUTCOMES
Child exhibits no evidence of either vessel obstruction or bleeding
Complications are identified early, and appropriate interventions are instituted

■ **PATIENT GOAL 2:** Will exhibit signs of adequate hydration

NURSING INTERVENTIONS/*RATIONALES*
*Maintain intravenous infusion as prescribed until PO fluids tolerated

Continued

Unit 4

The Child Who Undergoes Cardiac Catheterization—cont'd

Assess for nausea *since intravenous hydration and/or antiemetics may be necessary in older child if emesis persists*

Assess skin turgor and oral mucosa for signs of dehydration

Maintain accurate record of intake and output

EXPECTED OUTCOME

Child exhibits signs of adequate hydration

NURSING DIAGNOSIS: Altered family processes related to child undergoing diagnostic procedure

---

■ **PATIENT (FAMILY) GOAL 1:** Will receive adequate support

NURSING INTERVENTIONS/*RATIONALES*

Keep family informed of child's progress during procedure

Be with family when results of procedure are given

Answer any questions regarding child's care or diagnosis

Allow parents to hold and feed infant after procedure *to regain some aspect of caregiving role*

Assist family in providing comfort to child

EXPECTED OUTCOMES

Family members demonstrate an understanding of the procedural care and diagnosis

Family regains some aspect of caregiving role

■ **PATIENT (FAMILY) GOAL 2:** Will be prepared for home care

NURSING INTERVENTIONS/*RATIONALES*

Teach family signs of complications *so that they are identified early and treated promptly:*

Altered perfusion in the catheterized extremity (cold, pale leg or foot)

Infection (redness, swelling, or drainage from catheterization site)

Stress need to report these signs to practitioner

EXPECTED OUTCOMES

Family demonstrates understanding of signs of complications

(See also:

Nursing Care Plan: The Family of the Child Who Is Ill or Hospitalized, p. 282.)

Nursing Care Plan: The Child in the Hospital, p. 268.)

Nursing Care Plan: The High-Risk Newborn and Family, p. 350.)

NURSING CARE PLAN

The Child with Congenital Heart Disease

Congenital heart disease is a structural or functional defect of the heart or great vessels present at birth.

TYPES OF DEFECTS
The hemodynamic classification system classifies defects by blood flow patterns:

(1) Increased pulmonary blood flow
(2) decreased pulmonary blood flow
(3) obstruction to blood flow out of the heart
(4) mixed blood flow, in which saturated and desaturated blood mix within the heart or great arteries

ASSESSMENT
Perform physical assessment with special emphasis on color, pulse (apical and peripheral), respiration, blood pressure, and examination and auscultation of chest.

Take careful health history, including evidence of poor weight gain, poor feeding, exercise intolerance, unusual posturing, or frequent respiratory tract infections.

Observe child for manifestations of congenital heart disease:

Infants
Cyanosis—Generalized, especially mucous membranes, lips and tongue, conjunctiva; highly vascularized areas
Cyanosis during exertion such as crying, feeding, straining, or when immersed in water; peripheral or central
Dyspnea, especially following physical effort such as feeding, crying, straining
Fatigue
Poor growth and development (failure to thrive)
Frequent respiratory tract infections

Feeding difficulties
Hypotonia
Excessive sweating
Syncopal attacks such as paroxysmal hyperpnea, anoxic spells

Older children
Impaired growth
Delicate, frail body build
Fatigue
Effort dyspnea
Orthopnea
Digital clubbing
Squatting for relief of dyspnea
Headache
Epistaxis
Leg fatigue

(See also Assessment of the child with cardiovascular dysfunction, p. 432.)

Continued

GUIDELINES

Administering Digoxin at Home

Give digoxin at regular intervals (usually every 12 hours, such as at 8 AM and 8 PM).

Plan the times so that the drug is given *1 hour before* or *2 hours after* feedings.

Use a calendar to mark off each dose that is given; or post a reminder, such as a sign on the refrigerator.

Have the prescription refilled *before* the medication is completely used.

Administer the drug carefully by slowly directing it to the side and back of the mouth.

Do not mix it with other foods or fluids, since refusal to consume these results in inaccurate intake of the drug.

If the child has teeth, give water after administering the drug; whenever possible, brush the teeth to prevent tooth decay from the sweetened liquid.

If a dose is missed, and more than 4 hours have elapsed, withhold the dose and give the next dose at the regular time; if less than 4 hours have elapsed, give the missed dose.

If the child vomits, do not give a second dose.

If more than two consecutive doses have been missed, notify the physician or other designated practitioner.

Do not increase or double the dose for missed doses.

If the child becomes ill, notify the physician or other designated practitioner immediately.

Keep digoxin in a safe place, preferably a locked cabinet.

In case of accidental overdose of digoxin, call the nearest poison control center immediately; the number is usually listed in the front of the telephone directory.

Modified from Jackson PL: Digoxin therapy at home: keeping the child safe, *MCN* 4(2):105-109, 1979.

The Child with Congenital Heart Disease—cont'd

NURSING DIAGNOSIS: Risk for decreased cardiac output related to structural defect

■ **PATIENT GOAL 1:** Will exhibit improved cardiac output

NURSING INTERVENTIONS/*RATIONALES*
*Administer digoxin as ordered, using established precautions *to prevent toxicity* (See p. 438 and Guidelines box, p. 435.)
*Administer afterload reduction medications as ordered (See p. 438.)
*Administer diuretics as ordered (See p. 439.)

EXPECTED OUTCOMES
Heart rate, blood pressure, and peripheral perfusion are normal for age (See inside front cover.)
Urinary output is adequate (between 0.5 and 2 ml/kg, depending on age)

NURSING DIAGNOSIS: Activity intolerance related to imbalance between oxygen supply and demand

■ **PATIENT GOAL 1:** Will maintain adequate energy levels without additional stresses

NURSING INTERVENTIONS/*RATIONALES*
Allow for frequent rest periods and uninterrupted sleep periods
Encourage quiet games and activities
Help child select activities appropriate to age, condition, and capabilities
Avoid extremes of environmental temperature *because hyperthermia and hypothermia increase the need for oxygen*
Implement measures to reduce anxiety
Respond promptly to crying or other expressions of distress

EXPECTED OUTCOMES
Child determines and engages in activities commensurate with capabilities
Child receives appropriate amount of rest/sleep (specify)

NURSING DIAGNOSIS: Altered growth and development related to inadequate oxygen and nutrients to tissues; social isolation

■ **PATIENT GOAL 1:** Will follow growth curve for weight and height

NURSING INTERVENTIONS/*RATIONALES*
Provide well-balanced, highly nutritious diet *to achieve adequate growth*
Monitor height and weight; plot on growth charts *to determine growth trend*
*May administer iron supplements, if ordered, *to correct anemia*

EXPECTED OUTCOME
Child achieves adequate growth (specify)

■ **PATIENT GOAL 2:** Will have opportunity to participate in age-appropriate activities

NURSING INTERVENTIONS/*RATIONALES*
Encourage age-appropriate activities
Emphasize that child has same need for socialization as other children
Allow child to set own pace and activity limits *because child will rest when tired*

EXPECTED OUTCOMES
Child engages in age-appropriate activities
Child does not experience social isolation

NURSING DIAGNOSIS: Risk for infection related to debilitated physical status

■ **PATIENT GOAL 1:** Will exhibit no evidence of infection

NURSING INTERVENTIONS/*RATIONALES*
Avoid contact with infected persons
Provide for adequate rest
Provide optimum nutrition *to support body's natural defenses*

EXPECTED OUTCOME
Child remains free of infection

NURSING DIAGNOSIS: Altered family processes related to having a child with a heart condition

(See Nursing Care Plan: The Child with Chronic Illness or Disability, p. 287.)

■ **PATIENT (FAMILY) GOAL 1:** Will experience reduction of fear and anxiety

NURSING INTERVENTIONS/*RATIONALES*
Discuss with parents and child (if appropriate) their fears and concerns regarding child's cardiac defects and physical symptoms *since these frequently cause anxiety/fear*

EXPECTED OUTCOME
Family discusses their fears and anxieties

■ **PATIENT (FAMILY) GOAL 2:** Will exhibit positive coping behaviors

NURSING INTERVENTIONS/*RATIONALES*
Encourage family to participate in care of child while hospitalized *to better facilitate coping at home*
Encourage family to include others in child's care *to prevent their own exhaustion*
Assist family in determining appropriate physical activity and disciplining methods for child

EXPECTED OUTCOME
Family copes with child's symptoms in a positive way

■ **PATIENT (FAMILY) GOAL 3:** Will demonstrate knowledge of home care

NURSING INTERVENTIONS/*RATIONALES*
Teach skills needed for home care:
   Administration of medications

*Dependent nursing action.

Unit 4

The Child with Congenital Heart Disease—cont'd

Feeding techniques
Interventions to conserve energy and those directed toward relief of frightening symptoms
Signs that indicate complications
Where and whom to contact for help and guidance
Anticipate need for further information and support
Refer family to local chapter of the American Red Cross *for instruction in cardiopulmonary resuscitation*

EXPECTED OUTCOMES

Family demonstrates ability and motivation for home care
Family members learn cardiopulmonary resuscitation techniques

> **NURSING DIAGNOSIS:** Risk for injury (complications) related to cardiac condition and therapies

■ **PATIENT (FAMILY) GOAL 1:** Will recognize signs of complications early

NURSING INTERVENTIONS/*RATIONALES*

Teach family to recognize signs of complications:
Congestive heart failure (CHF) (For complete list, see assessment on p. 438.)
Early signs:
Tachycardia, especially during rest and slight exertion
Tachypnea
Profuse scalp sweating, especially in infants
Fatigue and irritation
Sudden weight gain
Respiratory distress
Digoxin toxicity:
Vomiting (earliest sign)
Nausea
Anorexia

Bradycardia
Dysrhythmias
Increased respiratory effort—Retraction, grunting, cough, cyanosis
Hypoxemia—Cyanosis, restlessness
Cardiovascular collapse—Pallor, cyanosis, hypotonia
Teach family to intervene during hypercyanotic spells
Place child in knee-chest position with head and chest elevated
Remain calm
Administer 100% oxygen by face mask (if available)
Call practitioner

EXPECTED OUTCOME

Family recognizes signs of complications and institutes appropriate action

■ **PATIENT (FAMILY) GOAL 2:** Will demonstrate understanding of diagnostic tests and surgery

NURSING INTERVENTIONS/*RATIONALES*

Explain or clarify information presented to the family by practitioner and surgeon
Prepare child and parents for the procedure
Assist with family's decision regarding surgery
Explore feelings regarding surgical options

EXPECTED OUTCOMES

Family demonstrates an understanding of procedures (e.g., tests, surgery) (specify learning and manner of demonstration)
(See also:
Nursing Care Plan: The Child in the Hospital, p. 268.)
Nursing Care Plan: The Family of the Child Who Is Ill or Hospitalized, p. 282.)
Nursing Care Plan: The Child Undergoing Surgery, p. 304.)
Nursing Care Plan: The High-Risk Newborn and Family, p. 350.)

Unit 4

NURSING CARE PLAN

The Child with Congestive Heart Failure

Congestive heart failure is the inability of the heart to pump an adequate amount of blood to the systemic circulation at normal filling pressures to meet the metabolic demands of the body.

ASSESSMENT

Perform a physical assessment. (See p. 28.)
Perform a cardiac assessment. (See p. 432.)
Take a careful health history, especially regarding previous cardiac problems.
Observe for manifestations of congestive heart failure:

Impaired myocardial function
Tachycardia
Sweating (inappropriate)
Decreased urine output
Fatigue
Weakness
Restlessness
Anorexia
Pale, cool extremities
Weak peripheral pulses
Decreased blood pressure
Gallop rhythm
Cardiomegaly

Pulmonary congestion
Tachypnea
Dyspnea
Retractions (infants)
Flaring nares
Exercise intolerance
Orthopnea
Cough, hoarseness
Cyanosis
Wheezing
Grunting

Systemic venous congestion
Weight gain
Hepatomegaly
Peripheral edema, especially periorbital
Ascites
Neck vein distention (children)

Assist with diagnostic procedures and tests (e.g., radiography, electrocardiography).

NURSING DIAGNOSIS: Decreased cardiac output related to structural defect, myocardial dysfunction

■ **PATIENT GOAL 1:** Will exhibit improved cardiac output

NURSING INTERVENTIONS/*RATIONALES*
*Administer digoxin (Lanoxin), as ordered, using established precautions *to prevent toxicity*
Make certain dosage is within safe limits
Infants rarely receive more than 1 ml (50 μg or 0.05 mg) in one dose; *a higher dose is an immediate warning of a dosage error*
Ascertain correct preparation for route
Check dosage with another nurse *to ensure safety*
Count apical pulse for 1 full minute before giving drug
    Withhold medication and notify practitioner if pulse rate is less than 90 to 110 beats/min (infants) or 70 to 85 beats/min (older children), depending on previous pulse readings
Recognize signs of digoxin toxicity (nausea, vomiting, anorexia, bradycardia, dysrhythmias)
Often an ECG rhythm strip is taken *to assess cardiac status before administration*
Ensure adequate intake of potassium
Observe for signs of hypokalemia (muscle weakness, hypotension, dysrhythmias, tachycardia or bradycardia, irritability, drowsiness) or hyperkalemia (muscle weakness, twitching, bradycardia, ventricular fibrillation, oliguria, apnea)
Monitor serum potassium levels *because decrease enhances digoxin toxicity*
*Administer medications to decrease afterload, as ordered
Check blood pressure
    Observe for signs of hypotension
Monitor electrolyte levels
Attach cardiac monitor if ordered

EXPECTED OUTCOMES
Heartbeat is strong, regular, and within normal limits for age (See inside back cover.)
Peripheral perfusion is adequate

NURSING DIAGNOSIS: Ineffective breathing pattern related to pulmonary congestion

■ **PATIENT GOAL 1:** Will exhibit improved respiratory function

NURSING INTERVENTIONS/*RATIONALES*
Place in inclined posture of 30 to 45 degrees *to encourage maximum chest expansion;* tilt mattress support of incubator; place older infant in infant seat
Avoid any constricting clothing or restraints around abdomen and chest
*Administer humidified oxygen as prescribed
Assess respiratory rate, ease of respiration, color, and oxygen saturations as measured by oximetry

EXPECTED OUTCOME
Respirations remain within normal limits, color is good, and child rests quietly (See inside front cover for normal variations in respirations.)

■ **PATIENT GOAL 2:** Will experience reduction of anxiety

NURSING INTERVENTIONS/*RATIONALES*
Employ flexible feeding schedule *to reduce fretfulness associated with hunger*
Handle child gently
Hold and comfort infant
Employ comfort measures found effective for individual child
Encourage family to provide comfort and solace
Explain equipment and procedures to child *to decrease anxiety*

---

*Dependent nursing action.

Unit 4

The Child with Congestive Heart Failure—cont'd

EXPECTED OUTCOME
Child rests quietly and breathes easily

> **NURSING DIAGNOSIS:** Fluid volume excess related to fluid accumulation (edema)

■ **PATIENT GOAL 1:** Will exhibit no evidence of fluid excess

NURSING INTERVENTIONS/*RATIONALES*
*Administer diuretics as prescribed
Maintain and record accurate intake and output
Weigh daily at same time and on same scale *to assess fluid gain or loss*
Assess for evidence of increased or decreased edema
Maintain fluid restriction, if ordered
Provide skin care for children with edema
    Change position frequently *to prevent skin breakdown associated with edema*
    Use alternating-pressure mattress

EXPECTED OUTCOME
Infant exhibits evidence of fluid loss (frequent urination, weight loss)

> **NURSING DIAGNOSIS:** Activity intolerance related to imbalance between oxygen supply and demand

■ **PATIENT GOAL 1:** Will exhibit no additional respiratory or cardiac stress

NURSING INTERVENTIONS/*RATIONALES*
Maintain neutral thermal environment *because hypothermia and hyperthermia increase need for oxygen*
    Place newborn in incubator or under warmer
    Keep infant warm
    Treat fever promptly
Feed small volumes, at frequent intervals (every 2 to 3 hours), using soft nipple with moderately large opening *since infants with CHF tire easily*
Implement gavage feeding if infant becomes fatigued before taking an adequate amount
Time nursing activities to disturb child as little as possible
Implement measures to reduce anxiety
Respond promptly to crying or other expressions of distress

EXPECTED OUTCOME
Child rests quietly

> **NURSING DIAGNOSIS:** Risk for infection related to reduced body defenses, pulmonary congestion

(See Nursing Care Plan: The Child at Risk for Infection, p. 341.)
(See also Nursing Care Plan: The Child with Congenital Heart Disease, p. 435.)

> **NURSING DIAGNOSIS:** Altered family processes related to a child with a life-threatening illness

■ **PATIENT (FAMILY) GOAL 1:** Will receive adequate support

**NURSING INTERVENTIONS/*RATIONALES*
AND EXPECTED OUTCOMES**
(See Nursing Care Plan: The Family of the Child Who Is Ill or Hospitalized, p. 282.)

■ **PATIENT (FAMILY) GOAL 2:** Will be prepared for home care

NURSING INTERVENTIONS/*RATIONALES*
Teach family:
    Medication administration and side/toxic effects
    Signs and symptoms of CHF and to report them to designated practitioner
    Feeding techniques and nutritional requirements
    Positioning
    Need for rest
    Growth and developmental considerations
        Growth is slowed
        Gross motor skills may be delayed more than fine motor skills
Refer to outpatient services and community resources as needed *for ongoing support*

EXPECTED OUTCOMES
Family demonstrates an understanding of the condition and the care required at home
Family uses appropriate community resources

*Dependent nursing action.

Unit 4

NURSING CARE PLAN

The Child with Rheumatic Fever

Rheumatic fever (RF) is an autoimmune reaction to group A, beta hemolytic, streptococcal pharyngitis that involves the joints, skin, brain, serous surfaces, and heart.

ASSESSMENT

Perform a routine physical assessment. (See p. 28.)

Take a health history, especially regarding evidence of antecedent streptococcus infections.

Observe for manifestations of rheumatic fever:

General

Positive throat culture or rapid streptococcal antigen test

Elevated or rising streptococcal antibody titer

Low-grade fever, usually spiking in late afternoon

Unexplained epistaxis

Abdominal pain

Arthralgia without arthritic changes

Weakness

Fatigue

Pallor

Loss of appetite

Weight loss

Specific manifestations

Carditis

Tachycardia out of proportion to degree of fever

Cardiomegaly

New murmurs or change in preexisting murmurs

Muffled heart sounds

Precardial friction rub

Precordial pain

Changes in ECG (especially prolonged P-R interval)

Migratory polyarthritis

Swollen, hot, red, painful joint(s)

After 1 to 2 days affects different joint(s)

Favors large joints—knees, elbows, hips, shoulders, wrists

Subcutaneous nodes

Nontender swelling

Located over bony prominences

May persist for some time, then gradually resolve

Chorea (St. Vitus dance, Sydenham chorea)

Sudden, aimless, irregular movements of extremities

Involuntary facial grimaces

Speech disturbances

Emotional lability

Muscle weakness (can be profound)

Muscle movements exaggerated by anxiety and attempts at fine motor activity; relieved by rest

Erythema marginatum

Erythemous macules with clear center and wavy, well-demarcated border

Transitory

Nonpruritic

Primarily affects trunk and proximal extremities (inner surfaces)

Assist with diagnostic procedures and tests (e.g., electrocardiography, throat culture, blood analysis for increased erythrocyte sedimentation rate, and antistreptolysin-O titer).

NURSING DIAGNOSIS: Risk for injury related to presence of streptococcal organisms, susceptibility to recurrence of RF, and bacterial endocarditis

■ **PATIENT (FAMILY) GOAL 1:** Will comply with therapeutic regimen

NURSING INTERVENTIONS/*RATIONALES*

Ask family and older child if child has ever had an allergic reaction to penicillin, *since penicillin is the drug of choice for RF*

*Administer penicillin, or erythromycin in penicillin-sensitive child, as ordered therapeutically and prophylactically *to eradicate hemolytic streptococci and to prevent recurrence of RF and bacterial endocarditis*

Teach family and older child proper administration of penicillin or erythromycin (See Community and Home Care Instructions, p. 598.)

Institute measures to encourage compliance with therapeutic regimen (See Nursing Care Plan: Child and Family Compliance p. 343.)

Explain to child and family importance of ongoing, long-term health supervision *since child is susceptible to recurrent RF*

Explain to child and family need for antibiotic prophylaxis for dental work, infection, and invasive procedures (Box 4-23)

EXPECTED OUTCOME

Child and family comply with therapeutic regimen

■ **PATIENT GOAL 2:** Will experience no or minimal complications or discomfort

NURSING INTERVENTIONS/*RATIONALES*

Encourage adequate rest and nutrition *to support body's natural defenses*

*Administer salicylates as ordered *to control inflammatory process and reduce fever and discomfort*

*Administer prednisone, if ordered, *to treat pancarditis and valvulitis*

If carditis is present, explain to child and family any activity restrictions and help them choose less strenuous activities

Recognize that chorea, if present, is usually disturbing and frustrating to child and family

Explain that chorea is a manifestation of RF *because it may be misinterpreted by child, family, and others* (e.g., teachers)

Stress that chorea is involuntary, transitory, and that all manifestations eventually disappear

Give child and family opportunity to verbalize feelings *to facilitate positive coping*

(For arthritis, see also Nursing Care Plan: The Child with Juvenile Rheumatoid Arthritis, p. 517.)

(For carditis, see also Nursing Care Plan: The Child with Congestive Heart Failure, p. 438.)

EXPECTED OUTCOMES

Child recovers from illness with no or minimum complications or discomfort

Child and family adjust to chorea and understand it is a temporary manifestation of RF

*Dependent nursing action.

Unit 4

The Child with Rheumatic Fever—cont'd

BOX 4-23

Endocarditis Prophylaxis Recommendations

Dental Procedures

Dental extractions

Periodontal procedures, including surgery, scaling and root planing, probing, and recall maintenance

Dental implant placement and reimplantation of evulsed teeth

Endodontic (root canal) instrumentation or surgery only beyond the apex

Subgingival placement of antibiotic fibers/strips

Initial placement of orthodontic bands but not brackets

Intraligamentary local anesthetic injections

Prophylactic cleaning of teeth or implants where bleeding is anticipated

Other Procedures

Respiratory Tract

Surgical operations that involve respiratory mucosa

Bronchoscopy with a rigid bronchoscope

Tonsillectomy and/or adenoidectomy

Gastrointestinal Tract

Sclerotherapy for esophageal varices

Esophageal stricture dilation

Endoscopic retrograde cholangiography with biliary obstruction

Biliary tract surgery

Surgical operations that involve intestinal mucosa

Genitourinary Tract

Prostatic surgery

Cystoscopy

Urethral dilation

From Dajani AS and others: Prevention of bacterial endocarditis: recommendations by the American Heart Association, *JAMA* 277:1794-1801, 1997.

NURSING CARE PLAN

The Child in Shock (Circulatory Failure)

Shock (circulatory failure) is a clinical syndrome characterized by tissue perfusion that is inadequate to meet the metabolic demands of the body, resulting in depressed vital cell function.

STAGES OF SHOCK

Compensated shock—Vital organ function is maintained by intrinsic compensatory mechanisms; blood flow is usually normal or increased but generally uneven or maldistributed in the microcirculation

Decompensated shock—Efficiency of the cardiovascular system gradually diminishes until perfusion in the microcirculation becomes marginal despite compensatory adjustments

Irreversible, or terminal shock—Damage to vital organs such as the heart or brain, of such magnitude that the entire organism will be disrupted regardless of therapeutic intervention; death occurs even if cardiovascular measurements return to normal levels with therapy

TYPES OF SHOCK

Hypovolemic shock

Characteristics

Reduction in size of vascular compartment

Falling blood pressure

Poor capillary filling

Low central venous pressure (CVP)

Most frequent causes

Blood loss (hemorrhagic shock)—Trauma, GI bleeding, intracranial hemorrhage

Plasma loss—Increased capillary permeability associated with sepsis and acidosis, hypoproteinemia, burns, peritonitis

Extracellular fluid loss—Vomiting, diarrhea, glycosuric diuresis, sunstroke

Distributive shock

Characteristics

Reduction in peripheral vascular resistance

Profound inadequacies in tissue perfusion

Increased venous capacity and pooling

Acute reduction in return blood flow to the heart

Diminished cardiac output

Most frequent causes

Anaphylaxis (anaphylactic shock)—Extreme allergy or hypersensitivity to a foreign substance

Sepsis (septic shock, bacteremic shock, endotoxic shock)—Overwhelming sepsis and circulating bacterial toxins

Loss of neuronal control (neurogenic shock)—Interruption of neuronal transmission (spinal cord injury)

Myocardial depression and peripheral dilation—Exposure to anesthesia or ingestion of barbiturates, tranquilizers, narcotics, antihypertensive agents, or ganglionic blocking agents

Cardiogenic shock

Characteristic

Decreased cardiac output

Most frequent causes

Following surgery for congenital heart disease

Primary pump failure—Myocarditis, myocardial trauma, biochemical derangements, congestive heart failure

Dysrhythmias—Paroxysmal atrial tachycardia, atrioventricular block, and ventricular dysrhythmias; secondary to myocarditis or biochemical abnormalities (occasionally)

ASSESSMENT

Maintain vigilance in situations that predispose the patient to shock (e.g., trauma, burns, overwhelming sepsis, diarrhea, vomiting).

Observe for manifestations of shock:

Early clinical signs

Apprehensiveness

Irritability

Unexplained tachycardia

Normal blood pressure

Narrowing pulse pressure

Thirst

Pallor

Diminished urinary output

Reduced perfusion of extremities

Advanced shock

Confusion and somnolence

Tachypnea

Moderate metabolic acidosis

Oliguria

Cool, pale extremities

Decreased skin turgor

Poor capillary filling

Impending cardiopulmonary arrest

Thready, weak pulse

Hypotension

Periodic breathing or apnea

Anuria

Stupor or coma

Monitor vital signs, central venous pressure, capillary filling, intake and output, and cardiac function, on admission and continuously or very frequently.

Assist with diagnostic procedures and tests (e.g., blood count, blood gases, pH, liver function tests, cultures, electrolytes, electrocardiography).

NURSING DIAGNOSIS: Impaired gas exchange related to diminished oxygen needed for impaired tissue perfusion

■ **PATIENT GOAL 1:** Will exhibit signs of adequate oxygenation

NURSING INTERVENTIONS/*RATIONALES*

*Administer oxygen as prescribed *to ensure adequate tissue oxygenation*

Position to maintain open airway (e.g., neck in neutral or "sniffing" position) *since critically ill child may not be able to maintain adequate airway*

Be prepared for intubation *since this may be necessary*

Monitor artificial airway and mechanical ventilation (if implemented) *to maintain airway and improve ventilation*

Monitor closely (e.g., vital signs, blood gases and pH, capillary filling, presence of pallor or cyanosis) *to assess efficacy of therapy*

Attach and monitor apnea and cardiac monitors *for ongoing assessment of child*

*Dependent nursing action.

The Child in Shock (Circulatory Failure)—cont'd

EXPECTED OUTCOME

Child exhibits signs of adequate oxygenation (specify)

NURSING DIAGNOSIS: Altered tissue perfusion related to reduced blood flow, decreased blood volume, reduced vascular tone

---

■ **PATIENT GOAL 1:** Will exhibit signs of improved cardiac output and circulation

NURSING INTERVENTIONS/*RATIONALES*

Position child flat on back with legs elevated *to promote venous return*

Avoid Trendelenburg position *because it tends to increase intracranial pressure, decrease diaphragmatic excursion and lung volume, and decrease venous return to the heart*

*Start (or help start) and monitor intravenous infusion of prescribed fluid and plasma expander *because rapid restoration of blood volume is essential in most shock situations*

Weigh child *in order to calculate drug dosages*

*Administer medications as prescribed (e.g., vasopressors) *to improve cardiac output and circulation*

*Administer medications as prescribed (e.g., antibiotics for septic shock) *to treat associated disorder*

Monitor closely (including hourly urine output, central venous pressure, level of consciousness) *to assess efficacy of therapy*

EXPECTED OUTCOME

Child exhibits evidence of improved cardiac output and circulation: pulse, respiration, blood pressure, oxygen saturation, and urinary output within acceptable limits (specify); skin warm, dry, and good color; alert and oriented

---

NURSING DIAGNOSIS: Fear/anxiety related to emergency care, ICU

■ **PATIENT GOAL 1:** Will remain calm

NURSING INTERVENTIONS/*RATIONALES*

*Administer sedation as ordered

Maintain calm demeanor *to decrease anxiety/fear*

Explain in simple terms what is being done to and for child *in order to not increase anxiety*

Assure child and family of close, continuous monitoring

Avoid conversations about the child in his or her presence *to reduce fear/anxiety and misconceptions*

Allow family to be with child as soon as condition and care permits

EXPECTED OUTCOME

Child will remain calm

NURSING DIAGNOSIS: Altered family processes related to a child in a life-threatening condition

---

■ **PATIENT (FAMILY) GOAL 1:** Will receive adequate support

NURSING INTERVENTIONS/*RATIONALES*

Keep family informed regarding child's status

Arrange for someone to remain with family and serve as a liaison between them and the critical care area (if possible)

Allow family to see child as soon as feasible

Encourage expression of feelings, especially regarding severity of condition and prognosis

Arrange for presence of family support systems (e.g., friends, clergy) if possible

EXPECTED OUTCOMES

Family demonstrates an attitude of assurance that the child is being given needed care

(See also:

Nursing Care Plan: The Family of the Child Who Is Ill or Hospitalized, p. 282.)

Nursing Care Plan: The Child in the Hospital, p. 268.)

Nursing care plans for specific disorders producing shock.)

Nursing Diagnosis: Anticipatory grieving, p. 495.)

*Dependent nursing action.

Unit 4

NURSING CARE OF THE CHILD WITH HEMATOLOGIC/IMMUNOLOGIC DYSFUNCTION

The **hematologic system** consists of the blood and blood-forming tissues: red bone marrow, lymph nodes, and spleen. The immune system includes the *primary lymphoid organs* (thymus, bone marrow, and liver) and the *secondary lymphoid organs* (lymph nodes, spleen, and gut-associated lymphoid tissue [GALT]).

NURSING CARE PLAN

The Child with Anemia

Anemia is a condition in which the number of red blood cells and/or the hemoglobin concentration is reduced below normal.

ASSESSMENT

Perform a physical assessment. (See p. 28.)

Take a health history, including a careful diet history, to identify any deficiencies (such as evidence of pica, the eating of nonfood substances such as clay, ice, or paste).

Observe for manifestations of anemia:

General manifestations

Muscle weakness

Easy fatigability

    Frequent resting

    Shortness of breath

    Poor sucking (infants)

Pale skin

    Waxy pallor seen in severe anemia

Pica

Central nervous system manifestations

Headache

Dizziness

Light-headedness

Irritability

Slowed thought processes

Decreased attention span

Apathy

Depression

Shock (blood loss anemia)

Poor peripheral perfusion

Skin moist and cool

Low blood pressure and central venous pressure

Increased heart rate

Assist with diagnostic tests (e.g., analysis of blood elements).

> **NURSING DIAGNOSIS:** Anxiety/fear related to diagnostic procedures/transfusion

- **PATIENT (FAMILY) GOAL 1:** Will become knowledgeable about the disorder, diagnostic tests, and treatment

NURSING INTERVENTIONS/*RATIONALES*

Prepare child for tests *to relieve anxiety/fear*

Allow child to play with the equipment on a doll and/or participate in the actual procedure (e.g., cleanse own finger with alcohol swab)

Remain with child during tests and initiation of transfusion *to provide support and observe for possible complications*

Explain purpose of blood components *to increase understanding of disorder, diagnostic tests, and treatment*

EXPECTED OUTCOMES

Child and family display minimal anxiety

Child and family demonstrate an understanding of the disorder, diagnostic tests, and treatment

---

> **NURSING DIAGNOSIS:** Activity intolerance related to generalized weakness, diminished oxygen delivery to tissues

- **PATIENT GOAL 1:** Will receive adequate rest

NURSING INTERVENTIONS/*RATIONALES*

Observe for signs of physical exertion (e.g., tachycardia, palpitations, tachypnea, dyspnea, shortness of breath, hyperpnea, breathlessness, dizziness, light-headedness, sweating, and change in skin color) and fatigue (sagging, limp posture, slow, strained movements, inability to tolerate additional activity, difficulty sucking in infants) *to plan appropriately for rest*

Anticipate and assist in those activities of daily living that may be beyond child's tolerance *to prevent exertion*

Provide diversional play activities *that promote rest and quiet but prevent boredom and withdrawal*

Choose appropriate roommate of similar age and interests who requires restricted activity *to encourage compliance with need for rest*

Plan nursing activities *to provide sufficient rest*

EXPECTED OUTCOMES

Child plays and rests quietly and engages in activities appropriate to capabilities

Child does not exhibit signs of physical exertion or fatigue

- **PATIENT GOAL 2:** Will exhibit normal respirations

NURSING INTERVENTIONS/*RATIONALES*

Maintain high Fowler position for *optimum air exchange*

*Administer supplemental oxygen, if needed, *to increase oxygen to tissues*

Take vital signs during periods of rest *to establish baseline for comparison during periods of activity*

EXPECTED OUTCOME

Patient breathes easily; respiratory rate and depth are normal (See inside front cover.)

---

*Dependent nursing action.

■ **PATIENT GOAL 3:** Will experience minimal emotional stress

NURSING INTERVENTIONS/*RATIONALES*

Anticipate child's irritability, short attention span, and fretfulness by offering to assist child in activities rather than waiting for a request for help

Encourage parents to remain with child *to minimize stress of separation*

Provide comfort measures (e.g., pacifier, rocking, music) *to minimize stress*

Encourage child to express feelings *to minimize anxiety/fear* (See also Nursing Care Plan: The Child in the Hospital, p. 268.)

EXPECTED OUTCOME

Child remains calm and quiet

■ **PATIENT GOAL 4:** Will receive appropriate blood elements

NURSING INTERVENTIONS/*RATIONALES*

*Administer blood, packed cells, platelets as prescribed (Table 4-31)

*Administer hematopoietic growth factors, as prescribed, *to stimulate blood cell formation*

EXPECTED OUTCOME

Child receives appropriate blood elements without incident

> **NURSING DIAGNOSIS:** Altered nutrition: less than body requirements related to reported inadequate iron intake (less than RDA); knowledge deficit regarding iron-rich foods

■ **PATIENT GOAL 1:** Will receive adequate supply of iron

NURSING INTERVENTIONS/*RATIONALES*

Provide diet counseling to caregiver, especially in regard to the following:

Food sources of iron (e.g., meat, liver, fish, egg yolks, green leafy vegetables, legumes, nuts, whole grains, and iron-fortified infant cereal and dry cereal) *to ensure that child receives adequate supply of iron*

Milk as supplemental food in infant's diet after solids are begun *because overingestion of milk decreases child's intake of iron-rich solid foods*

Teach older child about importance of adequate iron in the diet *to encourage compliance*

EXPECTED OUTCOME

Child receives at least minimum daily requirement of iron

■ **PATIENT GOAL 2:** Will consume iron supplements

NURSING INTERVENTIONS/*RATIONALES*

*Administer iron preparations as prescribed

Instruct family regarding correct administration of oral iron preparation:

Give in divided doses (specify) *for maximum absorption*

Give between meals *to increase absorption in upper gastrointestinal tract*

Administer with citrus fruit or juice preparation *because vitamin C reduces iron to its most soluble state*

Do not give with milk or antacids *since they decrease absorption*

Do not give with tea *because tannins in tea form an insoluble complex with iron from foods other than meat and because some herbal teas may affect iron absorption*

*Administer liquid preparation with dropper, syringe, or straw *to avoid contact with teeth and possible staining*

Assess characteristics of stools *because adequate dosage of oral iron turns stool a tarry green color*

Store iron preparation safely away from reach of children and keep no more than a 1 month supply in the home *because iron can be toxic*

EXPECTED OUTCOMES

Family relates a diet history that verifies child's compliance with these suggestions

Child is given iron supplement as evidenced by green, tarry stools

Child takes medication appropriately

(See also Nursing Care Plan: The Family of the Child Who Is Ill or Hospitalized, p. 282.)

*Dependent nursing action.

TABLE 4-31 Nursing Care of the Child Receiving Blood Transfusions

Complication	Signs/Symptoms	Precautions/Nursing Responsibilities
Immediate Reactions		
Hemolytic Reactions		
Most severe type, but rare	Chills	Verify patient identification
	Shaking	Identify donor and recipient blood types and groups before transfusion is begun; verify with another nurse or other practitioner
Incompatible blood	Fever	
Incompatibility in multiple transfusions	Pain at needle site and along venous tract	Transfuse blood slowly for first 15-20 minutes and/or initial ⅓ volume of blood; remain with patient
	Nausea/vomiting	Stop transfusion immediately in event of signs or symptoms, maintain patent IV line, and notify practitioner
	Sensation of tightness in chest	
	Red or black urine	Save donor blood to recrossmatch with patient's blood
	Headache	Monitor for evidence of shock
	Flank pain	Insert urinary catheter and monitor hourly outputs
	Progressive signs of shock and/or renal failure	Send samples of patient's blood and urine to laboratory for presence of hemoglobin (indicates intravascular hemolysis)
		Observe for signs of hemorrhage resulting from disseminated intravascular coagulation (DIC)
		Support medical therapies to reverse shock

Continued

Unit 4

TABLE 4-31   Nursing Care of the Child Receiving Blood Transfusions—cont'd

Complication	Signs/Symptoms	Precautions/Nursing Responsibilities
Immediate Reactions—cont'd		
Febrile Reactions		
Leukocyte or platelet antibodies	Fever	May give acetaminophen for prophylaxis
Plasma protein antibodies	Chills	Leukocyte-poor RBCs are less likely to cause reaction
		Stop transfusion immediately; report to practitioner for evaluation
Allergic Reactions		
Recipient reacts to allergens in donor's blood	Urticaria	Give antihistamines for prophylaxis to children with tendency toward allergic reactions
	Flushing	
	Asthmatic wheezing	Stop transfusion immediately
	Laryngeal edema	Administer epinephrine for wheezing or anaphylactic reaction
Circulatory Overload		
Too rapid transfusion (even a small quantity)	Precordial pain	Transfuse blood slowly
	Dyspnea	Prevent overload by using packed RBCs or administering divided amounts of blood
	Rales	
Excessive quantity of blood transfused (even slowly)	Cyanosis	Use infusion pump to regulate and maintain flow rate
	Dry cough	Stop transfusion immediately if signs of overload
	Distended neck veins	Place child upright with feet in dependent position to increase venous resistance
Air Emboli		
May occur when blood is transfused under pressure	Sudden difficulty in breathing	Normalize pressure before container is empty when infusing blood under pressure
	Sharp pain in chest	Clear tubing of air by aspirating air with syringe at nearest Y-connector if air is observed in tubing; disconnect tubing and allow blood to flow until air has escaped only if a Y-connector is not available
	Apprehension	
Hypothermia	Chills	Allow blood to warm at room temperatures (less than 1 hour)
	Low temperature	Use approved mechanical blood warmer or electric warming coil to rapidly warm blood; never use microwave oven
	Irregular heart rate	
	Possible cardiac arrest	Take temperature if patient complains of chills; if subnormal, stop transfusion
Electrolyte Disturbances		
Hyperkalemia (in massive transfusions or in patients with renal problems)	Nausea, diarrhea	Use washed RBCs or fresh blood if patient is at risk
	Muscular weakness	
	Flaccid paralysis	
	Paresthesia of extremities	
	Bradycardia	
	Apprehension	
	Cardiac arrest	
Delayed Reactions		
Transmission of Infection		
Hepatitis	Signs of infection (e.g., jaundice)	Blood is tested for antibodies to HIV, hepatitis C virus, and hepatitis B core antigen; in addition, blood is tested for hepatitis B surface antigen (HBsAg) and alanine aminotransferase (ALT), and a serology test is performed for syphilis; positive units are destroyed; individuals at risk for carrying certain viruses are deferred from donation
Human immunodeficiency virus (HIV)	Toxic reaction: high fever, severe headache or substernal pain, hypotension, intense flushing, vomiting/diarrhea	
Malaria		
Syphilis		
Bacteria or viruses		Report any sign of infection and, if occurring during transfusion, stop transfusion immediately, send sample for culture and sensitivity tests, and notify practitioner
Other		
Alloimmunization		
(Antibody formation)	Increased risk of hemolytic, febrile, and allergic reactions	Use limited number of donors
Occurs in patients receiving multiple transfusions		Observe carefully for signs of reaction
Delayed Hemolytic Reaction	Destruction of RBCs and fever 5 to 10 days after transfusion	Observe for posttransfusion anemia and decreasing benefit from successive transfusions

Unit 4

NURSING CARE PLAN

The Child with Sickle Cell Disease

Sickle cell anemia is a hereditary disorder in which normal adult hemoglobin (hemoglobin A[HgbA] is partly or completely replaced by an abnormal sickle hemoglobin (HgbS), causing distortion and rigidity of red blood cells under conditions of reduced oxygen tension.

ASSESSMENT

Perform a physical assessment.

Take a health history, especially regarding any evidence of sickling crisis and history of the disease in family members.

Observe for manifestations of sickle cell disease:

General

Growth retardation

Chronic anemia (Hgb 6.5 to 8 g/dl)

Delayed sexual maturation

Marked susceptibility to sepsis

Vaso-occlusive crisis

Pain in area(s) of involvement

Manifestations related to ischemia of involved areas:

Extremities—Painful swelling of hands and feet (sickle cell dactylitis, or "hand-foot syndrome"), painful joints

Abdomen—Severe pain resembling acute surgical condition

Cerebrum—Stroke, visual disturbances

Chest—Symptoms resembling pneumonia, protracted episodes of pulmonary disease

Liver—Obstructive jaundice, hepatic coma

Kidney—Hematuria

Sequestration crisis

Pooling of large amounts of blood

Hepatomegaly

Splenomegaly

Circulatory collapse

Effects of chronic vaso-occlusive phenomena

Heart—Cardiomegaly, systolic murmurs

Lungs—Altered pulmonary function, susceptibility to infections, pulmonary insufficiency

Kidneys—Inability to concentrate urine, progressive renal failure, enuresis

Genital—Priapism (painful, constant penile erection)

Liver—Hepatomegaly, cirrhosis, intrahepatic cholestasis

Spleen—Splenomegaly, susceptibility to infection, functional reduction in splenic activity progressing to autosplenectomy

Eyes—Intraocular abnormalities with visual disturbances, sometimes progressive retinal detachment and blindness

Extremities—Skeletal deformities, especially lordosis and kyphosis, chronic leg ulcers, susceptibility to salmonella osteomyelitis

CNS: hemiparesis, seizures

Assist with diagnostic procedures and tests (e.g., stained blood smear, sickle turbidity test (Sickledex), hemoglobin electrophoresis).

Observe for evidence of complications (crisis).

NURSING DIAGNOSIS: Risk for injury related to abnormal hemoglobin, decreased ambient oxygen, dehydration

- **PATIENT GOAL 1:** Will maintain adequate tissue oxygenation

NURSING INTERVENTIONS/*RATIONALES*

Explain measures to minimize complications related to physical exertion and emotional stress *to avoid additional tissue oxygen needs*

Prevent infection

Avoid low-oxygen environment

EXPECTED OUTCOME

Child avoids situations that reduce tissue oxygenation

- **PATIENT GOAL 2:** Will maintain adequate hydration

NURSING INTERVENTIONS/*RATIONALES*

Calculate recommended daily fluid intake (1600 ml/m^2/day) and base child's fluid requirements on this *minimum* amount (specify) *to ensure adequate hydration*

Increase fluid intake above minimum requirements during physical exercise/emotional stress and during a crisis *to compensate for additional fluid needs*

Give parents written instructions regarding specific quantity of fluid required *to encourage compliance*

Encourage child to drink *to encourage compliance*

Teach family signs of dehydration *to avoid delay in rehydration therapy* (See Nursing Care Plan: The Child with Fluid and Electrolyte Disturbance, p. 309.)

Stress importance of avoiding overheating *because it is a source of fluid loss*

EXPECTED OUTCOME

Child drinks an adequate amount of fluid and shows no signs of dehydration

- **PATIENT GOAL 3:** Will remain free of infection

NURSING INTERVENTIONS/*RATIONALES*

Stress importance of adequate nutrition; routine immunizations, including pneumococcal and meningococcal vaccines; protection from known sources of infection; and frequent health supervision

Report any sign of infection to practitioner immediately *to avoid delay in treatment*

Promote compliance with antibiotic therapy *to both prevent and to treat infection*

EXPECTED OUTCOME

Child remains free of infection

Continued

Unit 4

The Child with Sickle Cell Disease—cont'd

■ **PATIENT GOAL 4:** Will experience a decrease in risks associated with a surgical procedure

NURSING INTERVENTIONS/*RATIONALES*

Explain reason for preoperative blood transfusion (given to increase concentration of HgbA)

Keep child well hydrated *to prevent sickling*

Decrease fear through appropriate preparation *since anxiety increases oxygen needs*

*Administer pain medications *to keep child comfortable and reduce stress response*

Avoid unnecessary exertion *to avoid additional oxygen needs*

Promote pulmonary hygiene postoperatively *to prevent infection*

Use passive range-of-motion exercises *to promote circulation*

*Administer oxygen, if prescribed, *to saturate hemoglobin*

Monitor for evidence of infection *to avoid delay in treatment*

EXPECTED OUTCOME

Child undergoes a surgical procedure without crisis

NURSING DIAGNOSIS: Pain related to tissue anoxia (vaso-occlusive crisis)

■ **PATIENT GOAL 1:** Will have either no pain or a reduction of pain to level acceptable to child

NURSING INTERVENTIONS/*RATIONALES*

Plan preventive schedule of medication around the clock, not as needed, *to prevent pain*

Recognize that various analgesics, including opioids, and different medication schedules may need to be tried *to achieve satisfactory pain relief*

Avoid administration of meperidine (Demerol) *because of increased risk of normeperidine-induced seizures*

Reassure child and family that analgesics, including opioids, are medically indicated; that high doses may be needed; and that children rarely become addicted, *because needless suffering may result from these unfounded fears*

Apply heat to affected area *because this may be soothing*

Avoid applying cold compresses *because this enhances sickling and vasoconstriction*

EXPECTED OUTCOME

Child will experience no or minimal pain

NURSING DIAGNOSIS: Altered family processes related to a child with potentially life-threatening disease

■ **PATIENT (FAMILY) GOAL 1:** Will receive education regarding disease

NURSING INTERVENTIONS/*RATIONALES*

Teach family and older children characteristics of basic defect and measures *to minimize complications of sickling*

Stress importance of informing significant health personnel of child's disease *to ensure prompt and appropriate treatment* (e.g., for pain)

Explain signs of developing crisis (especially fever, pallor, respiratory distress, and pain) *to avoid delay in treatment*

Reinforce basics of trait transmission and refer to genetic counseling services *for family to make informed reproductive decisions*

Teach parents to be an advocate for their child *to secure the best care*

EXPECTED OUTCOME

Child and family demonstrate an understanding of the disease, its etiology, and its therapies

■ **PATIENT (FAMILY) GOAL 2:** Will receive adequate support

NURSING INTERVENTIONS/*RATIONALES*

Refer to special organizations and agencies *for ongoing support*

Refer child to comprehensive sickle cell clinic *for ongoing care*

Be especially alert to family's needs when two or more members are affected

(See also Nursing Care Plan: The Child with Chronic Illness or Disability, p. 287.)

EXPECTED OUTCOMES

Family takes advantage of community services (specify)

Child receives ongoing care from appropriate facility

(See also:

Nursing Care Plan: The Child in the Hospital, p. 268.)
Nursing Care Plan: The Family of the Child Who Is Ill or Hospitalized, p. 282.)

---

*Dependent nursing action.

NURSING CARE PLAN

The Child with Hemophilia

Hemophilia is a bleeding disorder caused by a hereditary deficiency of a blood factor essential for coagulation.

ASSESSMENT
Perform a physical assessment.

Take a family history, especially regarding evidence of the disease in male relatives.

Observe for manifestations of hemophilia:

Prolonged bleeding anywhere from or in the body

Hemorrhage from any trauma (e.g., loss of deciduous teeth, circumcision, cuts, epistaxis, injections)

Excessive bruising, even from a slight injury such as a fall

Subcutaneous and intramuscular hemorrhages

Hemarthrosis (bleeding into the joint cavities), especially of the knees, ankles, and elbows

Hematomas with pain, swelling, and limited motion

Spontaneous hematuria

Assist with diagnostic procedures and tests (e.g., coagulation tests, determination of specific factor deficiency, DNA testing).

NURSING DIAGNOSIS: Risk for injury related to hemorrhage

■ **PATIENT GOAL 1:** Will experience minimum or no bleeding

NURSING INTERVENTIONS/*RATIONALES*
Prepare and administer factor VIII concentrate or, for mild hemophilia, DDAVP (1-deamino-8-D-arginine vasopressin) as needed *to prevent bleeding*

Teach home administration of blood factor replacement *because treatment without delay results in more rapid recovery and decreased complications*

Institute supportive measures *to control bleeding:*

Apply pressure to area for 10 to 15 minutes *to allow clot formation*

Immobilize and elevate area above level of heart *to decrease blood flow*

Apply cold *to promote vasoconstriction;* encourage family to have plastic bags of ice or cold packs ready in freezer *for immediate use*

(See Table 4-32.)

EXPECTED OUTCOME
Child has minimum or no bleeding episodes

■ **PATIENT GOAL 2:** Will experience decreased risk of injury

NURSING INTERVENTIONS/*RATIONALES*
Make environment as safe as possible with close supervision *to minimize injuries without hampering development*

Encourage pursuit of intellectual/creative activities *to provide safe alternatives*

Encourage noncontact sports (e.g., swimming) and use of protective equipment (e.g., padding, helmet) *to decrease risk of injury*

Encourage older child to choose activities but to accept responsibility for his or her own safety *to encourage independence and sense of responsibility*

Involve teachers and school nurse in planning school activities *that promote normalization while decreasing risk of injury*

Discuss with parents appropriate limit-setting patterns *so that child's need for normal development is considered in addition to need for safety*

Teach methods of dental hygiene *that minimize trauma to gums and prevent bleeding*

Use soft, small toothbrush or sponge-tipped disposable toothbrush

Soften toothbrush in warm water before brushing

Use water irrigating device

Encourage adolescent to use electric shaver *to decrease risk of trauma*

Avoid passive range-of-motion exercises after an acute episode of bleeding *because joint capsule could easily be stretched and bleeding recur*

Advise patient to wear medical identification *for prompt, appropriate emergency care*

Encourage older children to recognize situations in which disclosing their condition is important (e.g., dental care, injections) *so that they receive appropriate care*

Discuss diet considerations *because excessive body weight can increase strain on joints and predispose to hemarthrosis*

Advise not to take aspirin or aspirin-containing ducts *because they inhibit platelet function;* use acetaminophen or ibuprofen for fever or discomfort

Teach family and older child how to recognize and control bleeding *so that prompt, appropriate care is instituted*

Take special precautions during nursing procedures such as injections (e.g., there is less bleeding after venipuncture than from finger/heel punctures; subcutaneous route is substituted for intramuscular injections when possible)

Continued

Unit 4

The Child with Hemophilia—cont'd

EXPECTED OUTCOMES

Child experiences few bleeding episodes

Child receives prompt, appropriate treatment

NURSING DIAGNOSIS: Pain related to bleeding into tissues and joints

■ **PATIENT GOAL 1:** Will experience either no pain or a reduction of pain to level acceptable to child

NURSING INTERVENTIONS/*RATIONALES* AND EXPECTED OUTCOMES

(See Nursing Care Plan: The Child in Pain, p. 315.)

NURSING DIAGNOSIS: Risk for impaired physical mobility related to effects of hemorrhages into joints and other tissues

■ **PATIENT GOAL 1:** Will experience reduced risk of impaired physical mobility

NURSING INTERVENTIONS/*RATIONALES*

Administer replacement therapy and use local measures *to control bleeding*

Elevate and immobilize joint during bleeding episodes *to control bleeding*

Institute active range-of-motion exercises after acute phase *because this allows child to control the degree of exercise according to level of discomfort*

Exercise unaffected joints and muscles *to maintain mobility*

Consult with physical therapist concerning exercise program *to promote maximum function of joint and unaffected body parts*

Refer to public health nurse and/or physical therapist for supervision at home

Explain to family serious long-range consequences of hemarthrosis *so that prompt treatment is instituted for bleeding episodes*

Support any orthopedic measures in joint rehabilitation

Assess need for pain management *to increase ease of mobility*

Discuss diet considerations *because excessive body weight can increase strain on joints and predispose to hemarthrosis*

EXPECTED OUTCOMES

Bleeding episodes are controlled sufficiently to prevent impaired physical mobility

Child participates in exercise program to maintain mobility

NURSING DIAGNOSIS: Altered family processes related to a child with a serious disease

■ **PATIENT GOAL 1:** Will receive adequate support

NURSING INTERVENTIONS/*RATIONALES*

Refer for genetic counseling, including identification of carrier offspring and other female relatives

Refer to special groups and agencies offering services to families with hemophilia

EXPECTED OUTCOMES

Family makes contact with appropriate support groups and agencies

Family receives genetic counseling

(See also:

Nursing Care Plan: The Family of the Child Who is Ill or Hospitalized, p. 282.)

Nursing Care Plan: The Child in the Hospital, p. 268.)

Nursing Care Plan: The Child with Chronic Illness or Disability, p. 287.)

Unit 4

TABLE 4-32   Adjunct Therapies for Hemophilia A

Site of Bleed	Treatment
Joint	Rest
	Ice
	Elevation
	Splint/Ace wrap/crutches
	Physical therapy
Soft tissue (substraneous)	Ice
	Elevation
	Splint/Ace wrap
Muscle	Rest
	Ice
	Elevation
	Splint/Ace wrap/crutches
	Physical therapy
	Complete bed rest for iliopsoas muscle bleed
Mucous membrane (e.g., nose, mouth)	Pressure to nares (for nosebleed)
	Topical antifibrinolytic agent (epsilon aminocaproic acid)
	Nasal pack (sometimes necessary)

NURSING CARE PLAN

The Child and Adolescent with Human Immunodeficiency Virus (HIV) Infection

Human immunodeficiency virus (HIV) is the causative agent for acquired immunodeficiency syndrome (AIDS). The virus has been found in blood and almost all body fluids (semen, saliva, vaginal secretions, urine, breast milk, and tears). The infection affects all organ systems.

ASSESSMENT

Perform a physical assessment.

Obtain an immunization history.

Obtain a history relative to risk factors for AIDS in children:
Exposure in utero to HIV-infected mother
Recipients of blood products, especially children with hemophilia (before testing began in 1985)
Adolescents engaging in high-risk behaviors

Observe for manifestations of AIDS in children:
Failure to thrive
Lymphadenopathy
Hepatosplenomegaly
Oral candidiasis

Recurrent bacterial infections

Pulmonary diseases (especially *Pneumocystis carinii* pneumonia, lymphocytic interstitial pneumonitis, and pulmonary lymphoid hyperplasia)

Chronic or recurrent diarrhea

Neurologic features:
Developmental delay
Loss of previously achieved motor milestones
Possible microcephaly
Abnormal neurologic examination

Assist with diagnostic procedures and tests (e.g., serum antibody tests).

NURSING DIAGNOSIS: Risk for infection related to impaired body defenses, presence of infective organisms

■ **PATIENT GOAL 1:** Will experience minimized risk of infection

NURSING INTERVENTIONS/*RATIONALES*

Use thorough handwashing technique *to minimize exposure to infective organisms*

Advise visitors to use good handwashing technique *to minimize exposure to infective organisms*

Place child in room with noninfectious children or in private room

Restrict contact with persons who have infections, including family, other children, friends, and members of staff; explain that child is highly susceptible to infection *to encourage cooperation and understanding*

Observe medical asepsis as appropriate *to decrease risk of infection*

Encourage good nutrition and adequate rest *to promote body's remaining natural defenses*

Explain to family and older child importance of contacting health professional if exposed to childhood illnesses (e.g., chickenpox, measles) *so that appropriate immunizations can be given*

*Administer appropriate immunizations as prescribed *to prevent specific infections*

*Administer antibiotics as prescribed

EXPECTED OUTCOMES

Child does not come in contact with infected persons or contaminated articles

Child and family apply good health practices

Child exhibits no evidence of infection

■ **PATIENT GOAL 2:** Will not spread virus to others

NURSING INTERVENTIONS/*RATIONALES*

Implement and carry out standard precautions *to prevent spread of virus* (See Nursing Care Plan: The Child at Risk for Infection, p. 341.)

Instruct others (e.g., family, members of staff) in appropriate precautions; clarify any misconceptions about communicability of virus *since this is a frequent problem and may interfere with use of appropriate precautions*

Teach affected children protective methods (e.g., handwashing, handling genital area, care after using bedpan or toilet) *to prevent spread of infection*

Endeavor to keep infants and small children from placing hands and objects in contaminated areas

Place restrictions on behaviors and contacts for affected children who bite or who do not have control of their bodily secretions

Assess home situation and implement protective measures as feasible in individual circumstances

EXPECTED OUTCOME

Others do not acquire the disease

NURSING DIAGNOSIS: Altered nutrition: less than body requirements related to recurrent illness, diarrheal losses, loss of appetite, oral candidiasis

■ **PATIENT GOAL 1:** Will receive optimum nourishment

NURSING INTERVENTIONS/*RATIONALES*

Provide high-calorie, high-protein meals and snacks *to meet body requirements for metabolism and growth*

Provide foods child prefers *to encourage eating*

Fortify foods with nutritional supplements (e.g., powdered milk or commercial supplements) *to maximize quality of intake*

Provide meals when child is most likely to eat well

Use creativity to encourage child to eat (See Nursing Care Plan: The Child with Special Nutritional Needs, p. 313.)

Monitor child's weight and growth *so that additional nutritional interventions can be implemented if growth begins to slow or weight drops*

*Administer antifungal medication as ordered *to treat oral candidiasis*

EXPECTED OUTCOME

Child consumes a sufficient amount of nutrients (specify)

---

*Dependent nursing action.

Continued

Unit 4

The Child and Adolescent with Human Immunodeficiency Virus (HIV) Infection—cont'd

NURSING DIAGNOSIS: Impaired social interaction related to physical limitations, hospitalizations, social stigma toward HIV

■ **PATIENT GOAL 1:** Will participate in peer-group and family activities

NURSING INTERVENTIONS/*RATIONALES*

Assist child in identifying personal strengths *to facilitate coping*

Educate school personnel and classmates about HIV *so that child is not unnecessarily isolated*

Encourage child to participate in activities with other children and family

Encourage child to maintain phone contact with friends during hospitalization *to lessen isolation*

EXPECTED OUTCOME

Child participates in activities with peer group and family

NURSING DIAGNOSIS: Altered sexuality patterns related to risk of disease transmission

■ **PATIENT GOAL 1:** Will exhibit healthy sexual behavior

NURSING INTERVENTIONS/*RATIONALES*

Educate adolescent about the following *so that adolescent has adequate information to identify safe, healthy expressions of sexuality:*

Sexual transmission

Risks of perinatal infection

Dangers of promiscuity

Abstinence, use of condoms

Avoidance of high-risk behaviors

Encourage adolescent to talk about feelings and concerns related to sexuality *to facilitate coping*

EXPECTED OUTCOMES

Adolescent exhibits a positive sexual identity

Adolescent does not infect other individuals

NURSING DIAGNOSIS: Pain related to disease process (e.g., encephalopathy, treatments)

■ **PATIENT GOAL 1:** Will exhibit minimal or no evidence of pain or irritability

NURSING INTERVENTIONS/*RATIONALES*

Assess pain (See Pain Assessment, p. 315.)

Use nonpharmacologic strategies *to help child manage pain*

For infants, may try general comfort measures (e.g., rocking, holding, swaddling, reducing environmental stimuli [may or may not be effective because of encephalopathy])

Use pharmacologic strategies (See Nursing Care Plan: The Child in Pain, p. 315.)

Plan preventive schedule if analgesics are effective in relieving continuous pain

Encourage use of premedication for painful procedures (e.g., use of EMLA; See p. 335.) *to minimize discomfort*

Child may benefit from use of adjunctive analgesics (e.g., antidepressants) that are effective against neuropathic pain

Use pain assessment record *to evaluate effectiveness of pharmacologic and nonpharmacologic interventions*

EXPECTED OUTCOME

Child exhibits absence of or minimal evidence of pain or irritability

NURSING DIAGNOSIS: Altered family processes related to having a child with a dreaded and life-threatening disease

■ **PATIENT (FAMILY) GOAL 1:** Will receive adequate support and will be able to meet needs of child

NURSING INTERVENTIONS/*RATIONALES* AND EXPECTED OUTCOMES

(See Nursing Care Plan: The Family of the Child Who Is Ill or Hospitalized, p. 282.)

NURSING DIAGNOSIS: Anticipatory grief related to having a child with a potentially fatal illness

(See Nursing Care Plan: The Child Who Is Terminally Ill or Dying, p. 296.)

NURSING CARE OF THE CHILD WITH RENAL DYSFUNCTION

NURSING CARE PLAN

The Child with Nephrotic Syndrome

Nephrotic syndrome is a clinical state characterized by an increased permeability of the glomerular membrane to protein, which results in massive urinary protein loss.

ASSESSMENT

Perform a physical assessment, including assessment of extent of edema.

Take a careful health history, especially relative to recent weight gain or renal dysfunction.

Observe for manifestations of nephrotic syndrome:

Weight gain

Edema

Puffiness of face:

Especially around the eyes

Apparent on arising in the morning

Subsides during the day

Abdominal swelling (ascites)

Respiratory difficulty (pleural effusion)

Labial or scrotal swelling

Edema of intestinal mucosa causes:

Diarrhea

Anorexia

Poor intestinal absorption

Extreme skin pallor (often)

Irritability

Easily fatigued

Lethargic

Blood pressure normal or slightly decreased

Susceptibility to infection

Urine alterations:

Decreased volume

Darkly opalescent

Frothy

Assist with diagnostic, procedures and tests (e.g., urine analysis for protein, casts, and red blood cells; blood analysis for serum protein [total, albumin/globulin ratio, cholesterol] serum sodium; and renal biopsy).

NURSING DIAGNOSIS: Fluid volume excess (total body) related to fluid accumulation in tissues and third spaces

■ **PATIENT GOAL 1:** Will exhibit no or minimal evidence of fluid accumulation

NURSING INTERVENTIONS/*RATIONALES*

Assess intake relative to output:

Measure and record intake and output accurately

Weigh daily (or more often, if indicated) *to assess fluid retention*

Assess changes in edema:

Measure abdominal girth at umbilicus *to assess ascites*

Monitor edema around eyes and dependent areas *because these are common sites of edema*

Note degree of pitting, if present

Note color and texture of skin

Test urine for specific gravity and albumin *because hyperalbuminuria is manifestation of nephrotic syndrome*

Collect specimens for laboratory examination

*Administer corticosteroids as prescribed (and immunosuppressive drugs, if ordered) *to reduce excretion of urinary protein*

*Administer diuretics if ordered *to provide temporary relief from edema*

Limit fluids as indicated *during massive edema*

EXPECTED OUTCOME

Child exhibits no or minimal evidence of fluid accumulation (specify parameters)

■ **PATIENT GOAL 2:** Will receive appropriate volume of fluid

NURSING INTERVENTIONS/*RATIONALES*

Regulate fluid intake carefully *so that child does not receive more than prescribed amount*

Monitor intravenous infusion *to maintain prescribed intake*

Employ strategies to prevent undesired intake:

Use small containers for fluid intake *so that volume does not appear so restricted*

Divide allowed intake into small volumes spread over entire day

Spray mouth with atomizer (mist) *to prevent feeling of dryness*

Offer chewing gum and sugarless hard candies

Keep lips lubricated *for comfort and to prevent cracking*

EXPECTED OUTCOME

Child receives no more fluid than prescribed

NURSING DIAGNOSIS: Risk for (intravascular) fluid volume deficit related to protein and fluid loss, edema

■ **PATIENT GOAL 1:** Will exhibit no or minimal evidence of intravascular fluid loss or hypovolemic shock

NURSING INTERVENTIONS/*RATIONALES*

Monitor vital signs *to detect physical evidence of fluid depletion*

Assess pulse quality and rate *for signs of hypovolemic shock*

Measure blood pressure *to detect hypovolemic shock*

Report any deviations from normal *so that prompt treatment is instituted*

*Administer salt-poor albumin if prescribed *as a plasma expander*

EXPECTED OUTCOME

Child exhibits no or minimal evidence of intravascular fluid loss or hypovolemic shock

---

NURSING DIAGNOSIS: High risk for infection related to lowered body defenses, fluid overload

*Dependent nursing action.

Continued

Unit 4

The Child with Nephrotic Syndrome—cont'd

■ **PATIENT GOAL 1:** Will exhibit no evidence of infection

NURSING INTERVENTIONS/*RATIONALES*

Protect child from contact with infected persons *to minimize exposure to infective organisms*

    Place in room with noninfectious children

    Restrict contact with persons who have infections, including family, other children, friends, and staff members

    Teach visitors appropriate preventive behaviors (e.g., handwashing)

Observe medical asepsis

Use good handwashing

Keep child warm and dry *because of vulnerability to upper respiratory infection*

Monitor temperature *for early evidence of infection*

Teach parents signs and symptoms of infection

EXPECTED OUTCOMES

Child and family apply good health practices

Child exhibits no evidence of infection

NURSING DIAGNOSIS: Risk for impaired skin integrity related to edema, lowered body defenses

■ **PATIENT GOAL 1:** Will maintain skin integrity

NURSING INTERVENTIONS/*RATIONALES*

Provide meticulous skin care

Avoid tight clothing *that may cause pressure areas*

Cleanse and powder opposing skin surfaces several times per day *to prevent skin breakdown*

Separate opposing skin surfaces with soft cotton *to prevent skin breakdown*

Support edematous organs, such as scrotum, *to relieve pressure areas*

Cleanse edematous eyelids with warm saline wipes

Change position frequently; maintain good body alignment *because child with massive edema is usually lethargic, easily fatigued, and content to lie still*

Use pressure-relieving or pressure-reducing mattresses or beds as needed *to prevent ulcers*

EXPECTED OUTCOME

Child's skin displays no evidence of redness or irritation

NURSING DIAGNOSIS: Altered nutrition: less than body requirements related to loss of appetite

■ **PATIENT GOAL 1:** Will receive optimum nutrition

NURSING INTERVENTIONS/*RATIONALES*

Offer nutritious diet

Avoid high protein diet if azotemia and renal failure are present

Restrict sodium during edema and steroid therapy

*Administer supplementary vitamins and iron as ordered

Enlist aid of child, parents, and dietitian in formulation of diet *to encourage optimum nutrition despite loss of appetite*

Provide cheerful, clean, relaxed atmosphere during meals *so that child is more likely to eat*

Serve small quantities initially *to stimulate appetite;* encourage seconds

Provide special and preferred foods *to encourage child to eat*

Serve foods in an attractive manner *to stimulate appetite*

(See also Nursing Care Plan: The Child with Special Nutritional Needs, p. 313.)

EXPECTED OUTCOME

Child consumes an adequate amount of nutritious food

NURSING DIAGNOSIS: Body image disturbance related to change in appearance

■ **PATIENT GOAL 1:** Will express feelings and concerns

NURSING INTERVENTIONS/*RATIONALES*

Explore feelings and concerns regarding appearance *to facilitate coping*

    Point out positive aspects of appearance and evidence of diminished edema *so that child feels encouraged*

    Explain to child and family that symptoms associated with steroid therapy will subside when medication is discontinued

Encourage activity within limits of tolerance

Encourage socialization with persons without active infection *so that child is not lonely and isolated*

Provide positive feedback *so that child feels accepted*

Explore areas of interest and encourage their pursuit

EXPECTED OUTCOMES

Child discusses feelings and concerns

Child engages in activities appropriate to interests and abilities

NURSING DIAGNOSIS: Activity intolerance related to fatigue

■ **PATIENT GOAL 1:** Will receive adequate rest

NURSING INTERVENTIONS/*RATIONALES*

Maintain bed rest initially if severely edematous

Balance rest and activity when ambulatory *to prevent fatigue*

Plan and provide quiet activities *to encourage rest*

Instruct child to rest when he or she begins to feel tired

Allow for periods of uninterrupted sleep

EXPECTED OUTCOMES

Child engages in activities appropriate to capabilities

Child receives adequate rest and sleep

NURSING DIAGNOSIS: Altered family processes related to a child with a serious disease

■ **PATIENT (FAMILY) GOAL 1:** Will receive adequate support

**NURSING INTERVENTIONS/*RATIONALES*
AND EXPECTED OUTCOMES**

(See Nursing Care Plan: The Family of the Child Who Is Ill or Hospitalized, p. 282.)

(See also Nursing Care Plan: The Child in the Hospital, p. 268.)

*Dependent nursing action.

Unit 4

NURSING CARE PLAN

The Child with Acute Renal Failure

Acute renal failure (ARF) is a condition that results when the kidneys suddenly are unable to excrete urine of sufficient volume or adequate concentration to maintain normal body fluid balance.

ASSESSMENT
Initial assessment
Perform a physical assessment.
Take a careful health history, especially regarding evidence of glomerulonephritis, obstructive uropathy, and exposure to or ingestion of toxic chemicals (including heavy metals, carbon tetrachloride, or other ~ganic solvents; and nephrotoxic drugs).
Observe for manifestations of acute renal failure:
Specific
    Oliguria
    Anuria uncommon (except in obstructive disorders)
Nonspecific (may develop)
    Nausea
    Vomiting
    Drowsiness
    Edema
    Hypertension
Ongoing assessment
Careful monitoring of the following:
    Urinary output (insert Foley catheter)
    Blood pressure, pulse, and respiration
    Cardiac function
    Neurologic function
    Observe for signs of fluid overload
    Manifestations of underlying disorder or pathology
Assist with diagnostic tests (e.g., urine analysis, blood urea nitrogen, nonprotein nitrogen, creatinine, serum electrolytes, complete blood count, blood gases, and specific tests to determine cause of renal failure).

NURSING DIAGNOSIS: Fluid volume excess related to failure or compromised renal regulatory mechanisms

■ **PATIENT GOAL 1:** Will maintain appropriate fluid volume

NURSING INTERVENTIONS/*RATIONALES*
*Assist with dialysis or continuous hemofiltration *to maintain excretory function*
Monitor progress *to assess adequacy of therapy and detect possible complications*

EXPECTED OUTCOME
Child exhibits no evidence of complications related to accumulated fluid and waste products between dialysis sessions

■ **PATIENT GOAL 2:** Will maintain appropriate fluid volume through regulation of fluid intake

NURSING INTERVENTIONS/*RATIONALES*
*Administer intravenous or oral fluids as prescribed
Closely monitor intravenous infusion *to maintain prescribed intake and prevent fluid overload*
Measure and record intake and output accurately
Weigh daily (or more often if indicated)
Employ strategies to prevent undesired intake:
    Remove fluids from access by child
    Use small containers for fluid intake *so that volume does not appear so restricted*
    Divide allowed intake into volumes spread over 24 hours to avoid period of no fluid allowance
    Spray mouth with atomizer (avoid excess use, which would increase intake) *to prevent feeling of dryness*
    Keep lips lubricated *for comfort and to prevent cracking*

EXPECTED OUTCOME
Child exhibits no evidence of fluid gain

NURSING DIAGNOSIS: Risk for injury related to accumulated electrolytes and waste products

■ **PATIENT GOAL 1:** Will maintain normal electrolyte levels

NURSING INTERVENTIONS/*RATIONALES*
*Assist with dialysis *to maintain excretory function*
*Administer Kayexalate as prescribed *to reduce serum potassium levels*
*Provide diet low in protein, potassium, and sodium, if prescribed, *to reduce excretory demand on kidneys*
Observe for evidence of accumulated waste products (e.g., hyperkalemia, hypernatremia, uremia) *to ensure prompt treatment*

EXPECTED OUTCOME
Child exhibits no evidence of waste product accumulation

■ **PATIENT GOAL 2:** Will maintain blood pressure within acceptable limits

NURSING INTERVENTIONS/*RATIONALES*
*Administer antihypertensive drugs as prescribed *to reduce blood pressure*
Avoid situations that increase child's anxiety and apprehension *since these factors can raise blood pressure*
Provide quiet, calm environment

EXPECTED OUTCOME
Child's blood pressure remains within acceptable limits (specify)

NURSING DIAGNOSIS: Potential for infection related to lowered body defenses, fluid overload

Unit 4

Continued

The Child with Acute Renal Failure—cont'd

- **PATIENT GOAL 1:** Will experience minimized risk of infection

NURSING INTERVENTIONS/*RATIONALES*

Protect child from contact with infected persons *to minimize exposure to infective organisms*
  Place in room with noninfectious children
  Restrict contact with persons who have infections, including family, other children, friends, and staff members
  Teach visitors appropriate preventive behaviors (e.g., handwashing)
Observe medical asepsis
  Practice good handwashing technique
Keep child warm and dry *because of vulnerability to upper respiratory infection*
Monitor temperature *for early evidence of infection*

EXPECTED OUTCOMES

Child and family apply good health practices
Child exhibits no evidence of infection

NURSING DIAGNOSIS: Altered family processes related to a child with a serious disease

- **PATIENT (FAMILY) GOAL 1:** Will receive adequate support

**NURSING INTERVENTIONS/*RATIONALES*
AND EXPECTED OUTCOMES**

(See Nursing Care Plan: The Family of the Child Who Is Ill or Hospitalized, p. 282.)
(See also Nursing Care Plan: The Child in the Hospital, p. 268.)

NURSING CARE PLAN

The Child with Chronic Renal Failure

Chronic renal failure (CRF) occurs when the diseased kidneys are unable to maintain the chemical composition of body fluids within normal limits under normal conditions.

The final stage is end-stage renal disease (ESRD), which is irreversible.

Various biochemical substances accumulate in the blood as a result of diminished renal function and produce complications such as the following:

Retention of waste products, especially blood urea nitrogen and creatinine

Water and sodium retention, which contribute to edema and vascular congestion

Hyperkalemia of dangerous levels; occurrence uncommon until the end stage

Metabolic acidosis of a sustained nature because of continual hydrogen ion retention and bicarbonate loss

Calcium and phosphorus disturbances resulting in altered bone metabolism, which in turn causes growth arrest or retardation, bone pain, and deformities known as *renal osteodystrophy*

Anemia caused by hematologic dysfunction, including shortened life span of red blood cells, impaired red blood cell production related to decreased production of erythropoietin, prolonged bleeding time, and nutritional anemia

Growth disturbance, probably caused by such factors as poor nutrition, anorexia, renal osteodystrophy, and biochemical abnormalities

ASSESSMENT

Initial assessment

Perform a routine physical assessment with special attention to measurements of growth parameters.

Take a health history, especially regarding renal dysfunction, eating behavior, frequency of infections, and energy level.

Observe for evidence of manifestations of chronic renal failure:

Early signs

Loss of normal energy

Increased fatigue on exertion

Pallor, subtle (may not be noticed)

Elevated blood pressure (sometimes)

As the disease progresses

Decreased appetite (especially at breakfast)

Less interest in normal activities

Increased or decreased urinary output with compensatory intake of fluid

Pallor more evident

Sallow, muddy appearance of skin

Child may complain of the following:

Headache

Muscle cramps

Nausea

Other signs and symptoms

Weight loss

Facial edema

Malaise

Bone or joint pain

Growth retardation

Dryness or itching of the skin

Bruised skin

Sensory or motor loss (sometimes)

Amenorrhea (common in adolescent girls)

Uremic syndrome (untreated)

Gastrointestinal symptoms:

Anorexia

Nausea and vomiting

Bleeding tendencies:

Bruises

Bloody, diarrheal stools

Stomatitis

Bleeding from lips and mouth

Intractable itching

Uremic frost (deposits of urea crystals on skin)

Unpleasant "uremic" breath odor

Deep respirations

Hypertension

Congestive heart failure

Pulmonary edema

Neurologic involvement:

Progressive confusion

Dulled sensorium

Coma (ultimately)

Tremors

Muscular twitching

Seizures

Ongoing assessment

Take a history for new or increasing symptoms.

Carry out frequent physical assessments with particular attention to blood pressure, signs of edema, and neurologic dysfunction.

Assess psychologic responses to the disease and its therapies.

Assist with diagnostic procedures and tests (e.g., urinalysis, complete blood count, blood chemistry, and renal biopsy).

NURSING DIAGNOSIS: Risk for injury related to accumulated electrolytes and waste products

■ **PATIENT GOAL 1:** Will maintain near-normal electrolyte levels

NURSING INTERVENTIONS/*RATIONALES*

*Assist with dialysis *to maintain excretory function*

Administer Kayexalate as prescribed *to reduce serum potassium levels*

Provide diet low in protein, potassium, sodium, and phosphorus, if prescribed, *to reduce excretory demand on kidneys*

Observe for evidence of accumulated waste products (hyperkalemia, hyperphosphatemia, uremia) *to ensure prompt treatment*

EXPECTED OUTCOME

Child exhibits no evidence of waste product accumulation

---

*Dependent nursing action.

Continued

The Child with Chronic Renal Failure—cont'd

NURSING DIAGNOSIS: Fluid volume excess related to failure of renal regulatory mechanisms

- **PATIENT GOAL 1:** Will maintain appropriate fluid volume

NURSING INTERVENTIONS/*RATIONALES*

Assist with dialysis *to maintain excretory function*
Monitor progress *to assess adequacy of therapy and detect possible complications*

EXPECTED OUTCOME

Child exhibits no evidence of complications related to accumulated fluid between dialysis sesssions

- **PATIENT GOAL 2:** Will maintain appropriate fluid volume through regulation of fluid intake

NURSING INTERVENTIONS/*RATIONALES*

*Administer oral fluids as prescribed
Use strategies to prevent undesirable intake:
   Review daily fluid restrictions with parents and child *to encourage cooperation*
   Suggest ways to divide total volume of fluid into small quantities to be spread over entire day
   Keep mouth moist by other means, such as hard candy, ice chips, or fine mist spray of cool water *to prevent feeling of dryness*

EXPECTED OUTCOME

Chlid exhibits no evidence of fluid gain

NURSING DIAGNOSIS: Altered nutrition: less than body requirements related to restricted diet

- **PATIENT GOAL 1:** Will consume appropriate diet

NURSING INTERVENTIONS/*RATIONALES*

Provide dietary instructions for foods *that reduce excretory demands on kidney and provide sufficient calories and protein for growth*
*Limit protein, phosphorus, salt, and potassium as prescribed
Encourage intake of carbohydrates *to provide calories for growth* and foods high in calcium *to prevent bone demineralization*
Recommend foods that are rich in folic acid and iron *because anemia is a complication of CRF*
Arrange for renal dietitian to meet with family to review allowable foods and assist in dietary planning *so that family understands dietary needs of child*
Help hemodialysis patients to fill out menu requests for meals (to be eaten while on dialysis)

EXPECTED OUTCOMES

Child consumes an adequate amount of appropriate foods
Child shows no evidence of deficiencies or weight loss

NURSING DIAGNOSIS: Body image disturbance related to chronic illness, impaired growth, and perception of being "different"

- **PATIENT GOAL 1:** Will develop positive self-esteem and understanding of disease

NURSING INTERVENTIONS/*RATIONALES*

Provide education about CRF, including management, treatment, and long-term outcome
Encourage child's independence with care and management of CRF *because independence helps child develop positive self-esteem*
   Allow child to participate in dialysis procedures
   Allow child to participate in making decisions when appropriate
Promote self-esteem in child with CRF
   Organize patient support group or suggest counseling as needed
   Provide positive reinforcement during dialysis procedures and follow-up visits

EXPECTED OUTCOMES

Child demonstrates an understanding of CRF and complies with therapies
Child exhibits signs of positive self-esteem

NURSING DIAGNOSIS: Altered family processes related to a child with a chronic disease

- **PATIENT (FAMILY) GOAL 1:** Will exhibit positive coping behaviors

NURSING INTERVENTIONS/*RATIONALES*

Assist parents in diet planning and support their efforts to adjust diet *to meet needs of all family members*
Provide anticipatory guidance regarding probable and expected events, such as symptoms, diet, and effects of medications
Assist parents in decision-making regarding dialysis and transplantation *because these are the alternatives once palliative care is no longer effective*
Prepare child and family for hemodialysis and/or kidney transplantation *because preparation is essential for positive coping*
Prepare child and family for home hemodialysis or continuous home peritoneal dialysis
Maintain periodic contact with family *for ongoing support*
Refer family to special agencies and support groups *for long-term support*

EXPECTED OUTCOMES

Child and family demonstrate ability to cope with stresses of illness (specify)
(See also:
   Nursing Care Plan: The Child with a Chronic Illness or Disability, p. 287.)
   Nursing Care Plan: The Child in the Hospital, p. 268.)
   Nursing Care Plan: The Family of the Child Who Is Ill or Hospitalized, p. 282.)
   Nursing Care Plan: The Child Who Is Terminally Ill or Dying, p. 296.)

*Dependent nursing action.

Unit 4

NURSING CARE OF THE CHILD WITH NEUROLOGIC DYSFUNCTION

Cerebral dysfunction concerns disorders affecting cerebral structure and function.

ASSESSMENT
Initial assessment
Take a careful history:

Family history, for evidence of genetic disorders with neurologic manifestations

Health history, especially for clues regarding the cause of dysfunction (e.g., injury, short febrile illness, encounter with an animal or insect, ingestion of neurotoxic substances, inhalation of chemicals, past illness, or known diabetes mellitus)

Sudden or progressive alterations in movement (e.g., ataxia, seizures) or mental ability

Headache, nausea, vomiting, double vision, bowel or bladder incontinence in a previously continent child

Unusual behavior, including the nature and frequency

Perform physical assessment with special emphasis on the following:

Neurologic assessment (See p. 64.)

Assessment of cranial nerves (See p. 68.)

Developmental assessment (See p. 127.)

Perform physical evaluation of infant:

Size and shape of the head

Spontaneous activity and postural reflex activity

Sensory responses

Attitude—Normal flexed posture, extreme extension, opisthotonos, hypotonia

Symmetry in movement of extremities

Excessive tremulousness or frequent twitching movements

Altered expiratory cycle:

Prolonged apnea

Ataxic breathing

Paradoxic chest movement

Hyperventilation

Skin and hair texture

Distinctive facial features

Presence of a high-pitched, piercing cry

Abnormal eye movements

Inability to suck or swallow

Lip smacking

Asymmetric contraction of facial muscles

Yawning (may indicate cranial nerve involvement)

Muscular activity and coordination

Level of development

Observe for speed of movement; and presence and location of any tremors, twitching, tics, or other unusual movements.

Observe gait (e.g., ataxia, spasticity, rigidity).

Note any unusual discharge from body orifices.

Note location, extent, and type of any wound.

Assess level of consciousness:*

Full consciousness—Awake and alert; oriented to time, place and person; behavior appropriate for age

Confusion—Impaired decision-making

Disorientation—Disoriented to time, place; decreased level of consciousness

Lethargy—Limited spontaneous movement, sluggish speech

Obtundation—Arousable with stimulation

Stupor—Remains in a deep sleep, responsive only to vigorous and repeated stimulation

Coma—No motor or verbal response to noxious or painful stimuli

Persistent vegetative state (PVS)—Permanently lost function of the cerebral cortex; eyes follow objects only by reflex or when attracted to the direction of loud sounds; all four limbs are spastic but can withdraw from painful stimuli; hands show reflexive grasping and groping; the face can grimace; some food may be swallowed; and the child may groan or cry, but utters no words

Observe for evidence of increased intracranial pressure:

Infants
Tense, bulging fontanel; lack of normal pulsations

Separated cranial sutures

Macewen sign (cracked-pot sound)

Irritability

High-pitched cry

Increased occipitofrontal circumference (OFC)

Distended scalp veins

Changes in feeding

Cries when held or rocked

Setting-sun sign

Children
Headache

Nausea

Vomiting, often without nausea

Diplopia, blurred vision

Seizures

Personality and behavior signs

Irritability (toddlers), restlessness

Indifference, drowsiness, or lack of interest

Decline in school performance

Diminished physical activity and motor performance

Increased complaints of fatigue, tiredness; increased time devoted to sleep

Significant weight loss possible from anorexia and vomiting

Memory loss if pressure is markedly increased

Inability to follow simple commands

Progression to lethargy and drowsiness

Late Signs

Lowered level of consciousness

Decreased motor response to command

Decreased sensory response to painful stimuli

Alterations in pupil size and reactivity

Sometimes decerebrate or decorticate posturing

Cheyne-Stokes respirations

Papilledema

Assist with diagnostic procedures and tests (e.g., lumbar puncture, subdural tap, ventricular puncture, electroencephalography, radiography, magnetic resonance imaging, computed tomography, nuclear brain scan, echoencephalography, positron emission transaxial tomography, real-time ultrasonography, digital subtraction angiography; blood biochemistry [pH, blood gases, ammonia, glucose]; and any special tests).

Ongoing assessment (extent of assessment depends on condition)
Monitor vital signs, especially noting changes in:

Temperature, pulse, blood pressure

Respirations—Regular or irregular, deep or shallow, pattern of breathing, odor of breath

Eye movements:

Position of globes—Divergence, conjugate deviation, skewed

---

*Modified from Hazinski MF, editor: *Care of the critically ill child*, ed 2, St Louis, 1992, Mosby, p. 544.

Continued

ASSESSMENT—CONT'D

Eye movements—cont'd:
Movement of globes—Extraocular palsy, nystagmus, fixed gaze
Pupil size—Dilated, pinpoint, unequal
Pupil reaction—Sluggish, absent, different

Motor function:
Voluntary movements of extremities (e.g., purposeful or random)
Changes in muscular tone
Changes in position of body and/or head
Tremor, twitching
Seizure activity (e.g., generalized or partial) (Box 4-24)
Signs of meningeal irritation (e.g., nuchal rigidity or opisthotonos)
Spontaneous—Normal but reduced, involuntary, evoked
Evoked—Purposeful, reflex withdrawal

Paresis—Decorticate, decerebrate; any lateralized difference in function
Crying and speech—Present or absent, conversant or confused, monosyllabic, jargon, type of cry (piercing, difficult to hear)
Level of consciousness
Monitor intracranial pressure device
Monitor central venous pressure device
Monitor fluid intake and output
Weigh daily or as ordered to detect fluid accumulation or reduction
Headache (if information can be elicited)—Presence or absence, type and location, continuous or intermittent

In infants:
Measure occipitofrontal circumference
Assess status of fontanel—Size and tension

BOX 4-24

Classification and Clinical Manifestations of Seizures

Partial Seizures

Simple Partial Seizures with Motor Signs

Characterized by:
Localized motor symptoms
Somatosensory, psychic, and autonomic symptoms
Combination of these
Abnormal discharges remain unilateral

Manifestations:
Aversive seizure (most common motor seizure in children)
Eye or eyes and head turn away from the side of the focus
Awareness of movement or loss of consciousness
Rolandic (Sylvian) seizure
Tonic-clonic movements involving the face
Salivation
Arrested speech
Most common during sleep
Jacksonian march (rare in children)
Orderly, sequential progression of clonic movements beginning in a foot, hand, or face and moving or "marching" to adjacent body parts

Simple Partial Seizures with Sensory Signs

Characterized by various sensations, including:
Numbness, tingling, prickling, paresthesia, or pain originating in one area (e.g., face or extremities) and spreading to other parts of the body
Visual sensations or formed images
Motor phenomena such as posturing or hypertonia
Uncommon in children under 8 years of age

Complex Partial Seizures (Psychomotor Seizures)

Observed more often in children from 3 years through adolescence

Characterized by:
Period of altered behavior
Amnesia for event (no recollection of behavior)
Inability to respond to environment
Impaired consciousness during event
Drowsiness or sleep usually follows seizure
Confusion and amnesia may be prolonged
Complex sensory phenomena (aura)
Most frequent sensation is strange feeling in the pit of the stomach that rises toward the throat
Often accompanied by:
Odd or unpleasant odors or tastes
Complex auditory or visual hallucinations
Ill-defined feelings of elation or strangeness (e.g., deja vu, a feeling of familiarity in a strange environment)
May be strong feelings of fear and anxiety, distorted sense of time and self
Small children may emit a cry or attempt to run for help

Patterns of motor behavior:
Stereotypic
Similar with each subsequent seizure
May suddenly cease activity, appear dazed, stare into space, become confused and apathetic, and become limp or stiff or display some form of posturing
May be confused
May perform purposeless, complicated activities in a repetitive manner (automatisms), such as walking, running, kicking, laughing, or speaking incoherently, most often followed by postictal confusion or sleep; may be oropharyngeal activities, such as smacking, chewing, drooling, swallowing, and nausea or abdominal pain followed by stiffness, a fall, and postictal sleep; rarely manifests such as rage or temper tantrums; aggressive acts uncommon during seizure

BOX 4-24

Classification and Clinical Manifestations of Seizures—cont'd

Generalized Seizures

Tonic-Clonic Seizues (Formerly Known as Grand Mal)

Most common and most dramatic of all seizure manifestations

Occur without warning

Tonic phase: lasts approximately 10 to 20 seconds

Manifestations:

Eyes roll upward

Immediate loss of consciousness

If standing, falls to floor or ground

Stiffens in generalized, symmetric tonic contraction of entire body musculature

Arms usually flexed

Legs, head, and neck extended

May utter a peculiar piercing cry

Apneic, may become cyanotic

Increased salivation and loss of swallowing reflex

Clonic phase: lasts about 30 seconds but can vary from only a few seconds to a half hour or longer

Manifestations:

Violent jerking movements as the trunk and extremities undergo rhythmic contraction and relaxation

May foam at the mouth

May be incontinent of urine and feces

As event ends, movements become less intense, occur at longer intervals, then cease entirely

Status epilepticus: series of seizures at intervals too brief to allow the child to regain consciousness between the time one event ends and the next begins

Requires emergency intervention

Can lead to exhaustion, respiratory failure, and death

Postictal state:

Appears to relax

May remain semiconscious and difficult to rouse

May awaken in a few minutes

Remains confused for several hours

Poor coordination

Mild impairment of fine motor movements

May have visual and speech difficulties

May vomit or complain of severe headache

When left alone, usually sleeps for several hours

On awakening is fully conscious

Usually feels tired and complains of sore muscles and headache

No recollection of entire event

Absence Seizures (Formerly Called Petit Mal or Lapses)

Characterized by:

Onset usually between 4 and 12 years of age

More common in girls than in boys

Usually cease at puberty

Brief loss of consciousness

Minimal or no alteration in muscle tone

May go unrecognized because little change in child's behavior

Abrupt onset; suddenly develops 20 or more attacks daily

Event often mistaken for inattentiveness or daydreaming

Events can be precipitated by hyperventilation, hypoglycemia, stresses (emotional and physiologic), fatigue, or sleeplessness

Manifestations:

Brief loss of consciousness

Appear without warning or aura

Usually last about 5 to 10 seconds

Slight loss of muscle tone may cause child to drop objects

Able to maintain postural control; seldom falls

Minor movements such as lip smacking, twitching of eyelids or face, or slight hand movements

Not accompanied by incontinence

Amnesia for episode

May need to reorient self to previous activity

Atonic and Akinetic Seizures (Also Known as Drop Attacks)

Characterized by:

Onset usually between 2 and 5 years of age

Sudden, momentary loss of muscle tone and postural control

Events recur frequently during the day, particularly in the morning hours and shortly after awakening

Manifestations:

Loss of tone causes child to fall to floor violently

Unable to break fall by putting out hand

May incur a serious injury to the face, head, or shoulder

Loss of consciousness only momentary

Myoclonic Seizures

A variety of convulsive episodes

May be isolated as benign essential myoclonus

May occur in association with other seizure forms

Characterized by:

Sudden, brief contractures of a muscle or group of muscles

Occur singly or repetitively

No postictal state

May or may not be symmetric

May or may not be loss of consciousness

Infantile Spasms

Also called: infantile myoclonus, massive spasms, hypsarrhythmia, salaam episodes or infantile myoclonic spasms

Most commonly occur during the first 6 to 8 months of life

Twice as common in males as in females

Child may have numerous seizures during the day without postictal drowsiness or sleep

Outlook for normal intelligence poor

Manifestations:

Possible series of sudden, brief, symmetric, muscular contractions

Head flexed, arms extended, and legs drawn up

Eyes may roll upward or inward

May be preceded or followed by a cry or giggling

May or may not be loss of consciousness

Sometimes flushing, pallor, or cyanosis

Infants who are able to sit but not stand:

Sudden dropping forward of the head and neck with trunk flexed forward and knees drawn up (the "salaam" or "jackknife" seizure)

Less often: alternate clinical forms observed

Extensor spasms rather than flexion of arms, legs, and trunk and head nodding

Lightning events involving a single, momentary, shock-like contraction of the entire body

NURSING CARE PLAN

The Unconscious Child

Unconsciousness is depressed cerebral function characterized by an inability to respond to sensory stimuli and have
subjective experiences.

ASSESSMENT

(See Assessment: The Child with Neurologic Dysfunction,
  p. 459.)
Assess state of consciousness (Fig. 4-3).

Assist with diagnostic procedures and tests.
Perform regular, frequent, ongoing neurologic assessments.

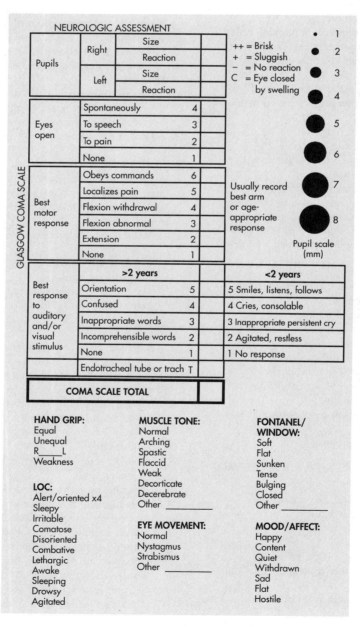

Fig. 4-3   Pediatric coma scale.

The Unconscious Child—cont'd

NURSING DIAGNOSIS: Risk for suffocation (aspiration): ineffective airway clearance related to depressed sensorium, impaired motor function

■ **PATIENT GOAL 1:** Will maintain patent airway

NURSING INTERVENTIONS/*RATIONALES*

Position for optimum ventilation:
Insert oral airway if indicated
Position with neck slightly extended and nose in "sniffing" position *to open trachea fully*
Avoid neck hyperextension, *which can block airway*
Place in semiprone or side-lying position *to prevent aspiration*
Remove accumulated secretions promptly *to prevent aspiration*
Administer care of endotracheal tube or tracheostomy if appropriate; have equipment available for emergency insertion if indicated for respiratory distress *to prevent delay in treatment*
Monitor artificial ventilation

EXPECTED OUTCOME
Airway remains patent

NURSING DIAGNOSIS: Risk for injury related to physical immobility, depressed sensorium, intracranial pathology

■ **PATIENT GOAL 1:** Will maintain stable ICP

NURSING INTERVENTIONS/*RATIONALES*

Elevate head of bed 15 to 30 degrees with child's head in midline position *to facilitate venous drainage and avoid jugular compression*
Avoid positions or activities that increase ICP:
Pressure on neck veins
Turning side-to-side is contraindicated *because of risk of jugular compression*
Flexion or hyperextension of neck
Head rotation
Valsalva maneuver
Painful stimuli
Respiratory procedures (especially suctioning, percussion)
Prevent constipation *because Valsalva maneuver increases ICP*
*Administer stool softener as prescribed
Closely monitor bowel elimination when child is receiving codeine *because of its constipating effect*
Minimize emotional stress and crying *because they cause increased ICP*
Provide quiet, subdued environment
Reduce environmental noise (e.g., by placing earphones over child's ears) *because this has been shown to lower ICP, heart rate, and blood pressure*
Provide pleasant auditory experiences
Use therapeutic touch
Avoid emotionally stressful conversation (e.g., about pain, condition, prognosis)
*Administer sedation, if ordered, for extreme agitation or restlessness

Prevent or relieve pain, *because pain causes increased ICP*
Closely observe child for signs of pain, especially changes in behavior (e.g., agitation); increased heart rate, respiratory rate, and blood pressure (usually increase with pain); and decreased oxygen saturation
Observe child's response during times of induced or suspected pain
Observe child's response following a painful procedure or the administration of analgesia
Use pain assessment record (See p. 323.)
*Administer paralyzing and analgesic agents if prescribed
Schedule disturbing procedures to take advantage of therapies that reduce ICP (e.g., bathe child after sedation or osmotherapy)
Monitor ICP monitoring device

EXPECTED OUTCOMES
ICP remains within safe limits
Child shows no evidence of sustained increased ICP

■ **PATIENT GOAL 2:** Will exhibit no signs of cerebral hypoxia

NURSING INTERVENTIONS/*RATIONALES*

Maintain patent airway *because respiratory obstruction leads to cardiac arrest, and cerebral hypoxia lasting longer than 4 minutes nearly always causes irreversible brain damage*
Provide oxygen as indicated by objective signs or as ordered
*Hyperventilate at prescribed intervals if ordered
Monitor blood gases and pH
If child is on mechanical ventilation:
Monitor for correct settings, proper functioning
Prepare to provide artificial ventilation in case of ventilatory failure; have manual resuscitation bag at bedside
*Administer medications as ordered *to prevent cerebral edema and improve cerebral circulation*

EXPECTED OUTCOME
Child breathes easily; respirations are within normal limits (See inside front cover.)

■ **PATIENT GOAL 3:** Will exhibit no evidence of cerebral edema

NURSING INTERVENTIONS/*RATIONALES*

Elevate head of bed to 15 to 30 degrees *to facilitate venous drainage*
Maintain IV fluids as prescribed
Avoid overhydration *to prevent cerebral edema*
Monitor intake and output
Monitor electrolyte balance and specific gravity *to detect signs of hypernatremia and hyperosmolality, because diabetes insipidus and the syndrome of inappropriate antidiuretic hormone commonly occur with CNS diseases and trauma*
*Administer hyperosmolar fluids as prescribed
*Administer corticosteroids as ordered

EXPECTED OUTCOME
Child exhibits no signs of sustained increased ICP

*Dependent nursing action.

Continued

Unit 4

The Unconscious Child—cont'd

■ **PATIENT GOAL 4:** Will experience no seizures

NURSING INTERVENTIONS/*RATIONALES*

Avoid stimulation that precipitates undesirable responses

Schedule nursing activities for minimum disturbance

*Administer antiepileptic drugs as prescribed

IV fosphenytoin (Cerebyx) is often used to treat seizures instead of IV phenytoin because of possible complications associated with IV phenytoin

If IV phenytoin is ordered, administer carefully and observe the following precautions:

Administer via slow IV push (not to exceed 50 mg/min) *because rapid administration may cause cardiac dysrhythmias*

Infuse completely in 1 hour *because drug tends to precipitate*

Never mix phenytoin with 5% dextrose *because drug will precipitate*

Dilute phenytoin with normal saline *to decrease vein irritation and pain*

EXPECTED OUTCOME

Child exhibits no seizure activity or undue restlessness and agitation

■ **PATIENT GOAL 5:** Will exhibit stable body temperature

NURSING INTERVENTIONS/*RATIONALES*

Closely monitor child's temperature *because elevations often occur with CNS dysfunction*

Remove excess coverings

*Administer antipyretics if prescribed for fever

Give tepid sponge bath if indicated, only for hyperthermia, not for fever, *because it may induce shivering*

Apply and monitor hypothermia blanket if indicated and ordered; administer antishivering agents, if ordered, *because shivering increases ICP and metabolic rate*

EXPECTED OUTCOME

Body temperature remains within safe limits (See inside front cover.)

■ **PATIENT GOAL 6:** Will exhibit no evidence of respiratory tract infection

NURSING INTERVENTIONS/*RATIONALES*

Turn frequently (at least every 2 hours, as tolerated) unless contraindicated by increased ICP

Keep persons with upper respiratory tract infection away from child

Use good handwashing technique

Keep all equipment in contact with child clean or sterile

Provide good oral hygiene *to decrease presence of infective organisms*

Perform chest physiotherapy if prescribed and as tolerated; avoid percussion *because it can increase ICP*

EXPECTED OUTCOME

Child exhibits no evidence of pulmonary dysfunction

■ **PATIENT GOAL 7:** Will experience no corneal irritation

NURSING INTERVENTIONS/*RATIONALES*

Patch eyes, if indicated, *for protection*

Keep lids completely closed *to protect corneas when corneal reflexes are absent*

Instill "artificial tears" *to lubricate eyes*

Assess eyes carefully for early signs of irritation or inflammation

EXPECTED OUTCOME

Corneas remain clear and moist

■ **PATIENT GOAL 8:** Will exhibit no breakdown in mucous membrane integrity

NURSING INTERVENTIONS/*RATIONALES*

Provide meticulous mouth care, *because mouth tends to become dry or coated with mucus*

Avoid drying products (e.g., lemon and glycerin)

EXPECTED OUTCOME

Mucous membranes remain clear, moist, and free of irritation

■ **PATIENT GOAL 9:** Will experience no physical injury

NURSING INTERVENTIONS/*RATIONALES*

Keep siderails up *to prevent falls*

Pad hard surfaces *that may injure extremities during spontaneous or involuntary movements*

EXPECTED OUTCOME

Child remains free of physical injury

■ **PATIENT GOAL 10:** Will maintain limb flexibility and full range of motion

NURSING INTERVENTIONS/*RATIONALES*

Perform passive range-of-motion exercises *to prevent contractures*

Position *to reduce contractures:*

Place small, rolled pad in palms to *maintain proper position of fingers*

Use foot board or ankle-high shoes to *prevent footdrop*

Splint joints, if needed, *to prevent severe contractures of wrists, knees, and ankles*

EXPECTED OUTCOME

Joints remain flexible and retain full range of motion

> **NURSING DIAGNOSIS:** Risk for impaired skin integrity related to immobility, bodily secretions, invasive procedures

■ **PATIENT GOAL 1:** Will maintain skin integrity

NURSING INTERVENTIONS/*RATIONALES*

Place child on pressure-reducing surface *to prevent tissue breakdown and pressure necrosis*

Change position frequently unless contraindicated by increased ICP

Protect pressure points (e.g., trochanter, sacrum, ankle, heels, shoulder, and occiput)

Inspect skin surfaces regularly for signs of irritation, redness, and evidence of pressure

Cleanse skin regularly, at least once daily

Protect skinfolds and surfaces that rub together *to prevent excoriation*

*Dependent nursing acion.

The Unconscious Child—cont'd

Keep clothing and linen clean, dry, and free of wrinkles
Carry out good perineal care
Gently massage skin with lotion or other lubricating substance (unless on existing reddened pressure areas) *to stimulate circulation and prevent drying*
Protect lips with cream or ointment *to prevent drying and cracking*

EXPECTED OUTCOME

Skin remains clean, intact, and free of irritation

NURSING DIAGNOSIS: Feeding, bathing/hygiene, toileting self-care deficits (level 4) related to physical immobility, perceptual and cognitive impairment

---

■ **PATIENT GOAL 1:** Will receive optimum nutrition

NURSING INTERVENTIONS/*RATIONALES*

Provide nourishment in manner suitable to child's condition
Monitor IV fluids when ordered
Record intake and output
*Feed prescribed formula by means of nasogastric or gastrostomy tube
Weigh daily or as ordered *to monitor nutritional adequacy*

EXPECTED OUTCOME

Child obtains sufficient nourishment

■ **PATIENT GOAL 2:** Will receive proper hygienic care

NURSING INTERVENTIONS/*RATIONALES*

Bathe daily or more often if indicated
Dress appropriately
Keep hair clean, combed, and styled

EXPECTED OUTCOME

Child appears clean and as well groomed as possible within limitations of condition

■ **PATIENT GOAL 3:** Will void and defecate adequately

NURSING INTERVENTIONS/*RATIONALES*

Provide sufficient liquid intake, unless contraindicated by cerebral edema or if overhydration is a threat
Apply urine-collecting device or insert indwelling catheter (if ordered)
Provide proper care of catheter
Clean skin well after each elimination *to prevent skin irritation*
Diaper as needed *to contain stool and urine*
Check abdomen for evidence of distention
    Measure abdominal girth *to detect enlargement*
*Administer stool softener *to prevent constipation*
*Administer suppositories or enema as indicated *to promote evacuation*

EXPECTED OUTCOMES

Child eliminates sufficient urine (specify)
Bowel is evacuated daily
Child's diaper area remains clean and free of irritation

NURSING DIAGNOSIS: Sensory/perceptual alterations (visual, auditory, kinesthetic, gustatory, tactile, olfactory) related to central nervous system impairment, bed rest

---

■ **PATIENT GOAL 1:** Will receive appropriate sensory stimulation

NURSING INTERVENTIONS/*RATIONALES*

Provide tactile stimulation as tolerated
Provide auditory stimulation (e.g., by voice, radio, music box)
Provide visual stimuli appropriate for age
Provide proprioceptive stimulation (e.g., by rocking, cuddling)
Encourage family to participate in stimulation program
Demonstrate for family how and where to touch child

EXPECTED OUTCOMES

Child receives sensory stimulation appropriate to age and condition
Child appears relaxed and rests quietly
Stimulation does not induce seizures or increase ICP

■ **PATIENT GOAL 2:** Will exhibit no evidence of pain

NURSING INTERVENTIONS/*RATIONALES*

Assess for evidence of pain
Use pain assessment record *to document effectiveness of interventions*
*Administer pain medication as needed

EXPECTED OUTCOME

Child exhibits no evidence of pain

NURSING DIAGNOSIS: Altered family processes related to a child hospitalized with a potentially fatal condition or permanent disability

---

■ **PATIENT (FAMILY) GOAL 1:** Will receive adequate support

**NURSING INTERVENTIONS/*RATIONALES*
AND EXPECTED OUTCOMES**

(See Nursing Care Plan: The Family of the Child Who Is Ill or Hospitalized, p. 282.)

■ **PATIENT (FAMILY) GOAL 2:** Will express feelings and concerns

NURSING INTERVENTIONS/*RATIONALES*

Provide needed information
Answer family's questions; encourage expression of feelings
Refer to persons or agencies for further information and clarification
Support parents' decisions

EXPECTED OUTCOME

Family verbalizes feelings and concerns

Unit 4

*Dependent nursing action.

NURSING CARE PLAN

The Child with a Head Injury

A head injury is a pathologic process involving the scalp, skull, meninges, or brain and resulting from mechanical force.

Concussion—A transient and reversible neuronal dysfunction, with instantaneous loss of awareness and responsiveness, that results from trauma to the head and persists for a relatively short time, usually minutes or hours.

Contusion—Petechial hemorrhages along superficial aspects of the brain at the site of impact (coup injury) and/or a lesion remote from the site of direct trauma (contrecoup injury)

ASSESSMENT

(See Assessment: The Child with Neurologic Dysfunction, p. 459.)

Assess airway, breathing, and circulation.

Examine head for evidence of injury—Bruises, lacerations, swelling, depression, drainage or bleeding from any orifice.

Perform a physical assessment of body for evidence of associated injuries.

Obtain a history of event and subsequent management.

Observe for manifestations of head injury:

Minor injury

May or may not lose consciousness

Transient period of confusion

Somnolence

Listlessness

Irritability

Pallor

Vomiting (one or more episodes)

Signs of progression

Altered mental status (e.g., difficulty rousing child)

Mounting agitation

Development of focal lateral neurologic signs

Marked changes in vital signs

Severe injury

Signs of increased ICP (See p. 459.)

  Increased head size (infant)

  Bulging fontanel (infant)

Retinal hemorrhage

Extraocular palsies (especially cranial nerve VI)

Hemiparesis

Quadriplegia

Elevated temperature (sometimes)

Unsteady gait (older child)

Papilledema (older child)

Associated signs

Skin injury (to area of head sustaining injury)

Other injuries (e.g., to extremities)

Observe for additional neurologic data:

  Bruises and wounds—Location, extent, type

  Unusual behavior—Note nature and frequency, related circumstances

  Incontinence in toilet-trained child (bowel, bladder); spontaneous or associated with other phenomena (e.g., seizure activity)

Assist with diagnostic procedures and tests (See Assessment: The Child with Neurologic Dysfunction, p. 459.)

Ongoing assessment

Perform frequent neurologic assessment including the following:

Level of consciousness

Position and movement

Presence of headache

Young child—Fussy and restless when handled; rolls head from side to side

Older child—Self-report

Presence of vertigo

Child assumes a position and vigorously resists efforts to be moved; forcible movement causes child to vomit and display spontaneous nystagmus

Seizures (relatively common in head injury) (See p. 474.)

Presence of drainage from any orifice—Amount and characteristics

Signs of increased intracranial pressure (See p. 459.)

> **NURSING DIAGNOSIS:** Risk for injury related to head injury, depressed sensorium, intracranial pathology

■ **PATIENT GOAL 1:** Will not experience further injury

NURSING INTERVENTIONS/*RATIONALES*

Stabilize child's spine until spinal cord injury is confirmed or ruled out *to prevent additional injury*

*Establish and maintain intravenous infusion as prescribed *for administration of medications and hydration*

Perform frequent assessments, especially of vital signs, neurologic signs, level of consciousness, and pain (using Pain Assessment Record; See p. 323.)

  Recognize that asymmetric pupils, or one dilated, unreactive pupil in a comatose child is a neurosurgical emergency requiring immediate treatment

  Recognize signs of brainstem involvement or other internal injuries that may require immediate intervention

Anticipate possibility of respiratory arrest in child with a severe head injury

Have emergency equipment and medications readily available *to prevent delay in treatment*

Maintain child NPO as ordered or needed *to prevent aspiration*

Give conscious child only clear liquids until no vomiting occurs for at least 6 hours

Place child on bed rest with siderails up during assessment period and as needed *to prevent injury if condition worsens*

Pad hard surfaces *to protect child during seizures or extreme restlessness*

Elevate head of bed, unless contraindicated, *to prevent increased ICP*

Avoid taking oral temperatures, *since seizures and vomiting are not uncommon*

Provide quiet environment *to reduce restlessness and irritability that may result in further injury*

Avoid suctioning through nares *to prevent catheter entering brain substance through a basal skull fracture*

Manage associated injuries appropriately (See specific injury.)

*Dependent nursing action.

The Child with a Head Injury—cont'd

EXPECTED OUTCOMES
Child exhibits no evidence of further injury
Child receives prompt, appropriate treatment for complications

NURSING DIAGNOSIS: Pain related to head injury

■ **PATIENT GOAL 1:** Will experience either no pain or a reduction of pain to level acceptable to child

NURSING INTERVENTIONS/*RATIONALES*
Provide ongoing pain assessment, especially differentiating between changing level of consciousness (LOC) and response to analgesics *since decreasing restlessness after administration of analgesic most likely reflects pain control rather than a decreasing LOC* (See Pain Assessment, p. 315.)
Communicate pain assessment with practitioner *so that appropriate analgesia can be provided*
*Administer analgesia *to provide pain relief*
*If there is a question regarding decreased LOC, or an order to give naloxone (Narcan), administer naloxone slowly *to differentiate between sedation from the opioid and the injury*
Apply cold compresses over site of injury *to reduce swelling and pain*
(See also Nursing Care Plan: The Child in Pain, p. 315.)

EXPECTED OUTCOME
Child rests quietly, reports, and/or exhibits no evidence of discomfort

NURSING DIAGNOSIS: Altered family processes related to a child with a head injury

■ **PATIENT (FAMILY) GOAL 1:** Will be prepared for child's home care

NURSING INTERVENTIONS/*RATIONALES*
Teach family skills needed for home observations (if child is not to be hospitalized) and to report any of the following:

Unusual drowsiness
Deviations in gait, coordination, and behavior
Symptoms such as headache, double vision, and nausea
Difficulty rousing from sleep (awaken twice during night to check level of consciousness)
Seizures
Change in pupil reaction (check every 4 hours including twice during night)
Teach skills such as changing dressings
Inform family of some manifestations of posttraumatic syndromes (Box 4-25)

EXPECTED OUTCOME
Family demonstrates the ability to provide needed care (specify skills and method of demonstration)

■ **PATIENT (FAMILY) GOAL 2:** Will receive adequate support

NURSING INTERVENTIONS/*RATIONALES*
AND EXPECTED OUTCOMES
(See Nursing Care Plan: The Family of the Child Who Is Ill or Hospitalized, p. 282.)

■ **PATIENT (FAMILY) GOAL 3:** Will be prepared for long-term care of child

NURSING INTERVENTIONS/*RATIONALES*
Refer family to support groups and agencies specializing in rehabilitation and long-term care
Maintain contact with family

EXPECTED OUTCOMES
Family contacts appropriate agencies
(See also:
    Nursing Care Plan: The Unconscious Child, p. 462.)
    Observation of Seizures, p. 474.)
    Nursing Care Plan: The Child in the Hospital, p. 268.)

*Dependent nursing action.

Unit 4

BOX 4-25

Clinical Manifestations of Posttraumatic Syndromes

Postconcussion Syndrome

Infants

Pallor
Sweating
Irritability
Sleepiness
Possible vomiting

Children

Behavioral disturbances
    Aggressiveness
    Disobedience

Withdrawal
Regression
Anxiety
Sleep disturbances
Phobias
Emotional lability
Irritability
Altered school performance
Seizures

Adolescents

Headache

Dizziness
Impaired concentration

Structural Complications

Hydrocephalus
Focal deficits
    Optic atrophy
    Cranial nerve palsies
    Motor deficits
    Diabetes insipidus
    Aphasia
Seizures

NURSING CARE PLAN

The Infant with Myelomeningocele

Myelomeningocele (meningomyelocele) is a hernial protrusion of a saclike cyst of meninges, spinal fluid, and a portion of the spinal cord with its nerves through a bony defect in the vertebral column.

Other terms used to describe spinal defects:

Myelodysplasia—All-inclusive term that refers to defective development of any part of the spinal cord

Spina bifida—Defect in closure of the vertebral column with or without varying degrees of tissue protrusion through the bony cleft

Spina bifida occulta—Fusion failure of posterior vertebral arches without accompanying herniation of spinal cord or meninges; not visible externally

Spina bifida cystica—Defect in closure with external saccular protrusion through the bony spine with varying degrees of nerve involvement

Meningocele—Form of spina bifida cystica; consists of a saclike cyst of meninges filled with spinal fluid, but involves no nerves or neurologic deficit

---

ASSESSMENT

Perform a physical assessment.
Observe for manifestations of myelomeningocele:
  Visible sac
  Sensory disturbances usually parallel motor dysfunction
    Below second lumbar vertebra:
      Flaccid, areflexic partial paralysis of lower extremities
      Varying degrees of sensory deficit
      Overflow incontinence with constant dribbling of urine
      Lack of bowel control
      Rectal prolapse (sometimes)
    Below third sacral vertebra:
      No motor impairment
      May be saddle anesthesia with bladder and anal sphincter paralysis

Joint deformities (sometimes produced in utero)
  Talipes valgus or varus contractures
  Kyphosis
  Lumbosacral scoliosis
  Hip dislocations
Perform or assist with neurologic examination to determine level of motor and sensory impairment.
Inspect myelomeningocele for any changes in appearance (e.g., abrasions, tears, signs of infection).
Observe for signs that indicate hydrocephalus. (See p. 470.)
Assist with diagnostic procedures and tests (e.g., radiography and tomography).

NURSING DIAGNOSIS: Risk for infection related to presence of infective organisms, nonepithelialized meningeal sac, paralysis

- **PATIENT GOAL 1:** Will experience minimized risk of central nervous system infection

NURSING INTERVENTIONS/RATIONALES
Position infant *to prevent contamination from urine and stool*
Cleanse myelomeningocele carefully with sterile normal saline if it becomes soiled or contaminated
*Apply sterile dressings and moisten with sterile solution as ordered (normal saline, antibiotic) *to prevent drying of sac*
*Administer antibiotics as prescribed
Monitor closely for signs of infection (elevated temperature, irritability, lethargy, nuchal rigidity) *to prevent delay in treatment*
Administer similar care to operative site postoperatively

EXPECTED OUTCOME
Meningeal sac remains clean, intact, and exhibits no evidence of infection

- **PATIENT GOAL 2:** Will experience minimized risk of urinary tract infection

NURSING INTERVENTIONS/RATIONALES
Avoid urethral contamination with stool *to prevent introduction of infective organisms into urinary tract*
Carry out meticulous perineal hygiene *to remove infective organisms*
Monitor urinary output for retention *to minimize risk of infection due to stasis of urine*
*Administer antibiotics as prescribed
*Administer urinary tract antiseptics if prescribed
Ensure adequate fluid intake *to increase urination and prevent bacterial growth*

EXPECTED OUTCOME
Infant exhibits no evidence of urinary tract infection

NURSING DIAGNOSIS: Risk for trauma related to delicate spinal lesion

- **PATIENT GOAL 1:** Will not experience trauma to spinal lesion/surgical site

NURSING INTERVENTIONS/RATIONALES
Handle infant carefully *to prevent damage to meningeal sac or surgical site*
Place infant in prone position, or side-lying position if permitted, *to minimize tension on the meningeal sac or surgical site*
Apply protective devices around sac (e.g., a surgical plastic drape, cut to fit and taped below the sac by the sacrum and loosely draped over the sac) *to provide a protective shield*
Modify routine nursing activities (e.g., feeding, making bed, comforting activities) *to prevent trauma*

EXPECTED OUTCOMES
Meningeal sac remains intact
Surgical site heals without trauma

NURSING DIAGNOSIS: Risk for impaired skin integrity related to paralysis, continual dribbling of urine, and feces

- **PATIENT GOAL 1:** Will not experience skin irritation

NURSING INTERVENTIONS/RATIONALES
Change diapers as soon as soiled, if diapered, *to keep skin clean, dry, and free of irritation*
Keep perianal area clean and dry
Place infant on pressure-reducing surface *to reduce pressure on knees and ankles during prone positioning*
Gently massage healthy skin during cleansing and application of lotion *to increase circulation*

EXPECTED OUTCOME
Skin remains clean and dry with no evidence of irritation

*Dependent nursing action.

Unit 4

The Infant with Myelomeningocele—cont'd

NURSING DIAGNOSIS: Risk for trauma related to impaired cerebrospinal fluid circulation

■ **PATIENT GOAL 1:** Will not experience adverse effects of increased intracranial pressure (ICP)

NURSING INTERVENTIONS/*RATIONALES*
Measure occipitofrontal circumference daily *to detect increased ICP and developing hydrocephalus*
Observe for signs of increased ICP, *which might indicate developing hydrocephalus:*
　Irritability
　Lethargy
　Infant:
　　Cries when picked up or handled; quiets when lies still
　　Increased occipitofrontal circumference
　　Separated sutures
　　Change in level of consciousness
　Child:
　　Headache (especially in morning)
　　Apathy
　　Confusion
Minimize stressful events (e.g., pain) *because stress increases blood pressure, a main determinant of ICP* (See Nursing Care Plan: The Child in Pain, p. 315.)

EXPECTED OUTCOME
Evidence of increased intracranial pressure and hydrocephalus is detected early, and appropriate interventions are implemented

NURSING DIAGNOSIS: Risk for injury related to repeated exposure to latex products and development of latex allergy

! PRACTICE ALERT !

Ask *all* patients, not only those at risk, about allergic reactions to latex. Ask this during the health interview with the parent and/or child. Be sure this is a routine part of all preoperative histories.

■ **PATIENT GOAL 1:** Will experience minimal exposure to latex

NURSING INTERVENTIONS/*RATIONALES*
Identify children with latex allergy (Practice Alert and Guidelines boxes)
Maintain a latex-free environment *to reduce exposure*
Educate family members and other caregivers (e.g., daycare workers, teachers) about the following:
　Risk of latex allergy, and items to avoid *to reduce exposure*
　Signs of allergy (from hives, rash, and wheezing, to anaphylaxis) *to detect a reaction quickly*
　Emergency treatment, including use of anaphylactic kit and summoning emergency medical services, *to prevent delay in treatment*

EXPECTED OUTCOME
Child does not develop allergic reactions to latex

NURSING DIAGNOSIS: Risk for injury related to neuromuscular impairment

■ **PATIENT GOAL 1:** Will experience no or minimized risk of hip and lower extremity deformity

NURSING INTERVENTIONS/*RATIONALES*
Carry out passive range-of-motion exercises *to prevent contractures;* do not push past point of resistance *to prevent trauma*
Carry out muscle stretching when indicated *to prevent contractures*
Maintain hips in slight to moderate abduction *to prevent dislocation;* maintain feet in neutral position *to prevent contractures*
Use diaper rolls, pads, small sandbags, or specially designed appliances *to maintain desired position*

EXPECTED OUTCOMES
Lower extremities maintain flexibility
Hips and lower extremities are maintained in correct articulation and alignment
(See also:
　Nursing Care Plan: The Child with Chronic Illness or Disability, p. 287.)
　Nursing Care Plan: The Child in the Hospital, p. 268.)
　Nursing Care Plan: The Family of the Child Who Is Ill or Hospitalized, p. 282.)

Unit 4

GUIDELINES

Identifying Latex Allergy

Does the child have any symptoms (such as sneezing, coughing, rashes, or wheezing) when handling rubber products (balloons, tennis or Koosh balls, adhesive bandage strips) or when in contact with rubber hospital products such as gloves and catheters?
Has your child ever had an allergic reaction during surgery?
Does the child have a history of rashes, asthma, or allergic reactions to medication or foods, especially milk, kiwi fruit, bananas, or chestnuts?

How would you identify or recognize an allergic reaction in your child?
What would you do if an allergic reaction occurred?
Has anyone ever discussed latex or rubber allergy or sensitivity with you?
Has the child had any allergy testing?
When did the child last come in contact with any type of rubber product? Were you present?

Modified from Romanczuk A: Latex use with infants and children: it can cause problems, *MCN* 18(4):208-212, 1993.

NURSING CARE PLAN

The Child with Hydrocephalus

Hydrocephalus is an excessive accumulation of cerebral spinal fluid (CSF) within the ventricular system, resulting in passive dilation of the ventricles.

Communicating hydrocephalus—Impaired absorption of CSF within the subarachnoid space (ventricles communicate)

Noncommunicating hydrocephalus—Obstruction to the flow of CSF within the ventricles (ventricles do not communicate)

ASSESSMENT

Obtain a health history, especially regarding a head injury or cerebral infection.

Perform a physical assessment, especially for evidence of repaired myelomeningocele and with occipitofrontal circumference measurement.

Observe for manifestations of hydrocephalus:

Early infancy

Abnormally rapid head growth

Bulging fontanels (especially anterior) sometimes without head enlargement:

Tense

Nonpulsatile

Dilated scalp veins

Separated sutures

Macewen sign (cracked-pot sound) on percussion

Thinning of skull bones

Later infancy

Frontal enlargement or "bossing"

Depressed eyes

Setting-sun sign (sclera visible above the iris)

Pupils sluggish, with unequal response to light

Infancy, general

Irritability

Lethargy

Infant cries when picked up or rocked and quiets when allowed to lie still

Early infantile reflex acts may persist

Normally expected responses fail to appear

May display the following:

Change in level of consciousness

Opisthotonos (often extreme)

Lower extremity spasticity

Advanced cases:

Difficulty in sucking and feeding

Shrill, brief, high-pitched cry

Cardiopulmonary embarrassment

Childhood

Headache on awakening; improvement following emesis or upright posture

Papilledema

Strabismus

Extrapyramidal tract signs (e.g., ataxia)

Irritability

Lethargy

Apathy

Confusion

Often incoherence

Assist with diagnostic procedures (e.g., magnetic resonance imaging, computed tomography, echoencephalography, transillumination, and ventricular puncture).

NURSING DIAGNOSIS: Risk for injury related to increased intracranial pressure (ICP)

■ **PATIENT GOAL 1:** Will not experience increased intracranial pressure

NURSING INTERVENTIONS/*RATIONALES*

Observe closely for signs of increased ICP (See p. 459.) *to prevent delay in treatment*

Obtain baseline neurologic assessment preoperatively *to serve as a guide for postoperative assessment and evaluation of shunt function*

Avoid placing intravenous infusion in a scalp vein if surgery is anticipated *since procedure will interfere with IV site*

*Position child as prescribed:

Place on unoperated side *to prevent pressure on shunt valve*

Elevate head of bed, if prescribed, *to enhance gravity flow through shunt*

Keep child flat, if prescribed, *to help prevent complications resulting from too rapid a reduction of intracranial fluid*

Avoid sedation *because level of consciousness is an important indicator of increased ICP*

*Pump the shunt to assess function according to surgeon's order and to manufacturer's recommendation

*Carry out postoperative care of shunt as prescribed

Teach family signs of increased ICP and when to notify health practitioner *to prevent delay in treatment*

EXPECTED OUTCOME

Child exhibits no evidence of increased ICP

NURSING DIAGNOSIS: Risk for infection related to presence of mechanical drainage system, surgical procedure

---

*Dependent nursing action.

The Child with Hydrocephalus—cont'd

■ **PATIENT GOAL 1:** Will exhibit no evidence of infection

NURSING INTERVENTIONS/*RATIONALES*

Assess child for signs of cerebral spinal fluid (CSF) infection, including elevated temperature, poor feeding, vomiting, decreased responsiveness, and seizure activity

Observe for redness, swelling *(signs of local inflammation)* at operative sites and along shunt tract

*Administer antibiotics as prescribed

*Assist practitioner with intraventricular instillation of antibiotics as needed

Inspect incision site for leakage; test drainage for glucose *because it is an indicator of CSF*

*Provide wound care as prescribed, using strict aseptic technique *to prevent contamination*

Keep child's diaper off peritoneal dressing site or suture line *to prevent contamination*

EXPECTED OUTCOME

Child exhibits no evidence of infection

NURSING DIAGNOSIS: Risk for impaired skin integrity related to pressure areas, paralysis, relaxed anal sphincter

■ **PATIENT GOAL 1:** Will maintain skin integrity

NURSING INTERVENTIONS/*RATIONALES*

Provide meticulous skin care *to prevent tissue damage from moisture and pressure*

(See also Patient Goal, Nursing Care Plan: The Unconscious Child, p. 462.)

EXPECTED OUTCOME

Skin remains clean, intact, and free of irritation

NURSING DIAGNOSIS: Altered family processes related to situational crisis (child with a physical defect)

■ **PATIENT (FAMILY) GOAL 1:** Will receive adequate support

**NURSING INTERVENTIONS/*RATIONALES*
AND EXPECTED OUTCOMES**

(See Nursing Care Plan: The Family of the Child Who Is Ill or Hospitalized, p. 282.)

(See also Nursing Care Plan: The Child with Chronic Illness or Disability, p. 287.)

Unit 4

NURSING CARE PLAN

The Child with Acute Bacterial Meningitis

Acute bacterial meningitis is a bacterial infection of the meninges and cerebrospinal fluid.

ASSESSMENT

Obtain a health history, especially regarding a previous infection, injury, or exposure.

Perform a physical assessment.

Observe for the following manifestations of bacterial meningitis:

Children and adolescents

Usually abrupt onset
Fever
Chills
Headache
Vomiting
Alterations in sensorium
Seizures (often the initial sign)
Irritability
Agitation
May develop:
  Photophobia
  Delirium
  Hallucinations
  Aggressive or maniacal behavior
  Drowsiness
  Stupor
  Coma
Nuchal rigidity
  May progress to opisthotonos
Positive Kernig and Brudzinski signs (See p. 66.)
Hyperactive but variable reflex responses
Signs and symptoms peculiar to individual organisms:
  Petechial or purpuric rashes (meningococcal infection), especially when associated with a shocklike state
  Joint involvement (meningococcal and *H. influenzae* infection)
  Chronically draining ear (pneumococcal meningitis)

Infants and young children

Classic picture rarely seen in children between 3 months and 2 years of age

Fever
Poor feeding
Vomiting
Marked irritability
Frequent seizures (often accompanied by a high-pitched cry)
Bulging fontanel
Nuchal rigidity may or may not be present
Brudzinski and Kernig signs are not helpful in diagnosis
  Difficult to elicit and evaluate in the age-group
Subdural empyema (*H. influenzae* infection)

Neonates: specific signs

Extremely difficult to diagnose
Manifestations vague and nonspecific
Well at birth but within a few days begins to look and behave poorly
Refuses feedings
Poor sucking ability
Vomiting or diarrhea
Poor tone
Lack of movement
Poor cry
Full, tense, and bulging fontanel may appear late in course of illness
Neck usually supple

Nonspecific signs that may be present in neonates

Hypothermia or fever (depending on the maturity of the infant)
Jaundice
Irritability
Drowsiness
Seizures
Respiratory irregularities or apnea
Cyanosis
Weight loss

Assist with diagnostic procedures and tests (e.g., lumbar puncture, spinal fluid examination, and cultures).

NURSING DIAGNOSIS: Risk for injury related to presence of infection

■ **PATIENT GOAL 1:** Will exhibit no signs of infection

NURSING INTERVENTIONS/*RATIONALES*

Assist health practitioner to obtain needed cultures *to identify causative organism*

*Administer antibiotic as prescribed, and as soon as it is ordered, *to prevent delay in treatment*

Maintain intravenous route for administration of medication

EXPECTED OUTCOME

Child exhibits evidence of diminishing symptoms

■ **PATIENT GOAL 2:** Will not spread infection to others

NURSING INTERVENTIONS/*RATIONALES*

Implement appropriate infection control:
  Place child in isolation for at least 24 hours after initiation of antibiotic therapy.
  (See also Nursing Care Plan: The Child at Risk for Infection, p. 341.)

© 2000 Mosby, Inc. All rights reserved.

*Dependent nursing action.

The Child with Acute Bacterial Meningitis—cont'd

Instruct others (family, members of staff) in appropriate precautions

Administer appropriate vaccinations:

Give routine, age-appropriate vaccines (e.g., vaccine to prevent *H. influenzae* type B [Hib])

Identify close contacts and high-risk children who might benefit from vaccinations (e.g., meningococci vaccination)

EXPECTED OUTCOME

Others remain free from infection

■ **PATIENT GOAL 3:** Will not experience complications

NURSING INTERVENTIONS/*RATIONALES*

Observe closely for signs of complications, especially increased ICP, shock, and respiratory distress, *so emergency treatment is initiated*

Measure head circumference of infant *because subdural effusions and obstructive hydrocephalus may develop*

*Maintain optimum hydration as prescribed

Monitor and record intake and output *to identify complications such as impending shock or increased fluid accumulation associated with cerebral edema or subdural effusion*

Reduce environmental stimuli, *since child may be sensitive to noise, bright lights, and other external stimuli*

Implement appropriate safety precautions *because child is often restless and subject to seizures*

Explain importance of follow-up care to parents *because neurologic sequelae, including hearing loss, may not be apparent during the acute illness*

EXPECTED OUTCOME

Child will not experience complications

NURSING DIAGNOSIS: Pain related to inflammatory process

■ **PATIENT GOAL 1:** Will experience either no pain or a reduction of pain to level acceptable to child

NURSING INTERVENTIONS/*RATIONALES*

Allow child to assume position of comfort

Use side-lying position, if tolerated, *because of nuchal rigidity*

Elevate head of bed slightly without using a pillow *because this is often the most comfortable position*

*Administer analgesics as prescribed, especially acetaminophen with codeine

EXPECTED OUTCOME

Child exhibits no or minimum signs of pain

NURSING DIAGNOSIS: Altered family processes related to a child with a serious illness

---

■ **PATIENT (FAMILY) GOAL 1:** Will receive adequate support

NURSING INTERVENTIONS/*RATIONALES*

Encourage family to discuss feelings *to minimize blame and guilt*

Reassure family that the onset of meningitis is sudden and that they acted responsibly in seeking medical assistance when they did *to minimize blame and guilt*

Keep family informed of child's condition, progress, procedures, and treatments *to reduce anxiety*

EXPECTED OUTCOMES

Family feels a sense of support

Family demonstrates understanding of the disease and its therapies (specify knowledge)

(See also:

Nursing Care Plan: The Family of the Child Who Is Ill or Hospitalized, p. 282.)

Nursing Care Plan: The Unconscious Child, p. 462.)

*Dependent nursing action.

Unit 4

NURSING CARE PLAN

The Child with Epilepsy

Seizures are brief malfunctions of the brain's electrical system resulting from cortical neuronal discharge. Seizures may manifest as **convulsions** (involuntary muscular contraction and relaxation); changes in behavior, sensations, or perception; visual and auditory hallucinations; and altered consciousness or unconsciousness.

Epilepsy is a chronic seizure disorder with recurrent and unprovoked seizures, which requires long-term treatment. Not every seizure is epileptic.

ASSESSMENT

Obtain a health history, especially regarding prenatal, perinatal, and neonatal events; any instances of infection, apnea, colic, or poor feeding; and any information regarding previous accidents or serious illnesses.

Obtain a history of seizure activity including the following:

Description of child's behavior during seizure

Age of onset

Time when seizure occurred—Time of day, while awake or during sleep, relationship to meals

Any triggering factors that might have precipitated seizure (e.g., fever, infection); falls that may have caused trauma to the head; anxiety; fatigue; activity (e.g., hyperventilation); environmental events (e.g., exposure to strong stimuli such as bright, flashing lights or loud noises)

Duration, progression, and any postictal feelings or behaviors

Perform a physical and neurologic assessment.

Observe seizure manifestations. (See Box 4-24, p. 460.)

Assist with diagnostic procedures and tests (e.g., electroencephalography, tomography, skull radiography, echoencephalography, brain scan; blood chemistry, serum glucose, blood urea nitrogen, ammonia; and specific tests for metabolic disorders).

Observe seizure

Describe the following:

Only what is actually observed

Order of events (before, during, and after)

Duration of seizure

Tonic-clonic: from first signs of event until jerking stops

Absence: from loss of consciousness until patient regains consciousness

Complex partial: from first sign of unresponsiveness, motor activity, or automatisms until there is responsiveness to environment

Onset

Time of onset

Significant preseizure events—Bright lights, noise, excitement, emotional outbursts

Behavior

Change in facial expression, such as for fear

Cry or other sound

Stereotypic or automatous movements

Random activity (wandering)

Position of head, body, extremities

Unilateral or bilateral posturing of one or more extremities

Body deviation to side

Movement

Change of position, if any

Site of commencement—Hand, thumb, mouth, generalized

Tonic phase, if present—Length, parts of body involved

Clonic phase—Twitching or jerking movements, parts of body involved, sequence of parts involved, generalized, change in character of movements

Lack of movement or muscle tone of any body part or entire body

Face

Color change—Pallor, cyanosis, flushing

Perspiration

Mouth—Position, deviation to one side, teeth clenched, tongue bitten, frothing at mouth, flecks of blood or bleeding

Lack of expression

Eyes

Position—Straight ahead, deviation upward, deviation outward, conjugate or divergent

Pupils (if able to assess)—Change in size, equality, reaction to light and accommodation

Respiratory effort

Presence and length of apnea

Presence of stertor

Other

Involuntary urination

Involuntary defecation

Observe postictally

Duration of postictal period

Method of termination

State of consciousness—Unresponsiveness, drowsiness, confusion

Orientation to time, persons

Sleeping but able to be aroused

Motor ability

Any change in motor power

Ability to move all extremities

Any paresis or weakness

Ability to whistle (if appropriate to age)

Speech—Changes, peculiarities, type and extent of any difficulties

Sensations

Complaint of discomfort or pain

Any sensory impairment of hearing, vision

Recollection of preseizure sensations, warning of attack

Awareness that attack was beginning

Recall of words spoken to child

NURSING DIAGNOSIS: Risk for injury related to type of seizure

■ **PATIENT GOAL 1:** Will not experience seizure activity

NURSING INTERVENTIONS/RATIONALES

*Administer antiepileptic medication

Teach family and child, when appropriate, the administration of medications

Stress importance of complying with therapeutic regimen

Avoid situations that are known to precipitate a seizure (e.g., blinking lights, fatigue)

EXPECTED OUTCOME

Child remains free of seizure activity

*Dependent nursing action.

Unit 4

The Child with Epilepsy—cont'd

- **PATIENT GOAL 2:** Will not experience complications from medication

NURSING INTERVENTIONS/RATIONALES

Be aware of and teach family to recognize unfavorable reactions to medications

Encourage periodic physical and laboratory assessment *to determine possible deviations from normal findings*

Encourage good dental care during phenytoin therapy *to reduce gingival hyperplasia from phenytoin*

Encourage adequate vitamin D and folic acid during phenytoin and phenobarbital therapy *to prevent deficiency*

EXPECTED OUTCOME

Child and family demonstrate an understanding of possible unfavorable responses to medications and the appropriate intervention (specify)

- **PATIENT GOAL 3:** Will not experience injury

NURSING INTERVENTIONS/RATIONALES

Educate parents and child regarding appropriate activities for child (depends on type, frequency, and severity of seizures)

Explore appropriate modifications or adaptations to situations that pose a danger during a seizure (e.g., climbing trees, playground apparatus)

Provide companionship during permissible activities, such as swimming, biking

Recommend showering or close supervision during bathing

Educate teachers and other persons who are associated with child regarding correct assistance during and after seizure

EXPECTED OUTCOMES

Child and family agree on appropriate activities or modifications of activities for child

Individuals in contact with child intervene appropriately during and after seizure

NURSING DIAGNOSIS: Risk for injury, hypoxia, and aspiration related to motor activity and loss of consciousness (tonic-clonic seizure)

- **PATIENT GOAL 1:** Will not experience injury, respiratory distress, or aspiration

NURSING INTERVENTIONS/RATIONALES

Time seizure *to determine duration of possible hypoxia and possible need for emergency care*

Protect child during seizure:

Do not attempt to restrain child or use force *because this may cause injury to child or self*

If child is standing or sitting in chair or wheelchair at beginning of episode, ease child to floor *to prevent falls*

Place small cushion or blanket or own hand under child's head *to prevent injury*

Do not put anything in child's mouth (e.g., tongue blades, food, or fluids) *because this can cause injury, obstruct breathing, or be aspirated*

Remove eyeglasses *to protect eyes from trauma*

Loosen clothing *that may restrict movement or breathing*

Prevent child from hitting head on sharp objects *that might cause injury during uncontrollable muscle jerks*

Remove hazards such as furniture

Pad objects such as crib, siderails, and wheelchair *to lessen injury from impact*

Keep siderails raised when child is sleeping, resting, or seizing *to avoid falls*

Allow seizure to end without interference

Position child with head in midline, not hyperextended, when possible *to promote adequate ventilation*

If child begins to vomit, turn to side as a unit *to prevent aspiration*

Protect child after seizure (postictal period)

Time postictal period

Maintain child in side-lying position

Call emergency medical service (EMS)

EXPECTED OUTCOME

Child exhibits no signs of physical or mental injury or aspiration

NURSING DIAGNOSIS: Risk for injury related to impaired consciousness and automatisms (complex partial seizure)

- **PATIENT GOAL 1:** Will not experience injury and will remain calm

NURSING INTERVENTIONS/RATIONALES

Time seizure *to establish duration and possible need for emergency care*

Protect child during seizure:

Do not restrain unless child is in danger *to prevent injury to child or self*

Remove hazards in immediate environment

Redirect child to safe area, especially away from windows, stairs, heating elements, or sources of water, *to prevent falls, burns, and drowning*

Do not agitate; rather, talk in calm voice and reassuring manner

Do not expect child to follow instructions *because of impaired consciousness*

Watch to see if seizure generalizes into a tonic-clonic seizure

Protect child after seizure (postictal)

Time postictal period

Stay and reassure child until fully alert *because child may be confused and frightened*

Call EMS

EXPECTED OUTCOME

Child exhibits no sign of physical injury and remains calm

NURSING DIAGNOSIS: Altered family processes related to a child with a chronic illness

- **PATIENT (FAMILY) GOAL 1:** Will receive adequate support

NURSING INTERVENTIONS/RATIONALES

(See Nursing Diagnosis: Risk for altered family processes, in Nursing Care Plan: The Child with Chronic Illness or Disability, p. 287.)

Refer to special support groups and agencies (e.g., Epilepsy Foundation of America)

EXPECTED OUTCOMES

Family becomes involved with special group

(See also:

Nursing Care Plan: The Child with Chronic Illness or Disability, p. 287.

Nursing Care Plan: The Unconscious Child, p. 462.)

Unit 4

NURSING CARE PLAN

The Child with Cerebral Palsy

Cerebral palsy is a nonspecific term applied to disorders characterized by impaired movement and posture and early onset. It is nonprogressive and may be accompanied by intellectual, perceptual, and language deficits.

Clinical classifications of cerebral palsy:

Spastic—May involve one side or both sides

Hypertonicity with poor control of posture, balance, and coordinated motion

Impairment of fine and gross motor skills

Active attempts at motion increase abnormal postures and overflow of movement to other parts of the body

Dyskinetic/athetoid—Abnormal involuntary movement

Athetosis—Characterized by slow, wormlike, writhing movements that usually involve all extremities, the trunk, neck, facial muscles, and tongue

Involvement of the pharyngeal, laryngeal, and oral muscles causes drooling and dysarthria (imperfect speech articulation)

Involuntary movements may take on choreoid (involuntary, irregular, jerking movements) and dystonic (disordered muscle tone) manifestations that increase in intensity under emotional stress and around adolescence

Ataxic

Wide-based gait

Rapid, repetitive movements performed poorly

Disintegration of movements of the upper extremities when the child reaches for objects

Mixed-type/dystonic—Combination of spasticity and athetosis

ASSESSMENT

Perform a physical assessment.

Obtain a health history, especially relative to prenatal and perinatal factors and circumstances surrounding birth that predispose to fetal anoxia.

Observe for warning signs of cerebral palsy*:

Physical signs:

Poor head control after 3 months of age

Stiff or rigid arms or legs

Pushing away or arching back

Floppy or limp body posture

Cannot sit up without support by 8 months

Uses only one side of the body, or only the arms, to crawl

Behavioral signs:

Extreme irritability or crying

Failure to smile by 3 months

Feeding difficulties:

Persistent gagging or choking when fed

After 6 months of age, tongue pushes soft food out of the mouth

Observe for manifestations of cerebral palsy, especially those related to attainment of developmental milestones:

Delayed gross motor development:

A universal manifestation

Delay in all motor accomplishments

Increases as growth advances

Abnormal motor performance:

Very early preferential unilateral hand use

Abnormal and asymmetric crawl

Standing or walking on toes

Uncoordinated or involuntary movements

Poor sucking

Feeding difficulties

Persistent tongue thrust

Alterations of muscle tone:

Increased or decreased resistance to passive movements

Opisthotonic postures (exaggerated arching of back)

Feels stiff on handling or dressing

Difficulty in diapering

Rigid and unbending at the hip and knee joints when pulled to sitting position (an early sign)

Abnormal postures:

Maintains hips higher than trunk in prone position with legs and arms flexed or drawn under the body

Scissoring and extension of legs, with the feet plantar flexed in supine position

Persistent infantile resting and sleeping posture:

Arms abducted at shoulders

Elbows flexed

Hands fisted

Reflex abnormalities:

Persistence of primitive infantile reflexes:

Obligatory tonic neck reflex at any age

Nonpersistence beyond 6 months of age

Persistence or hyperactivity of the Moro, plantar, and palmar grasp reflexes

Hyperreflexia, ankle clonus, and stretch reflexes elicited in many muscle groups on fast passive movements

Associated disabilities (may or may not be present):

Subnormal learning and reasoning (mental retardation in about two thirds of individuals)

Seizures

Impaired behavioral and interpersonal relationships

Sensory impairment (e.g., vision, hearing)

Assist with diagnostic procedures and tests if indicated (e.g., electroencephalography, tomography, screening for metabolic defects, and serum electrolyte values).

Perform developmental, hearing, or visual tests as indicated. (See Unit 1.)

*NOTE: These warning signs are not diagnostic. Data from Pathways Awareness Foundation: *Parents . . . if you see any of these warning signs . . . don't delay,* Chicago, 1991, The Foundation.

The Child with Cerebral Palsy—cont'd

NURSING DIAGNOSIS: Impaired physical mobility related to neuromuscular impairment

■ **PATIENT GOAL 1:** Will acquire locomotion within capabilities (per care plan of PT/OT)

NURSING INTERVENTIONS/*RATIONALES*

Encourage sitting, crawling, and walking as prescribed
Carry out therapies that strengthen and improve control *to facilitate optimum development*
Assist child in using reciprocal leg motion when learning to walk, if indicated in plan of care
Provide incentives to move (e.g., place toy out of child's reach)
Ensure adequate rest before attempting locomotion activities *to encourage success*
Incorporate play that encourages desired behavior, *because this encourages cooperation*
Employ aids such as parallel bars and crutches as prescribed *to facilitate locomotion*
Prepare child and family for surgical procedures if indicated

EXPECTED OUTCOME

Child acquires locomotion within capabilities (specify)

■ **PATIENT GOAL 2:** Will experience no or minimal deformity

NURSING INTERVENTIONS/*RATIONALES*

Apply and correctly use orthoses *for maximum benefit*
Carry out and teach family to perform stretching exercises as prescribed *to prevent deformities*
Employ appropriate range-of-motion exercises as prescribed *to facilitate muscle development and flexibility of joints*
Perform preoperative and postoperative care for child who requires corrective surgery

EXPECTED OUTCOME

Alignment and flexibility are maintained within child's limits

NURSING DIAGNOSIS: Bathing/hygiene, dressing/grooming, feeding, toileting self-care deficits related to physical disability

■ **PATIENT GOAL 1:** Will engage in self-help activities of daily living

NURSING INTERVENTIONS/*RATIONALES*

Encourage child to assist with care as age and capabilities permit *to facilitate optimum development*
Select toys and activities that allow maximum participation by child and that improve motor function and sensory input *so that child is more able to care for self*
Avoid undue persistence *because child may be unable or not ready to accomplish a goal*
Encourage activities that require both unimanual and bimanual actions *to encourage optimum development*
Assist with jaw control during feeding *to facilitate eating*

Encourage use of adapted utensils, foods, and clothing (e.g., large-bowled spoon with padded handle; finger foods and foods that adhere to, rather than slip from, utensil; clothing that opens from front with self-adhering closings rather than buttons) *to facilitate self-help*
Assist parents in toilet training child, *because methods may need to be individualized according to child's abilities*

EXPECTED OUTCOME

Child engages in self-help activities commensurate with capabilities

NURSING DIAGNOSIS: Risk for injury related to physical disability, neuromuscular impairment, perceptual and cognitive impairment

■ **PATIENT GOAL 1:** Will experience no physical injury

NURSING INTERVENTIONS/*RATIONALES*

Educate family to provide safe physical environment:
    Use padded furniture *for protection*
    Use siderails on bed *to prevent falls*
    Use sturdy furniture that does not slip *to prevent falls*
    Avoid scatter rugs and polished floors *to prevent falls*
Educate family to select toys appropriate to age and physical limitations *to prevent injuries*
Encourage sufficient rest *because fatigue can increase risk of injuries*
Use restraints when child is in chair or vehicle
Provide child who is prone to falls with protective helmet and enforce its use *to prevent head injuries*
Institute seizure precautions for susceptible child
*Administer antiepileptic drugs as prescribed *to prevent seizures*

EXPECTED OUTCOMES

Family provides a safe environment for child (specify)
Child is free of injury

NURSING DIAGNOSIS: Impaired verbal communication related to hearing loss, neuromuscular impairment, cognitive impairment

■ **PATIENT GOAL 1:** Will engage in communication process within limits of impairment

NURSING INTERVENTIONS/*RATIONALES*

Enlist the services of a speech therapist early *before child learns poor habits of communication*
Talk to child slowly *to give child time to understand speech*
Use articles and pictures *to reinforce speech and encourage understanding*
Use feeding techniques *that help facilitate speech,* such as using lips, teeth, and various tongue movements
Teach and use nonverbal communication methods (e.g., sign language) for child with severe dysarthria
Help family acquire electronic equipment (e.g., typewriter, microcomputer with voice synthesizer) *to facilitate nonverbal communication*

*Dependent nursing action.

Continued

Unit 4

The Child with Cerebral Palsy—cont'd

EXPECTED OUTCOME

Child is able to communicate needs to caregivers (specify desired communication and means of accomplishment)

NURSING DIAGNOSIS: Risk for altered nutrition: less than body requirements related to feeding and motor problems

---

■ **PATIENT GOAL 1:** Will receive optimum nutrition

NURSING INTERVENTIONS/*RATIONALES*

Provide extra calories *to meet energy demands of increased muscle activity*

Monitor weight gain *to evaluate adequacy of nutritional intake*

Provide vitamin, mineral, and/or protein supplements if eating habits are poor

Devise, with input from occupational/speech therapists, aids and techniques to facilitate feeding *so that child receives adequate nourishment*

EXPECTED OUTCOMES

Child eats a balanced diet

Weight remains within acceptable limits (specify)

NURSING DIAGNOSIS: Fatigue related to increased energy expenditure

---

■ **PATIENT GOAL 1:** Will receive optimum rest

NURSING INTERVENTIONS/*RATIONALES*

Maintain a well-regulated schedule that allows for adequate rest and sleep periods *to prevent fatigue*

Be alert for evidence of fatigue, which tends to aggravate symptoms

EXPECTED OUTCOME

Child is sufficiently rested

■ **PATIENT GOAL 2:** Will maintain good general health

NURSING INTERVENTIONS/*RATIONALES*

Ensure regular routine health maintenance *to promote general health:*

Physical assessment

Dental care

Immunizations

EXPECTED OUTCOMES

Child receives regular health assessments (specify schedule)

Child receives appropriate immunizations (specify) and dental care (specify)

NURSING DIAGNOSIS: Body image disturbance related to perception of disability

---

■ **PATIENT GOAL 1:** Will demonstrate positive body image

NURSING INTERVENTIONS/*RATIONALES*

Demonstrate acceptance of child through own behavior *because children are sensitive to affective attitude of the professional*

Capitalize on child's assets and provide compensation for liabilities *to encourage positive self-image*

Praise child for accomplishments and "near" accomplishments, such as partial completion of a task

Plan, *with* the child, activities and goals that provide opportunities for success *to encourage cooperation and positive self-image*

Encourage grooming and age-appropriate dress *to promote acceptance by others and positive body image*

(See also Nursing Diagnosis: Body image disturbance, in Nursing Care Plan: The Child with Chronic Illness or Disability, p. 294)

EXPECTED OUTCOME

Child exhibits behaviors that indicate positive body image (specify)

NURSING DIAGNOSIS: Risk for altered family processes related to a child with a lifelong disability

---

■ **PATIENT (FAMILY) GOAL 1:** Will receive adequate support

NURSING INTERVENTIONS/*RATIONALES*

(See Nursing diagnosis: Risk for altered family processes, in Nursing Care Plan: The Child with Chronic Illness or Disability, p. 287.)

Refer to special support group(s) and agencies *for ongoing support*

EXPECTED OUTCOMES

Family needs for support are met

(See also:

Nursing Care Plan: The Child with Chronic Illness or Disability, p. 287.)

Nursing Care Plan: The Child with Mental Retardation, p. 526.)

NURSING CARE PLAN

The Child Who Is Paralyzed

Paralysis is the loss or impairment of sensation and/or motor function, classified by cause, muscle tone, distribution, or parts of the body affected.
  Paraplegia—Paralysis in two extremities, usually the legs and lower part of the body
  Quadriplegia, or tetraplegia—Paralysis of four extremities

Hemiplegia—Paralysis of one side of the body
Flaccid paralysis—Paralysis with loss of muscle tone
Spastic paralysis—Paralysis with involuntary contraction of one or more muscles with associated loss of muscular function

ASSESSMENT

(See Neurologic Assessment, p. 64.)
(See also Assessment of Reflexes, p. 21; and Boxes 4-26, 4-27.)
Observe for manifestations of paralysis:
  Loss of sensation and/or motor function in affected areas:
    Limpness
    Loss of pinprick sensation in tested area
    Loss of position or vibration sense in tested area

Loss of reflexes
Constipation
Loss of anal sphincter control
Change in urinary patterns; enuresis
Assist with diagnostic procedures and tests (e.g., perform or assist with extensive neurologic examination that includes determining level of injury, residual sensory or motor function (if any), and autonomic function).

NURSING DIAGNOSIS: Impaired physical mobility related to nerve damage

(See Nursing Care Plan: The Child Who Is Immobilized, p. 503.)

NURSING DIAGNOSIS: Risk for injury related to paralysis, immobility

■ **PATIENT GOAL 1:** Will experience no physical injury

NURSING INTERVENTIONS/*RATIONALES*

Implement and maintain safety devices according to degree of dysfunction (specify) *to prevent injuries*
Employ correct techniques for moving, transporting, and otherwise manipulating paralyzed body part(s)
Implement appropriate safety measures to prevent thermal injuries *since there is loss of sensation in affected areas*

EXPECTED OUTCOME

Child remains free of physical injury

■ **PATIENT GOAL 2:** Will not experience circulatory complications

NURSING INTERVENTIONS/*RATIONALES*

Monitor peripheral pulses, skin temperature, and capillary filling *to evaluate circulation*
Ensure frequent position changes *to optimize circulation to all tissues*
Wrap legs in elastic bandage or stockings *to decrease pooling of blood when in upright position*
Perform range-of-motion exercises *to increase venous return*
Encourage child to be as active as condition and restrictive devices allow

EXPECTED OUTCOME

Peripheral circulation remains good as evidenced by color, capillary filling, and skin temperature

■ **PATIENT GOAL 3:** Will not experience loss of function of unaffected body parts

NURSING INTERVENTIONS/*RATIONALES*

Assist child and family to identify child's abilities *so that child does not lose function unnecessarily*
Encourage self-care activities within limitations of paralysis
Employ use of play and diversional activities *to encourage child to use unaffected body parts*

EXPECTED OUTCOME

Child uses unaffected body parts

■ **PATIENT GOAL 4:** Will maintain limb flexibility and range of motion without contractures

NURSING INTERVENTIONS/*RATIONALES*

Position *to maintain correct body alignment and reduce contractures*
Perform range-of-motion, active, passive, and stretching exercises *to maintain limb flexibility*
Employ joint splints and braces as indicated *to prevent contractures*
Carry out exercises with care *to avoid fracturing fragile bones*
Maintain hips in slight to moderate abduction *to prevent dislocation*

EXPECTED OUTCOMES

Joints remain flexible
Child exhibits no evidence of contractures

Unit 4

Continued

- **PATIENT GOAL 5:** Will not exhibit signs of bone demineralization

NURSING INTERVENTIONS/*RATIONALES*

Handle extremities carefully when turning and positioning *to prevent fractures*

Promote adequate fluid intake *to ensure adequate urinary output and to decrease risk of renal calculi*

Use upright posture on tilt table daily *to prevent bone demineralization*

Monitor serum calcium *for early detection of electrolyte imbalance*

*Administer ascorbic acid (1 to 4 g daily) and encourage drinking of cranberry juice *to acidify urine, decreasing likelihood of stone formation*

*Administer calcium-mobilizing drugs, if prescribed

EXPECTED OUTCOMES

Child develops no fractures

Serum calcium remains within normal limits

Lower extremities maintain flexibility

NURSING DIAGNOSIS: Risk for impaired skin integrity related to immobility

(See Nursing Care Plan: The Child Who Is Immobilized, p. 503.)

NURSING DIAGNOSIS: Risk for infection related to neuromuscular impairment, immobility

- **PATIENT GOAL 1:** Will exhibit no evidence of upper respiratory tract infection

NURSING INTERVENTIONS/*RATIONALES*

Maintain interventions that facilitate respiratory efforts

Place child in high Fowler position *to promote chest expansion and diaphragm excursion*

Ensure good body alignment when in sitting or standing position *for maximum chest expansion*

Avoid restriction of chest or abdominal musculature

Change position frequently *to facilitate drainage of secretions*

Perform chest physiotherapy as indicated *to facilitate drainage of secretions*

Encourage coughing and deep breathing

Use good handwashing technique *to prevent infection*

Keep all equipment in contact with child clean or sterile

Provide good oral hygiene *to decrease presence of infective organisms*

Keep persons with upper respiratory infections away from child

Monitor breath sounds *to assess for adequate ventilation in all lobes*

Monitor respirations and observe for signs of acute respiratory distress

EXPECTED OUTCOMES

Lungs remain clear

Respirations remain within normal limits (specify)

- **PATIENT GOAL 2:** Will exhibit no signs of urinary tract infection

NURSING INTERVENTIONS/*RATIONALES*

Implement bladder training in appropriate children *to promote normal bladder function as much as possible*

Teach self-catheterization to appropriate children (paraplegia)

Catheterize periodically to evaluate for retention (See Bladder catheterization, p. 235.)

*Administer ascorbic acid (1 to 4 g daily) and encourage drinking cranberry juice *to acidify urine for inhibition of bacterial growth*

Monitor urine cultures *for early detection of infection*

*Administer antispasmodics as prescribed for some children *to relax bladder musculature and promote more adequate emptying*

*Administer urinary antibiotics as prescribed *to either prevent or treat urinary tract infections*

EXPECTED OUTCOMES

Child does not develop urinary tract infection

Child voids regularly with complete emptying

NURSING DIAGNOSIS: Constipation related to neuromuscular impairment

- **PATIENT GOAL 1:** Will experience adequate bowel elimination

NURSING INTERVENTIONS/*RATIONALES*

Modify diet as appropriate *to prevent constipation:*

High-fiber diet (See Box 4-22 on p. 405.)

Adequate fluid intake

Provide individualized bowel training *to control defecation until an appropriate time and place are found*

*Administer stool softeners as prescribed

*Administer laxative and/or suppository as prescribed *for bowel evacuation*

EXPECTED OUTCOME

Child evacuates bowel daily

NURSING DIAGNOSIS: Sexual dysfunction related to inability to feel sexual stimuli, inability to attain and/or maintain an erection

- **PATIENT GOAL 1:** Will experience age-appropriate sexual gratification

NURSING INTERVENTIONS/*RATIONALES*

Teach alternative methods for sexual gratification

Refer to qualified sex therapist *for long-term sexual adjustment*

EXPECTED OUTCOME

Patient achieves some type of sexual gratification

NURSING DIAGNOSIS: Altered family processes related to a child with a physical disability

- **PATIENT (FAMILY) GOAL 1:** Will receive adequate support

**NURSING INTERVENTIONS/*RATIONALES*
AND EXPECTED OUTCOMES**

(See the following:

Nursing Care Plan: The Child with Chronic Illness or Disability, p. 287.)

Nursing Care Plan: The Child in the Hospital, p. 268.)

Nursing Care Plan: The Family of the Child Who Is Ill or Hospitalized, p. 282.)

Nursing Care Plan: The Child Who Is Immobilized, p. 503.)

*Dependent nursing action.

QUADRIPLEGIA

Special needs

> **NURSING DIAGNOSIS:** Ineffective breathing pattern related to diaphragmatic paralysis

■ **PATIENT GOAL 1:** Will exhibit signs of adequate respiratory function

NURSING INTERVENTIONS/*RATIONALES*

Monitor ventilatory device
Have resuscitation equipment at bedside *to use in case of malfunction of ventilator*
If the patient has a tracheostomy, change and maintain as needed *to maintain patent airway*
Monitor respiratory functions, including breath sounds, *to evaluate adequacy of ventilation*
(See Nursing Care Plan: The Child at Risk for Infection, p. 341.)

EXPECTED OUTCOMES

Lungs are well aerated
Child breathes for short periods without mechanical ventilation

> **NURSING DIAGNOSIS:** Ineffective thermoregulation related to absence of sweating, dilated blood vessels

■ **PATIENT GOAL 1:** Will maintain optimum body temperature

NURSING INTERVENTIONS/*RATIONALES*

Regulate environmental temperature *to maintain optimum body temperature*
Add or remove clothing and blankets according to body temperature

EXPECTED OUTCOME

Child maintains optimum body temperature (See inside front cover.)

> **NURSING DIAGNOSIS:** Risk for dysreflexia related to autonomic nerve dysfunction

■ **PATIENT GOAL 1:** Will not exhibit signs of autonomic dysreflexia

NURSING INTERVENTIONS/*RATIONALES*

Recognize autonomic dysreflexia (manifested by flushed face, sweating of forehead, pupillary constriction, marked hypertension, headache, bradycardia) *to ensure prompt, appropriate intervention to prevent encephalopathy and shock*
Rule out other causes (e.g., orthostatic hypertension)
Identify precipitating factor (e.g, constipation, full bladder)
Correct cause (e.g., empty bladder or bowel)
*Administer antihypertensives and/or antispasmodics as prescribed *to alleviate autonomic dysreflexia*

EXPECTED OUTCOME

Symptoms of autonomic dysreflexia are promptly identified and relieved

*Dependent nursing action.

BOX 4-26

Differences in Clinical Manifestations Between Upper and Lower Motor-Neuron Syndromes

Upper Motor Neuron Syndrome	Lower Motor Neuron Syndrome
Spastic paralysis in muscle groups below lesion (reflex arcs below lesion are intact)	Flaccid paralysis caused by muscle atonia (reflex arcs are permanently damaged)
Hyperreflexia with tendon reflexes exaggerated, Babinski reflex present	Reflex with associated muscle response absent
No wasting of muscle mass because of increased muscle tone	Marked atrophy of atonic muscle
Flexion contractures and spasms of muscle groups below lesion level common	Fasciculations (local twitching of muscle groups) common
No skin or tissue changes	No flexor spasms
	Loss of hair
	Skin and tissue changes
	Cornified nails

BOX 4-27

Significant Effects of Autonomic Disruption

Decreased muscle tone and impairment of vasoconstrictive effects of sympathetic innervation cause venous pooling, diminished venous return to the heart, decreased cardiac output, and hypotension, especially orthostatic hypotension.

Thermoregulatory disruption in the hypothalamus and skin receptors causes blood vessels to remain dilated during the initial stage, an inabiliy to sweat in response to increased environmental temperature, and possible rapid elevation in body temperature.

Voluntary bowel and bladder function is lost because of damage to nerve fibers that innervate these organs.

Altered sexual function (lack of erection, ejaculation, and orgasm) results from interference with numerous autonomic nerve fibers and plexuses.

NURSING CARE OF THE CHILD WITH METABOLIC DYSFUNCTION

NURSING CARE PLAN

The Child with Diabetes Mellitus

Diabetes mellitus (DM) is a disorder involving primarily carbohydrate metabolism and characterized by a deficiency (relative or absolute) of the hormone insulin.

DM can be classified into the following three major groups:

Insulin-dependent diabetes mellitus (IDDM), or type 1—Characterized by catabolism and the development of ketosis in the absence of insulin replacement therapy; onset is typically in childhood and adolescence, but can be at any age

Non–insulin-dependent diabetes mellitus (NIDDM), or type 2—Appears to involve resistance to insulin action and defective glucose-mediated insulin secretion; onset is usually after age 40, and there appears to be considerable heterogeneity; affected persons may or may not require daily insulin injections

Maturity-onset diabetes of youth (MODY)—Transmitted as an autosomal-dominant disorder in which there is formation of structurally abnormal insulin that has decreased biologic activity

ASSESSMENT

Perform a physical assessment.

Obtain a family history, especially regarding other members who have diabetes.

Obtain a health history, especially relative to weight loss, frequency of drinking and voiding, increased appetite, diminished activity level, behavior changes, and other manifestations of type 1 diabetes mellitus as follows:

The three polys (cardinal signs of diabetes):
Polyphagia
Polyuria
Polydipsia
Weight loss
Child may start bed-wetting
Irritability and "not himself" or "herself"
Shortened attention span
Temper tantrums in young children
Appears overly tired
Dry skin

Blurred vision
Poor wound healing
Flushed skin
Headache
Frequent infections, including perineal yeast infections and/or thrush
Hyperglycemia:
Elevated blood glucose levels
Glucosuria
Diabetic ketosis:
Ketones as well as glucose in urine
No noticeable dehydration
Diabetic ketoacidosis:
Dehydration
Electrolyte imbalance
Acidosis
Perform or assist with diagnostic procedures and tests (e.g., fasting blood sugar, serum insulin levels, urine for ketones, blood glucose, and serum islet cell antibody level).

HOSPITAL CARE

NURSING DIAGNOSIS: Risk for injury related to insulin deficiency

■ **PATIENT GOAL 1:** Will exhibit normal blood glucose levels

NURSING INTERVENTIONS/RATIONALES

Obtain blood glucose level *to determine most appropriate dose of insulin*

*Administer insulin as prescribed *to maintain normal blood glucose level*

Understand the action of insulin

Understand the differences in composition, time of onset, and duration of action for the various insulin preparations *to ensure accurate insulin administration*

Employ proper insulin techniques when preparing and administering insulin

Subcutaneous injection: use the appropriate size of syringe and needle length (considering thickness of subcutaneous tissue)

Rotate sites *to enhance absorption of insulin* and prevent lipohypertrophy

EXPECTED OUTCOME

Child demonstrates normal blood glucose levels

NURSING DIAGNOSIS: Risk for injury related to hypoglycemia

■ **PATIENT GOAL 1:** Will exhibit no evidence of hypoglycemia

NURSING INTERVENTIONS/RATIONALES

Recognize signs of hypoglycemia early

Be particularly alert at times when blood glucose levels are lowest (e.g., at 11:00 AM and 2:30 AM; after bursts of physical activity without additional food; or after a delayed, omitted, or incompletely consumed meal or snack) and based on estimated peak time of insulin given

Obtain blood glucose level

Offer 10 to 15 g of readily absorbed carbohydrates (simple sugars), such as orange juice, hard candy, or milk, *to elevate blood glucose level and alleviate symptoms of hypoglycemia*

Follow with complex carbohydrate and protein, such as bread or cracker spread with peanut butter or cheese, if more than an hour from regular meal or snack time, *to maintain blood glucose level*

*Administer glucagon to chlid who is unconscious, having seizures, or unable to swallow *to elevate blood glucose level;* position child *to minimize risk of aspiration, since vomiting may occur*

EXPECTED OUTCOMES

Child ingests an appropriate carbohydrate
Child exhibits no evidence of hypoglycemia

Unit 4

*Dependent nursing action.

The Child with Diabetes Mellitus—cont'd

PREPARATION FOR HOME CARE

> **NURSING DIAGNOSIS:** Knowledge deficit (diabetes management) related to care of a child with newly diagnosed diabetes mellitus

■ **PATIENT (FAMILY) GOAL 1:** Will understand teaching provided of basic survival skills

NURSING INTERVENTIONS/*RATIONALES*

Assess current ability to learn

Select methods, vocabulary, and content appropriate to the level of the learner *to maximize learning*

Allow 3 or 4 days for family and child to begin to adjust to the initial impact of the diagnosis

Select an environment conducive to learning

Allow ample time for the education process

Restrict length of teaching sessions *because this is how people learn best:*

Child, 15 to 20 minutes

Parents, 45 to 60 minutes

Involve all senses and employ a variety of teaching strategies, especially participation, *because it is usually the most effective method for learning*

Provide pamphlets or other supplementary materials *for future referral*

EXPECTED OUTCOME

Child and/or family understand basic survival skills

■ **PATIENT (FAMILY) GOAL 2:** Will demonstrate understanding of the disorder and its therapy

NURSING INTERVENTIONS/*RATIONALES*

Provide information regarding the pathophysiology of diabetes and the function and actions of insulin and glucagon in relation to caloric intake and exercise

Answer questions and clarify misconceptions *to ensure optimum learning*

Explain function and expected effects of procedures and tests *since these are a necessary part of diabetes management*

EXPECTED OUTCOME

Child and/or family demonstrate an understanding of the disease and its therapy (specify indicators)

■ **PATIENT (FAMILY) GOAL 3:** Will demonstrate understanding of meal plan and food selection

NURSING INTERVENTIONS/*RATIONALES*

Consult a dietitian *to develop and teach meal plan*

Emphasize the relationship between normal nutritional needs and the disease *to encourage a sense of normalcy*

Become familiar with family's cultural beliefs and food preferences *so that these are included in meal planning*

Teach or reinforce learners' understanding of the basic food groups and the diet plan prescribed (e.g., carbohydrate counting)

Help child and family estimate food weights by volume *since this is more practical than weighing food*

Suggest low-carbohydrate snack items

Guide family in assessment of food labels for carbohydrate content to incorporate into meal plan *since concentrated sugars are avoided in the diet*

Teach or reinforce an understanding of the concept of exchanges *since exchanges ensure day-to-day consistency in total intake while allowing a choice of foods*

Relate constant carbohydrate equivalents to familiar foods

Incorporate cultural patterns and family preferences as much as possible *so that child and family are more likely to adhere to diet requirements*

EXPECTED OUTCOME

Child and/or family demonstrate an understanding of diet planning and food selection (specify indicators)

■ **PATIENT (FAMILY) GOAL 4:** Will demonstrate knowledge of and ability to administer insulin

NURSING INTERVENTIONS/*RATIONALES*

Teach child and family the characteristics of the insulins prescribed for child *since there are several insulin preparations*

Teach proper mixing of insulins

Teach subcutaneous injection procedure:

Impress on learners that the procedure will be a routine part of child's life *in order to decrease anxiety and increase cooperation*

Involve caregivers and child, if old enough, *so that more than one person learns procedure*

Teach basic techniques using a rolled towel or teaching doll *so that learner can gain confidence before injecting a person*

Use demonstration and return demonstration techniques on one another before injecting child *because this is usually less stressful*

Help families and child develop a rotational pattern *because this is important for maximum absorption of insulin*

Teach proper care of insulin, supplies, and equipment including proper disposal of syringes and lancets

Teach management of continuous infusion pump (if applicable)

EXPECTED OUTCOMES

Child and/or family demonstrate an understanding of insulin, its various forms, and action (specify indicators)

Child and/or family demonstrate correct injection technique

Child and/or family develop a rotation plan

Child and/or family demonstrate correct use of infusion pump and care of injection site

■ **PATIENT (FAMILY) GOAL 5:** Will demonstrate ability to test blood glucose level

NURSING INTERVENTIONS/*RATIONALES*

Teach family (and child, if old enough):

Blood glucose monitoring and/or use of equipment selected for use

Interpretation of results *so that they learn how to adjust insulin based on blood glucose level*

Care and maintenance of equipment

EXPECTED OUTCOME

Child and/or family demonstrate correct use of the home blood glucose monitoring equipment

Unit 4

Continued

The Child with Diabetes Mellitus—cont'd

■ **PATIENT (FAMILY) GOAL 6:** Will demonstrate ability to test urine for ketones

NURSING INTERVENTIONS/*RATIONALES*

Teach family (and child, if old enough):
    Urine ketone testing and interpretation of results
    Proper care of test strips

EXPECTED OUTCOME

Child and/or family demonstrate urine/ketone testing and interpretation

■ **PATIENT (FAMILY) GOAL 7:** Will demonstrate understanding of importance of proper hygiene

NURSING INTERVENTIONS/*RATIONALES*

Emphasize the importance of personal hygiene *so that child establishes health practices that last a lifetime*
Encourage regular dental care and yearly ophthalmologic examinations *since these are important for child's general health*
Teach proper care of cuts and scratches *to minimize risk of infection*
Teach proper foot care because this must always be considered a high priority

EXPECTED OUTCOME

Child and family demonstrate understanding of importance of proper hygiene

■ **PATIENT (FAMILY) GOAL 8:** Will demonstrate understanding of importance of exercise regimen

NURSING INTERVENTIONS/*RATIONALES*

Work with child, family, and others (e.g., exercise physiologist, physical therapist, or coaches) to help plan a home exercise program *since this is an important part of diabetic management*
Reiterate practitioner's instructions regarding adjustment of food and/or insulin to meet child's activity pattern; reinforce with examples *so that child and family are adequately prepared*

EXPECTED OUTCOME

Child and family help child outline and carry out a regular exercise program

■ **PATIENT (FAMILY) GOAL 9:** Will demonstrate understanding and management of hyperglycemia and hypoglycemia

NURSING INTERVENTIONS/*RATIONALES*

Instruct learners in how to recognize signs of hyperglycemia and hypoglycemia (especially hypoglycemia) *to prevent delay in treatment* (Table 4-33)
Explain the relationship of insulin needs to illness, activity, and intense emotion (either positive or negative)
Teach how to adjust food, activity, and insulin at times of illness and during other situations that alter blood glucose levels
Suggest carrying source of carbohydrate, such as sugar cubes, glucose tablets or gel, or hard candy in pocket or handbag *so that it is readily available to treat hypoglycemia*

Instruct parents and child in how to treat hypoglycemia with food, simple sugars, or glucagon

EXPECTED OUTCOMES

Child and family demonstrate an understanding of the signs and symptoms of hyperglycemia and hypoglycemia
Child and family demonstrate an understanding of treatment of hypoglycemia

■ **PATIENT GOAL 10:** Will wear medical identification

NURSING INTERVENTIONS/*RATIONALES*

Encourage acquisition of emergency medical identification, such as an identification bracelet, *that explains child's condition in case of emergency*
Explain to child why identification is important *so that child is more likely to comply*

EXPECTED OUTCOME

Family acquires and child wears emergency medical identification

■ **PATIENT (FAMILY) GOAL 11:** Will keep proper records of insulin administration and testing procedures

NURSING INTERVENTIONS/*RATIONALES*

Help child and family to design a form for keeping records of the following *because this information is useful to both practitioner and family in managing diabetes:*
    Insulin administered
    Blood and urine tests
    Food intake
    Marked variations in exercise
    Illness

EXPECTED OUTCOME

Family and child keep accurate record of insulin administration, blood glucose levels, and urine for ketones

■ **PATIENT (FAMILY) GOAL 12:** Will engage in self-management

NURSING INTERVENTIONS/*RATIONALES*

Encourage honesty in recording, such as food intake not on prescribed meal plan, *so that record is accurate and useful*
Encourage independence in applying the concepts learned in teaching sessions *since diabetes management is a lifelong endeavor*
Instruct when to seek assistance from medical personnel *to prevent delay in treatment*

EXPECTED OUTCOME

Child takes responsibility for management of disorder commensurate with age and developmental level

> **NURSING DIAGNOSIS:** Altered family processes related to situational crisis (child with a chronic disorder)

(See Nursing Care Plan: The Child with Chronic Illness or Disability, p. 287.)

The Child with Diabetes Mellitus—cont'd

TABLE 4-33   Comparison of Manifestations of Hypoglycemia and Hyperglycemia

Variable	Hypoglycemia	Hyperglycemia
Onset	Rapid (minutes)	Gradual (days)
Mood	Labile, irritable, nervous, crying, combative	Lethargic
Mental status	Difficulty concentrating, speaking, focusing, coordinating	Dulled sensorium
		Confused
Inward feeling	Shaky feeling, hunger	Thirst
	Headache	Weakness
	Dizziness	Nausea/vomiting
		Abdominal pain
Skin	Pallor	Flushed
	Sweating	Signs of dehydration
Mucous membranes	Normal	Dry, crusty
Respirations	Shallow	Deep, rapid (Kussmaul)
Pulse	Tachycardia	Less rapid, weak
Breath odor	Normal	Fruity, acetone
Neurologic	Headache	Diminished reflexes
	Tremors	
	Late: hyperreflexia, dilated pupils, seizure	Paresthesia
Ominous signs	Shock, coma	Acidosis, coma
Blood:		
Glucose	Low: below 60 mg/dl	High: 240 mg/dl or more
Ketones	Negative/trace	High/large
Osmolarity	Normal	High
pH	Normal	Low (7.25 or less)
Hematocrit	Normal	High
HCO_3	Normal	Less than 15 mEq/L
Urine:		
Output	Normal	Polyuria (early) to oliguria (late)
Glucose	Negative	High
Acetone	Negative/trace	High

Unit 4

NURSING CARE OF THE CHILD WITH CANCER

NURSING CARE PLAN

The Child with Cancer

Cancer is a neoplasm characterized by the uncontrolled growth of anaplastic cells that invade adjacent tissues and tend to metastasize to distant sites within the body.

ASSESSMENT

Perform a physical assessment.

Obtain a health history with special attention to vague complaints (e.g., fatigue, pain in a limb, night sweating, lack of appetite, headache, and general malaise); any evidence of a lingering disorder; and parental concerns.

Assist with diagnostic procedures and tests (e.g., blood and urine examination, radiology, lumbar puncture, imaging techniques, biopsy, and bone marrow aspiration).

Assess family's coping capabilities and support system(s).

(See also nursing care plans for specific cancers.)

NURSING DIAGNOSIS: Risk for injury related to malignant process, treatment

■ **PATIENT GOAL 1:** Will experience partial or complete remission from disease

NURSING INTERVENTIONS/RATIONALES

*Administer chemotherapeutic agents as prescribed

Assist with radiation therapy as ordered

Assist with procedures for administration of chemotherapeutic agents (e.g., lumbar puncture for intrathecal administration)

†Prepare child and family for surgical procedure if appropriate

EXPECTED OUTCOME

Child achieves a partial or complete remission from disease

■ **PATIENT GOAL 2:** Will have minimal complications of chemotherapy

NURSING INTERVENTIONS/RATIONALES

Follow guidelines for administration of chemotherapeutic agents (Table 4-34)

Observe for signs of infiltration at intravenous site: pain, stinging, swelling, redness

Stop infusion immediately if any sign of infiltration occurs *to prevent severe tissue damage*

Implement policies of institution *to treat infiltration*

Obtain careful history for known allergies *to prevent anaphylaxis*

Observe child for 1 hour after infusion for signs of anaphylaxis (cyanosis, hypotension, wheezing, or severe urticaria)

Stop infusion of drug and flush intravenous line with normal saline if reaction is suspected

Have emergency equipment (especially blood pressure monitor and manual resuscitation bag and mask) and emergency drugs (especially oxygen, epinephrine, antihistamine, aminophylline, corticosteroids, and vasopressors) readily available *to prevent delay in treatment*

EXPECTED OUTCOMES

Child will have minimal complications of chemotherapy

Child will receive prompt, appropriate treatment of complications

---

NURSING DIAGNOSIS: Risk for infection related to depressed body defenses

■ **PATIENT GOAL 1:** Will experience minimized risk of infection

NURSING INTERVENTIONS/RATIONALES

Place child in private room when possible *to minimize exposure to infective organisms*

Advise all visitors and staff to use good handwashing technique *to minimize exposure to infective organisms*

Screen all visitors and staff for signs of infection *to minimize exposure to infective organisms*

Use scrupulous aseptic technique for all invasive procedures

Monitor temperature *to detect possible infection*

Evaluate child for any potential sites of infection (e.g., needle punctures, mucosal ulceration, minor abrasions, dental problems)

Provide nutritionally complete diet for age *to support body's natural defenses* (Community Focus box)

Avoid giving live attenuated virus vaccines (e.g., measles, varicella, mumps, rubella, and oral poliovirus) to child with depressed immune system *because these vaccines can result in overwhelming infection*

*Give inactivated virus vaccines (e.g., polio, influenza) as prescribed and indicated *to prevent specific infections*

*Administer antibiotics as prescribed

*Administer granulocyte colony–stimulating factor (GCSF) as prescribed

EXPECTED OUTCOMES

Child does not come in contact with infected persons or contaminated articles

Child consumes diet appropriate for age (specify)

Child does not exhibit signs of infection

NURSING DIAGNOSIS: Risk for injury (hemorrhage) related to interference with platelet production

■ **PATIENT GOAL 1:** Will exhibit no evidence of bleeding

NURSING INTERVENTIONS/RATIONALES

Use all measures to prevent infection, especially in ecchymotic areas, *because infection increases tendency toward bleeding*

Use local measures (e.g, apply pressure) to stop bleeding

Restrict strenuous activity *that could result in accidental injury*

Involve child in responsibility for limiting activity when platelet count drops *to encourage compliance*

Avoid skin punctures when possible *to prevent bleeding*

Observe for bleeding after procedures such as venipuncture and bone marrow aspiration

Nursing Care Plan text continued on p. 492.

*Dependent nursing action.

†Indicates content that is specific to a particular malignancy.

Unit 4

COMMUNITY FOCUS

Health Promotion for Children with Cancer

Important considerations for health care providers caring for the child in the community include:

Immunizations—Children on immunosuppressive therapy should receive no live virus vaccinations. Household contacts should receive inactivated polio virus.

Nutrition—Assessment of nutritional status should be ongoing.

Vision, hearing, and dental screening—These screenings should be continued throughout treatment.

School—Children should continue in school during therapy.

Discipline—Parents should be encouraged to maintain discipline.

TABLE 4-34   Summary of Chemotherapeutic Agents Used in the Treatment of Childhood Cancers*

Agent/Administration	Side Effects and Toxicity	Comments and Specific Nursing Considerations
ALKYLATING AGENTS		
Mechlorethamine (Nitrogen mustard, Mustargen) IV	N/V† (½-8 hours later) (severe) BMD‡ (2-3 weeks later) Alopecia Local phlebitis	Vesicant§ May cause phlebitis and discoloration of vein
Cyclophosphamide (Cytoxan, CTX Neosar) PO, IV, IM	N/V (3-4 hours later) (severe at high doses) BMD (10-14 days later) Alopecia Hemorrhagic cystitis Severe immunosuppression Stomatitis (rare) Hyperpigmentation Transverse ridging of nails Infertility	BMD has platelet-sparing effect Give dose early in day to allow adequate fluids afterward Force fluids before administering drug and for 2 days after to prevent chemical cystitis; encourage frequent voiding, even during night Mesna is given to reduce hemorrhagic cystitis Warn parents to report signs of burning on urination or hematuria to practitioner
Ifosfamide (Ifos, IFF) IV	Hemorrhagic cystitis BMD (10-14 days later) Alopecia Neurotoxicity—lethargy, disorientation, somnolence, seizures (rare)	Mesna is given to reduce hemorrhagic cystitis Hydrate as with CTX Myelosuppression less severe than with CTX
Melphalan (L-phenylalanine mustard, Alkeran, L-Pam) PO, IV	N/V (severe) BMD (2-3 weeks later) Diarrhea Alopecia	Vesicant Give over 1 hour

Procarbazine (Matulane) PO	N/V (moderate)
	 BMD (3-4 weeks later)
	 Lethargy
	 Dermatitis
	 Myalgia
	 Arthralgia
	 Less commonly:
	   Stomatitis
	   Neuropathy
	   Alopecia
	   Diarrhea
	 Azoospermia
	 Cessation of menses
		Central nervous system depressants (phenothiazines, barbiturates) enhance central nervous system symptoms
		 Monoamine oxidase (MAO) inhibition sometimes occurs, causing increased norepinephrine; foods containing high levels of tyramine may elevate norepinephrine to toxic levels; foods to avoid are *overripe* or aged products (e.g., cheddar, mozzarella, and parmesan cheeses, avocados, bananas, and figs; broad beans, fava beans; red wines; and excessive amounts of yogurt, chocolate, and soy sauce‖; to avoid drug interactions, all other drugs are avoided unless medically approved

*Table includes principal drugs used in the treatment of childhood cancers. Several other conventional and investigational chemotherapeutic agents may be employed in the treatment regimen.

IT, Intrathecal; *IV,* intravenous; *PO,* by mouth; *IM,* intramuscular; *SC,* subcutaneous.

†*N/V,* Nausea and vomiting. Mild = <20% incidence; moderate = 20% to 70% incidence; severe = >75% incidence.

‡*BMD,* Bone marrow depression.

§Vesicants (sclerosing agents) can cause severe cellular damage if even minute amounts of the drug infiltrate surrounding tissue. Only nurses experienced with chemotherapeutic agents should administer vesicants. These drugs must be given through a free-flowing intravenous line. The infusion is stopped *immediately* if any sign of infiltration (pain, stinging, swelling, or redness at needle site) occurs. Interventions for extravasation vary, but each nurse should be aware of the institution's policies and implement them at once.

‖McKenry LM, Salerno E: *Mosby's pharmacology in nursing,* ed 18, St Louis, 1992, Mosby.

Continued

TABLE 4-34 Summary of Chemotherapeutic Agents Used in the Treatment of Childhood Cancers—cont'd

Agent/Administration	Side Effects and Toxicity	Comments and Specific Nursing Considerations
ALKYLATING AGENTS—cont'd		
Dacarbazine (DTIC-Dome) IV	N/V (especially after first dose) (severe) BMD (7-14 days later) Alopecia Flulike syndrome Burning sensation in vein during infusion (not extravasation)	Vesicant (less sclerosive) Must be given cautiously in patients with renal dysfunction Decrease IV rate or use cold pack along vein to decrease burning
Cisplatin (Platinol) IV	Renal toxicity (severe) N/V (1-4 hours later) (severe) BMD (mild, 2-3 weeks later) Ototoxicity Neurotoxicity (similar to that for vincristine) Electrolyte disturbances, especially hypomagnesium, hypocalcemia, hypokalemia, and hypophosphatemia Anaphylactic reactions may occur	Renal function (creatinine clearance) must be assessed before giving drug Must maintain hydration before and during therapy (specific gravity of urine is used to assess hydration) Mannitol may be given IV to promote osmotic diuresis and drug clearance Monitor intake and output Monitor for signs of ototoxicity (e.g., ringing in ears) and neurotoxicity; report signs immediately; ensure that routine audiogram is done before treatment for baseline and routinely during treatment Do not use aluminum needle; reaction with aluminum decreases potency of drug Monitor for signs of electrolyte loss (i.e., hypomagnesium—tremors, spasm, muscle weakness, lower extremity cramps, irregular heartbeat, convulsions, delirium) Have emergency drugs at bedside*
Carboplatin (CBDCA) IV	BMD (14 days later) N/V (mild) Mild hepatotoxicity Alopecia	Do not use saline dilution Less nephrotoxic and ototoxic than cisplatin
Chlorambucil (Leukeran) PO	N/V (mild) BMD (7-14 days later) Diarrhea Dermatitis Less commonly may be hepatotoxicity	Usually slow onset of side effects; side effects related to high doses
ANTIMETABOLITES		
Cytosine arabinoside (Ara-C, Cytosar, cytarabine, arabinosyl cytosine) IV, IM, SC, IT	Alopecia N/V (mild) BMD (7-14 days later) Mucosal ulceration Immunosuppression Hepatitis (usually subclinical)	Crosses blood-brain barrier Use with caution in patients with hepatic dysfunction Conjunctivitis with high doses
5-Azacytidine (5-AzaC) IV	N/V (moderate) BMD (7-14 days later) Diarrhea	Infuse slowly via IV drip to decrease severity of N/V
Mercaptopurine (6-MP, Purinethol) PO, IV	N/V (mild) Diarrhea Anorexia Stomatitis BMD (4-6 weeks later) Immunosuppression Dermatitis Less commonly may be hepatotoxic	6-MP is an analog of xanthine; therefore allopurinol (Zyloprim) delays its metabolism and increases its potency, necessitating a lower dose (⅓ to ¼) of 6-MP

*Emergency drugs include oxygen and parenteral preparations of epinephrine 1:1000, diphenhydramine or similar antihistamine, aminophylline, corticosteroids, and vasopressors.

Unit 4

The Child with Cancer—cont'd

TABLE 4-34   Summary of Chemotherapeutic Agents Used in the Treatment of Childhood Cancers—cont'd

Agent/Administration	Side Effects and Toxicity	Comments and Specific Nursing Considerations
ANTIMETABOLITES—cont'd		

Methotrexate (MTX, amethopterin) PO, IV, IM, IT May be given in conventional doses (mg/m²) or high doses (g/m²)	N/V (severe at high doses)
	 Diarrhea
	 Mucosal ulceration (2-5 days later)
	 BMD (10 days later)
	 Immunosuppression
	 Dermatitis
	 Photosensitivity
	 Alopecia (uncommon)
	 Toxic effects include:
	     Hepatitis (fibrosis)
	     Osteoporosis
	     Nephropathy
	     Pneumonitis (fibrosis)
	 Neurologic toxicity with IT use—pain at injection site, meningismus (signs of meningitis without actual inflammation), especially fever and headache; potential sequelae—transient or permanent hemiparesis, convulsions, dementia, death
		Side effects and toxicity are dose related
		 Potency and toxicity increased by reduced renal function, salicylates, sulfonamides, and aminobenzoic acid; avoid use of these substances, such as aspirin
		 Use sunscreen
		 High-dose therapy:
		     Citrovorum factor (folinic acid or leucovorin) decreases cytotoxic action of MTX; used as an antidote for overdose and to enhance normal cell recovery following high-dose therapy; avoid use of vitamins containing folic acid during MTX therapy unless prescribed by physician
		 IT therapy:
		     Drug *must* be mixed with preservative-free diluent
		     Report signs of neurotoxicity immediately

6-Thioguanine (6-TG, Thioguan) PO	N/V (mild)
	 BMD (7-14 days later)
	 Stomatitis
	 Rarely:
	     Dermatitis
	     Photosensitivity
	     Liver dysfunction
		Side effects are unusual

PLANT ALKALOIDS		
Vincristine (Oncovin) IV	Neurotoxicity—Paresthesia (numbness); ataxia; weakness; footdrop; hyporeflexia; constipation (adynamic ileus); hoarseness (vocal cord paralysis); abdominal, chest, and jaw pain; mental depression Fever N/V (mild) BMD (minimal; 7-14 days later) Alopecia SIADH	Vesicant Report signs of neurotoxicity because may necessitate cessation of drug Individuals with underlying neurologic problems may be more prone to neurotoxicity Monitor stool patterns closely; administer stool softener Excreted primarily by liver into biliary system; administer cautiously to anyone with biliary disease Maximum dose is 2 mg
Vinblastine (Velban) IV	Neurotoxicity (same as for vincristine but less severe) N/V (mild) BMD (especially neutropenia; 7-14 days later) Alopecia	Same as for vincristine

Continued

Unit 4

TABLE 4-34 Summary of Chemotherapeutic Agents Used in the Treatment of Childhood Cancers—cont'd

Agent/Administration	Side Effects and Toxicity	Comments and Specific Nursing Considerations
PLANT ALKALOIDS—cont'd		
VP-16 (etoposide, VePesid) IV	N/V (mild to moderate) BMD (7-14 days later) Alopecia Hypotension with rapid infusion Bradycardia Diarrhea (infrequent) Stomatitis (rare) May reactivate erythema of irradiated skin (rare) Allergic reaction with anaphylaxis possible Neurotoxicity	Give slowly via IV drip with child recumbent Have emergency drugs available at bedside*
VM-26 (teniposide) IV	Same as for VP-16	Same as for VP-16
ANTIBIOTICS		
Actinomycin-D (dactinomycin, Cosmegen, ACT-D) IV	N/V (2-5 hours later) (moderate) BMD (especially platelets; 7-14 days later) Immunosuppression Mucosal ulceration Abdominal cramps Diarrhea Anorexia (may last a few weeks) Alopecia Acne Erythema or hyperpigmentation of previously irradiated skin Fever Malaise	Vesicant Enhances cytotoxic effects of radiation therapy but increases toxic effect May cause serious desquamation of irradiated tissue

Doxorubicin (Adriamycin) IV	N/V (moderate)
	 Stomatitis
	 BMD (7-14 days later)
	 Fever, chills
	 Local phlebitis
	 Alopecia
	 Cumulative-dose toxicity includes:
	   Cardiac abnormalities
	   ECG changes
	   Heart failure
		Vesicant (extravasation may *not* cause pain)
		 Observe for any changes in heart rate or rhythm and signs of failure
		 Cumulative dose must not exceed 550 mg/m^2, less with radiation
		 Warn parents that drug causes urine to turn red (for up to 12 days after administration); this is normal, not hematuria

Daunorubicin (Daunomycin, Rubidomycin) IV	Similar to doxorubicin	Similar to doxorubicin

Bleomycin (Blenoxane) IV, IM, SC	Allergic reactions—Fever, chills, hypotension, anaphylaxis
	 Fever (nonallergic)
	 N/V (mild)
	 Stomatitis
	 Cumulative dose effects include:
	   Skin—Rash, hyperpigmentation, thickening, ulceration, peeling, nail changes, alopecia
	   Lungs—Pneumonitis with infiltrate that can progress to fatal fibrosis
		Should give test dose (SC) before therapeutic dose administered
		 Have emergency drugs* at bedside
		 Hypersensitivity occurs with first one to two doses
		 May give acetaminophen before drug to reduce likelihood of fever
		 Concentration of drug in skin and lungs accounts for toxic effects
		 Follow pulmonary function tests

*Emergency drugs include oxygen and parenteral preparations of epinephrine 1:1000, diphenhydramine or similar antihistamine, aminophylline, corticosteroids, and vasopressors.

Unit 4

TABLE 4-34   Summary of Chemotherapeutic Agents Used in the Treatment of Childhood Cancers—cont'd

Agent/Administration	Side Effects and Toxicity	Comments and Specific Nursing Considerations
HORMONES		
Corticosteroids (prednisone most frequently used; many proprietary names, such as Meticorten, Deltasone, Paracort) PO; also IM or IV but rarely used	For short-term use, no acute toxicity Usual side effects are mild; moon face, fluid retention, weight gain, mood changes, increased appetite, gastric irritation, insomnia, susceptibility to infection Hyperglycemia	Explain expected effects, especially in terms of body image, increased appetite, and personality changes Monitor weight gain Recommend moderate salt restriction Administer with antacid and early in morning (sometimes given every other day to minimize side effects) May need to disguise bitter taste (crush tablet and mix with syrup, jam, ice cream, or other highly flavored substance; use ice to numb tongue before administration; place tablet in gelatin capsule if child can swallow it) Observe for potential infection sites; usual inflammatory response and fever are absent
	Long-term effects of chronic steroid administration are mood changes, hirsutism, trunk obesity (buffalo hump), thin extremities, muscle wasting and weakness, osteoporosis, poor wound healing, bruising, potassium loss, gastric bleeding, hypertension, diabetes mellitus, growth retardation	Same as for short-term use; in addition, encourage foods high in potassium (bananas, raisins, prunes, coffee, chocolate) Test stools for occult blood Monitor blood pressure Test blood for sugar and urine for acetone Observe for signs of abrupt steroid withdrawal; flulike symptoms, hypotension, hypoglycemia, shock
ENZYMES		
L-Asparaginase (Elspar) **Erwinia L-Asparaginase** **PEG L-Asparaginase** **IV, IM**	Allergic reactions (including anaphylactic shock) Fever N/V (mild) Anorexia Weight loss Arthralgia Toxicity: Liver dysfunction Hyperglycemia Renal failure Pancreatitis	Have emergency drugs at bedside* Record signs of allergic reaction, such as urticaria, facial edema, hypotension, or abdominal cramps Check weight daily Normally, blood urea nitrogen (BUN) and ammonia levels rise as a result of drug; not evidence of liver damage Check urine for sugar and blood amylase
NITROSOUREAS		
Carmustine (BCNU) IV **Lomustine (CCNU) PO**	N/V (2-6 hours later) (severe) BMD (3-4 weeks later) Burning pain along IV infusion (usually due to alcohol diluent) BCNU—Flushing and facial burning on infusion Alopecia	Prevent extravasation; contact with skin causes brown spots Oral form—give 4 hours after meals when stomach is empty Reduce IV burning by diluting drug and infusing slowing via IV drip Crosses blood-brain barrier
OTHER AGENTS		
Hydroxyurea (Hydrea) PO	N/V (mild) Anorexia Less commonly: Diarrhea BMD Mucosal ulceration Alopecia Dermatitis	Must be given cautiously in patients with renal dysfunction

*Emergency drugs include oxygen and parenteral preparations of epinephrine 1:1000, diphenhydramine or similar antihistamine, aminophylline, corticosteroids, and vasopressors.

Continued

Unit 4

The Child with Cancer—cont'd

Text continued from p. 486.

Turn frequently and use pressure-reducing or pressure-relieving mattress *to prevent decubitus ulcers*

Teach parents and older child measures to control nosebleeding

Prevent oral and rectal ulceration *because ulcerated skin is prone to bleeding*

Avoid aspirin-containing medications *because aspirin interferes with platelet function*

*Administer platelets as prescribed *to raise platelet count*

EXPECTED OUTCOME

Child exhibits no evidence of bleeding

NURSING DIAGNOSIS: Risk for hemorrhagic cystitis due to bladder irritation related to administration of chemotherapeutic agents

■ **PATIENT GOAL 1:** Will exhibit no evidence of hemorrhagic cystitis

NURSING INTERVENTIONS/RATIONALES

Observe for signs of cystitis (e.g., burning and pain on urination, blood in urine)

Report signs of cystitis to practitioner *since prompt medical evaluation is needed*

Give liberal (3000 ml/m²/day) fluid intake

*Administer mesna as prescribed *to reduce hemorrhagic cystitis*

Encourage frequent voiding, including during nighttime, *to minimize metabolites' contact with bladder mucosa*

Administer drugs irritating to bladder early in the day *to allow for sufficient fluid intake and voiding*

EXPECTED OUTCOMES

Child voids without discomfort

No hematuria is present

NURSING DIAGNOSIS: Risk of anemia related to chemotherapy and radiation therapy

■ **PATIENT GOAL 2:** Will experience minimal effects of anemia

NURSING INTERVENTIONS/RATIONALES AND EXPECTED OUTCOMES

(See Nursing Care Plan: The Child with Anemia, p. 444.)

NURSING DIAGNOSIS: Risk for fluid volume deficit related to nausea and vomiting

■ **PATIENT GOAL 1:** Will experience minimal nausea or vomiting

NURSING INTERVENTIONS/RATIONALES

*Administer initial dose of antiemetic before chemotherapy begins *to prevent child from ever experiencing nausea and vomiting, thus preventing an anticipatory response*

*Administer antiemetic around the clock for as long as nausea and vomiting typically last *to prevent any episodes from occurring*

Assess child's response to antiemetic *since no antiemetic drug is uniformly successful*

Avoid foods with strong odors *that may induce nausea and vomiting*

Uncover hospital food tray outside of child's room *to reduce food odors that may induce nausea*

Encourage frequent intake of fluids in small amounts *since small portions are usually better tolerated*

*Administer intravenous fluid, as prescribed, *to maintain hydration*

EXPECTED OUTCOME

Child retains food and fluid

Child does not experience nausea or vomiting

NURSING DIAGNOSIS: Altered oral mucous membrane related to administration of chemotherapeutic agents

■ **PATIENT GOAL 1:** Will not develop or will have minimal oral mucositis

NURSING INTERVENTIONS/RATIONALES

Inspect mouth daily for oral ulcers; report evidence of ulcers to practitioner *for early treatment*

Avoid oral temperatures *to prevent trauma*

Institute meticulous oral hygiene as soon as a drug is used that causes oral ulcers:

    Use soft-sponge toothbrush, cotton-tipped applicator, or gauze-wrapped finger *to avoid trauma*

    Administer frequent (at least every 4 hours and after meals) mouthrinses (normal saline with or without sodium bicarbonate solution) *to promote healing*

Apply local anesthetics to ulcerated areas before meals and as needed *to relieve pain*

    Avoid using viscous lidocaine for young children *because if applied to pharynx, it may depress gag reflex, increasing risk of aspiration, and may also cause seizures*

Apply lip balm *to keep lips moist and prevent cracking or fissuring*

Serve bland, moist, soft diet; offer food best tolerated by child

Encourage fluids; use a straw *to help bypass painful areas*

Encourage parents to relax any eating pressures *since stomatitis is a temporary condition*

Avoid juices containing ascorbic acid and hot or cold or spicy foods if they cause further discomfort

Avoid using lemon glycerin swabs (*irritate eroded tissue and can decay teeth*), hydrogen peroxide (*delays healing by breaking down protein*), and milk of magnesia (*dries mucosa*)

Explain to parents that child may require hospitalization for hydration, parenteral nutrition, and pain control (often with intravenous morphine) *if stomatitis interferes with food and fluid intake*

*Administer antiinfective medication as ordered *to prevent or treat mucositis*

*Administer analgesics, including opioids, *to control pain*

EXPECTED OUTCOMES

Mucous membranes remain intact

Ulcers show evidence of healing

Child reports and/or exhibits no evidence of discomfort

*Dependent nursing action.

The Child with Cancer—cont'd

■ **PATIENT GOAL 2:** Will not develop rectal ulceration

NURSING INTERVENTIONS/*RATIONALES*

Wash perianal area after each bowel movement *to lessen irritation*

Use warm sitz baths or tub baths *to promote healing*

Expose reddened but not ulcerated areas to air *to keep skin dry*

Apply protective skin barriers (transparent film dressings, occlusive ointment) to perineal area *to protect skin from direct contact with urine or feces and to promote healing*

Observe for constipation *because it may result from child's voluntary refusal to defecate or from chemotherapy or opioids*

Record bowel movements; use stool softener *to prevent constipation;* may need stimulants *for evacuation*

Avoid rectal temperatures and suppositories *to prevent rectal trauma*

EXPECTED OUTCOMES

Rectal mucosa remains clean and intact

Ulcerated areas heal without complications

Child has regular bowel movements

NURSING DIAGNOSIS: Altered nutrition: less than body requirements related to loss of appetite

---

■ **PATIENT GOAL 1:** Will receive adequate nutrition

NURSING INTERVENTIONS/*RATIONALES*

Encourage parents to relax pressures placed on eating; explain that loss of appetite *is a direct consequence of nausea and vomiting, and chemotherapy*

Allow child *any* food tolerated; plan to improve quality of food selections when appetite increases

Explain expected increase in appetite from steroids *to prepare child and parents for this change*

Take advantage of any hungry period: serve small "snacks" *since small portions are usually better tolerated*

Fortify foods with nutritious supplements, such as powdered milk or commercial supplements, *to maximize quality of intake*

Allow child to be involved in food preparation and selection *to encourage eating*

Make food appealing

Remember usual food practices of children in each age-group, such as food jags in toddlers or normal occurrence of physiologic anorexia, *to distinguish these expected changes from actual refusal to eat*

Assess family for additional problems (e.g., use of food by child as a control mechanism) if appetite does not improve despite improved physical status *to identify areas that require intervention*

EXPECTED OUTCOMES

Nutritional intake is adequate

Child maintains adequate weight

NURSING DIAGNOSIS: Impaired skin integrity related to administration of chemotherapeutic agents, radiation therapy, immobility

---

■ **PATIENT GOAL 1:** Will maintain skin integrity

NURSING INTERVENTIONS/*RATIONALES*

Provide meticulous skin care, especially in mouth and perianal regions *because these areas are prone to ulceration*

Change position frequently *to stimulate circulation and relieve pressure*

Encourage adequate caloric-protein intake *to prevent negative nitrogen balance*

EXPECTED OUTCOME

Skin remains clean and intact

■ **PATIENT GOAL 2:** Will experience minimal negative effects of therapy

NURSING INTERVENTIONS/*RATIONALES*

Select loose-fitting clothing over irradiated area *to minimize additional irritation*

Protect area from sunlight and sudden changes in temperature (avoid ice packs, heating pads) during radiotherapy or administration of methotrexate

EXPECTED OUTCOME

Child and family comply with suggestions (specify)

NURSING DIAGNOSIS: Impaired mobility related to neuromuscular impairment (neuropathy), GI immobility

---

■ **PATIENT GOAL 1:** Will experience minimal negative effects of neurotoxic chemotherapeutic drugs (e.g., Vincristine, Vinblastine)

NURSING INTERVENTIONS/*RATIONALES*

Encourage ambulation when child is able

Alter activity, including school attendance, *to prevent injuries if weakness occurs*

Use footboard or high-top shoes *to prevent footdrop*

Provide fluids and soft foods *to lessen chewing movements with jaw pain*

Evaluate bowel movements *to rule out constipation*

*Administer stool softeners as prescribed

EXPECTED OUTCOMES

Child ambulates without incident or difficulty

Child has no constipation

NURSING DIAGNOSIS: Body image disturbance related to loss of hair, moon face, debilitation

---

■ **PATIENT (FAMILY) GOAL 1:** Will exhibit positive coping behaviors

NURSING INTERVENTIONS/*RATIONALES*

Introduce idea of wig before hair loss

Encourage child to select a wig similar to child's own hairstyle and color before hair falls out *to foster later adjustment to hair loss*

Provide adequate covering during exposure to sunlight, wind, or cold *since natural protection is lost*

Suggest keeping thin hair clean, short, and fluffy *to camouflage partial baldness*

Unit 4

Explain that hair begins to regrow in 3 to 6 months and may be a slightly different color or texture *to prepare child and family for changes in appearance of new hair*

Explain that alopecia may be less severe during a second treatment with same drug

Encourage good hygiene, grooming, and sex-appropriate items (e.g., wig, scarves, hats, makeup, attractive sex-appropriate clothing) *to enhance appearance*

EXPECTED OUTCOMES

Child verbalizes concern regarding hair loss

Child helps determine methods to reduce effects of hair loss and applies these methods

Child appears clean, well-groomed, and attractively dressed

■ **PATIENT GOAL 2:** Will exhibit adjustment to altered facial appearance

NURSING INTERVENTIONS/*RATIONALES*

Encourage rapid reintegration with peers *to lessen contrast of changed facial appearance*

Stress that this reaction is temporary *to provide reassurance that usual appearance will return*

Evaluate weight gain carefully *(because with weight gain resulting from administration of steroids, extremities remain thin)*

Encourage visits from friends before discharge *to prepare child for reactions and questions*

EXPECTED OUTCOMES

Family demonstrates understanding of consequences of therapies

Child resumes former activities and relationships within capabilities

■ **PATIENT GOAL 3:** Will express feelings

NURSING INTERVENTIONS/*RATIONALES*

Provide opportunities for child to discuss feelings and concerns

Provide materials for nonverbal expression (e.g., play, art)

EXPECTED OUTCOME

Child expresses feelings regarding altered body in words, play, art (specify)

NURSING DIAGNOSIS: Pain related to diagnosis, treatment, physiologic effects of neoplasia

■ **PATIENT GOAL 1:** Will experience either no pain or a reduction of pain to level acceptable to child

NURSING INTERVENTIONS/*RATIONALES*

Whenever possible, make use of procedures (e.g., noninvasive temperature monitoring, venous access device) to minimize discomfort

Assess need for pain management

Evaluate effectiveness of pain relief with degree of alertness vs sedation *to determine need for change in dosage, in time of administration, or in drug*

Implement appropriate nonpharmacologic pain reduction techniques as adjunct to analgesics (See p. 339.)

*Administer analgesics as prescribed

Avoid aspirin or any of its compounds (e.g., other nonsteroidal antiinflammatory agents) *because aspirin increases bleeding tendency*

*Administer drugs on preventive schedule (around the clock) *to prevent pain from recurring*

Monitor effectiveness of therapy on pain assessment record

EXPECTED OUTCOME

Child rests quietly, reports and/or exhibits no evidence of discomfort, verbalizes no complaints of discomfort

---

NURSING DIAGNOSIS: Fear related to diagnostic tests, procedures, treatments

■ **PATIENT GOAL 1:** Will exhibit reduced fear related to diagnostic procedures and tests

NURSING INTERVENTIONS/*RATIONALES*

Explain procedure carefully at child's level of understanding *to reduce fear of the unknown*

Explain what will take place and what child will feel, see, and hear *to increase sense of control*

Use recall of each step *as method of distraction*

Explain special requests of child (e.g., need to remain motionless during test and/or radiation therapy) *to encourage cooperation*

Provide child with some means for involvement with procedure (e.g., holding a piece of equipment, such as bandage or tape, counting with the operator, answering questions) *to promote sense of control, encourage cooperation, and support child's coping skills*

Implement distracting techniques and pain reduction techniques as indicated

(See also Guidelines box: Selecting Nonthreatening Words or Phrases on p. 221.)

EXPECTED OUTCOMES

Child readily responds to verbal directives

Child repeats information accurately

Child discusses fears without evidence of stress

NURSING DIAGNOSIS: Fear related to diagnosis, prognosis

(See Nursing Care Plan: The Child Who is Terminally Ill or Dying, p. 296.)

NURSING DIAGNOSIS: Diversional activity deficit related to restricted environment (private room)

■ **PATIENT GOAL 1:** Will have opportunity to participate in diversional activities

NURSING INTERVENTIONS/*RATIONALES*

Provide age-appropriate toys that can be properly cleaned *to provide diversion without risk of infection*

Involve child-life specialist or other supportive services in planning diversional activities

EXPECTED OUTCOMES

Child engages in activities appropriate for age and interests

Suitable toys are provided

NURSING DIAGNOSIS: Altered family processes related to having a child with a life-threatening disease

- **PATIENT (FAMILY) GOAL 1:** Will demonstrate knowledge about diagnostic/therapeutic procedures

NURSING INTERVENTIONS/*RATIONALES*

Explain reason for each test and procedure

Explain reason for radiation therapy, chemotherapy

Explain operative procedure honestly (if appropriate)

Avoid overemphasis on benefits, which may not be immediately evident (applies primarily to brain tumors) *to avoid unrealistic expectations*

(See also Guidelines for Preparing Children for Procedures, p. 219.)

EXPECTED OUTCOME

Child and family demonstrate understanding of procedures (specify learning and manner of demonstration)

- **PATIENT (FAMILY) GOAL 2:** Will receive adequate support

NURSING INTERVENTIONS/*RATIONALES*

Teach parents about disease process

Explain all procedures that will be done to child

Schedule time for family to be together, without interruptions from staff, *to encourage communication and expression of feelings*

Help family plan for future, especially for helping child live a normal life, *to promote child's optimum development*

Encourage family to discuss feelings regarding child's course before diagnosis and child's prognosis

Discuss with family how they will tell child about outcome of treatment and need for additional treatment (if appropriate) *to maintain open and honest communication*

Refer to local chapter of American Cancer Society or other organizations

EXPECTED OUTCOMES

Family demonstrates knowledge of child's disease and treatments (specify methods of learning and evaluation)

Family expresses feelings and concerns and spends time with child

(See also:

Nursing Care Plan: The Child in the Hospital, p. 268.)

Nursing Care Plan: The Family of the Child Who Is Ill or Hospitalized, p. 282.)

NURSING DIAGNOSIS: Altered family processes relatd to a child undergoing therapy

- **PATIENT (FAMILY) GOAL 1:** Will demonstrate understanding of side effects and/or complications of treatment

NURSING INTERVENTIONS/*RATIONALES*

Advise family of expected side effects vs toxicities; clarify which side effects demand medical evaluation (e.g., mucosal ulceration, hemorrhagic cystitis, peripheral neuropathy, evidence of infection or dehydration) (Table 4-35) *to prevent delay in treatment*

Reassure family that such reactions are not caused by return of cancer cells *to minimize undue concern*

Interpret prognostic statistics carefully, realizing family's temporary need to interpret them as they see necessary, *to present a realistic, but hopeful, future*

Prepare family for expected mood changes from steroids

Interpret mood changes based on drugs or reactions to disease/treatment *to prevent any unwarranted negative reaction to child (e.g., punishment)*

EXPECTED OUTCOMES

Family demonstrates knowledge of instructions (specify method of learning and evaluation)

Family demonstrates understanding of behavior changes

- **PATIENT GOAL 2:** Will receive adequate support during treatment

NURSING INTERVENTIONS/*RATIONALES*

Explain reason for antibiotics and/or transfusions

Observe for signs of transfusion reaction (See Table 4-31, p. 445.)

Record appropriate time for hemostasis to occur after administration of platelets *to determine if transfusions are becoming less effective*

EXPECTED OUTCOME

Child demonstrates understanding of procedures and tests (specify method and learnings)

- **PATIENT (FAMILY) GOAL 3:** Will be prepared for home care

NURSING INTERVENTIONS/*RATIONALES*

Teach preventive measures at discharge (e.g., handwashing and isolation from crowds) *to prevent infection*

Stress importance of isolating child from any known cases of chickenpox or other childhood diseases; work with school nurse and physician to determine optimum time for reattendance *to prevent unnecessary absences or risk of infection*

Teach home care instructions specific to child's needs

EXPECTED OUTCOME

Family demonstrates ability to provide home care for child (specify)

NURSING DIAGNOSIS: Anticipatory grieving related to perceived potential loss of a child

- **PATIENT (FAMILY) GOAL 1:** Will acknowledge and cope with possibility of child's death

NURSING INTERVENTIONS/*RATIONALES*

Provide consistent contact with family *to establish a trusting relationship that encourages communication*

Clarify, refocus, and supply information as needed

Help family plan care of child, especially at terminal stage (e.g., extent of extraordinary lifesaving measures), *to ensure their wishes are implemented*

Provide or arrange for hospice care if family desires it

Arrange for spiritual support in accordance with family's beliefs and/or affiliations

EXPECTED OUTCOMES

Family remains open to counseling and nursing contact

Family and child discuss their fears, concerns, needs, and desires at terminal stage

Family investigates hospice care

Appropriate religious representative is contacted (specify)

- **PATIENT (FAMILY) GOAL 2:** Will receive adequate support

NURSING INTERVENTIONS/*RATIONALES* AND EXPECTED OUTCOMES

(See Nursing Care Plan: The Child Who is Terminally Ill or Dying, p. 296.)

---

*Dependent nursing action.

Continued

The Child with Cancer—cont'd

TABLE 4-35 Early Side Effects of Radiation Therapy

Site/Effects	Nursing Interventions	Site/Effects	Nursing Interventions
Gastrointestinal Tract		**Head**	
Nausea/vomiting	Give antiemetic around the clock	Nausea/vomiting (from stimulation of vomiting center in brain)	Same as for gastrointestinal tract
	Measure amount of emesis to assess for dehydration	Alopecia	Same as for skin
Anorexia	Encourage fluids and foods best tolerated, usually light, soft diet and small, frequent meals	Mucositis	Encourage regular dental care, fluoride treatments
	Monitor weight loss	Potential effects	May need analgesics to relieve discomfort

Mucosal ulceration	Use frequent mouthwashes and oral hygiene to prevent mucositis	Parotitis
		  Sore throat
		  Loss of taste	

Diarrhea	Can be controlled with antispasmodics and kaolin pectin preparations	Xerostomia (dry mouth)	Combat severe dryness of mouth with oral hygiene and liquid diet
	Observe for signs of dehydration	**Urinary Bladder**	
Skin		Rarely cystitis	More likely to occur with concomitant use of cyclophosphamide
Alopecia (within 2 weeks; begins to regrow by 3-6 months)	Introduce idea of wig		Encourage liberal fluid intake and frequent voiding
	Stress necessity of scalp hygiene and need for head covering in cold weather		Evaluate for hematuria
Dry or moist desquamation	Do not refer to skin change as a "burn" (implies use of too much radiation)	**Bone Marrow**	
	Keep skin clean	Myelosuppression	Observe for fever (temperature above 38.3° C [101° F])
	Wash daily, using mild soap (e.g., Tone, Dove) sparingly		Initiate workup for sepsis as ordered
	Do not remove skin marking for radiation fields		Administer antibiotics as prescribed
	Avoid exposure to sun		Avoid use of suppositories, rectal temperatures
	For dryness, apply lubricant		Institute bleeding precautions
	For desquamation, consult practitioner for skin hygiene and care		Observe for signs of anemia

NURSING CARE PLAN

The Child with a Brain Tumor

A **brain tumor** is a neoplasm originating from nerve cells, neuroepithelium, glial cells, cranial nerves, blood vessels, pineal gland, or hypophysis.

ASSESSMENT
Perform a physical assessment.
Perform a neurologic assessment.
Observe for signs of increased intracranial pressure (ICP).
Observe for manifestations of brain tumors (Table 4-36).
Assess child's physical capabilities.

Assess mental functioning by asking simple questions (e.g., name, age, residence).
Assist with diagnostic procedures and tests (e.g., tomography, magnetic resonance imaging, angiography, electroencephalography, lumbar puncture, and biopsy).

PREOPERATIVE CARE

(See Nursing Care Plan: The Child Undergoing Surgery, preoperative care, p. 304.)

NURSING DIAGNOSIS: Risk for injury related to altered neurologic functioning

■ **PATIENT GOAL 1:** Will not experience injury

NURSING INTERVENTIONS/RATIONALES
Maintain seizure precautions (See Nursing Care Plan: The Child with Epilepsy, p. 474.)
Keep siderails up on bed *to prevent falls*
Assist with ambulation and activities of daily living as appropriate *to prevent injury*

EXPECTED OUTCOME
Child remains free of injury

NURSING DIAGNOSIS: Pain related to increased intracranial pressure (ICP)

■ **PATIENT GOAL 1:** Will experience either no pain or a reduction of pain to level acceptable to child

NURSING INTERVENTIONS/RATIONALES
Provide pain relief with environmental manipulation (e.g., dimly lit room, no noise, sudden movement)
*Administer analgesics as prescribed; observe for side effects *that may mask level of consciousness and/or depress respiratory center*
(See also Nursing Care Plan: The Child in Pain, p. 315.)

EXPECTED OUTCOME
Child exhibits evidence of no or minimal discomfort

■ **PATIENT GOAL 2:** Will maintain stable ICP

NURSING INTERVENTIONS/RATIONALES
Prevent constipation *to avoid straining, which can increase ICP*
*Administer stool softeners as prescribed
Encourage older child to not cough or sneeze
(See also Patient Goal: Will maintain stable ICP, in Nursing Care Plan: The Unconscious Child, p. 463.)

EXPECTED OUTCOMES
ICP remains within safe limits
Child exhibits no evidence of increased ICP

NURSING DIAGNOSIS: Sensory/perceptual alterations (visual, auditory, kinesthetic, gustatory, tactile, olfactory) related to interference with reception, transmission, and/or integration of sensory input

■ **PATIENT GOAL 1:** Will exhibit signs of adjustment to sensory/perceptual deficits

NURSING INTERVENTIONS/RATIONALES
(See Nursing Care Plan: The Child with Impaired Vision, p. 519.)
(See also Nursing Care Plan: The Child with Impaired Hearing, p. 522.)
Provide attractively served meals to stimulate appetite
Offer favorite foods and fluids
(See also Nursing Care Plan: The Child with Special Nutritional Needs, p. 313.)
Assist child to orient to time and space, especially when ambulating, *to prevent injury*
Keep daily records of signs and symptoms *to assess child's physical capabilities and to assist family in adjusting to insidious or acute deterioration*

EXPECTED OUTCOME
Child adjusts to sensory/perceptual deficits

NURSING DIAGNOSIS: Risk for injury related to surgical procedure

■ **PATIENT GOAL 1:** Will receive proper preparation

NURSING INTERVENTIONS/RATIONALES
Prepare child and family for head shaving (may be done in OR after anesthesia)
If done in room or while awake:
    Provide absolute privacy *to protect child from teasing or ridicule by other children*
    Allow child to look into mirror at different stages *to lessen shock of total baldness, unless this increases anxiety*
    Emphasize that hair will regrow shortly after surgery
    Introduce idea of wearing a wig, especially if irradiation or chemotherapy is anticipated

*Dependent nursing action.

Continued

Unit 4

The Child with a Brain Tumor—cont'd

TABLE 4-36   Clinical Manifestations and Assessment of Brain Tumors

Signs and Symptoms	Assessment
Headache	
Recurrent and progressive	Record description of pain, location, severity, and duration
In frontal or occipital areas	Use pain rating scale to assess severity of pain (See p. 316.)
Usually dull and throbbing	Note changes in relation to time of day and activity
Worse on arising, less during day	Observe changes in behavior in infants (persistent irritability,
Intensified by lowering head and straining, such as during bowel movement, coughing, sneezing	crying, head rolling)
Vomiting	
With or without nausea or feeding	Record time, amount, and relationship to feeding, nausea,
Progressively more projectile	and activity
More severe in morning	
Relieved by moving about and changing position	
Neuromuscular Changes	
Incoordination or clumsiness	Test muscle strength, gait, coordination, and reflexes (See
Loss of balance (use of wide-based stance, falling, tripping, banging into objects)	Physical Assessment, p. 64.)
Poor fine motor control	
Weakness	
Hyporeflexia or hyperreflexia	
Positive Babinski sign	
Spasticity	
Paralysis	
Behavioral Changes	
Irritability	Observe behavior regularly
Decreased appetite	Compare observations with parental reports of normal
Failure to thrive	behavioral patterns
Fatigue (frequent naps)	Monitor growth and food intake
Lethargy	Monitor activity and sleep
Coma	
Bizarre behavior (staring, automatic movements)	
Cranial Nerve Neuropathy	
Cranial nerve involvement varies according to tumor location	Assess cranial nerves, especially VII (facial), IX (glossopha-
Most common signs	ryngeal), X (vagus), V (trigeminal, sensory roots), and VI
Head tilt	(abducens) (See Physical Assessment, p. 68.)
Visual defects (nystagmus, diplopia, strabismus, episodic "graying out" of vision, visual field defects)	Assess visual acuity, binocularity, and peripheral vision
Vital Sign Disturbances	
Decreased pulse and respiration	Measure vital signs frequently
Increased blood pressure	Monitor pulse and respirations for 1 full minute
Decreased pulse pressure	Record pulse pressure (difference between systolic and dia-
Hypothermia or hyperthermia	stolic blood pressure)
Other Signs	
Seizures	Record seizure activity (See p. 474.)
Cranial enlargement*	Measure head circumference daily (infant and young child)
Tense, bulging fontanel at rest*	Perform funduscopic examination (if skilled in procedure)
Nuchal rigidity	
Papilledema (edema of optic nerve)	

*Present only in infants and young children.

Unit 4

The Child with a Brain Tumor—cont'd

Provide an attractive covering (lacy nightcap or baseball cap)

Save long hair by brading it first

Shave head carefully *to avoid skin cuts, which can become infected*

Cleanse scalp as prescribed

Prepare child and parents for the large dressing; may help to show a picture or wrap gauze around a doll's head

EXPECTED OUTCOME

Head is shaved with a minimum of distress to child and family

---

NURSING DIAGNOSIS: Altered family processes related to having a child with a serious illness

---

■ **PATIENT (FAMILY) GOAL 1:** Will be prepared for diagnostic/operative procedures

NURSING INTERVENTIONS/*RATIONALES*

Explain reason for each test and radiation therapy

Explain responsibility of the child (e.g., need to remain motionless during test and/or radiation therapy) *to encourage cooperation*

Explain operative procedure honestly:

Avoid overpreparation, *which can increase fear*

Avoid overemphasis on positive benefits, which may not be evident for several days postoperatively or which may not occur

Arrange for child and parents to visit special intensive care unit where the child will be postoperatively

Explain to child common experiences after surgery (e.g., may be very sleepy, have a headache, and must remain quiet)

Explain to family what to expect postoperatively (e.g., child may be comatose) *to decrease anxiety*

Participate in preoperative conferences with family and physician *to give more explanations or support when needed*

(See also Preparation for Procedures, p. 219.)

(See also Nursing Care Plan: The Child with Cancer, p. 486.)

EXPECTED OUTCOMES

Family demonstrates an understanding of tests and procedures (specify learning and manner of demonstration)

Child and family visit the ICU

Child and family demonstrate an understanding of information presented (specify information and manner of demonstration)

POSTOPERATIVE CARE

(See:

Nursing Care Plan: The Child Undergoing Surgery, Postoperative Care, p. 305.)

Nursing Care Plan: The Unconscious Child, p. 462.)

NURSING DIAGNOSIS: Risk for injury related to intracranial trauma

---

■ **PATIENT GOAL 1:** Will experience minimal stress on operative site

NURSING INTERVENTIONS/*RATIONALES*

Consult with surgeon regarding positioning, including degree of neck flexion, which may differ from the following:

Infratentorial—Position child flat and on either side, not on back; neck is usually slightly extended *to prevent strain on sutures*

Supratentorial—Elevate head, usually above level of heart, *to facilitate drainage of cerebrospinal fluid and prevent hemorrhage;* do not lower head unless ordered by practitioner

Post sign above bed noting exact position of head *to ensure correct positioning*

Turn child cautiously *to maintain proper position*

Avoid Trendelenburg position *because it increases ICP and risk of hemorrhage,* for impending shock notify practitioner before lowering head

EXPECTED OUTCOMES

Minimal stress is applied to operative site

Child remains in desired position

NURSING DIAGNOSIS: Risk for injury related to surgical procedure

---

■ **PATIENT GOAL 1:** Will experience no complications; will receive appropriate therapy if complications occur

NURSING INTERVENTIONS/*RATIONALES*

Maintain integrity of dressings:

Observe dressings for drainage:

Reinforce with sterile gauze pads but do not remove bandage

Circle area of drainage as often as every hour *to identify continuous bleeding*

Report evidence of colorless drainage immediately *since it most likely is cerebrospinal fluid*

Restrain child's hands as necessary *to preserve intact dressing,* especially if child is disoriented or restless

Monitor temperature closely *because hyperthermia may result from brain surgery or anesthesia, and hypothermia may result when cooling measures are used*

Place hypothermia blanket on bed before child's return to room

View any temperature elevation, especially 1 to 2 days postoperatively, as potential sign of infection

Assess ocular signs at least hourly:

Report immediately sluggish, dilated, or unequal pupils *because they may indicate increased ICP and potential brainstem herniation*

If vomiting occurs, stop oral fluids *because vomiting may result in aspiration, increased ICP, and incisional rupture*

Calculate and monitor all fluids very carefully *to prevent overload, cerebral edema, and increased ICP*

Provide eye care, especially if child is unconscious or experiencing facial edema:

Apply ice compresses to eyes for short intervals *to relieve edema*

Keep eyes closed or apply eye dressings

May need to instill normal saline eye drops *to prevent corneal ulceration if blink reflex is depressed*

Suction oral secretions, if needed, using correct technique *since brain edema may depress gag reflex*

Give foods and fluids cautiously *to prevent aspiration:*

Monitor for presence of gag and swallowing reflexes and any sign of facial paralysis

EXPECTED OUTCOMES

Child exhibits no evidence of complications

Child will receive prompt, appropriate treatment for complications

Unit 4

The Child with a Brain Tumor—cont'd

NURSING DIAGNOSIS: Pain related to surgical procedure, cerebral edema

---

■ **PATIENT GOAL 1:** Will experience either no pain or a reduction of pain to level acceptable to child

NURSING INTERVENTIONS/*RATIONALES*

(See Nursing Care Plan: The Child in Pain, p. 315.)

Provide pain relief with environmental manipulation (e.g., quiet, dimly lit room; keep visitors to a minimum)

Prevent any sudden jarring movement, such as banging into bed, *which may increase headache*

Prevent increased ICP (See preoperative care, p. 497.) *since this causes increased pain*

Apply ice bag to forehead, *especially if facial edema is severe, to provide headache relief*

*Administer analgesics as prescribed *to relieve pain*

EXPECTED OUTCOME

Child will exhibit signs of either no pain or a reduction of pain to level acceptable to child

---

NURSING DIAGNOSIS: Altered family processes related to a child with critical surgery for a life-threatening disease

---

■ **PATIENT (FAMILY) GOAL 1:** Will receive adequate support

NURSING INTERVENTIONS/*RATIONALES*

Help family plan for the future, especially for helping child live a normal life

Encourage family to discuss feelings regarding child's course before diagnosis and prospects for survival

Discuss with family how they will tell the child about the outcome of surgery and need for additional treatment

Help family plan a realistic activity schedule:

Resumption of school attendance

Limited or modified physical activity (e.g., may have to wear a helmet) *to protect the skull until it is completely healed*

Encourage child to pursue academic goals

Help child prepare for questions from peers regarding "brain surgery," hair loss, or any residual neurologic deficit

Provide continuing support for family through comprehensive oncology clinic and/or community nursing service

EXPECTED OUTCOMES

Family discusses feelings and concerns

Family devises a realistic activity schedule

Child and family employ safety devices (specify)

Child attends school with reasonable regularity (specify)

Family receives continuing support (specify type and amount)

(See also:

Nursing Care Plan: The Child in the Hospital, p. 268.)

Nursing Care Plan: The Family of the Child Who Is Ill or Hospitalized, p. 282.)

Nursing Care Plan: The Child with Chronic Illness or Disability, p. 287.)

Nursing care plan for specific disability resulting from therapy.)

---

*Dependent nursing action.

NURSING CARE PLAN

The Child with a Bone Tumor

Osteosarcoma (osteogenic sarcoma)—Tumor arising from bone-forming mesenchyme

Ewing sarcoma—Primitive neuroectodermal tumor of the bone

ASSESSMENT

Perform a physical assessment.
Observe for manifestations of bone tumors:
Pain localized at affected site:
May be severe or dull
Often relieved by position of flexion
Frequently brought to attention when child does the following:
Limps
Curtails own physical activity
Is unable to hold heavy objects

Examine affected area for functional status, signs of inflammation, size of mass, regional lymph node involvement, and any evidence of systemic involvement (See Assessment: The Child with Cancer, p. 490.)
Obtain a health history, especially regarding pain (clues to duration and rate of tumor growth).
Assist with diagnostic procedures and tests (e.g., radiography, tomography, radioisotope bone scan, needle or surgical bone biopsy, lung tomography, other tests for differential diagnosis, and bone marrow aspiration [Ewing sarcoma]).

OSTEOSARCOMA

PREOPERATIVE CARE

(See Nursing Care Plan: The Child Undergoing Surgery, Preoperative Care, p. 304.)

NURSING DIAGNOSIS: Anticipatory grieving related to prospect of loss of limb

■ **PATIENT (FAMILY) GOAL 1:** Will be prepared for possible amputation or limb salvage procedure

NURSING INTERVENTIONS/*RATIONALES*

Employ straightforward approach *to gain trust and cooperation of child*
Avoid disguising diagnosis with terms such as "infection"
Discuss lack of alternatives for treatment *to encourage acceptance of surgery*
Answer questions regarding information presented by surgeon and clarify any misconceptions
Avoid overwhelming child or parents with too much information
Be available and willing to listen and to talk to child and parents about their concerns
Allow for and encourage expression of feelings *to facilitate grieving process*

EXPECTED OUTCOMES

Family and child express feelings regarding the potential loss
Family and child readily discuss concerns and ask appropriate questions

■ **PATIENT GOAL 2:** Will exhibit signs of adjustment to impending loss

NURSING INTERVENTIONS/*RATIONALES*

Allow child time and opportunity to go through grief process, *since this is part of adjustment*
Introduce, but do not elaborate on, information regarding need for chemotherapy
Reserve extensive discussion of chemotherapy and rehabilitation until after surgery *to avoid overwhelming child*

Allow for expression of feelings regarding the loss and the undesirable effects of chemotherapy
Recognize anger as a common reaction, *since child's behavior may be misinterpreted*
Assist child to cope with side effects
Encourage independence *to prepare for postoperative period when independence may be more difficult*

EXPECTED OUTCOME

Child expresses feelings about impending change in lifestyle

POSTOPERATIVE CARE

(See Nursing Care Plan: The Child Undergoing Surgery, p. 305.)

NURSING DIAGNOSIS: Impaired physical mobility related to amputation

■ **PATIENT GOAL 1:** Will not experience complications of amputation

NURSING INTERVENTIONS/*RATIONALES*

*Administer stump care as prescribed *to prevent infection and facilitate healing*
Maintain special bandaging, if employed, *to aid in shaping stump for prosthesis and to decrease stump edema and bleeding*
*Elevate stump during first 24 hours, if prescribed, *to reduce edema;* avoid prolonged elevation *because this can lead to contractures in proximal joint*
Maintain proper body alignment *to decrease risk of contractures*
Perform range-of-motion exercises of joints above amputation *to maintain flexibility*
Encourage child in activities such as play *that provide exercise*

EXPECTED OUTCOME

Child will not experience complications of amputation

■ **PATIENT GOAL 2:** Will adjust to loss of limb and regain mobility

NURSING INTERVENTIONS/*RATIONALES*

Assist with early ambulation

Continued

The Child with a Bone Tumor—cont'd

Assist with use of temporary prosthesis
*Arrange for physical therapy as prescribed
Arrange for preparation of permanent prosthesis
Teach use of auxiliary appliances such as wheelchair or crutches
Encourage self-care within limitations *to promote adjustment and normalization*

EXPECTED OUTCOMES
Child adjusts to loss of limb
Child regains mobility

NURSING DIAGNOSIS: Body image disturbance related to loss of limb

■ **PATIENT GOAL 1:** Will exhibit positive coping behaviors

NURSING INTERVENTIONS/*RATIONALES*
Encourage visits from friends before discharge *to prepare child for reactions and questions*
Encourage early and consistent interactions with peers
Assist child to become adept in use of appliances
Assist child to select clothing *to camouflage prosthesis*
Encourage good hygiene and grooming such as wig (for hair loss from chemotherapy), makeup, and attractive clothing *to enhance appearance*
Encourage child to express feelings and concerns *to facilitate coping*

EXPECTED OUTCOMES
Child resumes former contacts and activities within capabilities
Child appears clean, well-groomed, and attractively dressed
Child expresses feelings and concerns

NURSING DIAGNOSIS: Altered family processes related to having a child with a life-long disability, traumatic therapy

■ **PATIENT (FAMILY) GOAL 1:** Will receive adequate support

NURSING INTERVENTIONS/*RATIONALES*
Allow parents to express their feelings and concerns
Interpret the child's emotional reactions, such as depression, anger, and hostility, *because these may be misinterpreted*

EXPECTED OUTCOMES
Family verbalizes feelings and concerns
Family accepts and understands child's emotional reactions

■ **PATIENT (FAMILY) GOAL 2:** Will be prepared for supplemental therapies and their effects

NURSING INTERVENTIONS/*RATIONALES*
(See Preparation for Procedures, p. 219.)
Impress on child importance of therapy *to encourage acceptance and cooperation*
Explain probable side effects of chemotherapy

EXPECTED OUTCOME
Child and family demonstrate an attitude of understanding of therapies and their side effects

■ **PATIENT (FAMILY) GOAL 3:** Will be prepared for home care

NURSING INTERVENTIONS/*RATIONALES*
Answer questions regarding posthospital care
Explain phantom limb pain (e.g., tingling, itching, burning, cramping, and pain in amputated limb) *so that child does not hide sensations and seeks treatment*
Teach skills and give information necessary for home care
Teach stump care to parents, if appropriate, and to child if child is old enough to assume some responsibility
Assess home and school for environmental barriers such as stairs
Assist family to prepare environment
Arrange for and emphasize importance of maintaining physical therapy regimen
Arrange for acquisition of needed supplies such as dressings, crutches, wheelchair, and prosthesis
Encourage family to allow child to live as normal a life as possible *to facilitate long-term adjustment*
Refer to appropriate agencies and groups *to facilitate care and adjustment*
Maintain contact with family *for ongoing support*

EXPECTED OUTCOMES
Child and family demonstrate skills needed for home care (specify)
Child and family demonstrate an understanding of therapeutic regimen
Child attends school with reasonable regularity (specify)
Family receives continuing support (specify type and amount)
(See also:
Nursing Care Plan: The Child with Chronic Illness or Disability, p. 287.)
Nursing Care Plan: The Child in the Hospital, p. 268.)
Nusing Care Plan: The Family of the Child Who Is Ill or Hospitalized, p. 282.)
Nursing Care Plan: The Child with Cancer, p. 486.)

*Dependent nursing action.

NURSING CARE OF THE CHILD WITH MUSCULOSKELETAL DYSFUNCTION

Musculoskeletal dysfunction refers to disorders involving the bones, muscles, and joints of the body.

NURSING CARE PLAN

The Child Who Is Immobilized

Immobilization is a major therapy for injuries to soft tissues, long bones, ligaments, vertebrae, and joints.

Prolonged immobilization, whether for therapy or because of illness or disability, can produce severe complications, many of which are preventable.

ASSESSMENT

Assess for evidence of the physical effects of immobilization (Table 4-37).

Assess for evidence of the following psychologic responses to immobilization:

Immobility deprives the child of:

Means of communication, expression, and impulse control

Natural outlet for feelings

Means of stress reduction

Immobility restricts the amount and variety of environmental stimuli:

Decrease in tactile output

Restricted limbs transmit less than normal sensation

Proprioception impaired

Decreased sensorimotor activity

May feel isolated, bored, and forgotten

May express anger and aggression inappropriately

Restlessness

Prolonged immobilization can produce the following:

Sluggish intellectual and psychomotor responses

Decreased communication

Increased fantasizing

Depression

Regression—Greater reliance on others

Delayed development

> **NURSING DIAGNOSIS:** Impaired physical mobility related to mechanical restrictions, physical disability (specify level)

■ **PATIENT GOAL 1:** Will have opportunity for mobilization

NURSING INTERVENTIONS/*RATIONALES*

Transport child by gurney, stroller, wagon, bed, wheelchair, or other conveyance from confines of room *to provide for mobilization despite restrictions*

Change position of bed in room *to reduce monotony of immobilization*

Change position in bed when possible *to decrease feelings of being immobilized*

EXPECTED OUTCOMES

Child moves from confines of room or within room

Child's position is changed when possible

■ **PATIENT GOAL 2:** Will maintain optimum autonomy

NURSING INTERVENTIONS/*RATIONALES*

Instruct child in use of orthoses, crutches, or wheelchair *to facilitate independent mobility*

Provide mobilizing devices (orthoses, crutches, wheelchair)

Assist with acquisition of specialized equipment *to encourage independence*

Instruct in use of equipment *to ensure safety*

Encourage activities that require mobilization

Allow as much freedom of movement as possible and encourage normal activities *to maintain a sense of autonomy*

Encourage child to participate in own care as much as possible *to encourage sense of autonomy and independence*

Allow child to make choices (e.g., daily routine, food, clothes) *to encourage sense of autonomy despite limitations*

EXPECTED OUTCOMES

Child moves about without assistance

Child engages in activities appropriate to limitations and developmental level

---

> **NURSING DIAGNOSIS:** Risk for impaired skin integrity related to immobility, therapeutic appliances

■ **PATIENT GOAL 1:** Will maintain skin integrity

NURSING INTERVENTIONS/*RATIONALES*

Place child on pressure-reducing surface (mattress overlay or special bed) *to prevent tissue breakdown and pressure necrosis*

Change position frequently, unless contraindicated, *to prevent dependent edema and to stimulate circulation*

Protect pressure points (e.g., trochanter, sacrum, ankle, shoulder, occiput)

Inspect skin surfaces regularly for signs of irritation, redness, or evidence of pressure

Eliminate mechanical factors causing pressure, friction, or irritation (e.g., keep linen and clothing free of wrinkles)

Maintain meticulous skin cleanliness

Gently massage only *healthy* skin with lubricating substance *to stimulate circulation*

Continued

Unit 4

The Child Who Is Immobilized—cont'd

TABLE 4-37   Summary of Physical Effects of Immobilization with Nursing Interventions*

Primary Effects	Secondary Effects	Nursing Considerations
Muscular System		
Decreased muscle strength, tone, and endurance	Decreased venous return and decreased cardiac output	Use elastic stockings or wrap legs with Ace bandages to promote venous return
	Decreased metabolism and need for oxygen	Plan play activities to use uninvolved extremities
	Decreased exercise tolerance	Place in upright posture when possible
	Bone demineralization	
Disuse atrophy and loss of muscle mass	Catabolism	Perform range-of-motion, active, passive, and stretching exercises
	Loss of strength	Maintain correct body alignment
Loss of joint mobility	Contractures, ankylosis of joints	Use joint splints as indicated to prevent further deformity
Weak back muscles	Secondary spinal deformities	Maintain body alignment
Weak abdominal muscles	Impaired respiration	(See Nursing Considerations, Respiratory System.)
Skeletal System		
Bone demineralization— Osteoporosis, hypercalcemia	Negative calcium balance	In paralysis, use upright posture on tilt table
	Pathologic fractures	Handle extremities carefully when turning and positioning
	Calcium deposits	
	Extraosseous bone formation, especially at hip, knee, elbow, and shoulder	Administer calcium-mobilizing drugs (diphosphonates) if ordered
	Renal calculi	Ensure adequate intake of fluid; monitor output
		Acidify urine
		Promptly treat urinary tract infections
Negative calcium balance	Life-threatening electrolyte imbalance	Monitor blood levels of calcium electrolytes
		Provide electrolyte replacement as indicated
Metabolism		
Decreased metabolic rate	Slowing of all systems	Mobilize as soon as possible
	Decreased food intake	Perform active and passive resistance and deep breathing exercises
		Ensure adequate food intake
		Provide a high-protein diet
Negative nitrogen balance	Decline in nutritional state	Encourage small, frequent feedings with protein and preferred foods
	Impaired healing	Prevent pressure areas
Hypercalcemia	Electrolyte imbalance	(See Nursing Considerations, Skeletal System.)
Decreased production of stress hormones	Decreased physical and emotional coping capacity	Identify etiologies of stress
		Implement appropriate interventions to lower physical and psychosocial stresses

*Use measures that apply. Not all problems will be applicable in every situation.

The Child Who Is Immobilized—cont'd

TABLE 4-37   Summary of Physical Effects of Immobilization with Nursing Interventions*—cont'd

Primary Effects	Secondary Effects	Nursing Considerations
Cardiovascular System		
Decreased efficiency of orthostatic neurovascular reflexes	Inability to adapt readily to upright position	Monitor peripheral pulses and skin temperature changes
	Pooling of blood in extremities in upright posture	Wrap legs in elastic bandage or stockings to decrease pooling when upright
Diminished vasopressor mechanism	Orthostatic hypotension with syncope—Hypotension, decreased cerebral blood flow, tachycardia	Provide abdominal support
		In severe cases, use antigravitational suit
		Administer peripheral sympathetic stimulating agents such as ephedrine if ordered
		Position horizontally
Altered distribution of blood volume	Decreased cardiac workload	Monitor hydration and urine output
	Decreased exercise tolerance	
Venous stasis	Pulmonary emboli and/or thrombi	Have frequent position changes
		Elevate extremities without knee flexion
		Ensure adequate fluid intake
		Perform active or passive exercises or movement, if ordered
		Prescribe routine wearing of antiembolic stockings or wrap lower extremities from metatarsus to gluteal folds
		Measure circumference of extremities periodically
		Give anticoagulant drugs if ordered until mobilization possible
		Promptly intervene to maintain adequate oxygen if signs and symptoms of pulmonary emboli are noted
Dependent edema	Tissue breakdown and susceptibility to infection	Administer good skin care
		Turn every 2 hours
		Monitor skin for color, temperature, and integrity
Respiratory System		
Decreased need for oxygen	Altered oxygen–carbon dioxide exchange and metabolism	Exercise as tolerated
		Use position for optimum chest expansion
Decreased chest expansion and diminished vital capacity	Diminished oxygen intake	Use prone positioning without pressure on abdomen to allow gravity to aid in diaphragmatic excursion
	Dyspnea and inadequate arterial oxygen saturation; acidosis	When sitting, maintain proper alignment to prevent pressure on respiratory mechanism
Poor abdominal tone and distention	Interference with diaphragmatic excursion	Avoid restriction of chest and abdominal musculature
		Supply torso support to promote chest expansion
Mechanical or biochemical secretion retention	Hypostatic pneumonia	Change position frequently
	Bacterial and viral pneumonia	Carry out percussion, vibration, and drainage (or suctioning) as necessary
	Atelectasis	Monitor breath sounds

*Use measures that apply. Not all problems will be applicable in every situation.   *Continued*

The Child Who Is Immobilized—cont'd

TABLE 4-37 Summary of Physical Effects of Immobilization with Nursing Interventions*—cont'd

Primary Effects	Secondary Effects	Nursing Considerations
Respiratory System—cont'd		
Loss of respiratory muscle strength	Poor cough	Encourage coughing and deep breathing
		Support chest wall when coughing
		Use special devices such as a rocking bed, breathing bag, incentive spirometers
		Observe for signs of acute respiratory distress with blood gas levels measured as necessary
	Upper respiratory infection	Avoid contact with infected persons
		Provide adequate hydration
Gastrointestinal System		
Distention caused by poor abdominal muscle tone	Interference with respiratory movements	Monitor bowel sounds
	Difficulty in feeding in prone position	Encourage small, frequent feedings
		Sit in upright position if possible
No specific primary effect	Gravitation effect on feces through ascending colon or weakened smooth muscle tone may cause constipation	Carry out bowel-training program with hydration, stool softeners, and mild laxatives if necessary
	Anorexia	Stimulate appetite with favored foods
Urinary System		
Alteration of gravitational force	Difficulty in voiding in prone position	Position as upright as possible to void
Impaired ureteral peristalsis	Urinary retention in calyces and bladder	Hydrate to ensure adequate urinary output for age
	Infection	Collect specimens as needed
	Renal calculi	Stimulate bladder emptying with warm water, running water, striking suprapubic area
		Catheterize only for severe retention
		Administer urinary tract antiseptics as indicated
Integumentary System		
No specific primary effect	Decreased circulation and pressure leading to tissue injury	Turn and position at least every 2 hours
	Difficulty with personal hygiene	Frequently inspect total skin surface
		Eliminate mechanical factors causing pressure, friction, or irritation
		Assess ability to perform hygienic care and assist with bathing, grooming, and toileting as needed

*Use measures that apply. Not all problems will be applicable in every situation.

Unit 4

The Child Who Is Immobilized—cont'd

EXPECTED OUTCOME
Skin remains clean and intact with no evidence of irritation

NURSING DIAGNOSIS: Risk for injury related to impaired mobility

■ **PATIENT GOAL 1:** Will experience no physical activity

NURSING INTERVENTIONS/*RATIONALES*
Teach correct use of mobilizing devices and/or apparatus *to ensure safety*
Assist with moving and/or ambulating as needed *to ensure safety*
Remove hazards from environment (specify)
Modify environment as needed (specify)
Keep call button within reach
Keep siderails up at all times *to prevent falls*
Help child to use bathroom or commode, if possible
Implement safety measures appropriate to child's developmental age (specify)

EXPECTED OUTCOME
Child remains free of injury

NURSING DIAGNOSIS: Diversional activity deficit related to impaired mobility, musculoskeletal impairment, confinement to hospital or home

■ **PATIENT GOAL 1:** Will engage in diversional activity

**NURSING INTERVENTIONS/*RATIONALES*
AND EXPECTED OUTCOMES**
(See Nursing Care Plan: The Child in the Hospital, p. 268.)

NURSING DIAGNOSIS: Risk for altered family processes related to a child with disability, illness

■ **PATIENT (FAMILY) GOAL 1:** Will receive support as desired

**NURSING INTERVENTIONS/*RATIONALES*
AND EXPECTED OUTCOMES**
(See Nursing Care Plan: The Family of the Child Who Is Ill or Hospitalized, p. 282.)

Unit 4

NURSING CARE PLAN

The Child with a Fracture

A fracture is a break in the continuity of a bone caused when the resistance of the bone yields to a stress or force exerted on it.

Complete fracture—Fracture fragments are separated

Incomplete fracture—Fracture fragments remain attached

Simple or closed fracture—Fracture does not produce a break in the skin

Open or compound fracture—Fracture with an open wound through which the bone has protruded

Complicated fracture—Bone fragments cause damage to other organs or tissues (e.g., lung or bladder)

Comminuted fracture—Small fragments of bone are broken from fractured shaft and lie in surrounding tissue (very rare in children)

Most frequent fractures in children:

Bends—A child's flexible bone can be bent 45 degrees or more before breaking. However, if bent, the bone will straighten slowly, but not completely, to produce some deformity but without the angulation that exists when the bone breaks. Bends occur more commonly in the ulna and fibula, often associated with fractures of the radius and tibia.

Buckle fracture—Compression of the porous bone produces a *buckle* or *torus* fracture. This appears as a raised or bulging projection at the fracture site. Torus fractures occur in the most porous portion of the bone near the metaphysis (the portion of the bone shaft adjacent to the epiphysis) and are more common in young children.

Greenstick fracture—Occurs when a bone is angulated beyond the limits of bending; the compressed side bends and the tension side fails, causing an incomplete fracture similar to the break observed when a green stick is broken.

Complete fracture—Divides the bone fragments; they often remain attached by a periosteal hinge, which can aid or hinder reduction.

ASSESSMENT

Obtain a history of event, previous injury, and experience with health personnel.

Observe for manifestations of fracture:

Signs of injury:

Generalized swelling

Pain or tenderness

Diminished functional use of affected part (strongly suspect fracture in small child who refuses to walk or move an upper extremity)

Bruising

Severe muscular rigidity

Crepitus (grating sensation at fracture site)

Assess for location of fracture—Observe for deformity, instruct child to point to painful area.

Assess for circulation and sensation distal to fracture site.

Assist with diagnostic procedures and tests (e.g., radiography, and tomography).

THE CHILD IN A CAST

CATEGORIES OF CASTS:

Upper extremity cast—Immobilizes wrist and/or elbow

Lower extremity cast—Immobilizes ankle and/or knee

Spica cast—Immobilizes hip and knee

Spinal and cervical casts—Immobilizes the spine

ASSESSMENT OF CASTED EXTREMITY

Monitor cardiovascular status:

Monitor peripheral pulses.

Blanch skin on extremity distal to fracture to ascertain adequate circulation to the part.

Feel cast for tightness; cast should allow insertion of fingers between skin and cast after it has dried.

Assess for increase in the following:

Pain

Swelling

Coldness

Cyanosis or pallor

Assess finger or toe movement and sensation:

Request child to move fingers or toes.

Observe for spontaneous movement in children who are unable to respond to requests.

Report signs of impending circulatory impairment immediately

Instruct child to immediately report any feelings of numbness or tingling.

Check temperature (plaster cast):

Chemical reaction in cast drying process, which generates heat.

Water evaporation, which causes heat loss

Inspect skin for irritation or pressure areas.

Inspect skin for irritation or pressure areas.

Inspect inside cast for items that a small child may place there.

Observe for signs of infection:

Check for drainage.

Smell cast for foul odor.

Feel cast for "hot spots" indicating infection under the cast.

Be alert to increased temperature, lethargy, and discomfort.

Observe for respiratory impairment (spica cast):

Assess child's chest expansion.

Observe respiratory rate.

Observe color and behavior.

Assess for evidence of bleeding (surgical open reduction):

Outline area of bleeding; assess for increase.

Assess need for pain medication. (See p. 315.)

NURSING DIAGNOSIS: Risk for injury related to presence of cast, tissue swelling, possible nerve damage

- **PATIENT GOAL 1:** Will not experience neurologic or circulatory impairment

NURSING INTERVENTIONS/*RATIONALES*

Elevate casted extremity *to decrease swelling, since elevation increases venous return*

Place leg cast on pillows, making certain that leg is well supported and that there is no pressure on heel

Elevate arm on pillows or support in stockinette sling suspended from intravenous infusion pole, either in bed or during ambulation; triangular arm sling is adequate for lesser elevation and support

Assess exposed part(s) of casted extremity for pain, swelling, discoloration (cyanosis or pallor), pulsation, warmth, sensation, and ability to move

EXPECTED OUTCOME

Toes/fingers are warm, pink, sensitive, and demonstrate brisk capillary filling

- **PATIENT GOAL 2:** Will maintain cast integrity

NURSING INTERVENTIONS/*RATIONALES*

Handle damp cast with palms of hands; avoid indenting the cast with fingertips (plaster cast) *because indenting can create pressure areas*

Cover rough edges of cast with adhesive "petals" *to protect cast edges and prevent skin irritation*

Do not allow weight bearing until cast is completely dry, even if weight-bearing device is attached

Keep wet cast uncovered *to allow it to dry from the inside out*

Avoid drying cast with heated fan or dryer *because burns can result and cast will dry on outside but be wet inside*

Use regular fan if cast is in high-humidity environment *to circulate air*

Change position of child in body cast or hip spica cast periodically (small child can be managed easily; adolescent may require one or two persons to assist; eventually children become very adept at moving themselves) *because turning helps to dry cast evenly*

Do *not* use abduction stabilizer bar between legs of hip spica as handle for turning

Position with buttocks lower than shoulders during toileting (body can be supported on pillows) *to prevent urine from flowing under cast at the back*

Protect rim of cast around perineal area of body cast with plastic film *to prevent soiling during toileting*

Use plastic-backed disposable diaper with edges tucked underneath rim of cast for infants and small children who are not toilet trained or who are prone to "accidents"; a sanitary napkin can also be used if waterproof material is placed between pad and cast

Caution against activities that might cause physical damage to cast

Remove soiled areas of cast with damp cloth and small amount of white, low-abrasive cleaner; do not cover soiled areas with shoe polish or paint

EXPECTED OUTCOME

Cast dries evenly and remains clean and intact

- **PATIENT GOAL 3:** Will not experience physical injury

NURSING INTERVENTIONS/*RATIONALES*

Keep a clear path for ambulation *to prevent falls:*

Remove toys, hazardous floor rugs, pets, or other items over which the child might stumble

Teach child to use crutches appropriately if he or she has a lower limb fracture

The crutches should fit properly, have a soft rubber tip to prevent slipping, and be well padded at the axilla

EXPECTED OUTCOME

Child remains free of injury

NURSING DIAGNOSIS: Pain related to physical injury

- **PATIENT GOAL 1:** Will experience no or minimal discomfort

NURSING INTERVENTIONS/*RATIONALES*

(See Nursing Care Plan: The Child in Pain, p. 315.)

Restrict strenuous activities if necessary *to prevent pain*

Position for comfort; use pillows to support dependent areas

Alleviate itching underneath cast by cool air blown from Asepto syringe, fan, or hair dryer (on low or cool setting); or scratching or rubbing the unaffected extremity

Avoid using powder or lotion under cast *since these substances have tendency to "ball" and produce irritation*

EXPECTED OUTCOMES

Child exhibits no evidence of discomfort

Minor discomforts are eased

NURSING DIAGNOSIS: Risk for impaired skin integrity related to cast

- **PATIENT GOAL 1:** Will not experience skin irritation

NURSING INTERVENTIONS/*RATIONALES*

Make certain that all cast edges are smooth and free from irritating projections; trim and/or pad as necessary; petal cast edges if needed

Do not allow the child to put anything inside the cast *to prevent skin trauma*

Keep small items that might be placed inside the cast away from small children

Caution older children not to place items under cast; explain why this is important *to encourage compliance*

Keep exposed skin clean and free of irritants

Protect cast during bathing, unless synthetic cast is waterproof, *because skin can become irritated from water inside cast*

After cast is removed, soak and gently wash skin *because it will be caked with desquamated skin and sebaceous secretions;* caution child and family not to forcibly remove this material *because vigorous scrubbing can cause excoriation and bleeding*

EXPECTED OUTCOME

Skin remains intact with no evidence of irritation

NURSING DIAGNOSIS: Impaired physical mobility related to musculoskeletal impairment

- **PATIENT GOAL 1:** Will maintain muscle use of unaffected areas

NURSING INTERVENTIONS/*RATIONALES*

Encourage to ambulate as soon as possible *to regain mobility*

Support casted arm in sling

The Child with a Fracture—cont'd

Teach use of mobilizing devices such as crutches for casted leg (walking device is applied when weight bearing is allowed)

Encourage child with an ambulation device to ambulate as soon as general condition allows

Provide and encourage play activities and diversions *that exercise unaffected muscles*

Encourage child to use joints above and below cast *to maintain flexibility and joint function*

EXPECTED OUTCOMES
Unaffected extremities maintain good muscle tone

Child engages in activities appropriate to age, interests, and condition

---

NURSING DIAGNOSIS: Altered family processes related to child with a physical injury

---

■ **PATIENT (FAMILY) GOAL 1:** Will be prepared for home care

NURSING INTERVENTIONS/*RATIONALES*
(See Box 4-28: Family Home Care: Cast Care.)

(See Community and Home Care Instructions: Caring for the Child in a Cast, p. 593.)

EXPECTED OUTCOMES
Family demonstrates correct cast care

Family provides appropriate care of cast and seeks assistance when needed

---

NURSING DIAGNOSIS: Fear related to cast application and removal

---

■ **PATIENT GOAL 1:** Will receive adequate support during cast application and removal

NURSING INTERVENTIONS/*RATIONALES*
(See Preparation for procedures, p. 219.)

Explain what will take place and what the child can do to help *to alleviate fear and encourage cooperation*

Explain what child will experience during cast removal:
Noise of the saw
Tickling sensation from vibration

Explain unlikelihood of injury from procedure:
Demonstrate safety of saw on self or someone else *to relieve fear of skin being cut*

EXPECTED OUTCOME
Child submits to casting and cast removal with minimal distress and cooperates during procedure

---

BOX 4-28

Family Home Care: Cast Care

Expose the plaster cast to air until dry.

Keep the casted part of the body elevated on pillows or similar support for the first day, or as directed by the health professional.

Lift and support the wet cast with the palms of the hands only, to avoid indenting with the fingers.

Observe the fingers or toes for any evidence of swelling or discoloration (darker or lighter than a comparable extremity) and contact the health professional immediately if noted.

Check movement and sensation of the visible fingers and toes frequently and contact the health professional regarding any changes noted.

Follow health professional's orders regarding any restriction of activities.

Restrict strenuous activities for the first few days:
Engage in quiet activities but encourage use of muscles.
Move the joints above and below the cast on the affected extremity.
Specific exercises for the child should be demonstrated by hospital staff, and a written copy should be provided to the parents.

Encourage frequent rest for a few days, keeping the injured arm or leg elevated while resting.

Avoid allowing the affected limb to hang down for more than 30 minutes:
Keep an injured arm or hand elevated (e.g., in a sling) most of the time; supporting it on pillows at chest level is helpful.
Elevate a leg when sitting, and avoid standing for more than 30 minutes.

Do not allow the child to put anything inside the cast:
Keep small items that might be placed inside the cast away from young children.

Itching may be relieved by an ice pack, by visualizing the skin at the cast edges, and by administering medication as recommended by the physician.

Keep a clear path for ambulation:
Remove toys, hazardous floor rugs, pets, or other items over which the child might stumble.

Use crutches appropriately (if lower limb fracture):
The crutches should fit properly, have a soft rubber tip to prevent slipping, and be well padded at the axilla. The axilla should not rest on the crutches.

Instruct child and parents to avoid placing the cast in water (e.g., tub, shower, swimming pool).

If patient is incontinent, protect the cast with waterproof tape and plastic, diapers, pull-ups, or other guards.

*Dependent nursing action.

NURSING CARE PLAN

The Child in Traction

Purposes of traction

To realign bone fragments

To provide rest for an extremity

To help prevent or improve contracture deformity

To correct a deformity

To treat a dislocation

To allow preoperative or postoperative positioning and alignment

To provide immobilization of specific areas of the body

To reduce muscle spasms (rare in children)

Types of traction

Manual traction—Traction applied to the body part by the hand placed distally to the fracture site; nurses frequently provide manual traction during cast application.

Skin traction—Pull applied directly to the skin surface and indirectly to the skeletal structures; the pulling mechanism is attached to the skin with adhesive material or an elastic bandage; both types are applied over soft, foam-backed traction straps to distribute the traction pull.

Skeletal traction—Pull applied directly to the skeletal structure by a pin, wire, or tongs inserted into or through the diameter of the bone distal to the fracture.

Figs. 4-4 to 4-9 illustrate various types of traction.

ASSESSMENT OF TRACTION

Check desired line of pull and relationship of distal fragment to proximal fragment:

Check whether fragment is being directed upward, adducted, or abducted.

Check function of each component:

Position of bandages, frames, splints

Ropes:

In center track of pulley, taut, no fraying, knots tied securely

Pulleys:

In original position on attachment bar; have not slid from original site

Wheels freely movable

Weights:

Correct amount of weight

Hanging freely

In safe location

Check bed position—Head or foot elevated as directed for desired amount of pull and countertraction

Assess child's behavior to determine if traction causes pain or discomfort.

Skin traction:

Replace nonadhesive straps and/or elastic bandage on skin traction *when permitted* and/or absolutely necessary, but make certain that traction on limb is maintained by someone during procedure.

Assess bandages to ascertain if they are correctly applied (diagonal or spiral) and not too loose or too tight, which could cause slippage and malalignment of traction.

Skeletal traction:

Check pin sites frequently for signs of bleeding, inflammation, or infection.

Check pin screws to be certain that they are tight in metal clamp that attaches traction apparatus to pin.

Note pull of traction on pin; pull should be even.

Observe for correct body alignment with emphasis on alignment of shoulder, hip, and leg.

Check alignment after child has moved.

Assess circular dressings for excessive tightness.

Assess restraining devices if prescribed:

Make certain that they are not too loose or too tight.

Remove periodically and check for pressure areas.

Check pulse in affected area and compare with pulse in contralateral site.

Note if any tightness, weakness, or contractures are developing in uninvolved joints and muscles.

Note any neurovascular changes, such as:

Alterations in color of skin and nail beds

Alterations in sensation

Alterations in motor ability

Check beneath child for small objects (e.g., food, toys).

NURSING DIAGNOSIS: Risk for injury related to immobility and traction apparatus

■ **PATIENT GOAL 1:** Will not experience complications

NURSING INTERVENTIONS/*RATIONALES*

Encourage deep breathing frequently with maximum inspiratory chest expansion *to prevent respiratory complications*

Check pulse in affected area and compare with pulse in contralateral site *to assess circulatory status*

Assess circular dressings for excessive tightness *to prevent compromised circulation*

Note any neurovascular changes, such as:

Alterations in color of skin and nail beds

Alterations in sensation, increased pain

Alterations in motor ability

Take immediate action *to correct problem* or report to practitioner if neurovascular changes are found *to prevent delay in treatment*

Apply restraints only when indicated *to maintain traction:*

Make certain restraints are not too loose or too tight

Remove periodically and check for pressure areas

(See Restraining Methods and "Therapeutic Hugging," p. 229.)

Maintain correct angles at joints *for proper alignment*

Carry out passive, active, or active-with-resistance exercises of uninvolved joints *to preserve joint function*

Take measures to correct or prevent further development of deformities, such as applying foot plate *to prevent footdrop*

*Cleanse and dress pin sites on skeletal traction as ordered *to decrease risk of infection*

*Apply topical antiseptic or antibiotic daily as ordered

*Dependent nursing action.

Continued

Unit 4

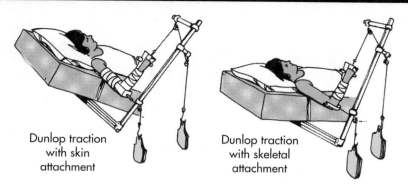

Fig. 4-4   Dunlop traction.

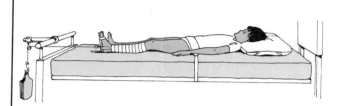

Fig. 4-5   Buck extension traction.

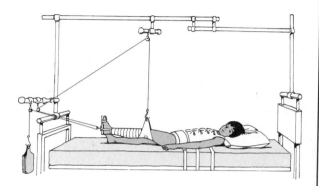

Fig. 4-6   Russell traction.

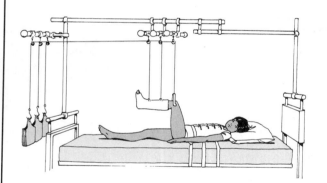

Fig. 4-7   Ninety degree–ninety degree traction.

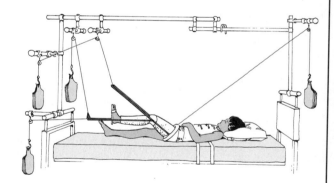

Fig. 4-8   Balance suspension with Thomas ring splint and Pearson attachment.

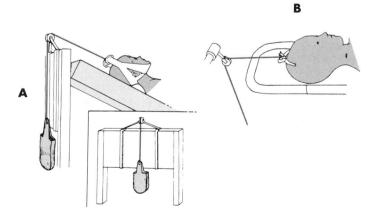

Fig. 4-9   Cervical traction. **A,** With chin strap. **B,** With Crutchfield tongs. (Figs. 4-4 to 4-9 redrawn from Hilt NE, Schitt EW: *Pediatric orthopedic nursing,* St Louis, 1975, Mosby.)

Unit 4

The Child in Traction—cont'd

Cover ends of pins with protective cord or padding *to prevent child from being scratched by pin*

Do not remove skeletal traction or adhesive traction straps on skin traction

*Administer stool softeners as indicated *to prevent constipation*

*Administer rectal suppository or mild laxative if indicated *to relieve constipation*

Make certain that child ingests sufficient amount of calcium-rich foods *for bone healing*

Encourage sufficient fluids and foods high in fiber *to prevent constipation*

EXPECTED OUTCOMES

Circulation in extremities remains satisfactory; movement, good (pink) color, sensation present

Child exhibits no signs of complications

Neurovascular status assessed for compromise (e.g., decrease in circulation, movement, or sensation)

NURSING DIAGNOSIS: Knowledge deficit related to use of traction

■ **PATIENT (FAMILY) GOAL 1:** Will verbalize understanding of purpose of traction

NURSING INTERVENTIONS/*RATIONALES*

Explain purpose and importance of traction (i.e., to decrease muscle spasm, reduce and stabilize a fracture or dislocation, maintain alignment, and immobilize a limb)

Encourage and answer all questions and concerns

EXPECTED OUTCOME

Child and/or family verbalizes understanding of purpose of traction as evidenced by verbal statements and compliance with therapeutic regimen

---

NURSING DIAGNOSIS: Pain related to physical injury

■ **PATIENT GOAL 1:** Will experience either no pain or a reduction of pain to level acceptable to child

(See Nursing Care Plan: The Child in Pain, p. 315.)

NURSING DIAGNOSIS: Risk for impaired skin integrity related to immobility, traction apparatus

■ **PATIENT GOAL 1:** Will not experience skin breakdown

NURSING INTERVENTIONS/*RATIONALES*

Provide pressure-reducing mattress underneath hips and back

Make total body skin checks for redness or breakdown, especially over areas that receive greatest pressure (a small hand mirror can be used to visualize inaccessible skin areas), *to prevent delay in treatment*

Wash and dry skin at least daily *to stimulate circulation and keep skin clean*

Gently massage over pressure areas *to stimulate circulation*

Change position at least every 2 hours, if possible, *to relieve pressure*

Check for small objects (e.g., toys, food) under child *since they can cause skin irritation*

EXPECTED OUTCOME

Skin remains clean and intact with no evidence of irritation

NURSING DIAGNOSIS: Impaired physical mobility (specify level) related to musculoskeletal impairment

■ **PATIENT GOAL 1:** Will maintain function of uninvolved muscles and joints

NURSING INTERVENTIONS/*RATIONALES*

Provide apparatus (e.g., overhead trapeze) and encourage child in activities *that provide exercise for uninvolved muscles and joints*

EXPECTED OUTCOME

Joints remain flexible; muscles retain tone

NURSING DIAGNOSIS: Fear related to discomfort, unfamiliar apparatus

■ **PATIENT GOAL 1:** Will exhibit signs of reduced fear

NURSING INTERVENTIONS/*RATIONALES*

Explain traction apparatus to child and family *to decrease fear/anxiety and increase cooperation*

Explain to child what nursing care will be *so that child knows what to expect*

Determine, with child, ways to participate in own care *to give child some measure of control*

Make certain that child knows how to call for help

Provide assurance that the child will not be left totally helpless

Have family bring child's favorite toy and/or security object

EXPECTED OUTCOMES

Child cooperates throughout procedures

Child remains calm

■ **PATIENT GOAL 2:** Will experience adequate comfort

NURSING INTERVENTIONS/*RATIONALES*

Use pads, pillows, and rolls *to position for comfort*

Encourage family to use favorite comfort measures (e.g., stroking, music, pacifier)

Touch and talk to child *to provide comfort while child cannot be held*

EXPECTED OUTCOMES

Child plays and interacts readily

Child exhibits no signs of discomfort

NURSING DIAGNOSIS: Bathing/hygiene, feeding, dressing/grooming, toileting self-care deficits related to impaired mobility

---

*Dependent nursing action.

Continued

Unit 4

The Child in Traction—cont'd

■ **PATIENT GOAL 1:** Will engage in self-help activities

NURSING INTERVENTIONS/RATIONALES

Allow child to help plan own daily routine and choose from alternatives when appropriate *to increase sense of control*

Devise means to facilitate self-help in daily activities

Assist with self-care activities where needed (e.g., bathe inaccessible parts, make food easy to eat without assistance, provide grooming)

EXPECTED OUTCOME

Child assists with self-care activities—Feeds self, washes reachable areas, attends to grooming within child's capabilities (specify)

■ **PATIENT GOAL 2:** Will exhibit normal elimination patterns

NURSING INTERVENTIONS/RATIONALES

Determine child's words for elimination needs *so that he or she receives assistance when needed*

Provide privacy *to promote relaxation needed for elimination*

Use fracture pan for bowel movements and voiding (for females)

Check frequency and consistency of bowel movements *to prevent delay in treating constipation*

Adjust fluid and food intake according to stool (e.g., increase fluids, fruits, grains for constipation)

EXPECTED OUTCOMES

Elimination is managed with minimum difficulty

Child has regular bowel movements

(See also:
Nursing Care Plan: The Child in the Hospital, p. 268.)
Nursing Care Plan: The Family of the Child Who Is Ill or Hospitalized, p. 282.)

Unit 4

NURSING CARE PLAN

The Child with Structural Scoliosis

Scoliosis is a complex spinal deformity in three planes, usually involving lateral curvature, spinal rotation causing rib asymmetry, and thoracic hypokyphosis. It can be caused by a number of conditions. In most cases, however, there is no apparent cause and it is called **idiopathic scoliosis.**

ASSESSMENT

Perform a physical assessment.

Observe for manifestations of scoliosis:

With the child standing erect, clothed only in underpants (and bra if older girl), observe from behind, noting asymmetry of the shoulders and hips.

With the child bending forward so that the back is parallel to the floor, observe from the side, noting asymmetry or prominence of the rib cage.

Assist with diagnostic procedures (e.g., radiography or MRI).

Surgical therapy for structural scoliosis

Harrington instrumentation—Implantation of metal rods by way of clips to hold the vertebrae and bone fragments for permanent fusion; child immobilized on a Stryker frame following surgery

Luque segmental instrumentation—A flexible L-shaped metal rod fixed by wires to the bases of the spinous processes; patient can walk within a few days and no postoperative immobilization is necessary

Dwyer instrumentation—A titanium cable through cannulated screws transfixed to each vertebra; child cared for in bed following surgery

Zielke procedure—A combination of Harrington and Dwyer procedures

Cotrel-Dubousset (CD) procedure—A form of bilateral segmental fixation that uses two knurled rods and multiple hooks; casting and bracing not needed

Texas Scottish Rite Hospital (TSRH) system—Use of bilateral rods, hooks, and cross-link plates; if needed, system allows for easier surgical revision than CD instrumentation

---

ASSESSMENT (PREOPERATIVE)

(See Nursing Care Plan: The Child Undergoing Surgery, Preoperative Care, p. 304.)

Assess status of child with progressive traction application: (See Nursing Care Plan: The Child in Traction, p. 511.)

Assess peripheral nerves both proximal and distal to curvature.

Assess cranial nerves and deep tendon reflexes in extremities.

ASSESSMENT (POSTOPERATIVE)

Perform postoperative assessments of circulation, vital signs, and wound.

Perform neurologic assessment, especially of extremities.

Assess for presence of bowel sounds.

Assess urinary output.

Assess pain.

| **NURSING DIAGNOSIS:** Risk for injury related to unaccustomed brace |

- **PATIENT GOAL 1:** Will not experience injury related to wearing brace

NURSING INTERVENTIONS/*RATIONALES*

Assess environment for hazards *to prevent injuries*

Teach safety precautions such as using handrails on stairways and avoiding slippery surfaces *to prevent falls*

Help develop safe methods of mobilization

EXPECTED OUTCOME

Child remains free of injury related to wearing brace

- **PATIENT GOAL 2:** Will adjust to restricted movement

NURSING INTERVENTIONS/*RATIONALES*

Demonstrate alternative modes of accomplishing tasks such as getting in and out of bed, dressing

Help devise alternatives for restricted activities and for coping with awkwardness

EXPECTED OUTCOME

Child demonstrates appropriate adaptation to corrective device (specify)

| **NURSING DIAGNOSIS:** Risk for impaired skin integrity related to corrective device |

- **PATIENT GOAL 1:** Will not experience skin irritation or breakdown

NURSING INTERVENTIONS/*RATIONALES*

Examine skin surfaces in contact with brace for signs of irritation *so that appropriate treatment is instituted*

Implement corrective action to treat or prevent skin breakdown

Suggest nonirritating fabrics and clothing, such as cotton T-shirts, that can be worn under brace *to minimize risk of skin irritation*

Recommend daily bath or shower followed by thorough drying *to maintain cleanliness and minimize risk of skin irritation*

EXPECTED OUTCOME

Skin remains clean with no evidence of irritation

| **NURSING DIAGNOSIS:** Body image disturbance related to perception of defect in body structure |

- **PATIENT GOAL 1:** Will exhibit signs of physical adjustment to appliance

NURSING INTERVENTIONS/*RATIONALES*

Plan *with* the child *to encourage compliance and adjustment*

Attempt to determine source of any discomfort *so that appropriate care is instituted*

Refer to orthotist for needed adjustment and service

Assist with plan for personal hygiene

Help in selection of appropriate and attractive apparel to wear over brace

Advise regarding selection of appropriate footwear *to maintain proper balance*

Reinforce teaching regarding removal and reapplication of appliance *so that child receives maximum benefit of appliance*

Continued

Unit 4

EXPECTED OUTCOMES

Brace fits well and produces no discomfort

Child complies with directions for wear and care of brace

Child is well-groomed and wears attractive attire and proper footwear

■ **PATIENT GOAL 2:** Will exhibit positive coping behaviors

NURSING INTERVENTIONS/RATIONALES

Encourage child to discuss feelings about wearing brace *to encourage coping*

Emphasize positive aspects and eventual outcome *to encourage acceptance of treatment*

EXPECTED OUTCOMES

Child verbalizes feelings and concerns

Child recognizes benefits of treatment

(See also Nursing Care Plan: The Child with Chronic Illness or Disability, p. 287.)

PREOPERATIVE CARE

(See Nursing Care Plan: The Child Undergoing Surgery: Preoperative Care, p. 304.)

POSTOPERATIVE CARE

(See Nursing Care Plan: The Child Undergoing Surgery: Postoperative Care, p. 305.)

NURSING DIAGNOSIS: Risk for injury related to surgery

■ **PATIENT GOAL 1:** Will attain ambulation without injury to surgical repair

NURSING INTERVENTIONS/RATIONALES

Place on special bed, if ordered (Harrington instrumentation), *which facilitates care and decreases risk of injury to surgical repair*

Maintain proper body alignment; avoid twisting movements, *which can cause indwelling instruments to twist the spine*

Logroll with care when moving child who is not on a Stryker frame

Keep flat for 12 hours before logrolling (Luque procedure)

Beginning activity—have child roll from side-lying to sitting position

Encourage child to exercise by contracting and relaxing thigh and calf muscles periodically *to maintain optimum movement of lower extremities in the immediate postoperative period*

Perform regular tests of neurologic integrity

Assist with physical therapy and range-of-motion exercises *to maintain muscle tone and joint flexibility*

Walk slowly with aid of safety belt and walker; unassisted ambulation usually allowed before discharge

EXPECTED OUTCOME

Child attains ambulation without injury

■ **PATIENT GOAL 2:** Will not experience abdominal distention (from paralytic ileus)

NURSING INTERVENTIONS/RATIONALES

*Insert and maintain nasogastric suction, if used, *to prevent abdominal distention*

Assess for returning bowel function (e.g., bowel sounds) *to aid in determining when nasogastric suction can be discontinued*

EXPECTED OUTCOME

Child exhibits no evidence of abdominal distention

NURSING DIAGNOSIS: Pain related to surgical procedure

■ **PATIENT GOAL 1:** Will experience either no pain or a reduction of pain to level acceptable to child

NURSING INTERVENTIONS/RATIONALES

Anticipate need for pain management *because of the nature of this surgery*

*Administer opioids on preventive schedule (around the clock) until pain can be controlled with nonopioids *to prevent pain from occurring*

Consider/encourage patient-controlled analgesia for child able to follow instructions *in order to give child more control in prevention and alleviation of pain*

EXPECTED OUTCOME

Child rests quietly, reports and/or exhibits no evidence of discomfort or minimal discomfort

---

NURSING DIAGNOSIS: Altered urinary elimination related to surgical procedure, loss of blood, renal hypoperfusion

---

■ **PATIENT GOAL 1:** Will exhibit signs of adequate urinary elimination

NURSING INTERVENTIONS/RATIONALES

*Insert indwelling catheter *because urinary retention is common with this surgery*

Encourage frequent voiding after catheter removal

Provide privacy *to encourage urination*

Monitor intake and output *to assess adequacy of kidney function*

*Maintain intravenous infusion, if ordered, *for adequate hydration and urinary output*

Encourage oral fluids when allowed

EXPECTED OUTCOME

Child has a sufficient urinary output

NURSING DIAGNOSIS: Impaired physical mobility related to spinal surgery and instrumentation

---

(See Nursing Care Plan: The Child Who Is Immobilized, p. 503.)

NURSING DIAGNOSIS: Risk for altered family processes related to a child with a physical disability

---

■ **PATIENT GOAL 1:** Will receive support as desired

NURSING INTERVENTIONS/RATIONALES

(See Nursing Care Plan: The Family of the Child Who Is Ill or Hospitalized, p. 282.)

EXPECTED OUTCOME

Family members have needed support

(See also Nursing Care Plan: The Child in the Hospital, p. 268.)

---

*Dependent nursing action.

NURSING CARE PLAN

The Child with Juvenile Rheumatoid Arthritis

Juvenile Rheumatoid Arthritis (JRA) is an inflammatory disease of joints with an unknown inciting agent. The disease takes the following three major courses:
Systemic onset—Associated with daily temperature spikes, with or without maculopapular rash

Pauciarticular—Involves few joints, usually fewer than four
Polyarticular—Simultaneous involvement of five or more joints

ASSESSMENT
Perform a physical assessment.
Obtain a health history, especially regarding symptoms related to illness and joint involvement.
Observe for manifestations of juvenile rheumatoid arthritis.
Involved joints:
Stiffness
Swelling
Tenderness
Painful to touch or relatively painless
Warm to touch (seldom red)
Loss of motion

Characteristic morning stiffness or "gelling" on arising in the morning or after inactivity
Extraarticular manifestations:
Systemic onset—Fever, malaise, myalgia, rash, pleuritis or pericarditis, adenomegaly, splenomegaly, hepatomegaly
Pauciarticular—Chronic or acute iridocyclitis, mucocutaneous lesions, sacroiliitis
Polyarticular—Possible low-grade fever, malaise, weight loss, rheumatoid nodules, vasculitis
Assist with diagnostic procedures and tests (e.g., white blood cells, erythrocyte sedimentation rate, tests for rheumatoid factors (not usually of value in children); and antinuclear antibodies, radiography, and joint aspiration).

NURSING DIAGNOSIS: Pain related to joint inflammation

■ **PATIENT GOAL 1:** Will exhibit signs of reduced joint inflammation

NURSING INTERVENTIONS/*RATIONALES*
*Administer antiinflammatory drugs as prescribed *to suppress inflammatory process of JRA*

EXPECTED OUTCOMES
Child exhibits no evidence of discomfort
Joints indicate no evidence of inflammation

■ **PATIENT GOAL 2:** Will experience either no pain or a reduction of pain to level acceptable to child

NURSING INTERVENTIONS/*RATIONALES*
Provide heat to painful joints *to relieve pain and stiffness:*
Tub baths, including whirlpool
Paraffin baths
Warm, moist pads
Soaks
*Maintain preventive schedule of drug administration *to reduce likelihood of pain occurring*
Avoid overexercising painful, swollen joints *because exercise at this time will aggravate pain*
Implement nonpharmacologic pain reduction techniques *to modify pain perception* (See p. 339.)
Provide well-balanced diet to avoid excess weight gain, *which can cause additional strain on inflamed joints*

EXPECTED OUTCOME
Child is able to move with no or minimum discomfort

NURSING DIAGNOSIS: Impaired physical mobility related to joint discomfort and stiffness

■ **PATIENT GOAL 1:** Will exhibit signs of adequate joint function

NURSING INTERVENTIONS/*RATIONALES*
Carry out or supervise physical therapy regimen, including:
Muscle-strengthening exercises
Joint mobilization exercises
Apply splints or sandbags, if needed, *to maintain position and reduce flexion deformity during rest*
Lay flat in bed on a firm mattress with joints extended *to reduce flexion deformity*
Use prone position frequently, with either no pillow or a very thin one, *to maintain good alignment of spine, hips, and knees*
Incorporate therapeutic exercises in play activities:
Swimming
Throwing a ball
Hanging from monkey bar
Riding tricycle or bicycle
Encourage child to be physically active but in a way that does not excessively strain affected joints (e.g., swimming)
Supervise and encourage activities of daily living *since these provide exercise*
Encourage child's natural tendency to be active
Frequently assess joint function *so that appropriate treatment is instituted to prevent deformity*

EXPECTED OUTCOMES
Joint flexibility improves in relation to baseline findings
Child develops no contractures
Child engages in activities suitable to interests, capabilities, and developmental level

NURSING DIAGNOSIS: Bathing/hygiene, dressing/grooming, feeding, or toileting self-care deficit related to discomfort, impaired joint mobility

---

*Dependent nursing action.

Continued

Unit 4

The Child with Juvenile Rheumatoid Arthritis—cont'd

■ **PATIENT GOAL 1:** Will perform activities of daily living

NURSING INTERVENTIONS/RATIONALES

Encourage maximum independence; avoid doing for child what child is capable of doing

Provide and/or help devise methods *to facilitate independent functioning:*

Select clothes for convenience in putting on and fastening

Modify utensils (spoons, toothbrush, comb, and so on) for easier grasp

Elevate toilet seat, if needed, *to facilitate independent toileting*

Install handrails for convenience and safety (in hallways, bathroom)

Teach application of splints (when able) and encourage responsibility for their use

EXPECTED OUTCOME

Child is involved in activities of daily living to maximum capabilities

■ **PATIENT GOAL 2:** Will maintain adequate energy level

NURSING INTERVENTIONS/RATIONALES

Schedule regular periods for sleep and rest, especially during acute flare-ups, *to conserve energy*

Include school nurse and teachers in planning for needed rest during school day

Encourage child to participate in activities *that do not cause excessive fatigue or overexertion*

EXPECTED OUTCOMES

Child engages in appropriate activities without undue fatigue

Child receives adequate rest, sleep

NURSING DIAGNOSIS: Knowledge deficit related to introduction of new medications and treatment modalities

■ **PATIENT (FAMILY) GOAL 1:** Will demonstrate knowledge of medications and treatment modalities

NURSING INTERVENTIONS/RATIONALES

Allow patient and parents to discuss concerns and fears *so that they are better able to learn*

Instruct in medication/treatment purpose, administration, side effects, and adverse reactions; repeat instructions as necessary *to ensure learning*

Provide written information/guidelines for all medications and treatments ordered *so that the family can refer to this as needed at home*

Involve patient/family in administration of medications and treatments

Document patient/family education

EXPECTED OUTCOMES

Patient/family will be knowledgeable about medication and treatment modalities

Patient/family will recognize signs of adverse drug reaction/side effects

NURSING DIAGNOSIS: Risk for body image disturbance related to disease process

■ **PATIENT GOAL 1:** Will express feelings and concerns

NURSING INTERVENTIONS/RATIONALES

Be available to child *so that there are opportunities for expression of feelings and concerns*

Use therapeutic communication techniques (e.g., reflection, active listening, silence) *to encourage expression of feelings and concerns*

Explore and develop activities in which child can succeed *to promote positive self-image*

Include child in therapy and treatment decisions *to promote positive self-image and decrease sense of powerlessness*

Refer child to a support group for children with JRA

EXPECTED OUTCOME

Child will express feelings and concerns

NURSING DIAGNOSIS: Risk for altered family processes related to a situational crisis (child with a chronic illness)

■ **PATIENT (FAMILY) GOAL 1:** Will receive adequate support as desired

NURSING INTERVENTIONS/RATIONALES AND EXPECTED OUTCOMES

Refer family to special support group(s) and agencies

(See also Nursing Care Plan: The Child with Chronic Illness or Disability, p. 287.)

NURSING CARE OF THE CHILD WITH SENSORY OR COGNITIVE IMPAIRMENT

Sensory and cognitive impairment includes problems of children with impaired vision and hearing and children with mental retardation.

NURSING CARE PLAN

The Child with Impaired Vision

Impaired vision refers to visual loss that cannot be corrected with regular prescription lenses.
Classifications of visual impairment:
> **Partially sighted**—Visual acuity above 20/200 but worse than 20/70 in the better eye, with correction

Legal blindness—Visual acuity of 20/200 or less and/or visual field of 20 degrees or less in the better eye

---

ASSESSMENT

Perform a physical assessment with special emphasis on assessment of the eyes. (See p. 44.)

(See vision screening, p. 134.)

Obtain a health history, especially relative to illness or injury that may have contributed to visual impairment; include prenatal history.

Obtain family history for diseases or defects with known hereditary predisposition.

At birth, assess neonate's response to visual stimuli (e.g., following light or object and cessation of body movements); observe for signs associated with congenital blindness.

Check for strabismus (lack of binocularity); refer to ophthalmologist for evaluation if malalignment persists past 4 months of age.

Test for visual acuity as soon as child is cooperative (sometimes by age 2 years).

Suspect blindness if infant does not react to light or in child of any age if parents express concern.

Observe for signs or behaviors that indicate eye problems (See p. 137.); include questions regarding behavioral indications of vision impairment in health histories.

Assume responsibility, as school nurse, for follow-up care of children who require corrective lenses or other types of treatments, such as patching.

Stress to parents importance of continued periodic eye examinations, since child's eyesight may change significantly in a short period.

Observe eye for manifestations of visual impairment. (See p. 46.)

NURSING DIAGNOSIS: Altered growth and development related to sensory/perceptual alterations (visual)

■ **PATIENT GOAL 1:** Will achieve optimum independence for age

NURSING INTERVENTIONS/*RATIONALES*

Provide visual-motor activities for infant (e.g., sitting in chair or swing, holding head up, standing, crawling, grasping for objects) *to promote optimum development*

Provide an environment that fosters familiarity and security; arrange furniture *to allow safe ambulation;* place identifying markers *to denote steps or other dangerous areas*

Enroll child in special programs for the blind as soon as possible *to learn independence skills, braille reading and writing, and navigational skills* (e.g., cane method, sighted guide, guide dog)

Encourage participation in active play *to promote optimum development*

Discuss need for experimenting with active play in safe environment and with other children *to encourage independence without compromising safety*

Discuss importance of discipline and limit-setting with family *since all children have this need*

EXPECTED OUTCOMES

Infant or child engages in appropriate activities for level of development (specify)

Child demonstrates an attitude of security in the environment

Appropriate discipline and limit-setting is provided

■ **PATIENT GOAL 2:** Will have opportunities for play/socialization

NURSING INTERVENTIONS/*RATIONALES*

Talk to child about the environment *to encourage play without compromising safety*

Guide family in selection of play materials *that encourage motor development and stimulate the senses of hearing and touch*

Discuss with family how play for visually impaired children differs from that for sighted children

Encourage family to initiate play activities and teach child how to use toys *because children with visual impairment do not automatically learn to play*

Assess adequacy of environmental stimulation if blindisms are present *because self-stimulatory activities develop to compensate for inadequate stimulation*

Use behavior modification to discourage blindisms *because such habits decrease child's social acceptance*

Discuss importance of consistent limit-setting *to help child learn acceptable behavior and tolerate frustration*

Discuss with child's family possible opportunities for socialization (e.g., preschools with sighted children)

EXPECTED OUTCOMES

Parents engage in appropriate activities with the child and have realistic expectations for child

Child engages in play and socialization activities appropriate to developmental level

---

NURSING DIAGNOSIS: Altered family processes related to diagnosis of blindness in a child

■ **PATIENT (FAMILY) GOAL 1:** Will adjust to child's loss of sight

NURSING INTERVENTIONS/*RATIONALES*

Anticipate grief reaction *as part of adjustment to loss*

Stress to family (and older child) that such feelings are normal and that grief takes time to resolve

Help family gain a realistic concept of child's disability and abilities *to encourage sense of hope*

Continued

Encourage formal rehabilitation as soon as realistically feasible *to promote optimum development of child*

Assist family in orienting newly blind child to environment and in making immediate surroundings safe *to encourage ambulation*

Listen to family's feelings and concerns regarding child's visual loss *to encourage coping*

Refer to community agencies and support groups *for ongoing support and assistance*

EXPECTED OUTCOMES

Parents express their feelings and concerns regarding child's loss of sight

Parents demonstrate an understanding of child's disability and its implications

■ **PATIENT (FAMILY) GOAL 2:** Will demonstrate parent-child attachment behaviors

NURSING INTERVENTIONS/*RATIONALES*

Help parents identify cues from infant, other than eye contact, that signify communication with them *since eye contact is normally important in facilitating attachment*

Encourage parents to discuss their feelings regarding lack of visual contact or smiling from child *since parents may misinterpret this as rejection*

Stress that lack of such responses is not an indication of child's rejection or dislike of parents *since parents may misinterpret this*

Demonstrate your own acceptance of child *to encourage family's acceptance of child*

Emphasize positive abilities or attributes *to encourage parent-child attachment and discourage rejection*

Encourage parents in their attempts to promote child's development

EXPECTED OUTCOME

Parents and child exhibit a positive relationship

NURSING DIAGNOSIS: Risk for injury related to environmental hazards, noncompliance with therapeutic plan

■ **PATIENT GOAL 1:** Will not experience visual impairment

NURSING INTERVENTIONS/*RATIONALES*

Participate in prenatal screening for pregnant women at risk (e.g., those with rubella, syphilis, family history of genetic disorders associated with visual loss) *for early identification and treatment of visual impairment*

Provide prophylactic eye care at birth *to prevent ophthalmia neonatorum*

Provide adequate prenatal care *to prevent prematurity*

Administer oxygen cautiously to premature infant *to prevent retinopathy of prematurity*

Periodically screen all children from birth through adolescence *for early identification and treatment of visual impairment*

Participate in immunization programs for children *to prevent visual impairment*

Teach safety regarding common causes of eye injuries (Guidelines box) *since trauma is the leading cause of blindness*

Recommend use of face mask and helmet for children playing baseball, softball, hockey, and football *to prevent eye trauma*

Stress importance of good eye care (e.g., use of proper lighting, avoidance of excessive close work, proper rest and nutrition, and yearly eye examinations)

Encourage compliance with corrective treatment for eye problems *to prevent further ocular damage*

EXPECTED OUTCOMES

Healthy child does not acquire visual defect

Child is properly immunized

Child complies with measures to prevent visual impairment

■ **PATIENT GOAL 2:** Will exhibit no complications from eye trauma

NURSING INTERVENTIONS/*RATIONALES*

Provide appropriate emergency care (emergency treatment, Box 4-29) *to prevent further eye injury*

Discuss eye injury in a sensitive manner *to avoid any implication of guilt*

Reassure parent and child but avoid giving false reassurance *to encourage realistic understanding of eye condition*

Apprise parents and child of each step of treatment, especially if therapy interferes with vision (e.g., patching eyes) *to encourage compliance*

Teach family correct procedure for instilling ophthalmic preparations (always in conjunctival cul-de-sac) *to prevent further eye injury*

EXPECTED OUTCOME

Child exhibits no evidence of complications from eye trauma

■ **PATIENT GOAL 3:** Will exhibit no complications of eye defects

NURSING INTERVENTIONS/*RATIONALES*

Encourage compliance with corrective therapies *so that child receives appropriate care and complications are prevented*

For strabismus:

Discuss with school-age child necessity of patch in preserving vision; allow child to verbalize feelings regarding altered facial appearance; help overcome visual difficulties imposed by seeing with weaker eye (favorable seating in school, large-print books, additional time to complete assignments) *because strabismus, if untreated, can result in blindness from amblyopia*

Teach parents correct procedures for instilling anticholinesterase drugs *to ensure adequate treatment*

For refractive errors:

Recommend glasses with rounded temporal pieces or attach elastic strap to handles and around back of head *for secure fit of glasses*

Include older child in selection of frames *to encourage child to wear glasses*

Encourage parents to compare value of more expensive, attractive frames and inducement for wearing them against cost

If glasses are recommended for continuous wearing, discuss possibility of temporary removal for special occasions *to encourage compliance*

Encourage use of protective shields during contact sports *to prevent eye trauma*

Stress improvement in visual acuity as reason for wearing glasses *to encourage compliance*

Discuss feasibility of contact lenses with selected families, *since they are a popular alternative to glasses*

Know procedures for care, insertion, and removal of contact lens; teach these to parents and older children *to prevent eye injury and complications*

EXPECTED OUTCOMES

Child and family comply with therapy and perform procedures correctly

Child wears corrective lenses and cares for equipment correctly

(See also Nursing Care Plan: The Child with Chronic Illness or Disability, p. 287.)

GUIDELINES

Preventing Eye Injuries

Infants and Toddlers

Avoid any toys with long, pointed handles, such as a pinwheel on a stick.

Keep pointed instruments and tools out of reach (e.g., scissors, knives, screwdrivers, rulers, pencils, sticks).

Do not allow child to *walk* or *run* with any pointed object in the hand (e.g., spoon, lollipop, toothbrush).

Keep child away from play of older children and adults that involves projectile activities (e.g., throwing a ball, golf, target shooting, swings).

Stress importance of fire safety and poison protection in preventing thermal/chemical burns to the eye.

Shield child's eyes when in direct sunlight.

Preschoolers

Supervise the use of sharp or pointed objects, especially scissors.

Teach proper use of pointed objects such as toy guns or scissors (namely, to always point them *away* from their face or from anyone else at close range).

Teach child to walk carefully (never run) while carrying any sharp or pointed object.

Keep child away from projectile activities.

Begin teaching respect for firearms.

Avoid play with mirrors, especially where they can reflect sunlight.

School-age Children and Adolescents

Teach proper use and respect for potentially dangerous equipment such as power tools (objects fly from them), firearms, firecrackers (where legally permitted), and racquet sports.

Stress use of eye protection when riding motorcycles or when using equipment such as power saws or chemistry sets.

Teach child to open soda bottles by pointing screw cap away from face.

Encourage safe use of curling iron.

Advise child of danger of excessive sunlight (ultraviolet burns).

Warn child to never look directly at the sun, even with sunglasses; and to avoid using mirror in sunlight.

Monitor duration of wear of contact lens to prevent corneal scratching and possible scarring.

BOX 4-29

Emergency Care of Eye Injuries

Foreign Object

Examine eye for presence of a foreign body (evert upper lid to examine upper eye).

Remove a freely movable object with pointed corner of gauze pad lightly moistened with water.

Do not irrigate eye or attempt to remove a penetrating object (see below).

Caution child against rubbing eye.

Chemical Burns

Irrigate eye copiously with tap water for 20 minutes.

Evert upper lid to flush thoroughly.

Hold child's head with eye under tap of running lukewarm water.

Take to emergency room.

Have child rest with eyes closed.

Keep room darkened.

Ultraviolet Burns

If skin is burned, patch both eyes (make sure lids are completely closed); secure dressing with Kling bandages wrapped around head rather than tape.

Have child rest with eyes closed.

Refer to an ophthalmologist.

Hematoma ("Black Eye")

Use a flashlight to check for gross hyphema (hemorrhage into anterior chamber; visible fluid meniscus across iris; more easily seen in light-colored than in brown eyes).

Apply ice for first 24 hours to reduce swelling if no hyphema is present.

Refer to an ophthalmologist immediately if hyphema is present.

Have child rest with eyes closed.

Penetrating Injuries

Take child to emergency room.

Never remove an object that has penetrated eye.

Follow strict aseptic technique in examining eye.

Observe for the following:

  Aqueous or vitreous leaks (fluid leaking from point of penetration)

  Hyphema

  Shape and equality of pupils, reaction to light

  Prolapsed iris (not perfectly circular)

Apply a Fox shield if available (not a regular eye patch) and apply patch over unaffected eye to prevent bilateral movement.

Maintain bed rest with child in 30-degree Fowler position.

Caution child against rubbing eye.

NURSING CARE PLAN

The Child with Impaired Hearing

For classification of complete or partial loss of hearing, see Table 4-38.

Hearing impairment—Disability that may range in severity from mild to profound

Deaf—Hearing disability precludes successful processing of linguistic information through audition, with or without a hearing aid

Hard-of-hearing—Residual hearing, with a hearing aid, sufficient to enable successful processing of linguistic information through audition

Types of hearing loss:

Conductive (middle ear)—Interference with transmission of sound to the middle ear; mainly involves interference with loudness of sound

Sensorineural (perceptive or nerve deafness)—Involves damage to the inner ear structures and/or auditory nerve; sounds are distorted, severely affecting discrimination and comprehension

Mixed conductive-sensorineural—Interference with transmission of sound in the middle ear and along neural pathways; frequently results from recurrent otitis media and its complications

Central auditory imperception—All hearing losses that do not demonstrate defects in the conductive or sensorineural structures

ASSESSMENT

Perform a physical assessment; note any associated anomalies (e.g., low-set ears).

(See also assessment of the ears, p. 16.)

Obtain a family history, especially regarding members with hearing impairment:

Prenatal and perinatal history, especially regarding illness or drugs during gestation, type and duration of delivery, Apgar score, hypoxia, hyperbilirubinemia, admittance to neonatal intensive care unit

Health history, especially regarding immunizations, serious illnesses, seizures, high fever, ototoxic drugs, ear infection

History of responses to auditory stimuli, previous audiometric testing

History of motor development, self-care, adaptive behaviors, socialization behaviors (e.g., temper tantrums, vibratory stimulation, stubbornness), recent behavioral/personality changes

Observe for manifestations of hearing impairment:

Infants

Lack of startle or blink reflex to a loud sound

Failure to be awakened by loud environmental noises

Failure to localize a source of sound by 6 months of age

Absence of babble or inflections in voice by age 7 months

General indifference to sound

Lack of response to the spoken word; failure to follow verbal directions

Response to loud noises as opposed to the voice

Children

Use of gestures rather than verbalization to express desires, especially after 15 months

Failure to develop intelligible speech by age 24 months

Monotone quality, unintelligible speech, lessened laughter

Vocal play, head banging, or foot stamping for vibratory sensation

Yelling or screeching to express pleasure, annoyance (tantrums), or need

Asking to have statements repeated or answering them incorrectly

Responding more to facial expressions and gestures than verbal explanations

Avoidance of social interactions; often puzzled and unhappy in such situations, prefers to play alone

Inquiring, sometimes confused facial expressions

Suspicious alertness, sometimes interpreted as paranoia, alternating with cooperation

Frequently stubborn because of lack of comprehension

Irritable at not making self understood

Shy, timid, and withdrawn

Child often appears "dreamy," "in a world of his or her own," or markedly inattentive

Refer for hearing evaluation if family expresses concern about child's hearing and speech development.

Perform or assist with audiometry testing, auditory evoked potential testing, tympanometry, or auditory acuity measurements.

The Child with Impaired Hearing—cont'd

TABLE 4-38   Classifications of Hearing Loss Based on Symptom Severity

Hearing Level (dB)	Effect
Slight: <30 (hard of hearing)	Has difficulty hearing faint or distant speech
	Usually is unaware of hearing difficulty
	Likely to achieve in school but may have problems
	No speech defects
Mild: 30-55 (hard of hearing)	Understands conversational speech at 3 to 5 feet but has difficulty if speech is faint or if not facing speaker
	May have speech difficulties
Moderate: 55-70 (hard of hearing)	Unable to understand conversational speech unless loud
	Considerable difficulty with group or classroom discussion
	Requires special speech training
Profound: 70-90 (deaf)	May hear a loud noise if nearby
	May be able to identify loud environmental noises
	Can distinguish vowels but not most consonants
	Requires speech training
Extreme: >90 (deaf)	May hear only loud sounds
	Requires extensive speech training

NURSING DIAGNOSIS: Sensory/perceptual alterations (auditory) related to hearing impairment

- **PATIENT GOAL 1:** Will experience maximum hearing potential

NURSING INTERVENTIONS/*RATIONALES*

Help family investigate hearing aid dealers *to locate a reliable one*

Discuss types of hearing aids and their proper care *to ensure maximum benefit*

Stress to family importance of storing hearing aid batteries safely, and of supervising young children or teaching older children not to remove the battery, *to prevent ingestion/aspiration of batteries*

Teach child how to regulate hearing aid *for maximum benefit*

Help child focus on all sounds in the environment and talk about them *to maximize hearing*

Encourage child to help select hearing aid (e.g., hearing aids in bright colors)

For older child, discuss methods of camouflaging the aid *to make it less conspicuous.*

For child with severe sensorineural loss, emphasize benefit of early use of cochlear implant

EXPECTED OUTCOMES

Child acquires and uses hearing aid properly

Child does not ingest/aspirate hearing aid battery

Family is aware of benefit of cochlear implant

NURSING DIAGNOSIS: Impaired verbal communication related to inability to hear auditory cues

- **PATIENT/FAMILY GOAL 1:** Will engage in communication process within limits of impairment

NURSING INTERVENTIONS/*RATIONALES*

Encourage family to attend rehabilitation program *to continue learning in the home;* encourage them to learn sign language *as a method of communication*

Teach language that serves a useful purpose *for communication*

Encourage use of language and books in the home *to stimulate verbal communication and promote normal development*

Encourage spontaneous language and correct speech *to promote speech development*

EXPECTED OUTCOMES

Child and family continue communication practices in home environment

Family provides stimulation to child

- **PATIENT GOAL 2:** Will demonstrate ability to lip-read

NURSING INTERVENTIONS/*RATIONALES*

Test child for visual problems *that may interfere with learning to lip-read or use sign language*

Teach family and others involved with child (e.g., teacher) behaviors that facilitate lipreading (Guidelines box) *to promote communication process*

EXPECTED OUTCOMES

Child communicates with others in manner taught (specify)

Persons communicating with child use good communication techniques

NURSING DIAGNOSIS: Altered growth and development related to impaired communication

- **PATIENT GOAL 1:** Will achieve optimum independence for age

NURSING INTERVENTIONS/*RATIONALES*

Help family transfer normal childrearing practices to this child *to promote optimum development*

Unit 4

Continued

The Child with Impaired Hearing—cont'd

Emphasize importance of attaining independence in self-care

Provide child with devices that foster independence (e.g., hearing ear dog, special signaling aids for telephone or doorbell)

Discuss with family importance of discipline and limit-setting *since all children have this need*

EXPECTED OUTCOMES

Child performs activities of daily living appropriate to level of development

Appropriate discipline and limit-setting is provided

■ **PATIENT GOAL 2:** Will have opportunity to participate in activities for play and socialization

NURSING INTERVENTIONS/*RATIONALES*

Guide family in selection of toys *to maximize visual and tactile senses, as well as residual hearing*

Encourage child to participate in group activities (e.g., Scouting, sports) *to promote socialization*

Help child follow group discussion by pointing out the speaker and arranging the group in a semicircle *to facilitate hearing and/or lipreading*

Help child develop friendships among hearing and deaf peers *to promote socialization*

Recommend closed-captioned TV *for child's enjoyment*

EXPECTED OUTCOMES

Child engages in activities appropriate to developmental level

Child has peer relationships and experiences

■ **PATIENT GOAL 3:** Will be provided educational opportunities within a regular classroom

NURSING INTERVENTIONS/*RATIONALES*

Discuss with teacher and other children ways of communicating effectively with child (e.g., through lipreading) *to facilitate child's education*

Promote socialization with classmates *to encourage enjoyment of education*

EXPECTED OUTCOMES

Child attends school regularly

Child communicates with others in the classroom

> **NURSING DIAGNOSIS:** Altered family processes related to diagnosis of deafness of a child

■ **PATIENT (FAMILY) GOAL 1:** Will adjust to child's hearing loss

NURSING INTERVENTIONS/*RATIONALES*

Anticipate grief reaction as part of adjustment to loss

Provide opportunities for family to express feelings and concerns *to promote adjustment*

Help family deal with feelings regarding previous responses to child when true nature of the problem was unknown *to minimize feelings of guilt*

Help family realize extent of child's disability and its tremendous influence on speech and language development

Discuss advantages and limitations of amplifying devices with different types of hearing loss *so that family can make informed decisions*

Encourage formal rehabilitation as soon as possible *to foster normal growth and development of child*

EXPECTED OUTCOMES

Family expresses feelings and concerns regarding child's loss of hearing

Family demonstrates an understanding of the implications of hearing loss

Family becomes involved in appropriate programs

■ **PATIENT (FAMILY) GOAL 2:** Will receive emotional support

NURSING INTERVENTIONS/*RATIONALES*

Be available to family *for assistance and support*

Encourage family members to discuss their feelings regarding the disability *to enhance coping*

Stress child's abilities rather than disability *to promote child's optimum development*

Become familiar with techniques used for communication if following the family on a long-term basis

Refer family to appropriate community agencies for medical, psychiatric, educational, vocational, or financial assistance *to ensure that their overall needs are met*

Involve parents in local parent groups for deaf children *for continuing support*

EXPECTED OUTCOMES

Family expresses feelings and concerns about the disability and its ramifications

Family members avail themselves of available resources

■ **PATIENT (FAMILY) GOAL 3:** Will demonstrate attachment to child

NURSING INTERVENTIONS/*RATIONALES*

Help family identify clues other than verbal ones that signify infant's communication with them *because communication is an important part of attachment process*

Encourage family to stimulate child with visual and tactile cues *since auditory cues are absent or diminished*

Stress importance of continuing to talk to child even though child may not hear their voices *to promote normalization*

EXPECTED OUTCOME

Parents and child demonstrate a positive relationship

> **NURSING DIAGNOSIS:** Risk for injury related to environmental hazards, infection

■ **PATIENT (OTHERS) GOAL 1:** Will not acquire or have greater hearing loss

NURSING INTERVENTIONS/*RATIONALES*

Infancy:

Encourage immunization at appropriate age *to prevent acquired sensorineural hearing loss from childhood diseases*

Minimize noise levels in intensive care unit *since this is associated with hearing loss*

Prevent ear infection; detect early *because this is the most common cause of impaired hearing*

Childhood:

Asses hearing ability of infants and children receiving ototoxic antibiotics *for early detection*

Promote compliance with treatment regimens for otitis media *since this is a common cause of impaired hearing*

The Child with Impaired Hearing—cont'd

Discuss with parents measures to prevent otitis media

Evaluate auditory ability of children prone to chronic ear or respiratory problems *for early detection of impaired hearing*

Assess sources of excessive noise in child's environment: institute appropriate measures to decrease sound levels (turn music lower, use ear protection) *because exposure to excessive noise is a cause of sensorineural hearing loss*

Participate in immunization programs for children *to prevent childhood diseases that may result in hearing loss*

EXPECTED OUTCOMES

Infant or child does not develop hearing loss

Child is not exposed to excessive noise levels

Child is properly immunized

(See also Nursing Care Plan: The Child with Chronic Illness or Disability, p. 287.)

GUIDELINES

Facilitating Lipreading

Attract child's attention before speaking: use light touch to signal speaker's presence.

Stand close to child.

Face child directly, or move to a 45-degree angle.

Stand still: do not walk back and forth or turn away to point or look elsewhere.

Establish eye contact and show interest.

Speak at eye level and with good lighting on speaker's face.

Be certain nothing interferes with speech patterns, such as chewing food or gum.

Speak clearly and with a slow and even rate.

Use facial expression to assist in conveying messages.

Keep sentences short.

Rephrase message if child does not understand the words.

NURSING CARE PLAN

The Child with Mental Retardation

Mental retardation (MR) is a subaverage intellectual functioning existing concurrently with deficits in adaptive behavior and onset before 18 years of age.*

Table 4-39 describes the classification of mental retardation.

ASSESSMENT

Perform a physical assessment.

Perform a developmental assessment.

Obtain a family history, especially regarding mental retardation and hereditary disorders in which mental retardation is a feature.

Obtain a health history for evidence of:
Prenatal, perinatal, or postnatal trauma or physical injury
Prenatal maternal infection (e.g., rubella), alcoholism, drug consumption
Inadequate nutrition
Deprived environment
Psychiatric disorders (e.g., autism)
Infections, especially those involving the brain (e.g., meningitis, encephalitis, measles) or a high body temperature
Chromosomal abnormality
Assist with diagnostic tests (e.g., chromosome analysis, metabolic dysfunction, radiography, tomography, electroencephalography).

Perform or assist with intelligence tests:
Bayley Mental and Motor Scales (infants)
Cattell Infant Intelligence Scale
Wechsler Preschool and Primary Scales of Intelligence (WPPSI-R) (preschoolers)
Wechsler Intelligence Scale for Children (WISC III) (school-age children)
Perform or assist with testing of adaptive behaviors:
Vineland Social Maturity Scale
AAMR Adaptive Behavior Scale
Observe for early manifestations of mental retardation:
Nonresponsiveness to contact
Poor eye contact during feeding
Diminished spontaneous activity
Decreased alertness to voice or movement
Irritability
Slow feeding

*American Association on Mental Retardation (AAMR).

TABLE 4-39 Classification of Mental Retardation

Level (IQ)	Preschool (Birth-5 Years)— Maturation and Development	School Age (6-21 Years)— Training and Education	Adult (21 Years and Older)— Social and Vocational Adequacy
Mild: 50-55 to approximately 70	Often not noticed as retarded by casual observer but is slower to walk, feed self, and talk than most children; follows same sequence in development as normal children	Can acquire practical skills and useful reading and arithmetic to a third to sixth grade level with special education; can be guided toward social conformity; achieves mental age of 8-12 years	Can usually achieve social and vocational skills adequate to self-maintenance; may need occasional guidance and support when under unusual social or economic stress; can adjust to marriage but not childrearing
Moderate: 35-40 to 50-55	Noticeable delays in motor development, especially in speech; responds to training in various self-help activities	Can learn simple communication, elementary health and safety habits, and simple manual skills; does not progress in functional reading or arithmetic; achieves mental age of 3-7 years	Can perform simple tasks under sheltered conditions; participates in simple recreation; travels alone in familiar places; usually incapable of self-maintenance
Severe: 20-25 to 35-40	Marked delay in motor development; little or no communication skills; may respond to training in elementary self-care (e.g., self-feeding)	Usually walks, barring specific disability; has some understanding of speech and some response; can profit from systematic habit training; achieves mental age of toddler	Can conform to daily routines and repetitive activities; needs continuing direction and supervision in protective environment
Profound: below 20-25	Gross retardation; minimum capacity for functioning in sensorimotor areas; needs total care	Obvious delays in all areas of development; shows basic emotional responses; may respond to skillful training in use of legs, hands, and jaws; needs close supervision; achieves mental age of young infant	May walk; needs complete custodial care; has primitive speech; usually benefits from regular physical activity

Data from American Psychiatric Association: *Diagnostic and statistical manual of mental disorders (DSM-IV)*, ed 4, Washington, DC, 1994, The Association.

The Child with Mental Retardation—cont'd

NURSING DIAGNOSIS: Altered growth and development related to impaired cognitive functioning

- **PATIENT GOAL 1:** Will achieve optimum growth and development potential

NURSING INTERVENTIONS/*RATIONALES*

Involve child and family in an early infant stimulation program *to help maximize child's development*

Assess child's developmental progress at regular intervals; keep detailed records to distinguish subtle changes in functioning *so that plan of care can be revised as needed*

Help family determine child's readiness to learn specific tasks *since readiness may not be easily recognized*

Help family set realistic goals for child *to encourage successful attainment of goals and to support self-esteem*

Employ positive reinforcement for specific tasks or behaviors *because this improves motivation and learning*

Encourage learning of self-care skills as soon as child is ready

Reinforce self-care activities *to facilitate optimum development*

Encourage family to investigate special daycare programs and educational classes as soon as possible

Emphasize that child has same needs as other children (e.g., play, discipline, social interaction)

Before adolescence, counsel child and parents regarding physical maturation, sexual behavior, marriage, and childrearing

Encourage optimum vocational training

EXPECTED OUTCOMES

Child and family are actively involved in infant stimulation program

Family applies developmental concepts and continues activities in home care of child

Child performs activities of daily living at optimum capacity

Family investigates special educational programs

Appropriate limit-setting, recreation, and social opportunities are provided

Adolescent issues are explored as appropriate

- **PATIENT GOAL 2:** Will achieve optimum socialization

NURSING INTERVENTIONS/*RATIONALES*

Emphasize that child has same need for socialization as other children

Encourage family to teach child socially acceptable behavior (e.g., saying "hello" and "thank you," manners, appropriate touch)

Encourage grooming and age-appropriate dress *to encourage acceptance by others and to support self-esteem*

Recommend programs that provide peer relationships and experiences (e.g., mainstreaming, Boy Scouts, Girl Scouts, Special Olympics) *to promote optimum socialization*

Provide adolescent with practical sexual information and a well-defined, concrete code of conduct *because child's easy persuasion and lack of judgment may place child at risk*

EXPECTED OUTCOMES

Child behaves in socially acceptable manner

Child has peer relationships and experiences

Child does not experience social isolation

NURSING DIAGNOSIS: Risk for altered family processes related to having a child with MR

- **PATIENT (FAMILY) GOAL 1:** Will receive adequate information and support

NURSING INTERVENTIONS/*RATIONALES*

Inform family at or as soon as possible after birth *since family may suspect a problem and need immediate support*

Have both parents present at informing conference *to avoid problem of one parent having to relay complex information to the other parent and deal with the initial emotional reaction of the other*

Give family, when possible, written information about the condition (e.g., a specific syndrome or disease) *for family to refer to later*

Discuss with family members the pros and cons of home care and other placement options; allow them opportunities to investigate all residential alternatives before making a decision

Encourage family to meet other families that have a child with a similar diagnosis *so that they can receive additional support*

Refrain from giving definitive answers about the degree of retardation; stress the potential learning abilities of each child, especially with early intervention, *to encourage hope*

Demonstrate acceptance of child through own behavior *because parents are sensitive to the affective attitude of the professional*

Emphasize normal characteristics of child *to help family see child as an individual with strengths as well as weaknesses*

Encourage family members to express their feelings and concerns *because this is part of the adaptation process and effective collaboration*

EXPECTED OUTCOMES

Family members' needs for information and support are met

Family expresses feelings and concerns regarding the birth of a child with MR and its implications

Family members make realistic decisions based on their needs and capabilities

Family members demonstrate acceptance of child

- **PATIENT (FAMILY) GOAL 2:** Will be prepared for long-term care of child

NURSING INTERVENTIONS/*RATIONALES*

Discuss with parents alternatives to home care, especially as child grows older and as parents near retirement or old age, *so that appropriate long-term care can be provided*

Encourage family to consider respite care as needed *to facilitate family's ability to cope with child's long-term care*

Help family investigate residential settings *since this may be needed for child's optimum care*

Encourage family to include affected member in planning and to continue meaningful relationships after placement

Refer to agencies that provide support and assistance

EXPECTED OUTCOMES

Family identifies realistic goals for future care of child

Family avails themselves of supportive services as desired

(See also Nursing Care Plan: The Child with Chronic Illness or Disability, p. 287.)

Unit 4

NURSING CARE PLAN

The Child with Down Syndrome

Down syndrome is a chromosomal abnormality characterized by varying degrees of mental retardation and associated physical defects; also known as *trisomy 21.*

ASSESSMENT

Perform a physical assessment.

Perform a developmental assessment.

Obtain a family history, especially relative to mother's age or
any similarly affected child in the family.

Observe for manifestations of Down syndrome:

Physical characteristics (most frequently observed)

Small, rounded skull with a flat occiput

Inner epicanthal folds and oblique palpebral fissures
(upward, outward slant of the eyes)

Small nose with a depressed bridge (saddle nose)

Protruding, sometimes fissured, tongue

Hypoplastic mandible (makes tongue appear large)

High-arched, narrow palate

Short, thick neck

Hypotonic musculature (protruding abdomen, umbilical
hernia)

Hyperflexible and lax joints

Simian line (transverse crease on the palmar side of the
hand)

Broad, short, and stubby hands and feet

Intelligence

Varies from severely retarded to low normal intelligence

Generally within mild to moderate range

Language delay more severe than cognitive delay

Congenital anomalies (increased incidence)

Most common is congenital heart disease

Other defects include:

Renal agenesis

Duodenal atresia

Hirschsprung disease

Tracheoesophageal fistula

Patella dislocation

Hip subluxation

Instability of the first and second cervical vertebrae
(atlantoaxial instability)

Sensory problems (frequently associated)

May include the following:

Conductive, mixed, or sensorineural hearing loss (very
common)

Strabismus

Myopia

Nystagmus

Cataracts

Conjunctivitis

Growth and sexual development

Growth in both height and weight reduced; obesity common

Sexual development delayed, incomplete, or both

Males infertile; females can be fertile

Premature aging common; lowered life expectancy

Assist with diagnostic tests (e.g., chromosome analysis).

NURSING DIAGNOSIS: Risk for infection related
to hypotonia, increased susceptibility to respiratory
infection

■ **PATIENT GOAL 1:** Will exhibit no evidence of respiratory
infection

NURSING INTERVENTIONS/*RATIONALES*

Teach family to use good handwashing technique *to minimize
exposure to infective organisms*

Stress importance of changing child's position frequently, especially use sitting postures *to prevent pooling of secretions and facilitate lung expansion*

Encourage use of cool-mist vaporizer *to prevent crusting of
nasal secretions and drying of mucous membranes*

Teach family suctioning of nose with bulb-type syringe (See
p. 629.) *because the child's underdeveloped nasal bone
causes a chronic problem of inadequate drainage of
mucus*

Stress importance of good mouth care (e.g., follow feedings
with clear water), brush teeth *to keep mouth as clean as
possible*

Encourage compliance with recommended immunizations *to
prevent infection*

Stress importance of completing full course of antibiotics, if
ordered, *for successful eradication of infection and prevention of growth of resistant organisms*

EXPECTED OUTCOME

Child exhibits no evidence of respiratory infection or distress

---

NURSING DIAGNOSIS: Impaired swallowing related
to hypotonia, large tongue, cognitive impairment

■ **PATIENT GOAL 1:** Feeding difficulties in infancy will be
minimized

NURSING INTERVENTIONS/*RATIONALES*

Suction nares before each feeding, if needed, *to remove
mucus*

Schedule small frequent feedings; allow child to rest during
feedings *because sucking and eating for any length of
time is difficult with mouth-breathing*

Explain to family that tongue thrust is a normal response
of child's protruding tongue and does not indicate refusal
of food

Feed solid food by pushing it to back and side of mouth; use
long, straight-handled infant spoon; if food is thrust out,
refeed

The Child with Down Syndrome—cont'd

Calculate caloric needs to meet energy requirements; base intake on height and weight, not chronologic age *since growth tends to be slower in children with Down syndrome*

Monitor height and weight at regular intervals *to evaluate nutritional intake*

Refer to specialists for specific feeding problems

EXPECTED OUTCOMES

Infant consumes an adequate amount of food for age and size (specify)

Family reports satisfactory feeding

Infant gains weight in accordance with standard weight tables

Family avails themselves of specialist services

NURSING DIAGNOSIS: Risk for constipation related to hypotonia

---

■ **PATIENT GOAL 1:** Will exhibit no evidence of constipation

NURSING INTERVENTIONS/*RATIONALES*

Monitor frequency and characteristics of bowel movements *to detect constipation*

Promote adequate hydration *to prevent constipation*

Provide child high-fiber diet (See Box 4-22, p. 405.) *to promote stool evacuation*

*Administer stool softener, suppository, or laxative as needed and as ordered *for bowel elimination*

EXPECTED OUTCOME

Child will not experience constipation

NURSING DIAGNOSIS: Risk for injury related to hypotonia, hyperextensibility of joints, atlantoaxial instability

---

■ **PATIENT GOAL 1:** Will not experience injuries associated with physical activity

NURSING INTERVENTIONS/*RATIONALES*

Recommend play and sports activities appropriate to child's physical maturation, size, coordination, and endurance *to avoid injuries*

Recommend that child who participates in sports that may involve stress on head and neck (e.g., high jump, gymnastics, diving) be evaluated radiologically for atlantoaxial instability

Teach family and other caregivers (e.g., teachers, coaches) symptoms of atlantoaxial instability (neck pain, weakness, torticollis) *so that appropriate care is received*

Report immediately signs of spinal cord compression (e.g., persistent neck pain, loss of established motor skills and bladder/bowel control, changes in sensation) *to prevent delay in treatment*

EXPECTED OUTCOMES

Child will participate in appropriate play activities and sports

Child will not experience injuries associated with physical activity

---

NURSING DIAGNOSIS: Altered family processes related to having a child with Down syndrome

---

(See Nursing Care Plan: The Child with Mental Retardation, p. 526.)

(See also Nursing Care Plan: The Child with Chronic Illness or Disability, p. 287.)

■ **PATIENT (FAMILY) GOAL 1:** Will exhibit parent-infant attachment behaviors

NURSING INTERVENTIONS/*RATIONALES*

Demonstrate acceptance of child through your own behaviors *because parents are sensitive to affective attitudes of others*

Explain to family that infant's lack of molding or clinging is a physical characteristic of Down syndrome *because this may be easily misinterpreted as a sign of detachment or rejection*

Encourage parents to swaddle or wrap infant tightly in a blanket *to provide security and compensate for lack of molding and clinging*

(See also Nursing Care Plan: The Normal Newborn and Family, p. 345.)

EXPECTED OUTCOME

Parent and child will demonstrate attachment behaviors (specify)

■ **PATIENT (FAMILY) GOAL 2:** Family will be prepared for care of associated defect(s) (specify)

NURSING INTERVENTIONS/*RATIONALES*

(See Nursing Care Plan: The Child with Congenital Heart Disease, p. 435.)

(See also Nursing Care Plan: The Child with Acute Respiratory Infection, p. 381.)

Refer family to community agencies and support groups

EXPECTED OUTCOME

Family is able to cope with the care needed by the specific health problem (specify)

■ **PATIENT (FAMILY) GOAL 3:** Will receive adequate support

NURSING INTERVENTIONS/*RATIONALES*

Refer to genetic counseling services, if indicated and/or desired, *for information and support*

Refer to organizations and parent groups designed for families with a child with Down syndrome *for continued support*

Emphasize positive aspects of rearing child at home *to help family maximize child's developmental potential*

EXPECTED OUTCOMES

Family members avail themselves of support groups

Family demonstrates positive attitude

---

*Dependent nursing action.

Continued

Unit 4

The Child with Down Syndrome—cont'd

NURSING DIAGNOSIS: Altered growth and development related to impaired cognitive functioning

- **PATIENT GOAL 1:** Will achieve optimum growth and development

**NURSING INTERVENTIONS/*RATIONALES*
AND EXPECTED OUTCOMES**
(See Nursing Care Plan: The Child with Mental Retardation, p. 526.)

NURSING DIAGNOSIS: Risk for injury (physical) related to parental age factors

- **PATIENT (OTHERS) GOAL 1:** Down syndrome will be prevented

NURSING INTERVENTIONS/*RATIONALES*
Discuss, with high-risk women, the hazards of giving birth to a child with Down syndrome *so that the family can make informed reproductive decisions*
Encourage all pregnant women at risk (i.e., over age 35, family history of Down syndrome, or previous birth of child with Down syndrome) to consider chorionic villus sampling or amniocentesis *to rule out Down syndrome in fetus*
Discuss options of elective abortion or proceeding with pregnancy with women who are carrying an affected fetus
Discuss with parents of adolescent children with Down syndrome the possibility of conception in a female and the need for contraceptive methods *for family to make informed reproductive decisions*

EXPECTED OUTCOMES
Pregnant women at risk seek evaluation for Down syndrome
Families demonstrate an understanding of options available to them
Families of an affected female child seek contraceptive advice

NURSING CARE OF THE CHILD WITH A COMMUNICABLE AND/OR SKIN DISEASE

Children are prone to a number of skin disorders, including those known as **childhood communicable diseases.**

NURSING CARE PLAN

The Child with a Communicable Disease

A **communicable disease** is an illness caused by a specific infectious agent or its toxic products through a direct or indirect mode of transmission of that agent from a reservoir.

ASSESSMENT

Perform a physical assessment.

Obtain an immunization history.

Obtain a history of exposure to disease and a history of past and current illnesses.

Observe for manifestations characteristic of each disease:

Type, configuration, and distribution of lesions

Type and characteristics of associated manifestations

Table 4-40 describes the major communicable diseases of childhood.

Assist with diagnostic procedures (e.g., collection of specimens).

Continued

Unit 4

The Child with a Communicable Disease—cont'd

TABLE 4-40   Communicable Diseases of Childhood

Disease

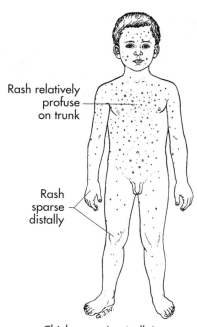

Rash relatively profuse on trunk

Rash sparse distally

Chickenpox (varicella)

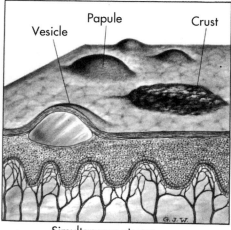

Vesicle   Papule   Crust

Simultaneous stages
of lesions in chickenpox

Chickenpox (Varicella)

Agent: Varicella zoster virus (VZV)

Source: Primary secretions of respiratory tract of infected person; to a lesser degree, skin lesions (scabs not infectious)

Transmission: Direct contact, droplet (airborne) spread, and contaminated objects

Incubation period: 2-3 weeks, usually 13-17 days

Period of communicability: Probably 1 day before eruption of lesions (prodromal period) to 6 days after first crop of vesicles when crusts have formed

Diphtheria

Agent: *Corynebacterium diphtheriae*

Source: Discharges from mucous membranes of nose and nasopharynx, skin, and other lesions of infected person

Transmission: Direct contact with infected person, a carrier, or contaminated articles

Incubation period: Usually 2-5 days, possibly longer

Period of communicability: Variable; until virulent bacilli are no longer present (identified by three negative cultures); usually 2 weeks but as long as 4 weeks

The Child with a Communicable Disease—cont'd

Clinical Manifestations	Therapeutic Management/Complications	Nursing Considerations
Prodromal stage: Slight fever, malaise, and anorexia for first 24 hours; rash highly pruritic; begins as macule, rapidly progresses to papule and then vesicle (surrounded by erythematous base, becomes umbilicated and cloudy, breaks easily and forms crusts); all three stages (papule, vesicle, crust) present in varying degrees at one time **Distribution:** Centripetal, spreading to face and proximal extremities but sparse on distal limbs and less on areas not exposed to heat (e.g., from clothing or sun) **Constitutional signs and symptoms:** Elevated temperature from lymphadenopathy, irritability from pruritus	**Specific:** Antiviral agent acyclovir (Zovirax), varicella-zoster immune globulin (VZIG) after exposure in high-risk children **Supportive:** Diphenhydramine hydrochloride or antihistamines to relieve itching; skin care to prevent secondary bacterial infection **Complications:** Secondary bacterial infections (e.g., abscesses, cellulitis, pneumonia, sepsis) Encephalitis Varicella pneumonia Hemorrhagic varicella (tiny hemorrhages in vesicles and numerous petechiae in skin) Chronic or transient thrombocytopenia	Maintain strict isolation in hospital Isolate child in home until vesicles have dried (usually 1 week after onset of disease) and isolate high-risk children from infected children Administer skin care: give bath and change clothes and linens daily; administer topical application of calamine lotion; keep child's fingernails short and clean; apply mittens if child scratches Keep child cool (may decrease number of lesions) Lessen pruritus; keep child occupied Remove loose crusts that rub and irritate skin Teach child to apply pressure to pruritic area rather than scratching it. If older child, reason with child regarding danger of scar formation from scratching Avoid use of aspirin; use of acetaminophen controversial
Vary according to anatomic location of pseudomembrane **Nasal:** Resembles common cold, serosanguineous mucopurulent nasal discharge without constitutional symptoms; may be frank epistaxis **Tonsillar/pharyngeal:** Malaise; anorexia; sore throat; low-grade fever; pulse increased above expected for temperature within 24 hours; smooth, adherent, white or gray membrane; lymphadenitis possibly pronounced (bull's neck); in severe cases, toxemia, septic shock, and death within 6-10 days **Laryngeal:** Fever, hoarseness, cough, with or without previous signs listed; potential airway obstruction, apprehensive, dyspneic retractions, cyanosis	Antitoxin (usually intravenously); preceded by skin or conjunctival test to rule out sensitivity to horse serum Antibiotics (penicillin or erythromycin) Complete bed rest (prevention of myocarditis) Tracheostomy for airway obstruction Treatment of infected contacts and carriers Complications: Myocarditis (second week) Neuritis	Maintain strict isolation in hospital Participate in sensitivity testing; have epinephrine available Administer antibiotics; observe for signs of sensitivity to penicillin Administer complete care to maintain bed rest Use suctioning as needed Observe respirations for signs of obstruction Administer humidified oxygen if prescribed

Unit 4

Continued

The Child with a Communicable Disease—cont'd

TABLE 4-40   Communicable Diseases of Childhood—cont'd

Disease

Erythema Infectiosum (Fifth Disease)
Agent: Human parvovirus B19 (HPV)
Source: Infected person
Transmission: Unknown; possibly respiratory secretions and blood
Incubation period: 4-14 days, may be as long as 20 days
Period of communicability: Uncertain but before onset of symptoms in most children; also for about 1 week after onset of symptoms in children with aplastic crisis

Exanthema Subitum (Roseola)
Agent: Human herpes virus type 6 (HHV-6)
Source: Unknown
Transmission: Unknown (virtually limited to children between 6 months and 2 years of age)
Incubation period: Usually 5-15 days
Period of communicability: Unknown

The Child with a Communicable Disease—cont'd

Clinical Manifestations	Therapeutic Management/Complications	Nursing Considerations
Rash appears in three stages: I—Erythema on face, chiefly on cheeks, "slapped face" appearance; disappears by 1-4 days II—About 1 day after rash appears on face, maculopapular red spots appear, symmetrically distributed on upper and lower extremities; rash progresses from proximal to distal surfaces and may last a week or more III—Rash subsides but reappears if skin is irritated or traumatized (sun, heat, cold, friction) In child with aplastic crisis, rash is usually absent and prodromal illness includes fever, myalgia, lethargy, nausea, vomiting, and abdominal pain	**Symptomatic and supportive:** Antipyretics, analgesics, antiinflammatory drugs Possible blood transfusion for transient aplastic anemia **Complications:** Self-limited arthritis and arthralgia (arthritis may become chronic) May result in fetal death if mother infected during pregnancy, but no evidence of congenital anomalies Aplastic crisis in child with hemolytic disease or immune deficiency Myocarditis (rare) Encephalitis (rare)	Isolation of child not necessary, except hospitalized child (immunosuppressed or with aplastic crisis) suspected of HPV infection is placed on respiratory isolation and standard precautions Pregnant women: need not be excluded from workplace where HPV infection; should not care for patients with aplastic crises; explain low risk of fetal death to those in contact with affected children
Presistent high fever for 3-4 days in child who appears well Precipitous drop in fever to normal with appearance of rash **Rash:** Discrete rose-pink macules or maculopapules appearing first on trunk, then spreading to neck, face, and extremities; nonpruritic, fades on pressure; appears 2-3 days after onset of fever and lasts 1-2 days **Associated signs and symptoms:** Cervical/postauricular lymphadenopathy, injected pharynx, cough, coryza	Nonspecific Antipyretics to control fever **Complications:** Recurrent febrile seizures (possibly from latent infection of central nervous system that is reactivated by fever) A mononucleosis-like illness— Fulminant hepatitis disseminated disease meningitis Encephalitis (rare)	Teach parents measures for lowering temperature (antipyretic drugs) If child is prone to seizures, discuss appropriate precautions, possibility of recurrent febrile seizures

Continued

Unit 4

The Child with a Communicable Disease—cont'd

TABLE 4-40   Communicable Diseases of Childhood—cont'd

	Disease
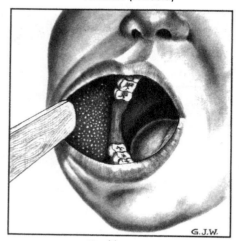**First day of rash** **Third day of rash** Koplik spots on buccal mucosa (see inset) Confluent maculopapules Rash discrete Discrete maculopapules Measles (rubeola) Koplik spots	**Measles (Rubeola)** **Agent:** Virus **Source:** Respiratory tract secretions, blood, and urine of infected person **Transmission:** Usually by direct contact with droplets from infected person **Incubation period:** 10-20 days **Period of communicability:** From 4 days before to 5 days after rash appears, but mainly during prodromal (catarrhal) stage
	Mumps **Agent:** Paramyxovirus **Source:** Saliva of infected person **Transmission:** Direct contact or droplet spread from an infected person **Incubation period:** 14-21 days **Period of communicability:** Most communicable immediately before and after swelling begins

The Child with a Communicable Disease—cont'd

Clinical Manifestations	Therapeutic Management/Complications	Nursing Considerations
Prodromal (catarrhal) stage: Fever and malaise, followed in 24 hours by coryza, cough, conjunctivitis, Koplik spots (small, irregular red spots with a minute, bluish-white center first seen on buccal mucosa opposite molars 2 days before rash); symptoms gradually increase in severity until second day after rash appears, when they begin to subside **Rash:** Appears 3-4 days after onset of prodromal stage; begins as erythematous maculopapular eruption on face and gradually spreads downward; more severe in earlier sites (appears confluent) and less intense in later sites (appears discrete); after 3-4 days assumes brownish appearance, and fine desquamation occurs over areas of extensive involvement **Constitutional signs and symptoms:** Anorexia, malaise, generalized lymphadenopathy	Vitamin A supplementation **Supportive:** Bed rest during febrile period; antipyretics Antibiotics to prevent secondary bacterial infection in high-risk children **Complications:** Otitis media Pneumonia Bronchiolitis Obstructive laryngitis and laryngotracheitis Encephalitis	Isolation until fifth day of rash; if hospitalized, institute respiratory precautions Maintain bed rest during prodromal stage; provide quiet activity **Fever:** Instruct parents to administer antipyretics; avoid chilling; if child is prone to seizures, institute appropriate precautions (fever spikes to 40° C [104° F] between fourth and fifth days) **Eye care:** Dim lights if photophobia present; clean eyelids with warm saline solution to remove secretions or crusts; keep child from rubbing eyes; examine cornea for signs of ulceration **Coryza/cough:** Use cool mist vaporizer; protect skin around nares with layer of petrolatum; encourage fluids and soft, bland foods **Skin care:** Keep skin clean; use tepid baths as necessary
Prodromal stage: Fever, headache, malaise, and anorexia for 24 hours, followed by "earache" that is aggravated by chewing **Parotitis:** By third day, parotid gland(s) (either unilateral or bilateral) enlarge and reach maximum size in 1-3 days; accompanied by pain and tenderness **Other manifestations:** Submaxillary and sublingual infection, orchitis, and meningoencephalitis	**Symptomatic and supportive:** Analgesics for pain and antipyretics for fever Intravenous fluid may be necessary for child who refuses to drink or who vomits because of meningoencephalitis **Complications:** Sensorineural deafness Postinfectious encephalitis Myocarditis Arthritis Hepatitis Epididymo-orchitis Sterility (extremely rare in adult males)	Isolation during period of communicability; institute respiratory precautions during hospitalization Maintain bed rest during prodromal phase until swelling subsides Give analgesics for pain; if child is unwilling to chew medication, use elixir form Encourage fluids and soft, bland foods; avoid foods requiring chewing Apply hot or cold compresses to neck, whichever is more comforting To relieve orchitis, provide warmth and local support with tight-fitting underpants (stretch bathing suit works well)

Unit 4

Continued

The Child with a Communicable Disease—cont'd

TABLE 4-40   Communicable Diseases of Childhood—cont'd

	Disease
	Pertussis (Whooping Cough) **Agent:** *Bordetella pertussis* **Source:** Discharge from respiratory tract of infected person **Transmission:** Direct contact or droplet spread from infected person; indirect contact with freshly contaminated articles **Incubation period:** 5-21 days, usually 10 **Period of communicability:** Greatest during catarrhal stage before onset of paroxysms and may extend to fourth week after onset of paroxysms
	Poliomyelitis **Agent:** Enteroviruses, three types: type 1—most frequent cause of paralysis, both epidemic and endemic; type 2—least frequently associated with paralysis; type 3—second most frequently associated with paralysis **Source:** Feces and oropharyngeal secretions of infected person, especially young child **Transmission:** Direct contact with person with apparent or inapparent active infection; spread is via fecal-oral and pharyngeal-oropharyngeal routes **Incubation period:** Usually 7-14 days, with range of 5-35 days **Period of communicability:** Not exactly known; virus is present in throat and feces shortly after infection and persists for about 1 week in throat and 4-6 weeks in feces

The Child with a Communicable Disease—cont'd

Clinical Manifestations	Therapeutic Management/Complications	Nursing Considerations
Catarrhal stage: Begins with symptoms of upper respiratory tract infection, such as coryza, sneezing, lacrimation, cough, and low-grade fever; symptoms continue for 1-2 weeks, when dry, hacking cough becomes more severe **Paroxysmal stage:** Cough most often occurs at night and consists of short, rapid coughs followed by sudden inspiration associated with a high-pitched crowing sound or "whoop"; during paroxysm cheeks become flushed or cyanotic, eyes bulge, and tongue protrudes; paroxysm may continue until thick mucus plug is dislodged; vomiting frequently follows attack; stage generally lasts 4-6 weeks, followed by convalescent stage	Antimicrobial therapy (e.g., erythromycin) Administration of pertussis-immune globulin **Supportive treatment:** Hospitalization required for infants, children who are dehydrated, or those who have complications Bed rest Increased oxygen intake and humidity Adequate fluids Intubation possibly necessary **Complications:** Pneumonia (usual cause of death) Atelectasis Otitis media Convulsions Hemorrhage (subarachnoid, subconjunctival, epistaxis) Weight loss and dehydration Hernia Prolapsed rectum	Isolation during catarrhal stage; if hospitalized, institute respiratory precautions Maintain bed rest as long as fever present Keep child occupied during day (interest in play associated with fewer paroxysms) Reassure parents during frightening episodes of whooping cough Provide restful environment and reduce factors that promote paroxysms (e.g., dust, smoke, sudden changes in temperature, chilling, activity, excitement); keep room well ventilated Encourage fluids; offer small amounts of fluids frequently; refeed child after vomiting Provide high humidity (humidifier or tent); suction gently to prevent choking on secretions Observe for signs of airway obstruction (e.g., increased restlessness, apprehension, retractions, cyanosis) Involve community health nurse if child cared for at home
May be manifested in three different forms: **Abortive or inapparent:** Fever, uneasiness, sore throat, headache, anorexia, vomiting, abdominal pain; lasts a few hours to a few days **Nonparalytic:** Same manifestations as abortive but more severe, with pain and stiffness in neck, back, and legs **Paralytic:** Initial course similar to nonparalytic type, followed by recovery and then signs of central nervous system paralysis	No specific treatment, including antimicrobials or gamma globulin Complete bed rest during acute phase Assisted respiratory ventilation in case of respiratory paralysis Physical therapy for muscles following acute stage **Complications:** Permanent paralysis Respiratory arrest Hypertension Kidney stones from demineralization of bone during prolonged immobility	Maintain complete bed rest Administer mild sedatives as necessary to relieve anxiety and promote rest Participate in physiotherapy procedures (use of moist hot packs and range-of-motion exercises) Position child to maintain body alignment and prevent contractures or decubiti; use footboard Encourage child to move; administer analgesics for maximum comfort during physical activity Observe for respiratory paralysis (difficulty in talking, ineffective cough, inability to hold breath, shallow and rapid respirations); report such signs and symptoms to practitioner; have tracheostomy tray at bedside

Unit 4

Continued

The Child with a Communicable Disease—cont'd

TABLE 4-40   Communicable Diseases of Childhood—cont'd

Disease

First day of rash

Third day of rash

Rash discrete

Rubella (German measles)

Rubella (German Measles)

Agent: Rubella virus

Source: Primarily nasopharyngeal secretions of person with apparent or inapparent infection; virus also present in blood, stool, and urine

Transmission: Direct contact and spread via infected person; indirectly via articles freshly contaminated with nasopharyngeal secretions, feces, or urine

Incubation period: 14-21 days

Period of communicability: 7 days before to about 5 days after appearance of rash

First day of rash

Third day of rash

Flushed cheeks

White strawberry tongue (see inset)

Increased density on neck

Transverse lines (Pastia sign)

Increased density in groin

Circumoral pallor

Red strawberry tongue (see inset)

Increased density in axilla

Positive blanching test (Schultz-Charlton)

Scarlet fever

Scarlet Fever

Agent: Group A beta hemolytic streptococci

Source: Usually from nasopharyngeal secretions of infected person or carrier

Transmission: Direct contact with infected person or droplet spread; indirectly by contact with contaminated articles or ingestion of contaminated milk or other food

Incubation period: 2-4 days, with range of 1-7 days

Period of communicability: During incubation period and clinical illness approximately 10 days; during first 2 weeks of carrier phase, although may persist for months

First day

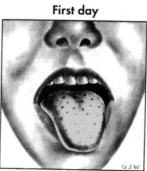

White strawberry tongue

Third day

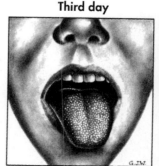

Red strawberry tongue

The Child with a Communicable Disease—cont'd

Clinical Manifestations	Therapeutic Management/Complications	Nursing Considerations
Prodromal stage: Absent in children, present in adults and adolescents; consists of low-grade fever, headache, malaise, anorexia, mild conjunctivitis, coryza, sore throat, cough, and lymphadenopathy; lasts for 1-5 days, subsides 1 day after appearance of rash **Rash:** First appears on face and rapidly spreads downward to neck, arms, trunk, and legs; by end of first day body is covered with a discrete, pinkish-red maculopapular exanthema; disappears in same order as it began and is usually gone by third day **Constitutional signs and symptoms:** Occasionally low-grade fever, headache, malaise, and lymphadenopathy	No treatment necessary other than antipyretics for low-grade fever and analgesics for discomfort **Complications:** Rare (arthritis, encephalitis, or purpura); most benign of all childhood communicable diseases; greatest danger is teratogenic effect on fetus	Reassure parents of benign nature of illness in affected child Employ comfort measures as necessary Isolate child from pregnant women
Prodromal stage: Abrupt high fever, pulse increased out of proportion to fever, vomiting, headache, chills, malaise, abdominal pain **Enanthema:** Tonsils enlarged, edematous, reddened, and covered with patches of exudate; in severe case appearance resembles membrane seen in diphtheria; pharynx is edematous and beefy red; during first 1-2 days tongue is coated and papillae become red and swollen (white strawberry tongue); by fourth or fifth day white coat sloughs off, leaving prominent papillae (red strawberry tongue); palate is covered with erythematous punctate lesions **Exanthema:** Rash appears within 12 hours after prodromal signs; red pinhead-sized punctate lesions rapidly become generalized but are absent on face, which becomes flushed with striking circumoral pallor; rash is more intense in folds of joints; by end of first week desquamation begins (fine, sandpaper-like on torso; sheet-like sloughing on palms and soles), which may be complete by 3 weeks or longer	Treatment of choice is a full course of penicillin (or erythromycin in penicillin-sensitive children); fever should subside 24 hours after beginning therapy Antibiotic therapy for newly diagnosed carriers (nose or throat cultures positive for streptococci) **Supportive measures:** Bed rest during febrile phase, analgesics for sore throat **Complications:** Otitis media Peritonsillar abscess Sinusitis Glomerulonephritis Carditis, polyarthritis (uncommon)	Institute respiratory precautions until 24 hours after initiation of treatment Ensure compliance with oral antibiotic therapy (intramuscular benzathine penicillin G [Bicillin] may be given if parents' reliability in giving oral drugs is questionable) Maintain bed rest during febrile phase; provide quiet activity during convalescent period Relieve discomfort of sore throat with analgesics, gargles, lozenges, antiseptic throat sprays (Chloraseptic), and inhalation of cool mist Encourage fluids during febrile phase; avoid irritating liquids (citrus juices) or rough foods; when child is able to eat, begin with soft diet Advise parents to consult practitioner if fever persists after beginning therapy Discuss procedures for preventing spread of infection

Unit 4

Continued

The Child with a Communicable Disease—cont'd

NURSING DIAGNOSIS: Risk for infection related to susceptible host and infectious agents

- **PATIENT GOAL 1:** Will not become infected

NURSING INTERVENTIONS/RATIONALES

Be highly suspicious of infectious diseases, especially in susceptible children

Identify high-risk children (e.g., those with an immunodeficiency or hemolytic disease) to whom communicable disease may be fatal; in case of an outbreak, advise parents to confine child to the home *to avoid exposure*

Participate in public education and service programs regarding prophylactic immunizations, method of spread of communicable diseases, proper preparation and handling of food and water supplies, control of animal vectors in regard to reservoirs of disease (not a factor in childhood communicable disease but in other infectious illness such as malaria), or screening programs to identify streptococcal infections

EXPECTED OUTCOME

Susceptible children do not contract the disease

- **PATIENT GOAL 2:** Will not spread disease

NURSING INTERVENTIONS/RATIONALES

Institute appropriate infection control practices (See Nursing Care Plan: The Child at Risk for Infection, p. 341.)

Make referral to community health nurse, when necessary, *to ensure appropriate procedures in the home*

Work with families *to ensure compliance with therapeutic regimens*

Identify close contacts who may require prophylactic treatment (e.g., specific immune globulin or antibiotics)

Report disease to local health department if appropriate

EXPECTED OUTCOME

Infection remains confined to original source

- **PATIENT GOAL 3:** Will exhibit no evidence of complications

NURSING INTERVENTIONS/RATIONALES

Ensure compliance with therapeutic regimen (e.g., bed rest, antiviral therapy, antibiotics, adequate hydration)

Avoid giving aspirin to children with varicella *because of the possible risk of Reye syndrome*

Institute seizure precautions if febrile convulsions are a possibility

Monitor temperature *because unexpected elevations may signal an infection*

Maintain good body hygiene *to reduce risk of secondary infection of lesions*

Offer small, frequent sips of water or favorite drinks *to ensure adequate hydration* and soft, bland foods (e.g., gelatin, pudding, ice cream, soups) *because many children are anorectic during an illness;* feed again after vomiting; observe for signs of dehydration

EXPECTED OUTCOME

Child exhibits no evidence of complications such as infection or dehydration

NURSING DIAGNOSIS: Pain related to skin lesions, malaise

- **PATIENT GOAL 1:** Will experience minimal discomfort

NURSING INTERVENTIONS/RATIONALES

Use cool-mist vaporizer, gargles, and lozenges *to keep mucous membranes moist*

Apply petrolatum to chapped lips or nares

Cleanse eyes with physiologic saline solution *to remove secretions or crusts*

Keep skin clean; change bedclothes and linens at least daily

Administer oral hygiene

Keep child cool *because overheating increases itching*

Give cools baths and apply lotion such as calamine *to decrease itching*

Assess need for pain medication

Employ nonpharmacologic pain reduction techniques (See p. 339.)

*Administer analgesics, antipyretics, and antipruritics as needed

EXPECTED OUTCOMES

Skin and mucous membranes are clean and free of irritants

Child exhibits minimal evidence of discomfort (specify)

NURSING DIAGNOSIS: Impaired social interaction related to isolation from peers

- **PATIENT GOAL 1:** Will have some understanding of reason for isolation

NURSING INTERVENTIONS/RATIONALES

Explain reason for confinement and use of any special precautions *to increase child's understanding of restrictions*

Allow child to play with gloves, mask, and gown (if used) *to facilitate positive coping*

EXPECTED OUTCOME

Child demonstrates understanding of restrictions

- **PATIENT GOAL 2:** Will have opportunity to participate in suitable activities

NURSING INTERVENTIONS/RATIONALES

Always introduce self to child; allow child to see face before donning protective clothing, if required

Provide diversionary activity

Encourage parents to remain with child during hospitalization *to decrease separation and to provide companionship*

Encourage contact with friends via telephone (in hospital, can use intercom between room and nurse's station)

Prepare child's peers for altered physical appearance, such as with chickenpox, *to encourage peer acceptance*

EXPECTED OUTCOMES

Child engages in suitable activities and interactions

Peers accept child

*Dependent nursing action.

The Child with a Communicable Disease—cont'd

NURSING DIAGNOSIS: Risk for impaired skin integrity related to scratching from pruritus

■ **PATIENT GOAL 1:** Will maintain skin integrity

NURSING INTERVENTIONS/*RATIONALES*

Keep nails short and clean *to minimize trauma and secondary infection*

Apply mittens or elbow restraints *to prevent scratching*

Dress in lightweight, loose, and nonirritating clothing *because overheating increases itching*

Cover affected areas (e.g., with long sleeves, pants, or one-piece outfit) *to prevent scratching*

Bathe in cool water with no soap, or apply cool compresses

Apply soothing lotions *to decrease pruritus;* use sparingly on open lesions *because absorption of drug is increased*

Avoid exposure to heat or sun, *which can aggravate rash* (e.g., chickenpox)

EXPECTED OUTCOME

Skin remains intact

NURSING DIAGNOSIS: Altered family processes related to child with an acute illness

■ **PATIENT GOAL 1:** Will receive adequate emotional support

NURSING INTERVENTIONS/*RATIONALES*

Inform parents of treatment options, especially use of acyclovir for varicella

Reinforce family's effort to carry out plan of care

Provide assistance, when necessary, such as visiting nurse *to help with home care*

Keep family aware of child's progress *to encourage optimistic attitude*

Stress rapidity of recovery in most cases *to decrease anxiety*

EXPECTED OUTCOMES

Family continues to comply with expectations

Family seeks needed support

Unit 4

NURSING CARE PLAN

The Child with a Skin Disorder

A **skin disorder** is a condition that causes alteration in the appearance and/or function of the skin.

ASSESSMENT

Perform a physical assessment with special regard for skin manifestations:

Erythema—Reddened area caused by increased amounts of oxygenated blood in the dermal vasculature

Ecchymoses—Localized red or purple discolorations caused by extravasation of blood into dermis and subcutaneous tissues

Petechiae—Pinpoint tiny and sharply circumscribed spots in the superficial layers of the epidermis

Primary lesions—Skin changes produced by some causative factor (Box 4-30)

Secondary lesions—Skin changes that result from alterations in the primary lesions, such as those caused by rubbing, scratching, medication, or by involution and healing (Box 4-31)

Describe distribution pattern of lesion (e.g., extensor surfaces, creases, exposed areas, entire body, diaper area).

Describe configuration and arrangement of any lesions (e.g., discrete, grouped or clustered, annular [ringed], confluent, linear, diffuse).

Describe any associated characteristics such as temperature, moisture, texture, elasticity, and hardness of skin in general or in area of lesion(s).

Observe for evidence of subjective manifestations associated with lesions (e.g., pruritis, pain or tenderness, burning, prickling, stinging, crawling, anesthesia, hyperesthesia, and hypesthesia or hypoesthesia; constant or intermittent; aggravated by specific activity or circumstance).

Observe for evidence of aggravating factor (e.g., foreign body such as a sliver, insect barb, cactus spine) or presence of insect (e.g., chiggers, fleas, ticks, mites).

Obtain a health history for previous skin reactions, allergies, and diseases associated with skin manifestations.

Obtain a recent history for onset, possible precipitating events, and course of development. Possible precipitating factors include exposure to infectious disease; contact with chemicals, plants, animals, insects, sunshine, allergenic toys or clothing (e.g., wool), metals, topical applications (e.g., soaps, makeup, lotions, bath salts); excess heat or cold; and visits to wooded areas or a beach.

Obtain a nutrition history, especially regarding foods known to be allergenic.

Assist with diagnostic procedures (e.g., skin testing, microscopic examination of scrapings, biopsy, culture, cytodiagnosis, patch testing, and blood tests).

The Child with a Skin Disorder—cont'd

BOX 4-30

Primary Skin Lesions

Flat, circumscribed area of color change (red, brown, purple, white, tan); less than 1 cm in diameter; nonpalpable
Example: Freckle, flat mole, rubella, rubeola

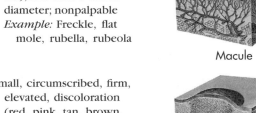

Macule

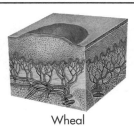

Wheal

Elevated, irregularly shaped area of cutaneous edema; transient, changing; variable diameter; pale pink with lighter center
Example: Insect bites, urticaria

Small, circumscribed, firm, elevated, discoloration (red, pink, tan, brown, bluish); less than 1 cm in diameter; the more superficial it is, the more distinct are the borders
Example: Wart, drug-related eruptions, pigmented nevi

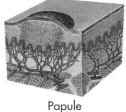

Papule

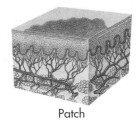

Patch

Flat, circumscribed, irregularly shaped, discoloration; nonpalpable; greater than 1 cm in diameter
Example: Vitiligo, port-wine marks

Circumscribed, firm elevation; round or ellipsoid; located deeper in dermis than papules; 1-2 cm in diameter
Example: Erythema nodosum, lipoma

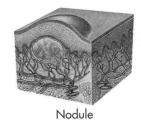

Nodule

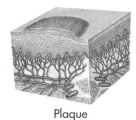

Plaque

Flattened, raised, firm, surface area relatively large in relation to height; greater than 1 cm in diameter
Example: Psoriasis, seborrheic and actinic keratoses

Elevated, circumscribed, palpable, encapsulated, filled with liquid or semisolid material
Example: Sebaceous cyst

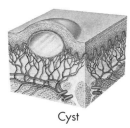

Cyst

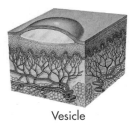

Vesicle

Small (less than 1 cm in diameter), superficial circumscribed elevation; contains serous fluid
Example: Varicella, blister

Elevated, superficial, similar to vesicle but filled with purulent fluid
Example: Acne, impetigo, variola

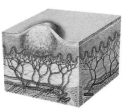

Pustule

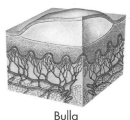

Bulla

Fluid-filled vesicle greater than 1 cm in diameter; a large vesicle; bleb; blister
Example: Blister, pemphigus vulgaris

Illustrations from Seidel HM and others: *Mosby's guide to physical examination*, ed 4, St Louis, 1999, Mosby.

Unit 4

The Child with a Skin Disorder—cont'd

BOX 4-31

Secondary Skin Lesions

Mound of keratinized cells; flaky exfoliation; irregular shape; variable thickness and diameter; dry or oily; silver, white, or tan
Example: Psoriasis, exfoliative dermatitis

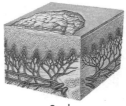

Scale

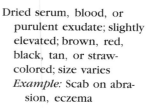

Crust

Dried serum, blood, or purulent exudate; slightly elevated; brown, red, black, tan, or straw-colored; size varies
Example: Scab on abrasion, eczema

Concave with loss of epidermis and dermis; variable size; exudative; red or reddish blue
Example: Decubiti, statis ulcers

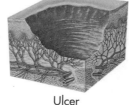

Ulcer

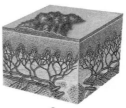

Fissure

Deep linear split through epidermis into dermis; small; deep; red
Example: Chapping, tinea pedis

Permanent thick to thin fibrous tissue that replaces damaged corium by production and deposition of collagen; irregular shape; red, pink, or white; atrophic or hypertrophic
Example: Vaccination, healed wound, abrasion, laceration

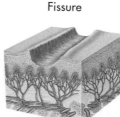

Scar

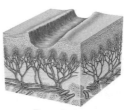

Excoriation

Loss of superficial epidermis, linear or punctate
Example: Scratch, abrasion

Rough, thickened epidermis; accentuated skin markings caused by rubbing or irritation; often involves flexor aspect of extremity
Example: Chronic dermatitis

Lichenification

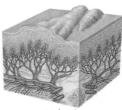

Keloid

Irregularly shaped, elevated, progressively enlarging scar; grows beyond boundaries of wound; caused by excessive collagen formation during healing
Example: Keloid from ear piercing or burn scar

Loss of all or part of epidermis; depressed; moist; glistening; follows rupture of vesicle or bulla; larger than fissure
Examples: Varicella; variola following rupture

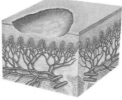

Erosion

Illustrations from Seidel HM and others: *Mosby's guide to physical examination,* ed 4, St Louis, 1999, Mosby.

The Child with a Skin Disorder—cont'd

NURSING DIAGNOSIS: Impaired skin integrity related to environmental agents, somatic factors, immunologic deficit

■ **PATIENT GOAL 1:** Will exhibit signs of skin healing

NURSING INTERVENTIONS/*RATIONALES*

Carry out therapeutic regimens as prescribed, or support and assist parents in carrying out treatment plan, *to promote skin healing*

Provide moist environment (dressing or ointment) *for optimum wound healing*

*Administer topical treatments and applications

*Administer systemic medications, if ordered

Prevent secondary infection and autoinoculation *since these delay healing*

Reduce external stimuli that aggravate condition, *causing delay in healing*

Encourage rest *to support body's natural defenses*

Encourage well-balanced diet *to support body's natural defenses*

Administer skin care and general hygiene measures *to promote skin healing*

EXPECTED OUTCOME

Affected area exhibits signs of healing

NURSING DIAGNOSIS: Risk for impaired skin integrity related to mechanical trauma, body secretions, increased susceptibility to infection

■ **PATIENT GOAL 1:** Will maintain skin integrity

NURSING INTERVENTIONS/*RATIONALES*

Keep intact skin clean and dry; cleanse skin at least once daily *to minimize risk of infection*

Inspect total skin area frequently for evidence of irritation or breakdown *so that appropriate therapy can be initiated*

Protect skinfolds and surfaces that rub together *to prevent mechanical trauma to skin*

Keep clothing and linen clean and dry *to prevent excoriation and infection of skin*

Apply protective lotion to anal and perineal areas, knees, elbows, ankles, and chin *since excoriation is most likely to occur in these areas*

Carry out good perineal care under urine collection device when applicable *to prevent impaired skin integrity*

Remove adhesives and occlusive dressings carefully *to prevent skin trauma*

EXPECTED OUTCOME

Skin remains clean, dry, and free of irritation

■ **PATIENT GOAL 2:** Will exhibit no evidence of secondary infection

NURSING INTERVENTIONS/*RATIONALES*

Maintain careful handwashing before handling affected child *to prevent infection*

Wear surgical gloves when handling or dressing affected parts, if indicated by nature of lesion, *to prevent contamination of lesions*

Teach child and family hygienic care and medical asepsis *to prevent secondary infection*

Devise methods to prevent secondary infection of lesions in small or uncooperative children:

Keep nails short and clean *to minimize trauma and secondary infection*

Apply mittens or elbow restraints *to prevent child from reaching skin lesions*

Dress in one-piece outfit with long sleeves and legs *to keep lesions covered and out of child's reach*

Observe skin lesions for signs of infection (e.g., increased erythema, edema, purulent exudate, pain, increased temperature) *so that appropriate therapy can be initiated*

EXPECTED OUTCOMES

Skin lesions remain confined to primary sites

Skin lesions exhibit no signs of secondary infection

■ **PATIENT GOAL 3:** Will maintain integrity of healthy skin

NURSING INTERVENTIONS/*RATIONALES*

Teach and impress on child importance of keeping hands away from lesions *to prevent spreading lesions and secondary infection*

Help child determine ways of preventing autoinoculation *to increase compliance*

Devise means for keeping small or uncooperative children from spreading infection to other areas

Keep healthy skin dry *to prevent maceration*

EXPECTED OUTCOMES

Healthy skin remains clean and intact

Skin lesions remain confined to primary sites

NURSING DIAGNOSIS: Risk for infection related to presence of infective organisms

■ **PATIENT GOAL 1:** Will not spread infection to self or others

NURSING INTERVENTIONS/*RATIONALES*

Implement standard precautions *to prevent spread of infection*

Isolate affected child from susceptible individuals if indicated *to prevent spread of infection*

Maintain careful handwashing after caring for child *to remove infective organisms*

Avoid unnecessary close contact with affected child during infective stage of disease

Use correct technique for disposal of dressings, solutions, and other fomites in contact with lesions *to safely dispose of infective organisms*

Teach and reinforce positive habits of hygienic care *to decrease risk of infection*

EXPECTED OUTCOMES

Infection remains confined to primary site

Child and family comply with preventive measures

NURSING DIAGNOSIS: Risk for impaired skin integrity related to allergenic factors

*Dependent nursing action.

Continued

Unit 4

The Child with a Skin Disorder—cont'd

■ **PATIENT GOAL 1:** Will experience no occurrence or recurrence of skin lesions

NURSING INTERVENTIONS/*RATIONALES*

Avoid or reduce contact with agents or circumstances known to precipitate skin reaction *to prevent occurrence or recurrence of lesions*

Teach child to recognize agents or circumstances that produce reaction *to prevent occurrence or recurrence of lesions*

EXPECTED OUTCOME

Child avoids precipitating agents

NURSING DIAGNOSIS: Pain related to skin lesions, pruritus

■ **PATIENT GOAL 1:** Will exhibit optimum comfort level

NURSING INTERVENTIONS/*RATIONALES*

Avoid or reduce external stimuli, such as clothing and bed linen, that aggravate discomfort

Implement other appropriate nonpharmacologic pain reduction techniques (See p. 339.)

*Apply soothing treatments and topical applications as ordered *to relieve pain or pruritus*

*Administer medications *to relieve discomfort and/or restlessness and irritability*

Advocate for child regarding appropriate topical anesthesia and/or sedation/analgesia for wound suturing or cleansing *to prevent unnecessary pain and emotional trauma*

EXPECTED OUTCOME

Child remains calm and exhibits no evidence of discomfort or pruritus

---

NURSING DIAGNOSIS: Body image disturbance related to perception of appearance

---

■ **PATIENT GOAL 1:** Will demonstrate positive self-image

NURSING INTERVENTIONS/*RATIONALES*

Encourage child to express feelings about personal appearance and perceived reactions of others *to facilitate coping*

Discuss with child improvement in skin condition *to instill hope*

EXPECTED OUTCOME

Child verbalizes feelings and concerns

■ **PATIENT GOAL 2:** Will receive tactile contact

NURSING INTERVENTIONS/*RATIONALES*

Hold child; remember that there is no substitute for the stimulation and comfort of human contact

Touch and caress unaffected areas *to provide tactile contact without risk of spreading infection*

EXPECTED OUTCOMES

Child exhibits signs of comfort

Child responds positively to tactile stimulation

■ **PATIENT GOAL 3:** Will receive adequate support

NURSING INTERVENTIONS/*RATIONALES*

Teach self-care where appropriate *to encourage sense of adequacy*

Involve child in planning treatment schedules *to give child some control*

Support and encourage child in efforts to deal with multiple problems that may be associated with disorder, including discomfort, rejection, discouragement, and feelings of self-revulsion, *to facilitate coping*

Encourage child to maintain usual activities *so that child experiences normalcy in situation*

Help child improve appearance (e.g., attractive clothing) *to promote positive self-image*

EXPECTED OUTCOMES

Child collaborates in determining means for improving appearance

Child maintains customary activities and relationships

Child participates in own care and treatment

NURSING DIAGNOSIS: Altered family processes related to having a child with a severe skin condition (e.g., eczema, psoriasis, ichthyosis)

■ **PATIENT (FAMILY) GOAL 1:** Will receive adequate support

NURSING INTERVENTIONS/*RATIONALES*

Teach family skills needed *to carry out therapeutic program*

Provide written instructions *to increase compliance*

Inform family of expected and unexpected results of therapy and a course of action to follow

Help devise special techniques to carry out therapy *to increase compliance and cooperation*

Be aware of overprotectiveness and restrictiveness *to prevent stifling child's emotional growth*

Allow and encourage family members, particularly the one who cares for the child most of the time, to express negative feelings such as anger, frustration, and perhaps guilt, *to facilitate coping*

Stress that negative feelings are normal, acceptable, and expected but that they must have an outlet if family members are to remain healthy

Encourage family in efforts to carry out plan of care *to provide support*

Provide assistance when appropriate

Refer to agencies and services that assist with social, financial, and medical problems *to provide ongoing support*

EXPECTED OUTCOME

Family demonstrates necessary skills (specify)

---

*Dependent nursing action.

NURSING CARE PLAN

The Child with Atopic Dermatitis (Eczema)

Eczema or **eczematous inflammation** of the skin refers to a descriptive category of dermatologic diseases and not to a specific cause.

Atopic dermatitis (AD) is a type of pruritic eczema that usually begins during infancy and is associated with allergy with a hereditary tendency.

ASSESSMENT

Perform a physical assessment with special emphasis on characteristics and distribution of skin manifestations.

Obtain a family history for evidence of skin lesions and allergies.

Obtain a health history, especially relative to previous involvement and environmental or dietary factors associated with present and previous exacerbations.

Observe for manifestations of ezcema:

Distribution of lesions

Infantile form—Generalized, especially cheeks, scalp, trunk, and extensor surfaces of extremities

Childhood form—Flexural areas (antecubital and popliteal fossae, neck), wrists, ankles, and feet

Preadolescent and adolescent form—Face, sides of neck, hands, feet, face, and antecubital and popliteal fossae (to a lesser extent)

Appearance of lesions

Infantile form:

Erythema

Vesicles

Papules

Weeping

Oozing

Crusting

Scaling

Often symmetric

Childhood form:

Symmetric involvement

Clusters of small erythematous or flesh-colored papules or minimally scaling patches

Dry and may be hyperpigmented

Lichenification (thickened skin with accentuation of creases)

Keratosis pilaris (follicular hyperkeratosis) common

Adolescent/adult form:

Same as childhood manifestations

Dry, thick lesions (lichenified plaques) common

Confluent papules

Other manifestations

Intense itching

Unaffected skin dry and rough

Black children likely to exhibit more papular and/or follicular lesions than white children

May exhibit one or more of the following:

Lymphadenopathy, especially near affected sites

Increased palmar creases (many cases)

Atopic pleats (extra line or groove of lower eyelid)

Prone to cold hands

Pityriasis alba (small, poorly defined areas of hypopigmentation)

Facial pallor (especially around nose, mouth, and ears)

Bluish discoloration beneath eyes ("allergic shiners")

Increased susceptibility to unusual cutaneous infections (especially viral)

Restlessness

Irritability

Observe lesions for type, distribution, and evidence of secondary infection.

Perform or assist with diagnostic procedures (e.g., skin testing, elimination diet).

NURSING DIAGNOSIS: Impaired skin integrity related to eczematous lesions

■ **PATIENT GOAL 1:** Will experience either no itching or a reduction of itching to level acceptable to child

NURSING INTERVENTIONS/*RATIONALES*

Eliminate any woolen or rough clothes or blankets or furry stuffed animals *since these increase itching*

Dress for climatic conditions *to avoid overheating and increased itching*

Avoid nylon clothing *because it encourages perspiration, which will increase itching*

Wear soft, cotton fabrics *because they usually decrease itching*

Avoid heat and humidity when possible (e.g., use air-conditioning) *because perspiration intensifies itching*

Launder all clothes and bedsheets in mild detergent and rinse thoroughly in clear water (without fabric softeners and antistatic chemicals) *to avoid exposure to irritants*

Bathe in tepid water *to minimize itching*

Avoid using soap (except as indicated), bubble bath, oils, powder, or perfumes *which can be skin irritants*

Provide colloid bath (e.g., cornstarch in warm water) *for temporary relief at bedtime*

Apply cool compresses if needed *to minimize itching*

*Administer oral antihistamines, if prescribed, *for itching*

*Administer topical corticosteroids, if prescribed, *to decrease inflammation*

*Administer mild sedative, if prescribed, *since itching increases at night*

EXPECTED OUTCOMES

Child does not scratch and rests or plays quietly

Child verbalizes that itching is absent or minimal

■ **PATIENT GOAL 2:** Will exhibit signs of adequate skin hydration

NURSING INTERVENTIONS/*RATIONALES*

*Carry out prescribed therapeutic regimen *to encourage skin hydration*

*Dependent nursing action.

Continued

Unit 4

The Child with Atopic Dermatitis (Eczema)—cont'd

Dry method:
  Bathe infrequently
  Cleanse skin with nonlipid, hydrophilic agent (e.g., Cetaphil)
Wet method:
  Bathe frequently, up to four times per day
  Follow immediately with application of lubricant (while skin is still damp) *to trap moisture in the skin*
  Use no soap or a very mild nonperfumed soap (e.g., Neutrogena, Lowila, Dove) *because soap has a drying effect*
  Provide oil or oilated oatmeal baths, if prescribed *for a protective, oily film on skin*
  Avoid showers *because of their drying effect*
  *Apply hydrating preparations as prescribed
  Use room humidifier *to minimize dry skin*
*Provide hypoallergenic diet as prescribed *since food allergies may contribute to lesions in some children*

EXPECTED OUTCOMES
Child appears comfortable and rests and plays quietly
Skin does not appear dry or inflamed

■ **PATIENT GOAL 3:** Will exhibit signs of no or minimum scratching

NURSING INTERVENTIONS/*RATIONALES*
Keep fingernails and toenails short and clean *to minimize trauma and secondary infection*
Wrap hands in soft cotton gloves or stockings; pin to shirt cuffs *to prevent scratching*
Use elbow restraints when absolutely necessary (e.g., at night when itching is intensified) *to prevent scratching*
Encourage adequate sleep and rest *because tired and irritable children are more likely to scratch*

EXPECTED OUTCOMES
Child does not scratch lesions
Affected areas remain free of irritation and infection

■ **PATIENT GOAL 4:** Will receive adequate rest/sleep

NURSING INTERVENTIONS/*RATIONALES*
Plan meals, baths, medications, and treatments around naps or bedtime *so child receives adequate rest/sleep*
Make child as comfortable as possible before sleep (e.g., give sedation and bath before bedtime) *to enhance restfulness*

EXPECTED OUTCOME
Child receives an adequate amount of rest/sleep for age

NURSING DIAGNOSIS: Altered family processes related to child's discomfort and lengthy therapy

■ **PATIENT (FAMILY) GOAL 1:** Will be prepared for home care

NURSING INTERVENTIONS/*RATIONALES*
Encourage play activities that are suitable to skin condition and child's developmental age *to facilitate normal development*
Provide kinesthetic, moving toys; large toys, *which require less fine motor skills if hands are covered;* and quiet musical or visual toys
Demonstrate proper procedure for dilution of soaks and applying wet dressings *so that therapeutic regimen is carried out at home*
Suggest applying dressings at quiet times when child is well rested and has received medication for itching *to encourage cooperation*

EXPECTED OUTCOME
Family demonstrates correct performance of procedures (specify procedures)

■ **PATIENT (FAMILY) GOAL 2:** Will be prepared to avoid causative allergens

NURSING INTERVENTIONS/*RATIONALES*
Avoid any furry, hairy stuffed toys or dolls *that may cause itching*
Avoid play materials that contain allergens (e.g., wheat-based paste or finger paint)
Encourage child and family to express feelings *since stress tends to aggravate severity of condition*
Stress reason for hypoallergenic diet or removal of inhalants, especially that positive results are not immediate, *to encourage compliance*
Give written list of foods restricted as well as those allowed
Assess home environment *before* suggesting ways to eliminate inhalants *to increase effectiveness of interventions*
Make community health referral for long-term home care follow-up

EXPECTED OUTCOME
Family eliminates irritating substances from diet and environment of child

*Dependent nursing action.

NURSING CARE PLAN

The Adolescent with Acne

Acne is an inflammatory process involving the pilosebaceous unit, which consists of the sebaceous glands and hair follicles. It is most commonly found on the face, neck, shoulders, back, and upper chest.

ASSESSMENT
Perform a physical assessment.
Obtain a family history and health history.
Observe for manifestations of acne:
Noninflamed
　Comedones—Compact masses of keratin, lipids, fatty acids, and bacteria that dilate the follicular duct producing:

　　　Closed comedones or "whiteheads"
　　　Open comedones or "blackheads"
Inflamed
　Papules
　Pustules
　Nodules
　Cysts

NURSING DIAGNOSIS: Impaired skin integrity related to presence of secretions, presence of infective organisms

■ **PATIENT GOAL 1:** Will exhibit signs of reduced inflammation and scarring

NURSING INTERVENTIONS/*RATIONALES*
Carefully cleanse skin once or twice a day with mild soap and water *to reduce risk of infection*
*Caution patient not to pick, squeeze, or otherwise manipulate lesions *because this perpetuates acne and increases risk of infection*
Caution against too vigorous scrubbing *to prevent skin damage*
Impress the importance of following instructions, such as using only prescribed preparations
Instruct about shampooing, hairstyling, and the selection and use of cosmetics *because this can reduce number of lesions*
*Apply topical medications such as tretinoin (Retin-A) and benzoyl peroxide as prescribed *to reduce inflammation*
*Administer oral antibiotics as prescribed *for inflammatory acne*
*Administer isotretinoin 13-cis-retinoic acid (Accutane) as prescribed for severe, cystic acne that has not responded to other treatments
　Monitor closely for side effects (e.g., dry skin and mucous membranes, nasal irritation, dry eyes, photosensitivity, arthralgia, headaches, mood changes, depression, and elevated cholesterol and triglyceride levels)
　Advise sexually active women that they must use an effective contraception method during treatment and for 1 month afterwards *because of the teratogenic effects of the medication*
*Administer oral contraceptive pill (in selected female cases) as prescribed
Stress to those on retinoic acid therapy and/or tetracycline the importance of avoiding exposure to sun; apply sunscreen for protection and wear hat or sun visor

EXPECTED OUTCOME
Lesions heal with minimum scarring

■ **PATIENT GOAL 2:** Will exhibit signs of reduced number of lesions

NURSING INTERVENTIONS/*RATIONALES*
Avoid oily applications to the skin *because they aggravate acne by plugging pilosebaceous ducts*
Shampoo hair and scalp frequently (if prescribed)
Style hair off the forehead *because this is often beneficial in reducing forehead lesions*
Avoid use of cosmetic preparations, if possible; remove cosmetics at bedtime
Avoid face contact with other areas of the body (e.g., chin resting on hands, lying with face on arm)

EXPECTED OUTCOMES
Adolescent uses appropriate precautions
Adolescent exhibits signs of reduced number of lesions

■ **PATIENT GOAL 3:** Will comply with measures that promote general health

NURSING INTERVENTIONS/*RATIONALES*
Encourage adequate rest and moderate exercise *since this is important for general health*
Help adolescent plan a well-balanced diet *to support body's natural defenses*
Help adolescent find mechanisms to reduce emotional stress *since stress can contribute to acne*
Assess for any foci of infection and initiate measures to eliminate them
Eliminate any food the adolescent has found that aggravates the symptoms *to assess its influence on acne*

EXPECTED OUTCOME
Adolescent complies with measures that promote general health

---

NURSING DIAGNOSIS: Body image disturbance related to perception of facial lesions

■ **PATIENT GOAL 1:** Will demonstrate knowledge about acne and its treatment

NURSING INTERVENTIONS/*RATIONALES*
Dispel myths regarding the cause of the condition *because myths associated with acne are common*
Reassure adolescent regarding unfounded fears
Provide accurate information about acne and the therapy to be implemented

*Dependent nursing action.

Continued

Unit 4

The Adolescent with Acne—cont'd

EXPECTED OUTCOME

Adolescent demonstrates an understanding of acne and its treatment

■ **PATIENT GOAL 2:** Will seek treatment for acne

NURSING INTERVENTIONS/*RATIONALES*

Be alert to cues that the adolescent wants to discuss the skin problem

Introduce the subject of therapy for the adolescent with obvious skin lesions

Refer to health practitioner (e.g., dermatologist) who is sympathetic to the special needs of the adolescent

Discourage self-treatment with over-the-counter preparations *because these are usually not effective*

EXPECTED OUTCOMES

Adolescent discusses feelings and concerns

Adolescent complies with suggestions

Adolescent seeks treatment

■ **PATIENT GOAL 3:** Will assume responsibility for care of skin

NURSING INTERVENTIONS/*RATIONALES*

Emphasize importance of gentle cleansing *because this is essential in treatment of acne*

Provide written instructions, including the cause of the lesions and the therapeutic regimen outlined, *to reinforce verbal instructions and provide for future referral*

Motivate the adolescent to assume responsibility for following through on instructions

Teach medication administration and other therapeutic and hygienic measures

Discourage "picking" at lesions *because this can increase the number of lesions and the risk of infection*

EXPECTED OUTCOME

Adolescent assumes responsibility for care of skin lesions and complies with preventive measures

■ **PATIENT GOAL 4:** Will receive adequate support

NURSING INTERVENTIONS/*RATIONALES*

Allow the adolescent to express feelings about the disorder, its effect on his or her appearance, and the length of time required for therapy

Provide positive reinforcement for compliance *so that adolescent continues to comply with therapy*

Encourage maintenance of normal activities and interactions with peers *so that adolescent does not become isolated because of self-consciousness*

Explore job opportunities and after-school interests with the adolescent

Reinforce the efficacy of therapy and improvement in appearance

Assist adolescent with grooming *to enhance appearance and improve body image*

EXPECTED OUTCOME

Adolescent discusses feelings and concerns regarding appearance and identifies positive aspects of appearance

---

NURSING DIAGNOSIS: Altered family processes related to the child with a troublesome skin problem

---

■ **PATIENT (FAMILY) GOAL 1:** Will demonstrate an understanding of adolescent's skin problem and therapy

NURSING INTERVENTIONS/*RATIONALES*

Explain acne and therapy prescribed *to increase family's understanding*

Assist family in helping adolescent assume greater responsibility for acne management

Explain the nature of adolescent development and the effect acne has on self-image and identify formation *so that family is more understanding and supportive*

EXPECTED OUTCOMES

Family demonstrates an understanding of the adolescent's skin problem and therapy

Family shows a supportive attitude

Unit 4

NURSING CARE PLAN

The Child with Burns

Burns are the destruction of skin caused by thermal, chemical, electric, or radioactive agents.

Burn severity criteria:

Minor burns

Partial-thickness burns of less than 10% of body surface area (BSA)

Moderate burns

Partial-thickness burns of 10% to 20% of BSA (age-related; see Major, or Critical, Burns)

Major, or critical, burns

Burns complicated by respiratory tract injury

Partial-thickness burns of 20% of BSA or greater

Burns of face, hands, feet, or genitalia, even if they appear to be partial thickness

All full-thickness burns

Any child younger than 2 years of age, unless the burn is very small and very superficial (20% of BSA or greater considered critical in child younger than 2 years of age)

Electric burns that penetrate

Deep chemical burns

Respiratory tract damage

Burns complicated by fractures or soft tissue injury

Burns complicated by concurrent illness, such as obesity, diabetes, epilepsy, or cardiac and renal diseases

---

ASSESSMENT

Initial assessments

Assess respiratory status.

Asses for extent of burn injury based on percentage of body surface area involved (Fig. 4-10).

Assess for depth of burn injury:

Superficial (first-degree) burns:

Dry, red surface

Blanches on pressure and refills

Minimal or no edema

Painful; sensitive to touch

Partial-thickness (second-degree) burns:

Blistered, moist

Serous drainage

Edema

Mottled pink or red

Blanches on pressure and refills

Very painful; sensitive to touch

Full-thickness (third-degree) burns:

Tough, leathery

Dull, dry surface

Marbled, pale white, brown, tan, red, or black

Does not blanch on pressure

Edema

Variable pain, often severe

Assess for evidence of associated injuries:

Check eyes for injury or irritation.

Check nasopharynx for edema or redness.

Check for singed hair, including nasal hair.

Assess for other injuries (e.g., bruises, fractures, internal injuries).

Observe for evidence of respiratory distress.

Assess need for pain medication.

Weigh child on admission; take vital signs.

Assess level of consciousness. (See p. 459.)

Obtain history of burn injury, especially time of injury, nature of burning agent, duration of contact, if injury occurred in an enclosed area, any medication given.

Obtain pertinent history relative to preburn condition—Weight, preexisting illnesses, any allergies, tetanus immunization.

Assist with diagnostic procedures and tests (e.g., blood count, urinalysis, wound cultures, hematocrit).

Ongoing assessments

Monitor vital signs, including blood pressure.

Measure intake and output.

Monitor intravenous infusion; observe for evidence of over-hydration.

Assess circulation of areas peripheral to burns.

Assess for evidence of healing, stability of temporary cover or graft, infection.

Observe for evidence of complications—Pneumonia, wound sepsis, Curling (stress) ulcer, central nervous system dysfunction (hallucinations, personality changes, delirium, seizures, alterations in sensorium), hypertension.

NURSING DIAGNOSIS: Impaired skin integrity related to thermal injury

■ **PATIENT GOAL 1:** Will exhibit evidence of wound healing

NURSING INTERVENTIONS/*RATIONALES*

Shave hair to a 2-inch margin from the wound and area immediately surrounding the burn *to remove a reservoir for infection*

Thoroughly cleanse the wound and surrounding skin *to decrease the risk of infection;* debride devitalized tissue *to promote healing*

Keep child from scratching and picking at the wound:

Provide distraction appropriate to child's age

Older child: explain reasons *to encourage cooperation*

Young child: supervise activity as needed

Maintain care in handling the wound *to avoid damaging epithelializing and granulating tissues*

Offer high-calorie, high-protein meals and snacks *to meet augmented protein and calorie requirements caused by increased metabolism and catabolism*

Prevent infection, which can delay healing and convert partial-thickness wounds to full-thickness wounds

Administer supplementary vitamins and minerals (e.g., vitamins A, B, C, iron, and zinc) *to facilitate wound healing and epithelialization*

Pad burned ears *to prevent tissue necrosis due to minimal blood flow to cartilage*

Monitor for signs/symptoms of wound infection *to ensure prompt recognition and treatment*

Wrap fingers and toes separately *to avoid tissue adherence from prolonged contact*

Continued

The Child with Burns—cont'd

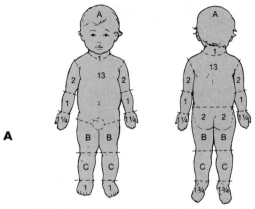

RELATIVE PERCENTAGES OF AREAS AFFECTED BY GROWTH

AREA	BIRTH	AGE 1 YR	AGE 5 YR
A = ½ of head	9½	8½	6½
B = ½ of one thigh	2¾	3¼	4
C = ½ of one leg	2½	2½	2¾

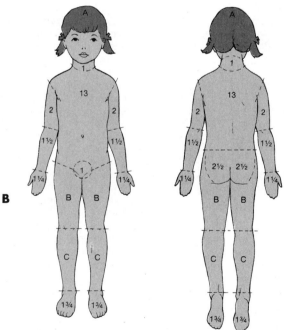

RELATIVE PERCENTAGES OF AREAS AFFECTED BY GROWTH

AREA	AGE 10 YR	AGE 15 YR	ADULT
A = ½ of head	5½	4½	3½
B = ½ of one thigh	4½	4½	4¾
C = ½ of one leg	3	3¼	3½

Fig. 4-10 Estimation of distribution of burns in children. **A,** Children from birth to age 5 years. **B,** Older children.

The Child with Burns—cont'd

EXPECTED OUTCOME
Wounds heal without evidence of damage or inflammation

■ **PATIENT GOAL 2:** Will maintain integrity of skin graft

NURSING INTERVENTIONS/*RATIONALES*
Position for minimal mechanical disturbance of graft site
Restrain if necessary *to prevent graft from being dislodged*
Maintain splints or dressings *if needed for protection of the graft*
Observe grafts for evidence of hematoma/fluid accumulation; aspirate or express fluids *to ensure contact of the graft with the base*

EXPECTED OUTCOME
Skin graft remains intact

NURSING DIAGNOSIS: Risk for altered tissue perfusion related to circumferential burns

---

■ **PATIENT GOAL 1:** Will retain optimal circulation to distal regions of the affected extremity

NURSING INTERVENTIONS/*RATIONALES*
Monitor closely for signs/symptoms of circulation compression related to edema (assess numbness, tingling, color, or temperature changes q 1-2 hr × 72 hours) *to ensure adequate circulation perfusion*
Assess diminished Doppler pulses and prolonged capillary refill (Doppler checks q 1-2 hr × 72 hours) *to indicate diminished distal perfusion*
Elevated extremity above the level of the heart *to prevent decreased circulation to the extremity*
Avoid restrictive dressings over the injured extremity *to prevent decreased circulation to the extremity*

EXPECTED OUTCOME
Adequate distal perfusion to the affected extremity is maintained

---

NURSING DIAGNOSIS: Pain related to skin trauma, therapies

■ **PATIENT GOAL 1:** Will experience reduction of pain to a level acceptable to the child

NURSING INTERVENTIONS/*RATIONALES*
Assess need for medication (See pain assessment, p. 315.)
Recognize that burn pain is often overwhelming, engulfing, and irrepressible
Position in extension *to minimize pain resulting from exercising to regain extension*
Implement passive and active exercising *to minimize contracture formation*
Reduce irritation *to prevent increased pain*
Touch/stroke unburned areas *to provide physical contact and comfort*
Employ appropriate nonpharmacologic pain reduction techniques (See Nursing Care Plan: The Child in Pain, p. 339.)
Promote control and predictability during painful procedures (Atraumatic Care box)

Anticipate the need for pain medication and administer before the onset of severe pain and at regular intervals *to prevent recurrence* (See Nursing Care Plan: The Child in Pain, p. 315.)

EXPECTED OUTCOME
Child exhibits reduction of pain to level acceptable to child

---

NURSING DIAGNOSIS: Risk for infection related to denuded skin, presence of pathogenic organisms, altered immune response

---

■ **PATIENT GOAL 1:** Will exhibit no evidence of wound infection

NURSING INTERVENTIONS/*RATIONALES*
Implement and maintain infection control precautions according to unit policy
Maintain careful handwashing by members of staff and visitors *to minimize exposure to infectious agents*
Wear clean or sterile gown, cap, mask, and gloves when handling wound area *to minimize exposure to infectious agents*
Debride eschar, crust, and blisters *to eliminate these reservoirs for organisms*
Avoid patient contact with persons who have upper respiratory or skin infections
Cover the wound and/or patient according to the protocol of the unit *to provide a barrier to organisms*
Administer good oral hygiene
*Apply prescribed topical antimicrobial preparation and dressings to the wound *to control bacterial proliferation*
Obtain baseline and serial wound cultures *to ascertain any increase or changes in wound flora*
Monitor closely for signs of sepsis and infection (disorientation, tachypnea, temperature above 39.5° C [103° F], hypothermia, distention of the abdomen or intestinal ileus, change in wound appearance)

EXPECTED OUTCOMES
Possible sources of infection are eliminated
Wound displays minimal or no evidence of infection

NURSING DIAGNOSIS: Risk for ineffective thermoregulation related to heat loss and disruption of skin's defense mechanism to maintain body temperature

---

■ **PATIENT GOAL 1:** Will maintain normal thermal regulation as evidenced by normal body temperatures ranging from 37° to 38° C (98.6° to 100.4° F)

NURSING INTERVENTIONS/*RATIONALES*
Assess patient skin for coolness, color changes, and capillary refill (acrocyanosis, nail bed color, and mottling) *to identify vascular accommodation of heat loss*
Monitor vital signs, especially temperature, *to identify significant trends*
Observe for chilling and shivering *to identify signs of heat loss*
Avoid exposure to cold stress procedures (limiting tubbing to 20 minutes, bundling child, covering the head of a child <6 months of age, artificial heat) *to maintain body temperature*

*Dependent nursing action.

Continued

Unit 4

The Child with Burns—cont'd

EXPECTED OUTCOME
Child's temperature remains within normal limits for age

> **NURSING DIAGNOSIS:** Risk for fluid volume deficit related to normal fluid loss from tissues because of burn insult

■ **PATIENT GOAL 1:** Will maintain adequate fluid hydration status during the acute postburn period

NURSING INTERVENTIONS/*RATIONALES*
*Administer crystalloid and/or colloid fluid per protocol, monitoring effect and maintaining IV, *to replace fluid loss related to burn injury*
Assess fluid replacement status: inadequate (skin turgor, increased pulse, decreased urine output, decreased circulation status, or change in mental status [restlessness, disorientation]) or excessive (pulmonary congestion or pulmonary edema) *to recognize appropriate fluid balance*
Monitor daily weights *to evaluate status of fluid retention or diuresis*
Observe and monitor hemodynamic parameters for changes in stability related to hypovolemia or overload *because change in blood pressure is a late sign*
Monitor laboratory results (Hbg, Hct, glucose, serum potassium, serum sodium, serum protein, phosphorus, and magnesium) *to identify fluid and electrolyte imbalance*
*Administer potassium-rich or potassium-restricted fluids or foods if child is hypokalemic or hyperkalemic, respectively, *to supplement IV therapy*

EXPECTED OUTCOME
Adequate fluid resuscitation is maintained as evidenced by adequate tissue perfusion and maintenance of urine output

> **NURSING DIAGNOSIS:** Altered nutrition: less than body requirements related to increased catabolism and metabolism, loss of appetite

■ **PATIENT GOAL 1:** Will receive optimum nourishment

NURSING INTERVENTIONS/*RATIONALES*
Encourage oral feeding (See Nursing Care Plan: The Child with Special Nutritional Needs, p. 313.)
Provide high-calorie, high-protein meals and snacks *to avoid protein breakdown and to meet augmented caloric requirements*
Provide foods child likes *to stimulate appetite*
Allow self-help *to encourage cooperation*
Provide meals when child is most likely to eat well
Provide attractive meals and surroundings *to encourage eating*
Provide companionship at meals *to create a more homelike environment*
Use "contract" with older children *to encourage compliance*
*Administer supplemental enteral feedings as prescribed *to meet calculated needs*
Obtain weekly weight *to monitor nutritional status*
Record accurate intake and output *to evaluate sufficiency of intake*
Monitor for diarrhea/constipation and institute prompt treatment *to avoid feeding intolerance*

EXPECTED OUTCOME
Child consumes a sufficient amount of nutrients (specify) and maintains preburn weight

> **NURSING DIAGNOSIS:** Risk for constipation and risk for diarrhea related to opioid administration, inadequate intake of nutrients, and the need for tube feedings

■ **PATIENT GOAL 1:** Will have routine bowel patterns

NURSING INTERVENTIONS/*RATIONALES*
Monitor for diarrhea/constipation and institute prompt treatment:
Record amount and consistency of stool daily
Administer antidiarrhea agents
Administer bulk laxative, stool softener, or cathartic *to avoid feeding intolerance*
Assess fluid hydration status to correlate dehydration with development of constipation
Monitor electrolyte panel, replacing lost electrolytes via IV or tube feeding, *to detect electrolyte imbalance*
In acute episodes of diarrhea, hold oral intake *to rest bowel*
Increase activity and ambulation *to increase peristalsis and motility*

EXPECTED OUTCOME
Normal bowel elimination pattern returns as evidenced by soft, formed stools q 1-2 days

> **NURSING DIAGNOSIS:** Impaired physical mobility (specify level) related to pain, impaired joint movement, scar formation

■ **PATIENT GOAL 1:** Will achieve optimum physical functioning

NURSING INTERVENTIONS/*RATIONALES*
Carry out range-of-motion exercises *to maintain optimum joint and muscle function*
Encourage mobility if child is able to move extremities
Ambulate as soon as feasible
Splint involved joints in extension at night and during rest periods *to minimize contracture formation*
Encourage and promote self-help activities *to increase mobility*
Administer analgesia before painful activity (e.g., physical therapy) *so that child is more likely to cooperate and be mobile*
Encourage participation in activities of daily living and play activities *to incorporate exercise into enjoyable events*
Use lotion and massage on healed areas before exercise *to soften tissues and promote relaxation*

EXPECTED OUTCOME
Child achieves functioning to level of ability

■ **PATIENT GOAL 2:** Will exhibit minimal scarring

NURSING INTERVENTIONS/*RATIONALES*
Position in a functional attitude for minimal deformity and optimum functioning
*Apply splints as ordered and designed *to minimize contracture*

*Dependent nursing action.

Unit 4

The Child with Burns—cont'd

*Wrap healing tissue with elastic bandage or dress in elastic garments as ordered *to help reduce scar hypertrophy by compressing collagen and decreasing vascularity*

Carry out physical therapy *to minimize deformity related to scar contracture formation*

Provide treatment for pruritus *to minimize scratching and irritation of newly healed tissue*

EXPECTED OUTCOME

Wound heals with minimal scar formation; joints remain flexible and functional

> **NURSING DIAGNOSIS:** Body image disturbance related to perception of appearance and mobility

■ **PATIENT GOAL 1:** Will receive adequate emotional support

NURSING INTERVENTIONS/RATIONALES

Convey positive attitude toward child *to demonstrate acceptance and so that child expects to get better*

Encourage parents to participate in care *to prevent the stress of separation and prepare for reintegration into the community*

Encourage as much independence as condition allows *to give child a sense of control*

Arrange for continued schooling *to encourage optimum development and sense of normalcy*

Promote peer contact where possible *to decrease isolation*

Be honest with child and family *to create a trusting nurse-patient relationship*

Encourage activities appropriate to age and capabilities *to promote normalcy and increase self-esteem*

Prepare peers for child's appearance *to encourage acceptance and support*

Provide opportunities for child and family to discuss the impact of the change in appearance and lifestyle *to increase coping*

Support behaviors suggesting adaptation *to build on strengths*

EXPECTED OUTCOMES

Child accepts efforts of family and caregivers

Child engages in activities with others according to age and capabilities

■ **PATIENT GOAL 2:** Will demonstrate improved body image

NURSING INTERVENTIONS/RATIONALES

Explore feelings concerning physical appearance *to facilitate coping with body image changes*

Discuss feelings about returning to home, family, school, and friends *to build coping mechanisms*

Provide reinforcement of positive aspects of appearance and capabilities *to recognize and build on strengths*

Point out evidence of healing *to encourage a sense of hope*

Discuss aids that camouflage disfigurement *to facilitate coping:*
Wigs
Clothing (e.g., turtleneck sweaters)
Makeup

Provide recreational and diversional activities *to promote a sense of normalcy*

Promote constructive thinking in child *to encourage positive coping*

Help child devise a plan to address and cope with the reactions of others *to increase the sense of control*

EXPECTED OUTCOMES

Child discusses feelings and concerns regarding appearance and the perceived reactions of others

Child verbalizes positive suggestions for adjusting to appearance and community/peer response

■ **PATIENT GOAL 3:** Will engage in self-care activities

NURSING INTERVENTIONS/RATIONALES

Assist with self-care activities as needed

Encourage self-care according to capabilities

Begin to discuss "going home" early in hospitalization *so that child expects to get better*

Accept regressive behavior where appropriate *because this is how child is coping with stress*

Help child develop independence and self-help capabilities *to increase self-esteem*

EXPECTED OUTCOMES

Child verbalizes and otherwise demonstrates interest in going home

Child engages in self-help activities

> **NURSING DIAGNOSIS:** Altered family processes related to situational crisis (child with a serious injury)

■ **PATIENT (FAMILY) GOAL 1:** Will be prepared for discharge and home care

NURSING INTERVENTIONS/RATIONALES

Teach wound care to caregiver *to achieve proficiency and increase confidence*

Discuss diet, rest, and activity *to assist in planning for a home care regimen*

Explore attitudes toward child's reentry into the family *to facilitate coping and identify a possible need for intervention*

Explore family's concepts regarding child's capabilities and the possible restrictions and freedom they will allow *to assist them in planning realistically for an altered lifestyle*

Help family set realistic goals for themselves, the child, and other family members *to clarify and validate the plan of home care*

Help family acquire needed equipment and supplies *to reduce anxiety*

EXPECTED OUTCOMES

Family demonstrates an understanding of child's needs and the impact child's condition will have on them

Family members set realistic goals for themselves, child, and others

■ **PATIENT (FAMILY) GOAL 2:** Will participate in follow-up care

NURSING INTERVENTIONS/RATIONALES

Coordinate team management of child and family for ongoing care *to provide continuity*

---

*Dependent nursing action.

Continued

The Child with Burns—cont'd

Arrange for return visits

Assess the needs of the family *to determine appropriate plan of care*

Arrange for referral agencies based on needs assessment

Collaborate with school nurse *to help with child's reintegration into school and the world of peers*

Visit the school, if possible, to prepare teacher and peers *to encourage acceptance of child*

EXPECTED OUTCOMES

Family maintains contact with health providers

Child attends school regularly and interacts with age-mates

(See also:

Nursing Care Plan: The Child in the Hospital, p. 268.)

Nursing Care Plan: The Family of the Child Who Is Ill or Hospitalized, p. 282.)

ATRAUMATIC CARE

Reducing the Stress of Burn Care Procedures

Have all materials ready before beginning.

Administer appropriate analgesics.

Remind the child of the impending procedure to allow sufficient time to prepare.

Allow the child to test and approve the temperature of the water.

Allow the child to select the area of the body on which to begin.

Allow the child to request a short rest period during the procedure.

Allow the child to remove the dressings if desired.

Provide something constructive for the child to do during the procedure (e.g., holding a package of dressings or a roll of gauze).

Inform the child when the procedure is near completion.

Praise the child for his or her cooperation.

NURSING CARE OF THE CHILD WITH PSYCHOPHYSIOLOGIC DYSFUNCTION

Psychophysiologic dysfunction refers to those disorders in which psychologic factors play an important, if not primary, role in producing a physiologic problem.

NURSING CARE PLAN

The Child with Nonorganic Failure to Thrive

Nonorganic failure to thrive (NFTT) is caused by factors unrelated to organic dysfunction and most often the result of psychosocial factors, such as inadequate nutritional information by the parent; deficiency in maternal care or a disturbance in maternal-child attachment; or a disturbance in the child's ability to separate from the parent, leading to food refusal to maintain attention.

ASSESSMENT

Perform a physical assessment, especially regarding growth.
Obtain a detailed history, especially regarding feeding behavior.
Observe for manifestations of NFTT:
  Growth failure—Below 5th percentile in weight only or in weight and height
  Developmental retardation—Social, motor, adaptive, language
  Apathy
  Poor hygiene
  Withdrawn behavior
  Feeding or eating disorders such as vomiting, anorexia, pica, rumination
  No fear of strangers (at age when stranger anxiety is normal)
  Avoidance of eye contact
  Wide-eyed gaze and continual scan of the environment ("radar gaze")
  Stiff and unyielding or flaccid and unresponsive
  Minimum smiling
Observe for evidence of parental maladaptive behaviors toward infant:
  Persistent ambivalence or negative feelings about the fetus and the pregnancy during the prenatal period
  Makes no plans for obtaining basic infant supplies
  Appears indifferent to infant at time of delivery; may appear sad or angry; is expressionless
  Makes no effort to establish contact with infant
  Handles infant only when necessary
  Does not talk to infant
  Makes few or no spontaneous movements with infant
  Asks few questions about care
  Sees infant as ugly, fat, or unattractive
  Displays disgust with infant's drooling and sucking sounds; is revolted by infant's body fluids
  Annoyed by diaper changing
  Perceives infant's odor as revolting

Holds infant with little support to head and body
Holds infant away from body during feeding, or props bottle for feeding; seldom cuddles infant
Does not coo or talk to infant
Refers to infant in an impersonal manner
Develops inappropriate responses to infant's needs (e.g., leaving infant in one place for long periods, leaving infant alone in room, overfeeding or underfeeding, ovestimulating or understimulating infant, forcing or refusing eye contact, bouncing or tickling infant when infant is fatigued)
Cannot discriminate between infant's signals for hunger, comfort, rest, body contact
Is convinced the infant has a defect or disease even when reassured to the contrary
Makes negative statements regarding parenting role
Believes the infant is judging him or her as an adult might
Believes the infant does not love him or her
Develops paradoxical attitudes and behaviors toward infant
Assess parent-child interaction during feedings.
Assess infant's feeding behaviors, temperament.
Assess family for marital stress, physical or mental illness, death or illness in a previous child, alcoholism, drug use, financial crises, mental retardation.
Determine if pregnancy was planned or unplanned; and any disturbing events associated with pregnancy or delivery of the child.
Perform developmental tests.
Assist with diagnostic procedures and tests, including those to rule out organic disease.
Observe for evidence of parental characteristics such as:
  History of maternal deprivation as a child
  Low self-esteem; feelings of inadequacy
  Desire for dependency
  Loneliness, isolation
  Limited support system
  Multiple life crises and stress

NURSING DIAGNOSIS: Altered nutrition: less than body requirements related to deprivation of necessities, emotional deprivation

■ **PATIENT GOAL 1:** Will experience weight gain

NURSING INTERVENTIONS/*RATIONALES***
Introduce a positive feeding environment (Guidelines box)
Provide unlimited feedings of a regular diet for child's age (preferably foods to which child is accustomed) *to encourage acceptance of foods*
Avoid interrupting feedings with other activities, such as laboratory examinations or radiography, *to maintain feeding routine*

Keep accurate record of intake *to ensure ingestion of calculated daily calories*
Weigh daily and record *to ascertain weight gain*

EXPECTED OUTCOMES
Responds positively to feeding practices (specify)
Child gains weight (specify) (usually a minimum of 1 to 2 oz/day)

NURSING DIAGNOSIS: Altered growth and development related to socially restricted environment (infant deprivation), physical neglect

Continued

The Child with Nonorganic Failure to Thrive—cont'd

- **PATIENT GOAL 1:** Will demonstrate positive response to developmental intervention

NURSING INTERVENTIONS/*RATIONALES*

Apply primary care concepts with a minimum number of care-givers *to ensure continuity of care*

Provide gentle, confident, and loving handling *to meet infant's emotional needs*

Perform physical care with as much holding, rocking, and cuddling as child will respond to *in order to provide tactile stimulation*

Encourage eye contact *to discourage child's withdrawal*

Employ consistent schedule in meeting child's needs for food, hygiene, care, and rest

Assign a foster grandparent or child life specialist to child *to provide appropriate stimulation*

Provide sensory stimulation and play appropriate to child's developmental level *to promote optimum growth and development*

EXPECTED OUTCOMES

Child displays a positive response to interventions (e.g., social smile)

Child exhibits developmental achievement (specify)

> **NURSING DIAGNOSIS:** Altered parenting related to (specify, e.g., knowledge deficit, poverty)

- **PATIENT (FAMILY) GOAL 1:** Will experience reduction of anxiety

NURSING INTERVENTIONS/*RATIONALES*

Welcome parents; encourage, but do not pressure them to become involved in child's care *to avoid creating additional stresses*

Teach parents about child's physical care, developmental skills, and emotional needs through example, not lecture, *to avoid decreasing self-esteem*

Afford parents the opportunity to discuss their lives and feelings toward child *to provide understanding and empathy*

Supply emotional nurturance without encouraging dependency *to encourage sense of adequacy*

Praise parents' achievements with child to promote their self-esteem and confidence

Prepare parents for adjustments with anticipatory guidance *to enhance coping skill*

EXPECTED OUTCOME

Parents demonstrate ability to provide appropriate care to child

- **PATIENT (FAMILY) GOAL 2:** Will be prepared for home care

NURSING INTERVENTIONS/*RATIONALES*

Assess home environment and relationships *to identify need for intervention*

Continue interventions begun in the hospital *to ensure adequate care following discharge*

Establish system for follow-up care (e.g., community health nurse) *so plan of care continues at home*

Establish a stimulation program *to promote child's optimum growth and development*

Provide for stress-relieving services to family *to help family cope*

Refer to appropriate agencies for assistance with financial, social, mental health, or other family needs *to ensure that their overall needs are met*

EXPECTED OUTCOMES

Child exhibits continued weight gain appropriate for age

Family follows through on programs and activities

Other agencies are involved as needed

GUIDELINES

Feeding Children with Nonorganic Failure to Thrive

Provide a primary core of staff to feed the child. The same nurses are able to learn the child's cues and respond consistently.

Provide a quiet, unstimulating atmosphere. A number of these children are very distractible, and their attention is diverted with minimum stimuli. Older children do well at a feeding table; younger children should always be held.

Maintain a calm, even temperament throughout the meal. Negative outbursts may be commonplace in this child's habit formation. Limits on eating behavior definitely need to be provided, but they should be stated in a firm, calm tone. If the nurse is hurried or anxious, the feeding process will not be optimized.

Talk to the child by giving directions about eating. "Take a bite, Lisa" is appropriate and directive. The more distractible the child, the more directive the nurse should be to refocus attention on feeding. Positive comments about feeding are actively given.

Be persistent. This is perhaps one of the most important guidelines. Parents often give up when the child begins

negative feeding behavior. Calm perseverance through 10 to 15 minutes of food refusal will eventually diminish negative behavior. Although forced feeding is avoided, "strictly encouraged" feeding is essential.

Maintain a face-to-face posture with the child when possible. Encourage eye contact and remain with the child throughout the meal.

Introduce new foods slowly. Often these children have been exclusively bottle-fed. If acceptance of solids is a problem, begin with pureed food and, once accepted, advance to junior and regular solid foods.

Follow the child's rhythm of feeding. The child will set a rhythm when the previous conditions are met.

Develop a structured routine. Disruption in the child's other activities of daily living has great impact on feeding responses, so bathing, sleeping, dressing, and playing, as well as feeding, are structured. The nurse should feed the child in the same way and place as often as possible. The length of the feeding should also be established (usually 30 minutes).

Unit 4

NURSING CARE PLAN

The Child Who Is Maltreated

Child maltreatment is a broad term that includes intentional physical abuse or neglect, emotional abuse or neglect, and sexual abuse of children, usually by an adult.

Physical abuse—The deliberate infliction of physical injury

Physical neglect—The deprivation of necessities, such as food, clothing, shelter, supervision, medical care, and education

Emotional abuse—The deliberate attempt to destroy or significantly impair a child's self-esteem or competence

Emotional neglect—Failure to meet the child's needs for affection, attention, and emotional nurturance

Sexual abuse—Contacts or interactions between a child and an adult when the child is being used for the sexual stimulation of that adult or another person

Munchausen syndrome by proxy—Physical abuse inflicted on a child, usually by the mother, to fabricate an illness that requires medical care for her child

ASSESSMENT

Perform a physical assessment with special attention to manifestations of potential abuse or neglect (Box 4-32).

Obtain a history of event, being alert for discrepancies in descriptions by caregiver and observations:

Note sequence of events, including times, especially time lapse between occurrence of injury and initiation of treatment.

Interview child when appropriate, including verbal quotations and information from drawings or other play activities.

Interview parents, witnesses, and other significant persons, including their verbal quotations.

Observe parent-child interactions (e.g., verbal interactions, eye contact, touching, evidence of parental concern).

Observe or obtain information regarding names, ages, and conditions of other children in the home (if possible).

Perform a developmental test.

Assist with diagnostic procedures and tests (e.g., radiology, collection of specimens for examination).

BOX 4-32

Clinical Manifestations of Potential Child Maltreatment

Physical Neglect

Suggestive Physical Findings

Failure to thrive

Signs of malnutrition, such as thin extremities, abdominal distention, lack of subcutaneous fat

Poor personal hygiene, especially of teeth

Unclean and/or inappropriate dress

Evidence of poor health care, such as nonimmunized status, untreated infections, frequent colds

Frequent injuries from lack of supervision

Suggestive Behaviors

Dull and inactive; excessively passive or sleepy

Self-stimulatory behaviors, such as finger-sucking or rocking

In older child:

Begging or stealing food

Absenteeism from school

Drug or alcohol addiction

Vandalism or shoplifting

Emotional Abuse and Neglect

Suggestive Physical Findings

Failure to thrive

Feeding disorders, such as rumination

Enuresis

Sleep disorders

Suggestive Behaviors

Self-stimulatory behaviors, such as biting, rocking, sucking

During infancy, lack of social smile and stranger anxiety

Withdrawal

Unusual fearfulness

Antisocial behavior, such as destructiveness, stealing, cruelty (Community Focus box)

Extremes of behavior, such as overcompliant and passive or aggressive and demanding

Lags in emotional and intellectual development, especially language

Suicide attempts

Physical Abuse

Suggestive Physical Findings

Bruises and welts:

On face, lips, mouth, back, buttocks, thighs, or areas of torso

Regular patterns descriptive of object used, such as belt buckle, hand, wire hanger, chain, wooden spoon, squeeze or pinch marks

May be present in various stages of healing

Continued

Unit 4

The Child Who Is Maltreated—cont'd

BOX 4-32

Clinical Manifestations of Potential Child Maltreatment—cont'd

Physical Abuse—cont'd

Suggestive Physical Findings—cont'd

Burns:

On soles of feet, palms of hands, back, or buttocks

Patterns descriptive of object used, such as round cigar or cigarette burns, "glovelike" sharply demarcated areas from immersion in scalding water, rope burns on wrists or ankles from being bound, burns in the shape of an iron, radiator, or electric stove burner

Absence of "splash" marks and presence of symmetric burns

Stun gun injury—Lesions circular, fairly uniform (up to 0.5 cm), and paired about 5 cm apart

Fractures and dislocations:

Skull, nose, or facial structures

Injury may denote type of abuse, such as spiral fracture or dislocation from twisting of an extremity or whiplash from shaking the child

Multiple new or old fractures in various stages of healing

Lacerations and abrasions:

On backs of arms, legs, torso, face, or external genitalia

Unusual symptoms, such as abdominal swelling, pain, and vomiting from punching

Descriptive marks such as from human bites or pulling the hair out

Chemical:

Unexplained repeated poisoning, especially drug overdose

Unexplained sudden illness, such as hypoglycemia from insulin administration

Suggestive Behaviors

Wary of physical contact with adults

Apparent fear of parents or of going home

Lying very still while surveying environment

Inappropriate reaction to injury, such as failure to cry from pain

Lack of reaction to frightening events

Apprehensive when hearing other children cry

Indiscriminate friendliness and displays of affection

Superficial relationships

Acting-out behavior, such as aggression, to seek attention

Withdrawal behavior

Sexual Abuse

Suggestive Physical Findings

Bruises, bleeding, lacerations or irritation of genitalia, anus, mouth, or throat

Torn, stained, or bloody underclothing

Pain on urination; or pain, swelling, and itching of genital area

Penile or vaginal discharge

Sexually transmitted disease, nonspecific vaginitis, or venereal warts

Difficulty in walking or sitting

Unusual odor in the genital area

Recurrent urinary tract infections

Presence of sperm

Pregnancy in young adolescent

Suggestive Behaviors

Sudden emergence of sexually related problems, including excessive or public masturbation, age-inappropriate sexual play, promiscuity, or overtly seductive behavior

Withdrawn, excessive daydreaming

Preoccupied with fantasies, especially in play

Poor relationships with peers

Sudden changes, such as increased anxiety, weight loss or gain, clinging behavior

In incestuous relationships, excessive anger at mother for not protecting daughter

Regressive behavior, such as bed-wetting or thumb-sucking

Sudden onset of phobias or fears, particularly fears of the dark, men, strangers, or particular settings or situations (e.g., undue fear of leaving the house or staying at the daycare center or the baby-sitter's house)

Running away from home

Substance abuse, particularly of alcohol or mood-elevating drugs

Profound and rapid personality changes, especially extreme depression, hostility, and aggression (often accompanied by social withdrawal)

Rapidly declining school performance

Suicidal attempts or ideation

Unit 4

The Child Who Is Maltreated—cont'd

NURSING DIAGNOSIS: Risk for trauma related to characteristics of child, caregiver(s), environment

■ **PATIENT GOAL 1:** Will experience no further abuse or neglect

NURSING INTERVENTIONS/*RATIONALES*

Implement measures *to prevent abuse:*
  Report suspicions to appropriate authorities
  Assist in removing child from unsafe environment and establishing a safe environment
  Establish protective measures for the hospitalized child as indicated *to prevent continued abuse in hospital*
Refer family to social agencies for assistance with finances, food, clothing, housing, and health care *to help prevent neglect*
Keep factual, objective records *for documentation,* including:
  Child's physical condition
  Child's behavioral response to parents, others, and environment
  Interviews with family members
Collaborate efforts of multidisciplinary team *to continually evaluate progress of child in foster home or in return to own family*
Be alert for signs of continued abuse or neglect
Help parents identify those circumstances that precipitate an abusive act and alternative ways to deal with the release of anger other than attacking child
Refer for alternative placement when indicated *to prevent further injury or neglect*

EXPECTED OUTCOME

Child experiences no further injury or neglect

NURSING DIAGNOSIS: Fear/anxiety related to negative interpersonal interaction, repeated maltreatment, powerlessness, potential loss of parents

■ **PATIENT GOAL 1:** Will experience reduction or relief of anxiety and stress

NURSING INTERVENTIONS/*RATIONALES*

Provide consistent caregiver and therapeutic environment during hospitalization *in order to relieve child's stress and to be a role model for family*
Demonstrate acceptance of child while not expecting same in return
Show attention while not reinforcing inappropriate behavior *since all children have this need*
Plan appropriate activities for attention with nurse, other adults, and other children; use play *to work through relationships*
Praise child's abilities *in order to promote self-esteem*
Treat child as one who has a specific physical problem for hospitalization, not as "abused" victim
Avoid asking too many questions *since this can upset child and interfere with other professionals' interrogations*

Use play, especially family or dollhouse activity, *to investigate types of relationships perceived by child*
Provide one person to whom child can consistently relate regarding events of abuse *so that child is not overwhelmed*
Help child grieve for loss of parents, if their rights are terminated, *because child may be very attached to parents despite abuse*
Encourage child to talk about feelings toward parents and future placement *to facilitate coping*
Encourage introduction to foster parents before placement, if possible, *to give child time to adjust*

EXPECTED OUTCOMES

Child exhibits minimal or no evidence of distress
Child engages in positive relationships with caregivers
Child grieves for loss of parent(s)

NURSING DIAGNOSIS: Altered parenting related to child, caregiver, or situational characteristics that precipitate abusive behavior

■ **PATIENT (FAMILY) GOAL 1:** Will exhibit evidence of positive interaction with children

NURSING INTERVENTIONS/*RATIONALES*

Identify families at risk for potential abuse *so that appropriate intervention is instituted*
Promote parental attachment to child *since all children have this need*
Emphasize childrearing practices, especially effective methods of discipline, *since parents may lack knowledge about nonviolent discipline methods*
Increase parents' feelings of adequacy and self-esteem
Encourage support systems *that lessen stress and total responsibility of child care on one or both parents*
Teach children to recognize situations that place them at risk for sexual abuse, and teach assertive responses *to discourage abuse*

EXPECTED OUTCOME

Families exhibit evidence of positive interaction with children

■ **PATIENT (FAMILY) GOAL 2:** Will receive adequate support

NURSING INTERVENTIONS/*RATIONALES*

Provide "mothering" by directing attention to parent, taking over child care responsibilities until parent feels ready to participate, and focusing on parent's needs *so that parents can eventually meet child's needs*
Convey an attitude of genuine concern, not one of accusation and punishment, *since this serves only to further alienate family*
Refer parents to special support groups and/or counseling *for long-term support*
Help identify a support group for parents, such as extended family or nearby neighbors; help these significant others understand their important role in also preventing further abuse

Unit 4

Continued

The Child Who Is Maltreated—cont'd

Refer to social agencies that can provide assistance in areas such as financial support, adequate housing, and employment

EXPECTED OUTCOMES

Parents demonstrate appropriate parenting activities

Parents seek group and individual support

Parents receive assistance with problems

■ **PATIENT (FAMILY) GOAL 3:** Will exhibit knowledge of normal growth and development

NURSING INTERVENTIONS/*RATIONALES*

Teach realistic expectations of child's behavior and capabilities

Emphasize alternate methods of discipline, such as reward, time-out, consequences, and verbal disapproval, *so that parents learn nonviolent discipline methods*

Suggest methods of handling developmental problems or goals, such as toddler negativism, toilet training, and independence, *because these situations may precipitate abuse*

Teach through demonstration and role modeling, rather than lecture; avoid authoritarian approach *because family may be sensitive to criticism or domination and lack self-esteem*

EXPECTED OUTCOME

Parents demonstrate an understanding of normal expectations for their child

NURSING CARE PLAN

The Adolescent with Anorexia Nervosa

Anorexia nervosa is a disorder characterized by a refusal to maintain a minimally normal body weight and by severe weight loss in the absence of obvious physical cause.

ASSESSMENT

Perform a physical assessment.

Obtain a history of eating behaviors; explore body image perception.

Assess family interpersonal relationships.

Observe for early signs of anorexia nervosa:

Consumes an inappropriate diet (excessively strict) or may refuse to eat altogether

Develops peculiar eating habits such as toying with food, food "rituals," preparing and forcing food on family members without personally eating any

Engages in excessive exercise, such as compulsive jogging, running up and down stairs, rigorous calisthenics to burn off calories, often to the point of exhaustion

Withdraws from social interaction; starts to spend all of his or her time in own room studying, exercising, or otherwise occupied

Ceases to have menstrual periods after sudden or excessive weight loss, sometimes almost as soon as dieting begins

Takes laxatives, diuretics, or enemas to speed intestinal transit time to lose added weight and empty intestines to flatten abdomen

Vomits deliberately; may go to bathroom after a meal and turn on faucets to avoid being heard

Denies hunger even after eating practically nothing for days or even weeks

Develops a distorted body image; states he or she "feels fat" while becoming increasingly thinner

Loses weight; growing adolescents fail to achieve the 25th percentile on normal growth curves

Observe for manifestations of anorexia nervosa:

Severe and profound weight loss

Signs of altered metabolic activity:

Secondary amenorrhea (if menarche attained)

Primary amenorrhea (if menarche not attained)

Bradycardia

Lowered body temperature

Decreased blood pressure

Cold intolerance

Dry skin and brittle nails

Appearance of lanugo hair

Assist with diagnostic procedures and tests, including assessment based on the diagnostic criteria for anorexia nervosa (Box 4-33).

Continued

BOX 4-33

Diagnostic Criteria for Anorexia Nervosa

1. Refusal to maintain body weight at or above a minimally normal weight for age and height (e.g., weight loss leading to maintenance of body weight less than 85% of that expected; or failure to make expected weight gain during period of growth, leading to body weight less than 85% of that expected)
2. Intense fear of gaining weight or becoming fat, even though underweight
3. Disturbance in the way in which one's body weight or shape is experienced, undue influence of body weight or shape on self-evaluation, or denial of the seriousness of the current low body weight
4. In postmenarcheal females, amenorrhea (i.e., the absence of at least three consecutive menstrual cycles). A woman is considered to have amenorrhea if her periods occur only following hormone (e.g., estrogen) administration.

Specify type:

Restricting type: During the current episode of anorexia nervosa, the person has not regularly engaged in binge-eating or purging behavior (e.g., self-induced vomiting or the misuse of laxatives, diuretics, or enemas)

Binge-eating/purging type: During the current episode of anorexia nervosa, the person has regularly engaged in binge-eating or purging behavior (e.g., self-induced vomiting or the misuse of laxatives, diuretics, or enemas)

From American Psychiatric Association: *Diagnostic and statistical manual of mental disorders,* ed 4, (DSM-IV), Washington, DC, 1994, The Association.

The Adolescent with Anorexia Nervosa—cont'd

NURSING DIAGNOSIS: Altered nutrition: less than body requirements related to self-starvation

■ **PATIENT GOAL 1:** Will consume nourishment adequate for weight gain

NURSING INTERVENTIONS/*RATIONALES*

Implement high-calorie diet as prescribed *to ensure nourishment adequate for gradual weight gain*

Explain nutritional plan to adolescent and family *to encourage compliance*

With dietitian and patient, select balanced diet with the prescribed incremental increase in calories; *rapid weight gain is avoided because it can cause cardiovascular overload and give child an overwhelming sense of being out of control*

Help patient prepare an eating-habits diary *to assess adequacy of nutrition*

EXPECTED OUTCOME

Adolescent evidences gradual weight gain

■ **PATIENT GOAL 2:** Will follow behavior modification plan (if implemented)

NURSING INTERVENTIONS/*RATIONALES*

Ensure that all members of the health team determine an approach, understand the plan, and adhere to it consistently

Involve all team members, including the patient

Ensure continuity of caregivers (team members)

Provide for clear communication among team members and with the patient *so that patient understands precisely what is expected*

Consult with patient regarding progress

Avoid coercive techniques *because coercion is usually ineffective for long-term success*

Support patient in efforts (e.g., positive feedback for accomplishments)

EXPECTED OUTCOME

Expectations are met consistently (specify)

■ **PATIENT GOAL 3:** Will reduce energy expenditure

NURSING INTERVENTIONS/*RATIONALES*

Monitor physical activity *to evaluate appropriateness for child's condition*

Supervise selection and performance of activity

Be alert to evidence of secretive exercising *because child may use exercising as a weight loss strategy*

EXPECTED OUTCOME

Adolescent engages in quiet and specified activities

NURSING DIAGNOSIS: Body image disturbance related to altered perception

■ **PATIENT GOAL 1:** Will express self in acceptable ways

NURSING INTERVENTIONS/*RATIONALES*

Channel need for control and feeling of effectiveness in appropriate directions (rather than control of weight)

Obtain psychiatric referral as indicated *because psychotherapy is essential in treatment*

Encourage patient to monitor own care as appropriate *to provide a sense of control*

EXPECTED OUTCOME

Adolescent expresses self in acceptable ways

■ **PATIENT GOAL 2:** Will receive adequate support

NURSING INTERVENTIONS/*RATIONALES*

Maintain open communications with adolescent *so that adolescent is able to express feelings and concerns*

Convey an attitude of caring and protection to adolescent

Avoid conveying an attitude of intrusion

Encourage participation in own care *so that adolescent has an appropriate sense of control*

EXPECTED OUTCOMES

Adolescent expresses feelings and concerns

Adolescent becomes actively involved in own care and management

■ **PATIENT GOAL 3:** Will receive assistance in altering distorted self-image

NURSING INTERVENTIONS/*RATIONALES*

Support psychiatric plan of care *because this is essential in helping adolescent alter distorted self-image*

EXPECTED OUTCOMES

Adolescent receives appropriate psychiatric care

Adolescent displays evidence of developing a positive self-image

NURSING DIAGNOSIS: Ineffective individual coping related to unrealistic perceptions

■ **PATIENT (FAMILY) GOAL 1:** Will conform to therapeutic program

NURSING INTERVENTIONS/*RATIONALES*

Maintain consistency in therapeutic approach selected

Maintain vigilance to detect signs of sabotaging the therapeutic plan, such as self-induced vomiting, laxative or enema use, hoarding food, disposing of food, placing weighted material in clothing for weigh-in, *because adolescent may use these methods to prevent weight gain*

Provide positive reinforcement for progress

Be alert for signs of depression

Support psychotherapeutic measures

Help arrange for follow-up care *because treatment requires long-term care*

The Adolescent with Anorexia Nervosa—cont'd

EXPECTED OUTCOME
Adolescent and family conform to therapeutic program
(specify behaviors)

> **NURSING DIAGNOSIS:** Family coping: potential for growth related to ambivalent family relationships

■ **PATIENT (FAMILY) GOAL 1:** Will recognize disturbed pattern of family interaction

NURSING INTERVENTIONS/*RATIONALES*
Observe family interaction *for assessment of coping patterns*
Explore feelings and attitudes of family members
Support psychotherapeutic measures for redirecting malfunctioning family processes
Help arrange for referral to individuals and groups that further therapeutic goals

EXPECTED OUTCOME
Family patterns of interaction are recognized and evaluated

■ **PATIENT (FAMILY) GOAL 2:** Will be prepared for home care

NURSING INTERVENTIONS/*RATIONALES*
Make certain both patient and family understand therapeutic plan
Arrange for follow-up care *because treatment needs to be long-term*
Refer to special agencies for additional information and support

EXPECTED OUTCOMES
Family demonstrates an understanding of the etiology of the disorder and conforms to therapeutic program
Family uses available resources

Unit 4

NURSING CARE PLAN

The Adolescent Who Is Obese

Obesity is an increase in body weight resulting from an excessive accumulation of body fat relative to lean body mass.

Overweight refers to the state of weighing more than average for one's height and body build, which may or may not include an increased amount of fat. It is possible for two children to have the same height and weight and for one to be obese whereas the other is not.

ASSESSMENT

Perform a physical assessment.
Observe for manifestations of obesity:
    Child appears overweight
    Weight over established standards
    Skinfold thickness greater than established standard (See p. 31.)
    Body fat increased above established standards
Obtain a family history regarding obesity, diet habits, and food preferences.
Obtain a health history, including analysis of weight charts, eating habits, and behaviors, especially relative to physical activity.

Interview child and family to elicit psychologic factors that might contribute to obesity (e.g., cultural standards, use of food for pacification, peer and family interpersonal relationships, use of food as a reward).
Assist with diagnostic procedures and tests (e.g., body weight, weight-height ratios, weight-age ratios, hydrostatic [underwater] weight, skinfold measurements, body mass index, bioelectric analysis, computed tomography, magnetic resonance imaging, neutron activation, and tests for metabolic and endocrine disorders).

NURSING DIAGNOSIS: Altered nutrition: more than body requirements related to dysfunctional eating patterns, hereditary factors

■ **PATIENT (FAMILY) GOAL 1:** Will identify eating patterns and behaviors

NURSING INTERVENTIONS/*RATIONALES*

Guide adolescent and, at times, family to:
    Keep a record of everything eaten, including:
        Time eaten
        Amount eaten
        Where food was consumed
        Activity engaged in while eating
        With whom the food was eaten or if it was eaten alone
        Feelings at the time food was eaten (e.g., angry, depressed, lonely, elated)
    Identify food stimuli *because this often contributes to obesity:*
        Feelings of hunger
        Television commercials
        Smell or sight of food
    Assess eating environments *to determine possible effect on obesity:*
        Where food is eaten
        With whom food is eaten, or eaten alone
        Feelings at time of food consumption
        Activity engaged in while eating
    Analyze preceding data for patterns of eating and relationships of other factors as a basis for making adjustments

EXPECTED OUTCOME

Adolescent's eating patterns and behaviors become apparent

■ **PATIENT GOAL 2:** Will demonstrate how to control food stimuli

NURSING INTERVENTIONS/*RATIONALES*

Encourage adolescent to do the following *to decrease temptation to overeat:*
    Separate eating from other activities
    Minimize food cues
    Get rid of "junk" food
    Prepare and serve only amounts to be eaten
    Put snacks out of sight
    Avoid purchase of problem foods such as "fast foods"
    Serve food from stove or other place out of reach of the established eating place

EXPECTED OUTCOME

Adolescent demonstrates an understanding of eating patterns and endeavors to alter destructive patterns

■ **PATIENT GOAL 3:** Will change eating patterns

NURSING INTERVENTIONS/*RATIONALES*

Encourage adolescent to do the following *because changes in eating patterns can lessen risk of overeating:*
    Eat at a specific place reserved just for eating
    Eat orderly meals at regular hours
    Use smaller plates to make amounts of food appear larger
    Eat at slow pace
    Leave a small amount of food on plate
    Eliminate eating during television viewing
    Substitute healthy snacks such as raw vegetables for "junk" food snacks

EXPECTED OUTCOME

Adolescent alters eating behaviors

Unit 4

The Adolescent Who Is Obese—cont'd

■ **PATIENT GOAL 4:** Will alter activity patterns

NURSING INTERVENTIONS/*RATIONALES*

Encourage adolescent to do the following:

Use activities other than eating to deal with emotional stress, boredom, and fatigue *since eating at these times often contributes to obesity*

Engage in hobby activity, take a walk, straighten up room *to avoid overeating*

Become involved in activities away from food

EXPECTED OUTCOME

Adolescent engages in suitable activities according to age and interest

■ **PATIENT GOAL 5:** Will eat the prescribed diet

NURSING INTERVENTIONS/*RATIONALES*

Assist adolescent with planning the diet so that it provides for:

Weight maintenance or slow weight loss

Meeting nutrient and energy needs

Lack of hunger

Preservation of lean body mass

Increased physical activity

Growth

Assist adolescent with meal planning

Employ strategies outlined above *so that child is more likely to adhere to prescribed diet*

EXPECTED OUTCOMES

Adolescent will participate in planning the diet

Adolescent adheres to prescribed diet plan

Adolescent evidences a steady weight loss (or weight maintenance in a growing child)

NURSING DIAGNOSIS: Activity intolerance related to sedentary lifestyle, physical bulk

■ **PATIENT GOAL 1:** Will increase physical activity

NURSING INTERVENTIONS/*RATIONALES*

Assess activity patterns and interests of adolescent

Arrange programmed activity such as running, swimming, cycling, aerobics, or after-school sports

Encourage routine activity such as walking, climbing stairs

Encourage activities that stress self-improvement rather than competition *to avoid sense of failure and feelings of rejection*

EXPECTED OUTCOME

Adolescent engages in preferred exercise and activities regularly (specify)

NURSING DIAGNOSIS: Ineffective individual coping related to little or no exercise, poor nutrition, personal vulnerability

■ **PATIENT GOAL 1:** Will receive adequate support

NURSING INTERVENTIONS/*RATIONALES*

Implement a school weight-loss program *to encourage attainment of goals*

Employ a buddy system

Use peers as sponsors and positive reinforcers

Employ frequent weigh-ins conducted by involved adult, nurse, teacher, physical education instructor

Provide reinforcement for weight change:

Social—Praise

Tangible—Contract that earns simple rewards

Graph positive weight changes and display graph where others in program can see it

Provide nutrition education

Have a family member serve as a monitor at home *to help in progress toward goals and to encourage adolescent with positive statements daily*

EXPECTED OUTCOME

Adolescent engages in school-based program (specify)

NURSING DIAGNOSIS: Self-esteem disturbance related to perception of physical appearance, internalization of negative feedback

■ **PATIENT GOAL 1:** Will have an opportunity to discuss feelings and concerns

NURSING INTERVENTIONS/*RATIONALES*

Encourage adolescent to discuss his or her feelings and concerns *because this can facilitate coping*

Reinforce accomplishments *so that child is not discouraged in attainment of goals*

EXPECTED OUTCOMES

Adolescent expresses feelings and concerns regarding problems

Adolescent maintains a positive attitude toward the weight-loss program

■ **PATIENT GOAL 2:** Will recognize ways to improve appearance

NURSING INTERVENTIONS/*RATIONALES*

Encourage good grooming, hygiene, and posture *to enhance appearance and promote self-esteem*

Assist with exploring positive aspects of appearance and ways to enhance these aspects

EXPECTED OUTCOME

Adolescent shows measurable efforts to improve appearance (specify)

■ **PATIENT GOAL 3:** Will exhibit signs of improved self-esteem

NURSING INTERVENTIONS/*RATIONALES*

Relate to adolescent as an important, worthwhile individual *because this encourages development of self-esteem*

Unit 4

Continued

The Adolescent Who Is Obese—cont'd

Encourage adolescent to set small, attainable goals

Encourage and support positive thinking (overweight persons are often negative thinkers) *to increase self-esteem*

Encourage activities *to relieve boredom*

Encourage interaction with peers *because isolation and feelings of rejection may decrease self-esteem*

EXPECTED OUTCOMES

Adolescent sets realistic short-term goals for self-improvement (specify)

Adolescent voices positive attitudes toward self

Adolescent engages in appropriate activities and interactions with peers (specify)

NURSING DIAGNOSIS: Altered family processes related to management of an obese adolescent

■ **PATIENT (FAMILY) GOAL 1:** Will become involved in adolescent's weight-loss program

NURSING INTERVENTIONS/*RATIONALES*

Educate family regarding weight-loss program, including nutrition, relationship of food intake and exercise, psychologic support

Encourage family to do the following:

Use appropriate reinforcement

Alter food and eating environment

Maintain proper attitudes regarding program

Assist in monitoring eating behavior, food intake, physical activity, weight change

Eliminate food as a reward *since this can contribute to obesity*

Encourage adolescent with positive statements *to increase self-esteem*

EXPECTED OUTCOMES

Family becomes actively involved in adolescent's weight-loss program

Family supports adolescent in attainment of goals

Unit 4

NURSING CARE OF THE CHILD WITH POISONING

Nonintentional poisoning is common in young children and demands immediate attention to prevent injury or death.

NURSING CARE PLAN

The Child with Poisoning

Poisoning is the condition or physical state produced when a substance, in relatively small amounts, is applied to body surfaces, ingested, injected, inhaled, or absorbed and subsequently causes structural damage or disturbance of function.

ASSESSMENT

Perform a physical assessment with particular attention to vital signs, breath odor, state of consciousness, skin changes, and neurologic signs.

Obtain a careful and detailed history regarding what, when, and how much of a toxic substance has entered the body.

Look for evidence of poison (e.g., container, plant, vomitus).

Observe for evidence of ingestion, inhalation, or absorption of toxic substances:

Skin manifestations
  Pallor
  Redness
  Evidence of burning
  Pain
Mucous membrane manifestations
  Evidence of irritation
  Red discoloration
  White discoloration
  Swelling
Gastrointestinal manifestations
  Salivation
  Dry mouth
  Nausea and vomiting
  Diarrhea
  Abdominal pain
Cardiovascular manifestations
  Arrhythmias
  Increased blood pressure
  Decreased blood pressure
  Tachycardia
  Bradycardia
  Evidence of shock
Respiratory manifestations
  Gagging, choking, coughing
  Tachypnea
  Bradypnea
  Unexplained cyanosis
  Grunting
Renal manifestations
  Oliguria
  Hematuria
Metabolic/autonomic manifestations
  Sweating
  Hyperthermia
  Hypothermia
  Metabolic acidosis
Neuromuscular manifestations
  Weakness
  Involuntary movements
  Teeth gnashing
  Ataxia
  Dilated pupils
  Constricted pupils
  Seizures
Altered sensorium
  Anxiety, agitation
  Hallucinations
  Sudden loss of consciousness
  Dizziness
  Confusion
  Lethargy, stupor
  Coma

Observe for clinical manifestations characteristic of specific poison (Box 4-34).

Assist with diagnostic tests (e.g., blood levels of toxins, radiograph to determine presence of masses of undissolved tablets remaining in GI tract).

Observe for latent symptoms of poisoning.

NURSING DIAGNOSIS: Risk for poisoning related to presence of toxic substance, immature judgment of child

■ **PATIENT GOAL 1:** Will not experience occurrence and/or recurrence of poisoning

NURSING INTERVENTIONS/*RATIONALES*

Assess possible contributing factors in occurrence of injury, such as discipline, parent-child relationship, developmental ability, environmental factors, and behavior problems

Institute anticipatory guidance for possible future injuries based on child's age and maturational level

Refer to visiting nurse agency *to evaluate home environment and need for safe-proofing measures*

Provide assistance with environmental manipulation when necessary, such as lead removal

Educate parents regarding safe storage of toxic substances (See Child Safety Home Checklist on p. 194.)

Advise parents to take drugs out of sight of children *because child may mimic adult, resulting in poisoning*

Advise parents to replace *immediately* all toxic substances to safe storage

Teach children the hazards of ingesting nonfood items without supervision

Advise parents against using plants for teas or medicine *since many plants are poisonous*

Discuss problems of discipline and children's noncompliance and offer strategies for effective discipline

Continued

Unit 4

The Child with Poisoning—cont'd

BOX 4-34

Selected Poisonings in Children

Corrosives (Strong Acids or Alkalis)

Drain, toilet, or oven cleaners
Electric dishwasher detergent (liquid, because of higher pH, is more hazardous than granular)
Mildew remover
Batteries
Clinitest tablets
Denture cleaners

Clinical Manifestations

Severe burning pain in mouth, throat, and stomach
White, swollen mucous membranes; edema of lips, tongue, and pharynx (respiratory obstruction)
Violent vomiting (hemoptysis)
Drooling and inability to clear secretions
Signs of shock
Anxiety and agitation

Comments

Household bleach is a commonly ingested corrosive but rarely causes serious damage
Liquid corrosives cause more damage than granular preparations

Treatment

Inducing emesis is contraindicated (vomiting redamages the mucosa)
Dilute corrosive with water or milk (usually no more than 120 ml [4 oz])
Do not neutralize: Neutralization can cause an exothermic reaction (which produces heat and causes increased symptoms or produces a thermal burn in addition to a chemical burn)
Provide patent airway, if needed
Administer analgesics
Do not allow oral intake
Esophageal stricture may require repeated dilations and/or surgery

Hydrocarbons

Gasoline
Kerosene
Lamp oil
Mineral seal oil (found in furniture polish)
Lighter fluid
Turpentine
Paint thinner and remover (some types)

Clinical Manifestations

Gagging, choking, and coughing
Nausea
Vomiting
Alterations in sensorium, such as lethargy
Weakness
Respiratory symptoms of pulmonary involvement:
   Tachypnea
   Cyanosis
   Retractions
   Grunting

Comments

Immediate danger is aspiration (even small amounts can cause bronchitis and chemical pneumonia)
Gasoline, kerosene, lighter fluid, mineral seal oil, and turpentine cause severe pneumonia

Treatment (Controversial)

Inducing emesis is generally contraindicated
Gastric decontamination and gastric emptying are questionable, even when the hydrocarbon contains a heavy metal or pesticide; if gastric lavage must be performed, a cuffed ET tube should be in place before lavage because of a high risk of aspiration
Symptomatic treatment of chemical pneumonia includes high humidity, oxygen, hydration, and antibiotics for secondary infection

Acetaminophen

Clinical Manifestations

Occurs in four stages:
1. Initial period (2-4 hours after ingestion):
   Nausea
   Vomiting
   Sweating
   Pallor
2. Latent period (24-36 hours):
   Patient improves
3. Hepatic involvement (may last up to 7 days and be permanent):
   Pain in right upper quadrant
   Jaundice
   Confusion
   Stupor
   Coagulation abnormalities
4. Patients who do not die during hepatic stage gradually recover

The Child with Poisoning—cont'd

BOX 4-34

Selected Poisoning in Children—cont'd

Comments

Most common drug poisoning in children

Occurs primarily from acute ingestion

Toxic dose is 150 mg/kg or greater in children

Toxicity from chronic therapeutic use is rare but may occur with ingestion of approximately 150 mg/kg/day, or about double the recommended maximum therapeutic dose (90 mg/kg/day) of acetaminophen, for several days*; toxicity is more likely in children with hepatic dysfunction†

Treatment

Antidote *N*-acetylcysteine (NAC) can usually be given orally but is first diluted in fruit juice or soda because of the antidote's offensive odor

   Given as one loading dose and usually 17 maintenance doses in different dosages

   May be given intravenously, but use is investigational

Aspirin (ASA)

Clinical Manifestations

Acute poisoning:

   Nausea

   Disorientation

   Vomiting

   Dehydration

   Diaphoresis

   Hyperpnea

   Hyperpyrexia

   Oliguria

   Tinnitus

   Coma

   Convulsions

Chronic poisoning:

   Same as above but subtle onset (often confused with illness being treated)

Dehydration, coma, and seizures may be more severe

Bleeding tendencies

Comments

May be caused by acute ingestion (severe toxicity occurs with 300-500 mg/kg)

May be caused by chronic ingestion (i.e., more than 100 mg/kg/day for 2 or more days); can be more serious than acute ingestion

Time to peak serum salicylate can vary with enteric aspirin or the presence of concretions (bezoars)

Treatment

Home use of ipecac for moderate toxicity

Hospitalization for severe toxicity

Emesis, lavage, activated charcoal, and/or cathartic

Lavage will not remove concretions of ASA

Activated charcoal is important early in ASA toxicity

Sodium bicarbonate transfusions to correct metabolic acidosis, and urinary alkalinization may be effective in enhancing elimination; urinary alkalinization is very difficult to achieve; be cautious about putting the patient into fluid overload and pulmonary edema (a common complication)

External cooling for hyperpyrexia

Diazepam for seizures

Oxygen and ventilation for respiratory depression

Vitamin K for bleeding

In severe cases, hemodialysis (not peritoneal dialysis) may be used

Iron

Mineral supplement or vitamin containing iron

Clinical Manifestations

Occurs in five stages:

1. Initial period (½-6 hours after ingestion) (if child does not develop gastrointestinal symptoms in 6 hours, toxicity is unlikely):
   Vomiting
   Hematemesis
   Diarrhea
   Hematochezia (bloody stools)
   Gastric pain
2. Latency (2-12 hours):
   Patient improves
3. Systemic toxicity (4-24 hours after ingestion):
   Metabolic acidosis
   Fever
   Hyperglycemia
   Bleeding
   Shock
   Death (may occur)
4. Hepatic injury (48-96 hours):
   Seizures
   Coma
5. Rarely, pyloric stenosis develops at 2-5 weeks

---

*Douidar SM, Al-Khalil I, Habersang RW: Severe hepatotoxicity, acute renal failure, and pancytopenia in a young child after repeated acetaminophen overdosing, *Clin Pediatr* 33(1):42-45, 1994.

†Cheung L, Potts RG, Meyer KC: Acetaminophen treatment nomogram, *N Engl J Med* 330(26):1907-1908, 1994.

Continued

Unit 4

BOX 4-34

Selected Poisoning in Children—cont'd

Iron—cont'd

Comments

Factors related to frequency of iron poisoning include:
Widespread availability
Packaging of large quantities in individual containers
Lack of parental awareness of iron toxicity
Resemblance of iron tablets to candy (e.g., M&Ms)
Toxic dose is based on the amount of elemental iron in various salts (sulfate, gluconate, fumarate), which ranges from 20%-33%; ingestions of 60 mg/kg are considered dangerous

Treatment

Emesis or lavage
For toxic doses lavage may be necessary for all chewable tablets or liquids if spontaneous vomiting has not occurred
Chelation therapy with deferoxamine in severe intoxication (may turn urine a red to orange color)
If intravenous deferoxamine is given too rapidly, hypotension, facial flushing, rash, urticaria, tachycardia, and shock may occur; stop the infusion, maintain the intravenous line with normal saline, and notify the practitioner immediately

Plants

(See Box 4-35.)

Clinical Manifestations

Depends on type of plant ingested
May cause local irritation of oropharynx and entire gastrointestinal tract
May cause respiratory, renal, and central nervous system symptoms
Topical contact with plants can cause dermatitis

Comments

Some of the most commonly ingested substances
Rarely cause serious problems, although some plant ingestions can be fatal
Can also cause choking and allergic reactions

Treatment

Remove plant parts (emesis)
Wash from skin or eyes
Supportive care as needed

BOX 4-35

Poisonous and Nonpoisonous Plants

Poisonous Plants	Toxic Parts	Nonpoisonous Plants
Apple	Leaves, seeds	African violet
Apricot	Leaves, stem, seed pits	Aluminum plant
Azalea	Foliage and flowers	Asparagus fern
Buttercup	All parts	Begonia
Cherry (wild or cultivated)	Twigs, seeds, foliage	Boston fern
Daffodil	Bulbs	Christmas cactus
Dumb cane, dieffenbachia	All parts	Coleus
Elephant ear	All parts	Gardenia
English ivy	All parts	Grape ivy
Foxglove	Leaves, seeds, flowers	Jade plant
Holly	Berries	Piggyback begonia
Hyacinth	Bulbs	Piggyback plant
Ivy	Leaves	Poinsettia†
Mistletoe*	Berries, leaves	Prayer plant
Oak tree	Acorn, foliage	Rubber tree
Philodendron	All parts	Snake plant
Plum	Pit	Spider plant
Poison ivy, poison oak	Leaves, fruit, stems, smoke from burning plants	Swedish ivy
Pothos	All parts	Wax plant
Rhubarb	Leaves	Weeping fig
Tulip	Bulbs	Zebra plant
Water hemlock	All parts	
Wisteria	Seeds, pods	
Yew	All parts	

*Eating one or two berries or leaves is probably nontoxic.

†Mildly toxic if ingested in massive quantities.

The Child with Poisoning—cont'd

Instruct parents regarding correct administration of drugs for therapeutic purposes and to discontinue drug if there is evidence of mild toxicity

Have syrup of ipecac available—two doses for each child in the family *since more than one child may ingest toxic substance*

Encourage grandparents or other frequent caregivers to keep syrup of ipecac in the home *so that it is readily available for emergencies*

Post number of local poison control center with emergency phone list by the telephone

EXPECTED OUTCOMES

Child does not swallow potentially poisonous substance

Family is prepared in the event poisoning occurs

NURSING DIAGNOSIS: Risk for injury related to presence of toxic substance

---

INGESTED POISONS

■ **PATIENT GOAL 1:** Will not experience complications from ingestion of poison

NURSING INTERVENTIONS/*RATIONALES*

Save any evidence of ingested substance (e.g., empty container, tablets in child's mouth, parts of plants) *to determine that a poisoning has occurred*

Call local poison control center, emergency facility, or health practitioner *for immediate advice regarding treatment*

Empty mouth of pills, plant parts, or other material *to terminate exposure to poison*

Give water, unless contraindicated, *to dilute poisonous substance*

Do not induce vomiting if any one of the following is true:
   Child is comatose, in severe shock, convulsing, or has lost the gag reflex *because of risk of aspiration*
   Poison is a low-viscosity hydrocarbon (unless it contains a more toxic substance [e.g., pesticide or heavy metal]) *because of risk of aspiration*
   Poison is a corrosive (strong acid or alkali) *because vomiting redamages the mucosa of esophagus and pharynx*

*Administer ipecac, if ordered, *to induce vomiting for removal of poison,* using the following guidelines:
   †6 to 12 months: 10 ml; do not repeat
   1 to 12 years: 15 ml; repeat dosage once if vomiting has not occurred within 20 minutes
   Over 12 years: 30 ml; repeat dosage once if vomiting has not occurred within 20 minutes
   Give 10 to 20 ml/kg of clear fluids after ipecac, but forcing fluids is not necessary

Place child in side-lying, sitting, or knee-chest position with head below chest *to prevent aspiration during vomiting*

*Administer activated charcoal (usual dose 1 g/kg) 30 to 60 minutes *after* vomiting from ipecac, if ordered, *to absorb any poison remaining in stomach*

If preparation is not sweetened, mix it with flavoring or a sweetener *to increase palatability*

Serve through a straw and covered, opaque glass *to increase child's acceptance of preparation, which resembles black mud*

*Perform or assist with gastric lavage, if ordered, *to remove poison in situations where vomiting is contraindicated or if poison is rapidly absorbed* (e.g., strychnine or cyanide)

*Administer specific antidote, if available and ordered, *to counteract the poison*

Assist with measures (e.g., cathartics, exchange transfusion, hemodialysis, hemoperfusion, chelation therapy) *that may be necessary to eliminate toxins from child's body*

EXPECTED OUTCOMES

Child's stomach is emptied without aspiration

Child swallows activated charcoal

Child receives antidote (if one is available)

Child does not experience complications from poisoning

TOPICALLY ABSORBED POISONS

■ **PATIENT GOAL 1:** Will exhibit signs of reduced absorption of poison

NURSING INTERVENTIONS/*RATIONALES*

Flush eyes continuously with normal saline (room-temperature tap water at home) for 15 to 20 minutes *to remove poison and decrease absorption*

Flush skin and wash with soap and a soft cloth *to remove poison and decrease absorption*

Remove contaminated clothes, especially if a pesticide, acid, alkali, or hydrocarbon is involved, *to reduce exposure to poison*

Wear protective gloves during handling of child *to protect yourself from exposure to poison*

EXPECTED OUTCOMES

Harmful substance is removed from child's eyes, skin

Child exhibits signs of reduced absorption of poison (specify)

INHALED POISONS

■ **PATIENT GOAL 1:** Will exhibit signs of reduced absorption of inhaled poison

NURSING INTERVENTIONS/*RATIONALES*

Remove child from source of inhalant *to decrease exposure to poison*

Have emergency equipment and medications readily available *to prevent delay in treatment*

*Assist ventilation as needed (humidified air, oxygen)

*Assist with intubation and/or respiratory support as indicated

EXPECTED OUTCOME

Respirations are within normal limits (See inside front cover for normal variations.)

---

*Dependent nursing action.

†Emesis of children at home is generally contraindicated between ages 6 to 10 months. Ipecac can be administered safely only in a health care facility because of the high risk of aspiration.

Continued

The Child with Poisoning—cont'd

NURSING DIAGNOSIS: Fear/anxiety related to sudden hospitalization and treatment

■ **PATIENT GOAL 1:** Will receive adequate support

NURSING INTERVENTIONS/*RATIONALES*

Explain procedures and tests according to developmental level of the child

Allow for expression of feelings *to facilitate coping*

Provide comfort measures appropriate to child's age and condition

Encourage parents to remain with child *to provide support and prevent separation*

EXPECTED OUTCOMES

Child expresses feelings and concerns

Child cooperates with procedures

Family remains with child as much as possible

NURSING DIAGNOSIS: Altered family processes related to sudden hospitalization and emergency aspects of illness

■ **PATIENT (FAMILY) GOAL 1:** Will receive adequate support

NURSING INTERVENTIONS/*RATIONALES*

Keep child and parents calm

Do not admonish or accuse child or parent of wrongdoing *because this is usually not helpful and serves to increase stress at an already stressful time*

Allow expression of feelings regarding circumstances related to the poisoning *to facilitate coping*

Provide reassurance as appropriate

Explain therapies and tests

Keep family informed of child's progress *to decrease fear and anxiety*

Avoid placing blame

Delay discussing prevention until child's condition stabilizes *because family's anxiety will block out any suggestions or guidance*

Make arrangements for follow-up care and prevention guidance after discharge (e.g., public health referral)

EXPECTED OUTCOMES

Family members express feelings and concerns

Family seeks needed support

Follow-up care and prevention will be discussed at an appropriate time

NURSING CARE PLAN

The Child with Lead Poisoning

Lead poisoning is the chronic ingestion or inhalation of lead-containing substances, resulting in physical and mental dysfunction.

ASSESSMENT

Perform a physical assessment.

Obtain a history of possible sources of lead in the child's environment:

Ingested

*Lead-based paint
  Interior: walls, windowsills, floors, furniture
  Exterior: door frames, fences, porches, siding
Plaster, caulking
Unglazed pottery
Colored newsprint
Painted food wrappers
Cigarette butts and ashes
Water from leaded pipes, water fountains
Foods or liquids from cans soldered with lead
Household dust
Soil, especially along heavily trafficked roadways
Food grown in contaminated soil
Urban playgrounds
Folk remedies
Pewter vessels or dishes
Food or drinks stored in lead crystal
Lead bullets
Lead fishing sinkers
Lead curtain weights
Hobby materials (e.g., leaded paint or solder for stained glass windows)

Inhaled

*Sanding and scraping of lead-based painted surfaces
Burning of leaded objects:
  Automobile batteries
  "Logs" made of colored newspaper
Automobile exhaust
Cigarette smoke
Sniffing leaded gasoline
Dust
  Poorly cleaned urban housing
Contaminated clothing and skin of household members working in smelting factories or construction

Obtain a history of pica or look for evidence of this behavior during assessment.

Obtain a diet history, especially regarding intake of iron and calcium.

Observe for manifestations of lead poisoning:

General signs
  Anemia
  Acute crampy abdominal pain
  Vomiting
  Constipation
  Anorexia
  Headache
  Fever
  Lethargy
  Impaired growth

Central nervous system signs (early)
  Hyperactivity
  Aggression
  Impulsiveness
  Decreased interest in play
  Lethargy
  Irritability
  Loss of developmental progress
  Hearing impairment
  Learning difficulties
  Short attention span
  Distractibility
  Mild intellectual deficits

Central nervous system signs (late)
  Mental retardation
  Paralysis
  Blindness
  Convulsions
  Coma
  Death

Signs of gasoline sniffing
  Irritability
  Tremor
  Hallucinations
  Confusion
  Lack of impulse control
  Depression
  Impaired perception and coordination
  Sleep disturbances

Assist with diagnostic procedures and tests (e.g., blood-lead concentration, erythrocyte-protoporphyrin level, bone radiography, urinalysis, hemoglobin and complete blood count, lead mobilization test).

Continued

© 2000 Mosby, Inc. All rights reserved.

*Most common sources.

Unit 4

The Child with Lead Poisoning—cont'd

NURSING DIAGNOSIS: Risk for poisoning related to sources of lead in the environment

- **PATIENT GOAL 1:** Will not experience further exposure to lead

NURSING INTERVENTIONS/*RATIONALES*
(See Box 4-36.)

EXPECTED OUTCOME
Child no longer ingests or inhales lead from environment

NURSING DIAGNOSIS: Risk for injury related to ingested or inhaled lead

- **PATIENT GOAL 1:** Will exhibit signs of reduced lead in body

NURSING INTERVENTIONS/*RATIONALES*
Ask family if child is allergic to peanuts; if so, child should not be given chelating agents such as dimercaprol (also called BAL [British antilewisite]) or D-penicillamine
*Administer chelating agents as prescribed *to reduce high blood lead levels*
Observe for and control seizures *for which child is at risk*
Implement measures to reduce nausea *since it is a side effect of some chelating agents*
Monitor intake, output, and serum electrolyte levels
Maintain adequate hydration, especially when chelating agent succimer is given
Monitor absolute neutrophil count *because neutropenia may occur if child is receiving succimer*
*Administer cleansing enemas or cathartic, if ordered, *for acute lead ingestion*
Avoid giving iron during chelation *because of possible interactive effects*
Rotate injection sites if chelating agent is given intramuscularly
If home oral chelation therapy is used, teach family proper administration of medication

EXPECTED OUTCOMES
Child receives chelation therapy without complications
Child exhibits signs of reduced lead in body (specify)

NURSING DIAGNOSIS: Fear related to multiple injections, venipunctures

- **PATIENT GOAL 1:** Will experience reduced fear of injections

NURSING INTERVENTIONS/*RATIONALES*
Prepare child for injections and/or venipunctures if required for chelation therapy (See p. 244.)
Reassure child that injections are a treatment, not a punishment for lead ingestion, *since child may misinterpret reason for injections/venipunctures*
Administer medication in place other than that perceived as "safe" (e.g., treatment room or space, instead of room or play area)
Encourage play activities (e.g., playing with syringes, pounding clay) that allow child to express feelings associated with therapy
Administer the local anesthetic procaine with IM injection of CaNa$_2$ EDTA *to reduce discomfort*
Apply EMLA cream over puncture site 2½ hours before the injection *to reduce discomfort*
(See Administration of Medications, p. 241, for other measures to reduce discomfort from injections.)

EXPECTED OUTCOME
Child receives injections or venipunctures with minimal distress

NURSING DIAGNOSIS: Altered family processes related to child's access to lead in the environment

- **PATIENT (FAMILY) GOAL 1:** Will receive adequate support

NURSING INTERVENTIONS/*RATIONALES*
Avoid blame or criticism regarding the child's exposure to lead sources
Assist family to obtain sources of help *for removing lead from the environment*
Offer praise for positive behaviors in directing child's activity away from pica
Be available to answer questions and offer suggestions

EXPECTED OUTCOME
Family demonstrates a positive attitude toward the child and toward reducing the risk of lead poisoning

*Dependent nursing action.

Unit 4

The Child with Lead Poisoning—cont'd

BOX 4-36

Parent Guidelines for Reducing Blood Lead Levels

Make sure child does not have access to peeling paint or chewable surfaces painted with lead-based paint, especially windowsills and window wells.

If a house was built before 1960 (and possibly before 1980) and has hard-surface floors, wet mop them at least once a week with a high-phosphate solution (e.g., trisodium phosphate [available in hardware stores]). Wipe other hard surfaces (such as windowsills and baseboards) with the same kind of solution. If there are loose paint chips in an area, such as a window well, use a disposable cloth soaked with the high phosphate (5% to 8%) solution to pick up and discard them. Do not vacuum hard-surfaced floors or windowsills or window wells, since this spreads dust. Use vacuum cleaners with agitators to remove dust from rugs rather than vacuum cleaners with suction only. If a rug is known to contain lead dust and cannot be washed, it should be discarded.

Wash and dry child's hands and face frequently, especially before eating.

Wash toys and pacifiers frequently.

If soil around home is or is likely to be contaminated with lead (e.g., if home was built before 1960 or is near a major highway), plant grass or other ground cover; plant bushes around outside of house so that child cannot play there.

During remodeling of older homes, be sure to follow correct procedures. Be certain children and pregnant women are not in the home, day or night, until process is completed. Following deleading, thoroughly clean house using high-phosphate cleaning solution to damp mop and dust before inhabitants return.

In areas where lead content of water exceeds the drinking water standard, run cold water until it is as cold as it will get before using for drinking, cooking, and making formula; may use first-flush water for other purposes.

Do not store food in open cans, particularly if cans are imported.

Do not use for food storage or service pottery or ceramic ware that was inadequately fired or that is meant for decorative use.

Do not store drinks or food in lead crystal.

Avoid folk remedies or cosmetics that contain lead.

Make sure that home exposure is not occurring from parental occupations or hobbies. Household members employed in occupations such as lead smelting should shower and change into clean clothing before leaving work. Construction and abatement workers may also bring home lead contaminants.

Make sure child eats regular meals, since more lead is absorbed on an empty stomach.

Make sure child's diet contains plenty of iron and calcium and not excessive fat.

Modified from Centers for Disease Control: *Preventing lead poisoning in young children,* Atlanta, GA, 1991, Centers for Disease Control.

Unit 4

Community and Home Care Instructions

PREPARING THE FAMILY FOR COMMUNITY AND HOME CARE

The Community and Home Care Instructions (CHCI) in this unit are provided as a supplement to assist the nurse in preparing the family to manage the child's care at home or in a setting in the community, such as a school or daycare facility. These instructions provide a written reference that the family can use when performing the procedure in the absence of a health professional or when entrusting their child's care to someone else. Each CHCI can be used as a teaching aid in preparing the patient for discharge from an acute care setting or a long-term care facility, clinic, or in the home when increasing the family's participation in the child's care.

The process of patient education involves giving the family information about the child's condition; the regimen that must be followed, and why; and other health teaching, as indicated. The goal of this education is to enable the family to modify behaviors and adhere to the regimen that has been mutually established.

One common problem with patient education is that the health professional delivers the information and the family listens. This one-way flow of material may not achieve the goal of the education. It is estimated that there is only a 50% compliance rate following patient education. Research has also shown that if the family is provided with written information that they can understand, they are more likely to comply with the regimen. The CHCI are written in clear, simple language to accommodate those with about a fifth grade reading level.

To avoid sexist language, but to also retain a personal and casual writing tone, the use of masculine and feminine pronouns is alternated. Unless otherwise indicated, the CHCI apply to both genders.

Every effort has been made to base the instructions on currently available evidence-based practice. For example, the sections on CPR, choking, and suctioning reflect the latest research and guidelines. However, most of the content is based on traditional practice because research is not available to define standards of practice. Information on taking rectal temperatures and using the dorsogluteal site for intramuscular injections is included because these practices persist, even though the authors believe strongly that unwarranted risks exist with these procedures. The choice has been made to provide instructions for the safest guidelines possible, but practitioners are encouraged to recognize the availability of safer alternatives. The practitioner should be aware that new information available after this publication may significantly change the content included in this unit. This is particularly relevant for the instructions on CPR and choking.

HOW TO USE THE CHCI

To maximize the benefits of patient teaching, these general guidelines should be followed:

1. Establish a rapport with the family.
2. Avoid using *any* specialized terms or jargon. Clarify all terms with the family.
3. When possible, allow the family to decide how they want to be taught (for example, all at once or over a day or two). This gives the family a chance to incorporate the information at a rate that is comfortable.
4. Teach the family about the illness.
5. Assist the family in identifying obstacles to their ability to comply with the regimen, and in identifying the means to overcome those obstacles. Then help the family find ways to incorporate the plan into their daily lives.

The CHCI represent commonly accepted guidelines for performing a procedure, but they may differ from those used in various settings. For this reason, review the instructions carefully and clarify any differences in protocol before giving them to the family. Complete any blanks, such as names of medication or the frequency of dressing changes. To document discharge teaching, make two copies of the CHCI, one for the family, and one to attach to the patient record or care plan.

If equipment will be needed at home (for example, suction machines or syringes), begin making the necessary arrangements in advance so that discharge can proceed smoothly. Whenever possible, make arrangements for the family to use the same equipment in the home that they are using in the hospital. This allows them to become familiar with the items. In addition, the staff can help "troubleshoot" the equipment in a controlled environment. When the family is being taught at home, individualize the instructions, encourage the family to write notes, and include any adaptations that will be necessary for the family. Plan the teaching sessions well in advance of the time the family will be responsible for performing the care. The more complex the procedure, the more time is needed for training.

Review the instructions with the family. Encourage note taking if they desire. Allow ample practice time under supervision. At least one family member, but preferably two members, should demonstrate the procedure before they are expected to care for the child at home. Provide the family with the telephone numbers of resource individuals who are available to assist them in the event of a problem.

Unit 5

INSTRUCTIONS RELATED TO HYGIENE AND CARE

COMMUNITY AND HOME CARE INSTRUCTIONS

Eliminating Extra Feedings at Sleep Times

Sleep problems in infants and young children can be very disruptive to the family. Sleep disturbances with a physiological basis are rare, with the exception of colic. The more common sleep problems are a learned pattern or developmental characteristic of some children. These instructions may be useful if your infant or young child:

- Goes to sleep at the breast or with a bottle
- Has a prolonged need for middle-of-night bottle- or breast-feeding
- Has frequent awakenings (may be hourly)
- Returns to sleep only after feeding; other comfort measures (e.g., rocking or holding) are usually ineffective

Day	Ounces in Each Bottle or Minutes Nursing	Minimum Hours Between Feedings
1	7	2
2	6	2.5
3	5	3
4	4	3.5
5	3	4
6	2	4.5
7	1	5
8	No more bottles or nursing at sleep times	

- The ounces and times in this chart are general guidelines. You will want to alter them to fit your own routines.
- If your child takes less than 8 ounces in the bottle, start with 1 ounce less than he or she usually takes and continue reducing from there.
- If you are breast-feeding, use the time spent nursing as an approximation of volume. Begin by nursing 1 or 2 minutes less than you usually nurse and continue decreasing the times from that point.
- If you prefer, you may follow this chart but decrease every other day instead of every day. It will just take a little longer.

This section may be photocopied and distributed to families.

From Wong DL, Hess CS: *Wong and Whaley's Clinical manual of pediatric nursing,* ed 5. Copyright © 2000, Mosby, St Louis.

Unit 5

COMMUNITY AND HOME CARE INSTRUCTIONS

Helping Your Child Learn to Fall Asleep with the Proper Associations—The Progressive Approach

These home care instructions may be helpful if your child has sleep problems that are disruptive to the family. Sleep disturbances are usually a learned pattern or developmental characteristic of some children. This chart shows the number of minutes to wait before going in if your child is crying at bedtime or after nighttime wakings.

NUMBER OF MINUTES TO WAIT BEFORE GOING IN TO YOUR CHILD BRIEFLY

| Day | At First Wait | If Your Child is Still Crying | | |
		Second Wait	Third Wait	Subsequent Waits
1	5	10	15	15
2	10	15	20	20
3	15	20	25	25
4	20	25	30	30
5	25	30	35	35
6	30	35	40	40
7	35	40	45	45

1. Each time you go in to your child, spend only 2 to 3 minutes. Remember, you are going in briefly to reassure the child and yourself, not necessarily to help the child stop crying and certainly not to help him or her fall asleep. The goal is for the child to learn to fall asleep alone, without being held, rocked, nursed, or using a bottle or pacifier.

2. When you get to the maximum number of minutes to wait for that night, continue leaving for that amount of time until your child finally falls asleep during one of the periods you are out of the room.

3. If your child wakes during the night, begin the waiting schedule at the minimum waiting time for that day and again work up to the maximum.

4. Continue this routine after all wakings until reaching a time in the morning (usually 5:30 to 7:30 AM) that you have previously decided to be reasonable to start the day. If your child wakes after that time, or is still awake then after waking earlier, get your child up and begin the morning routines.

5. Use the same schedule for naps; but if your child has not fallen asleep after 1 hour, or is awake again and crying vigorously after getting some sleep, end that naptime period.

6. The number of minutes listed to wait are ones that most families find workable. If they seem too long for you, use the times shown on the chart on p. 584 (though without closing the door). In fact, any schedule will work as long as the times increase progressively.

7. Be sure to follow your schedule carefully and chart your child's sleep patterns daily so you can monitor his or her progress accurately.*

8. By day 7 your child will most likely be sleeping very well, but if further work is necessary, just continue to add 5 minutes to each time on successive days.

From Ferber R: *Solve your child's sleep problems,* New York, 1985, Simon & Schuster, Inc. Used with permission.

*A 2-week sleep record is on p. 106.

This section may be photocopied and distributed to families.

From Wong DL, Hess CS: *Wong and Whaley's Clinical manual of pediatric nursing,* ed. 5. Copyright © 2000, Mosby, St Louis.

Unit 5

COMMUNITY AND HOME CARE INSTRUCTIONS

Helping Your Child Learn to Stay in Bed

Sleep problems can be very disruptive to the family. These home care instructions may be helpful if your child has difficulty staying in bed. This chart shows the number of minutes to close your child's door if your child will not stay in bed at bedtime or after nighttime wakings.

NUMBER OF MINUTES TO CLOSE THE DOOR IF YOUR CHILD WILL NOT STAY IN BED

		If Your Child Continues to Get Out of Bed			
Day	First Closing	Second Closing	Third Closing	Fourth Closing	Subsequent Closings
1	1	2	3	5	5
2	2	4	6	8	8
3	3	5	7	10	10
4	5	7	10	15	15
5	7	10	15	20	20
6	10	15	20	25	25
7	15	20	25	30	30

1. When you get to the maximum number of minutes for that night, continue closing the door for that amount of time until your child finally stays in bed.

2. Keep the door closed for the number of minutes listed, even if your child goes back to bed sooner. However, you may talk to your child through the door and tell him or her how much time remains.

3. When you open the door, speak to your child briefly if he or she is in bed, offer encouragement, and leave. If he or she is still out of bed, restate the rules, put your child back in bed (if it can be done easily), and shut the door for the next amount of time listed. If your child lets you put him or her back easily, and you are convinced the child will stay there, you may try leaving the door open; but if you are wrong, do not keep making the same mistake.

4. If your child wakes during the night and won't stay in bed, begin the door-closing schedule at the minimum time for that day and again work up to the maximum.

5. Continue this routine as necessary after all wakings until reaching a time in the morning (usually 5:30 to 7:00 AM) previously decided to be reasonable to start the day.

6. Use the same routine at naptimes, but if your child has not fallen asleep after 1 hour, or if he or she is awake again and out of bed after getting some sleep, end that naptime period.

7. If your child wakes and calls or cries but does not get out of bed, switch to the progressive routine described in the chart on p. 583.

8. The number of minutes listed to close the door are ones that most families find workable. However, you may change the schedule as you think best as long as the times increase progressively.

9. Be sure to follow your schedule carefully and chart your child's sleep patterns daily so you can monitor his or her progress accurately.*

10. Remember, your goal is to help your child learn to sleep alone. You are using the door as a controlled way of enforcing this, not to scare or punish him or her. So reassure your child by talking through the door; do not threaten or scream. By progressively increasing time of door closure, starting with short periods, your child does not have to be shut behind a closed door unsure of when it will be opened. Your child will learn that having the door open is entirely under his or her control.

11. By day 7 your child will most likely be staying in bed, but if further work is necessary, just continue to add 5 minutes to each time on successive days.

12. If you prefer, you may use a gate instead of a closed door as long as your child can't open or climb over it. In this case you must be out of his view during the periods of gate closure, but you can still talk to your child reassuringly from another room.

From Ferber R: *Solve your child's sleep problems,* New York, 1985, Simon & Schuster, Inc. Used with permission.

*A 2-week sleep record is on p. 106.

This section may be photocopied and distributed to families.

From Wong DL, Hess CS: *Wong and Whaley's Clinical manual of pediatric nursing,* ed. 5. Copyright © 2000, Mosby, St Louis.

COMMUNITY AND HOME CARE INSTRUCTIONS

Caring for Your Child's Teeth

Begin regular visits to the dentist soon after the first teeth erupt, usually around 1 year of age, and no later than 18 months.

Plan the first examination to be a "friendly visit"—meeting the dentist, seeing the room and equipment, and sitting in the chair.

BRUSHING AND FLOSSING

Begin cleaning the teeth as soon as the first tooth erupts. This is done by wiping it with a cloth.

Begin regular brushing and flossing soon after several "baby" teeth have erupted. Make mouth care pleasant by talking or singing to child.

Use a small toothbrush with soft, rounded, multitufted nylon bristles that are short and even. Change the toothbrush *often,* as soon as the bristles are bent or frayed.

For young children, place the tips of the bristles firmly at a 45-degree angle against the teeth and gums and move them back and forth in a vibratory motion. Do not move the ends of the bristles forcefully back and forth because this can damage the gums and enamel.

For children whose permanent teeth have erupted, place the sides of the bristles firmly against the gums and brush the gums and teeth in the direction the teeth grow, using a rolling action.

Clean all surfaces of the teeth in this manner, except the inner surfaces of the front teeth. To clean these areas, place the toothbrush vertical to the teeth and move it up and down.

Brush only a few teeth at one time, using six to eight strokes for each section.

Use a systematic approach so that all surfaces are thoroughly cleaned.

In brushing young children's teeth, use any of these positions:

Stand with the child's back toward you.

Sit on a couch or bed with the child's head in your lap.

Sit on a floor or stool with the child's head resting between your thighs.

Use one hand to cup the chin and the other hand to brush the teeth.

When child wants to begin brushing his or her own teeth, let him or her "help" by brushing before or after.

Floss the teeth after brushing. Wrap a piece of dental floss (about 18 inches long) around the middle finger and grasp it between the index finger and thumb of both hands. With about 1 inch of floss held firmly between the thumbs, insert the floss between two teeth and wrap it around the base of the tooth and below the gum in a C shape. Move the floss toward the top of the tooth in a sweeping motion. Repeat this a few times on every tooth, using a clean piece of floss. Children may find it easier to tie the floss in a circle, rather than wrapping it around the middle finger.

Check the thoroughness of the cleaning by having the child chew a special dental disclosing tablet (available commercially or from dentists) that stains any remaining plaque red. Rebrush any colored areas.

Form the habit of cleaning the teeth after each meal and especially before bedtime. Give the child nothing to eat or drink (except water) after the night brushing.

Use the "swish and swallow" method of cleaning the mouth at times when brushing is impractical. Have child rinse mouth with water and swallow, repeating this three or four times.

FLUORIDE

Use a fluoridated toothpaste, but supervise the amount used by the child. Use only a "pea-sized" amount on the brush and teach child not to eat toothpaste.

Use a fluoridated mouthrinse if the child is older than 6 years and can safely rinse and spit out the rinse without swallowing. Use only the recommended amount; time the 1-minute rinse with a clock. Give the child nothing to eat or drink for 30 minutes afterward.

If the local water supply is fluoridated, make sure that the child is drinking the water—plain, in juices, soups, or in other foods prepared with tap water.

If the local water supply is not fluoridated or if the infant after 6 months of age is exclusively breast-fed or given commercial ready-to-feed formula, make sure fluoride supplements are prescribed by a health professional.

When supplemental fluoride is prescribed:

- Give supplements on an empty stomach.
- Place the drops directly on the tongue to allow them to mix with saliva and come in contact with the teeth.
- Encourage older children to chew the tablet and swish it around the teeth for 30 seconds before swallowing.
- Give the child nothing to eat or drink for 30 minutes afterward.
- Store fluoride supplements and fluoridated toothpaste and mouthrinse in a safe place away from small children.

DIET

Keep sweet foods to a minimum, especially sticky or chewy candy and dried fruits (raisins, "fruit rolls"), chewing gum, and hard candy (lollipops, "lifesavers"). Read labels on packaged foods (e.g., dry cereals) for hidden sources of sugar, including honey, molasses, and corn syrup.

Remember: *It is how often children eat sweets, rather than the amount of sweets eaten at one time,* that is most important. Plan sweets to follow a meal when the child is likely to brush immediately afterward. Discourage frequent snacking with sweets.

Encourage snacks that are less likely to cause cavities (caries), such as cheese, fresh fruit, raw vegetables, crackers, pretzels, potato or corn chips, popcorn, peanuts, and artificially sweetened candy, gum, and soda. When choosing snacks for young children, avoid those foods (e.g., grapes, popcorn, and nuts) that can cause choking.

If the child takes a bottle to bed, fill it only with water, *never* formula, breast milk, cow's milk, or juice. Avoid frequent or prolonged breast-feeding during sleep.

If the child routinely takes any medicine in sweetened liquid or chewable tablet form, clean the teeth immediately afterward or at least have the child drink water to rinse the mouth.

Unit 5

Measuring Your Child's Temperature

Body temperature changes during the day; it is usually higher in the afternoon than in the early morning. If you are very active, your temperature may be higher than normal. Fever helps protect the body. A rise in body temperature above normal (usually 98.6° F) may mean an infection somewhere. Fever also helps the body fight the infection. Someone has a fever if the body temperature is higher than 100° F (oral or axillary temperature) or 100.4° F (rectal temperature). If you use the Centigrade (°C) system, the conversions from Fahrenheit (°F) are in Box 5-1.

You should measure a child's temperature:
1. When the skin feels warm to your touch.
2. When the child is not acting like his or her usual self.
3. Before calling your health professional to say that the child is sick.

BOX 5-1

Conversion of Degrees Fahrenheit (F) to Degrees Centigrade (C)

°F	°C	°F	°C	°F	°C
96.8	36.0	100.4	38.0	104.0	40.0
97.7	36.5	101.3	38.5	104.9	40.5
98.6	37.0	102.2	39.0	105.8	41.1
99.5	37.5	103.1	39.5	107.6	42.0

TYPES OF THERMOMETERS

There are many ways to measure your child's temperature. When you buy a thermometer, you should choose one that is easy to use. Because some are more accurate than others, tell your health professional how you measured your child's temperature.

Glass Mercury Thermometers

The most common way to measure temperature has been the use of a glass mercury thermometer. This thermometer is inexpensive but is hard for many people to read. It can break, and the mercury inside the thermometer can be dangerous if it leaks. If this happens, wipe up the mercury with a paper towel and throw the towel away. The instructions that begin with "How to measure axillary temperature" are for using the glass mercury thermometer. If you use the digital thermometer, the directions are the same, except that the thermometer will beep to tell you that the temperature is recorded on a small screen.

There are two types of glass thermometers, oral and rectal (Fig. 1). The only difference between the two kinds is the shape of the silver tip. A rectal thermometer has a short, rounded tip. It is shaped this way to prevent any damage to the rectum. The oral thermometer has a longer, slender tip. Either type of thermometer can be used for an axillary temperature.

While holding the clear (or white)

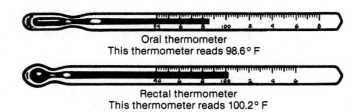

Oral thermometer
This thermometer reads 98.6° F

Rectal thermometer
This thermometer reads 100.2° F

Fig. 1 Comparison of oral (*top,* narrow tip) and rectal (*bottom,* rounded tip) thermometers.

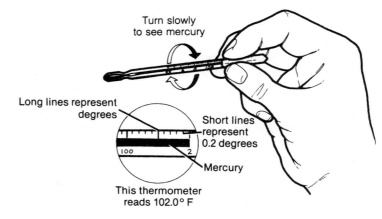

Turn slowly to see mercury

Long lines represent degrees

Short lines represent 0.2 degrees

Mercury

This thermometer reads 102.0° F

Fig. 2 Reading a glass mercury thermometer.

end of the thermometer at eye level, slowly turn the thermometer until you can see the silver line of mercury (Fig. 2). The lower numbers on the thermom-

From Wong DL, Hess CS: *Wong and Whaley's Clinical manual of pediatric nursing,* ed 5. Copyright © 2000, Mosby, St Louis.

Unit 5

Measuring Your Child's Temperature—cont'd

eter will be on the left. The amount the mercury moves from left to right will depend on your child's temperature. The highest number that the silver line reaches is the temperature. Before using the thermometer, make sure it reads 96° F or less. If not, while holding the clear end, shake the thermometer sharply in the air above a soft surface, such as a bed or sofa, in case it should fall. Look at the reading again. If it is below 96° F, measure the temperature. If not, repeat the shaking until the reading is below 96° F.

Digital Thermometers

Digital thermometers are used just like glass mercury thermometers, but they are safer and much easier to read. They have a button battery–powered heat sensor that measures temperature in less than 1 minute. The temperature is displayed in numbers on a small screen. Digital thermometers are also available within a pacifier. As your child sucks on the pacifier, the temperature is shown on a screen. Read the manufacturer's directions for the length of time to keep the pacifier in the mouth.

Ear Thermometers

Ear thermometers use a probe that is placed in the opening of the ear to measure the temperature of the eardrum. Although this device is expensive, it is easy to use, rapidly measures temperature (about 1 second), causes no discomfort to your child, and does not need your child's cooperation. However, an ear thermometer must be used correctly for accurate results. Read the manufacturer's instructions for how to place the probe in the ear canal and how to tug the earlobe. Tugging the earlobe straightens the ear canal so the probe can measure the temperature of the eardrum. As a general rule, for children less than 3 years, pull the bottom of the earlobe down and back. For children over 3 years, pull the top of the earlobe up and back.

Chemical Dot Thermometers

Several types of thermometers have a series of dots that change color as the body temperature goes up or down. Each dot has a specific degree of temperature marked under it; the dot that

gets brighter is your child's temperature. Plastic strip thermometers are placed on the child's skin (usually the forehead) and can be kept there to measure temperature continuously without disturbing your child. Another type, Tempa-Dot, is a plastic strip with dots at one end; this end is placed in the child's mouth or under the arm to measure temperature. Read the directions for the length of time to keep the thermometer in the mouth or armpit.

HOW TO MEASURE AXILLARY TEMPERATURE

Measuring temperature in the axilla (armpit) is the safest way to check if your child has a fever.

1. Tell the child that you are going to measure his temperature.
2. Wash your hands.
3. Look at the thermometer to make sure it is reading below 96° F.
4. Place the thermometer under the child's arm. The thermometer's tip should rest in the center of your child's armpit (Fig. 3).
5. Hold the child's arm firmly against his body.
6. Look at the time.
7. The glass mercury thermometer must remain in place for 3 to 4 minutes. To help make the time seem to go faster, read a story or watch TV with the child. Make sure you hold the thermometer securely.
8. Remove the thermometer and read.
9. PRAISE THE CHILD FOR HELPING.
10. Write down the thermometer reading and the time of day.
11. Clean the thermometer with cool water and soap.

HOW TO MEASURE ORAL TEMPERATURES

By 5 or 6 years of age, a child can understand how to safely hold the thermometer in his mouth. If the child has had something to eat or drink, wait 15 minutes before you measure an oral temperature.

1. Tell the child why you want to measure his temperature.
2. Wash your hands.

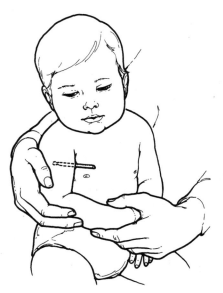

Fig. 3 Position for measuring axillary temperature.

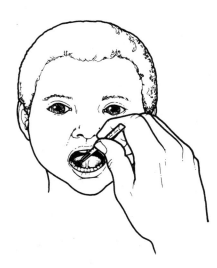

Fig. 4 Placement of thermometer under tongue, toward back of mouth.

3. Place the thermometer in the mouth, far back under the tongue (Fig. 4). Tell the child to keep the mouth closed, breathe through the nose, and not talk.
4. Make sure the child does not bite the thermometer.
5. Look at the time.

Unit 5

Continued

Measuring Your Child's Temperature—cont'd

6. Tell the child that the glass mercury thermometer must stay in place for 2 to 3 minutes. Read a story or watch TV with him.
7. Remove the thermometer and read it.
8. PRAISE THE CHILD FOR HELPING.
9. Write down the thermometer reading and the time of day.
10. Clean the thermometer with cool water and soap.

HOW TO MEASURE RECTAL TEMPERATURES

Note that rectal temperatures should not be taken if the child has diarrhea or is less than 1 year old. In taking a child's temperature, use the following procedure:

1. Tell the child that you are going to measure his temperature.
2. Wash your hands.
3. Measure 1 inch on the thermometer or ⅙ of the thermometer's length.
4. Place the child on his stomach (Fig. 5), on one side with the upper leg bent, or on his back with both legs up.
5. Dip the thermometer's tip in a lubricant such as petroleum jelly (Vaseline).
6. Place the end of the thermometer into the child's anus. Do not insert the thermometer any farther than 1 inch.

7. Hold the glass mercury thermometer in place for 2 to 3 minutes. Always hold the child so that he cannot twist around.
8. Remove the thermometer and read.
9. PRAISE THE CHILD FOR HELPING.
10. Clean the thermometer with cool water and soap.
11. Wash your hands with soap and water. Count to 10 while washing, then rinse with clear water and dry with a clean paper or cloth towel.
12. Write down the thermometer reading and the time of day.

WHEN A FEVER IS PRESENT

Call your health professional at _____ *as soon as possible* if (1) the child has a temperature higher than 105° F or (2) a fever (oral or axillary temperature above 100° F or 100.4° F rectally) is present and the child:

- Is less than 2 months of age.
- Has a stiff neck, severe headache, stomach pain, persistent vomiting, purplish spots on the skin, or earache along with the temperature.
- Has a serious illness in addition to the fever.
- Is confused or delirious.
- Has had a seizure.
- Has trouble breathing after you have cleaned his nose.
- Is hard to awaken.

- Seems sicker than you would expect.
- Cannot be comforted.
- Has a temperature that continues to rise after medicine has been given.

    Call your health professional *during office hours* if:

- The temperature is between 104° F and 105° F, especially if the child is less than 2 years old.
- The child has burning or pain with urination.
- The fever has been present for more than 72 hours.
- The fever has been present for more than 24 hours without a known cause.
- The fever went away for more than 24 hours, then returned.
- The child has a history of febrile seizures.
- You have some questions.

The most important thing to remember is not to bundle up the child with extra clothes and blankets, unless the child is shivering. Dress him in light clothing. This will help cool the child by letting air circulate and heat leave the body.

Do not bathe or give the child a sponge bath in cool water. If the temperature is lowered too quickly, the child may shiver, causing the temperature to go up. If shivering occurs, keep the child warm until it stops.

The presence of a fever increases the amount of liquid that is needed by the body. It is important to encourage the sick child to drink fluids. Some things that may help encourage drinking are using straws and small cups instead of a big glass; and giving Popsicles, jello, and soft drinks with the fizz removed (flat). The carbonation can be removed by leaving the soft drink uncovered, by warming the soda in a microwave or on a stove, or by stirring in ¼ teaspoon sugar.

Medicines should not be used routinely to lower the temperature. If the child is uncomfortable, and the fever needs to be treated with more than light clothes and increased fluids, then drugs can be used.

Be sure to give the right amount (dose) and type of medicine. Use the child's weight as a guide to the right dose. If using infant drops, do not replace with the syrup (elixir) because the amount of medicine in these bottles are different.

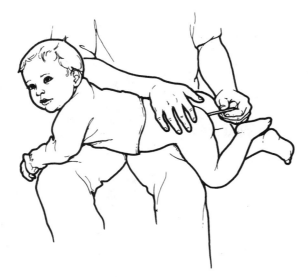

Fig. 5 Position for measuring rectal temperature. The thermometer is inserted no more than 1 inch into the rectum.

COMMUNITY AND HOME CARE INSTRUCTIONS

Measuring Your Child's Temperature—cont'd

RECOMMENDED DOSAGES OF ACETAMINOPHEN FOR EACH AGE/WEIGHT CHILD*

Age	3 mo	4-11 mo	12-23 mo	2-3 yr	4-5 yr	6-8 yr	9-10 yr	11 yr	12 yr and over
Weight (lb)	6-11	12-17	18-23	24-35	36-47	48-59	60-71	72-95	96 and over
Dose (mg)	40	80	120	160	240	320	400	480	650

TYPE OF MEDICINE

Liquids

Type	3 mo	4-11 mo	12-23 mo	2-3 yr	4-5 yr	6-8 yr	9-10 yr	11 yr	12 yr and over
Drops (1 dropper = 80 mg/0.8 ml)	½	1	1-1½	2	—	—	—	—	—
Elixir/suspension 160 mg/5 ml (1 tsp)	—	½ tsp	¾ tsp	1 tsp	1½ tsp	2 tsp	2½ tsp	3 tsp	

Tablets

Type	3 mo	4-11 mo	12-23 mo	2-3 yr	4-5 yr	6-8 yr	9-10 yr	11 yr	12 yr and over
Chewable tablets (80 mg/tablet)	—	—	—	2	3	4	—	—	—
Swallowable or chewable caplets/ tablets (160 mg/ tablet)	—	—	—	1	1½	2	2½	3	4
Capsules (80 mg)	—	—	—	2	3	4	—	—	—
Capsules (160 mg)	—	—	—	1	—	2	—	3	4

Suppository

Type	3 mo	4-11 mo	12-23 mo	2-3 yr	4-5 yr	6-8 yr	9-10 yr	11 yr	12 yr and over
Infant strength (80 mg)	½	1	—	—	—	—	—	—	—
Child strength (120 mg)	—	½†	1	1	2	—	—	—	—
Junior strength (325 mg)	—	—	—	—	—	1	1	1½†	2

Some Acetaminophen Brand Names:

Drops	*Tablets*	*Suppository*
Panadol	Chewable Anacin 3	Fever-all
Tylenol	Chewable Tylenol	
Tempra	St. Joseph Aspirin Free Chewable	
Liquiprin	Junior Strength Tylenol	

*If your child's weight is higher or lower than the weight listed for age, give the dose that is recommended for the weight. For example, if your child is 11 months old and weighs 20 pounds, give the dose (120 mg) listed under the column for 18-23 pounds. (To change kilograms to pounds, multiply kilograms by 2.2.) The dose may be repeated every 4 hours, but not more than five times a day.

†Cut suppository in half *lengthwise*.

Continued

Unit 5

COMMUNITY AND HOME CARE INSTRUCTIONS

Measuring Your Child's Temperature—cont'd

RECOMMENDED DOSAGES OF IBUPROFEN FOR EACH AGE/WEIGHT CHILD*

Age	6-11 mo	12-23 mo	2-3 yr	4-5 yr	6-8 yr	9-10 yr	11 yr	12 yr and over
Weight (lb)	12-17	18-23	24-35	36-47	48-59	60-71	72-95	96 and over
Dose (mg)	50	75	100	150	200	250	300	400
TYPE OF MEDICINE								
Drops (50 mg per dropper)	1	1½	2	3	4	—	—	—
Suspension 100 mg/5 ml (1 tsp)	½	¾	1	1½	2	2½	3	4
Chewable 50-mg tablets	—	—	2	3	4	5	6	8
Swallowable or chewable 100 mg caplets/tablets	—	—	—	1	2	2½	3	4
Swallowable 200 mg gelcaps/ tablets	—	—	—	—	1	1½	1½	2

Some Ibuprofen Brand Names:

Children's Motrin
Children's Advil

*If your child's weight is higher or lower than the weight listed for age, give the dose that is recommended for the weight. For example, if your child is 11 months old and weighs 20 pounds, give the dose (75 mg) listed under the column for 18-23 pounds. (To change kilograms to pounds, multiply kilograms by 2.2.) Your health professional may prescribe doses that are higher than those in the table if your child's fever is above 102.5° F. The dose may be repeated every 6-8 hours, but not more than three times a day.

COMMUNITY AND HOME CARE INSTRUCTIONS

Obtaining a Urine Sample

Children who are 8 years of age and older may be able to obtain the sample by themselves. Tell the child how to clean herself and how to obtain the sample. Help the child if needed. Children under 8 years of age will need your help. Young children may not be able to urinate on request. Use the child's words and usual place for urinating to obtain the sample, if possible. To help the child urinate, have her blow through a straw or listen to running water while you hold the specimen cup. Do not give the child more than one glass of liquid to drink. Large amounts of liquid can affect the result of the urine test. If you think the child does not understand, have her practice one time, then collect the specimen the next time.

INSTRUCTIONS FOR THE TOILET-TRAINED CHILD

Equipment
Urine cup
Potty chair or toilet
Soap and water
Washcloth or paper wipes

Routine Urine Sample (Boys and Girls)

1. Tell the child that you need to get some urine. Use the child's word for urine.
2. If the child is able to obtain the sample of urine, have the child wash her hands.
3. Wash your hands.
4. Gather the equipment needed.
5. Open the urine container, being careful not to touch the inside of the cup or lid.
6. Have the child urinate directly into the cup.
7. Replace the lid on the cup.
8. Label the cup with the child's first and last name.
9. PRAISE THE CHILD FOR HELPING.
10. Wash your hands with soap and water. Count to 10 while washing, then rinse with clear water and dry with a clean paper or cloth towel.
11. Have the child wash her hands (if she helped).

Urine Sample for Culture (Boys)

If you are told that a "clean catch" specimen is needed, follow steps 1 through 5 for routine urine sample, then do the following:

1. If paper wipes are provided, use these instead of a washcloth; rinsing is not necessary with the wipes.
2. Wash the tip of the penis with a wipe or soap and water. Rinse well if soap is used. If the child is uncircumcised, pull back the foreskin only as far as it will easily go and then wash and rinse the tip of the penis with a clean part of the washcloth. Make sure the foreskin is pushed back toward the tip after cleaning.
3. Have the child begin to urinate in the potty chair or toilet.
4. Tell him to stop.
5. Have the child begin to urinate into the cup. If he cannot stop the flow of urine, place the urine cup so that you can "catch" some of the urine.
6. Replace the lid on the cup.

7. Label the cup with the child's first and last name.
8. PRAISE THE CHILD FOR HELPING.
9. Wash your hands with soap and water. Count to 10 while washing, then rinse with clear water and dry with a clean paper or cloth towel.

Urine Sample for Culture (Girls)

If you are told that a "clean catch" specimen is needed, follow steps 1 through 5 for routine urine sample, then do the following:

1. If paper wipes are provided, use them instead of a washcloth; rinsing is not necessary with the wipes.
2. Spread the child's labia (lips) (Fig. 1) with your fingers. Wash the area with a paper wipe or soap and water; rinse well if soap is used. Wash from front to back, rinsing well with a clean part of the washcloth.
3. Have the child begin to urinate into the potty chair or toilet.
4. Tell her to stop.

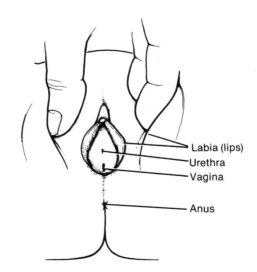

Labia (lips)
Urethra
Vagina
Anus

Fig. 1 Finger position to spread labia for cleaning before obtaining a urine sample for culture.

This section may be photocopied and distributed to families.

Continued

Unit 5

COMMUNITY AND HOME CARE INSTRUCTIONS

Obtaining a Urine Sample—cont'd

5. Hold the cup in place and tell her to start to urinate into the cup. If she cannot stop the flow of urine, place the cup so that you can "catch" some of the urine.
6. Replace the lid on the cup.
7. Label the cup with the child's first and last name.
8. PRAISE THE CHILD FOR HELPING.
9. Wash your hands with soap and water. Count to 10 while washing, then rinse with clear water and dry with a clean paper or cloth towel.

INSTRUCTIONS FOR THE CHILD WHO IS NOT TOILET TRAINED
Equipment
Urine cup
Urine collection bag
Soap and water
Washcloths or paper wipes
Clean diaper

Instructions
If the child is very active, you will need help to put on the urine bag.
1. Wash your hands with soap and water. Count to 10 while washing, then rinse with clear water and dry with a clean paper or cloth towel. Your helper should also wash his or her hands.
2. Tell the child what you are going to do.
3. Gather the needed equipment.
4. Place the child on her back.
5. Remove the child's diaper.
6. If the urine sample is for culture, clean the child's genital area with soap and water as described on the previous page.
7. Rinse thoroughly and pat dry.
8. Have your helper hold the child's legs apart while you apply the bag.
9. Hold the urine collector with the bag portion downward.
10. Remove the bottom half of the adhesive protector.

For Girls
1. Spread the labia and buttocks, keeping the skin tight.
2. Begin with the bottom of the adhesive. Place the sticky portion of the bag as flat as possible against the skin (Fig. 2).
3. Smooth the plastic to avoid any wrinkles.
4. Remove the top half of the adhesive protector and smooth it also on the labia.

For Boys
1. Place the boy's penis and scrotum into the bag if possible. If not, put the sticky part of the bag on the scrotum (Fig. 3).
2. Smooth the sticky portion of the bag on the skin, taking care to avoid making any wrinkles.
3. Remove the top half of the adhesive protector and smooth the top part on the skin to remove any wrinkles.

Check the bag often and remove it as soon as the child urinates.

To remove the bag, hold it against the child's skin at the bottom and carefully peel it off from top to bottom. Cut a corner of the bag to pour the urine into the urine cup.

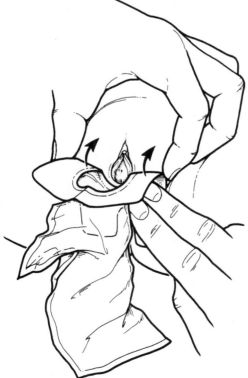

Fig. 2 Putting the urine bag on a girl, starting from back and proceeding to front.

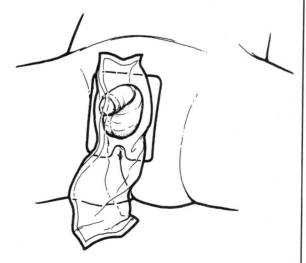

Fig. 3 Putting the urine bag on a boy, with the penis and scrotum inside the bag.

Unit 5

COMMUNITY AND HOME CARE INSTRUCTIONS

Caring for the Child in a Cast

Casts are made from many different types of material and used on different parts of the body. A cast was put on your child so that the injured area could heal well. The care of the cast will vary slightly, depending on the type of cast that was put on.

Before the cast is applied, a smooth material is used to protect the skin. The cast is then put on over this material. At first, the cast will feel warm; this will last for about 10 to 15 minutes. A plaster cast will remain damp for many hours, whereas a fiberglass cast will dry within 30 minutes. Do not put anything in the cast while it is drying or afterwards. During the drying time, touch the cast as little as possible. If you have to touch the cast, use the palms of your hands, not the fingers (Fig. 1). Turning the child in a plaster body cast at least every 2 hours will help the cast dry. Do not use a heated fan or dryer. A regular fan can be used in humid weather to circulate the air.

Check the skin around the cast frequently. Notify your health professional at _____ if any of these occur:

- Numbness
- Tingling
- Unrelieved pain
- Burning
- Odor
- Strange feelings

- Temperature change
- Fluid coming through cast
- Cast becomes soft, broken, or cracked
- Toes cannot be seen at edge of cast after correction of club foot

If it is a leg or arm cast, check the color of the toes or fingers. They should be pink and warm to the touch. When the skin in these areas is lightly pressed and released, the color should return quickly. To help prevent swelling, raise the arm/leg in the cast above the level of the child's heart (Fig. 2) by resting the cast on several pillows or blankets. If an arm is casted, a sling helps support the arm during the day and pillows can be used at night. For leg casts, loosen the covers on the bed at nighttime and place some pillows by the feet to keep the blanket from putting pressure on the toes.

Some leg casts are made so that the child can walk with the cast. If this type of cast (i.e., weight bearing) cannot be used, the older child can be taught how to walk with crutches. When crutches are needed, follow your health professional's guidelines for the correct size and padding of the crutches.

The cast will be on for about _____ weeks. During this time, the child should exercise the joints and muscles that are not casted. Games like "Simon says" can make movement fun. Your health professional can suggest some exercises for your child.

SKIN CARE

During the time the cast is on, special care is needed to keep the skin around the cast healthy. The back of the leg may be irritated when the child is in a short leg cast, and the skin between the thumb and the index finger is often a problem with an arm cast. If the cast rubs against the skin, tape can be used to cover the rough edges of a cast. This is called petalling and includes these steps (Fig. 3):

1. Use adhesive bandages for strips or cut several 3-inch strips of 1 to 2 inch wide adhesive or duct tape.

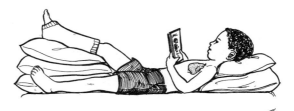

Fig. 2 Position cast above level of heart to prevent swelling.

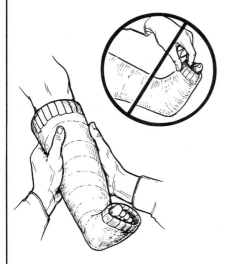

Fig. 1 When the cast is drying, lift it with the palms of the hands, not the fingers (inset), to avoid making dents in the cast.

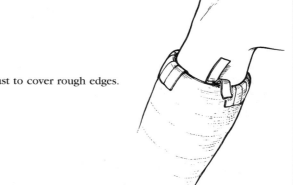

Fig. 3 "Petalling" the cast to cover rough edges.

Unit 5

Continued

Caring for the Child in a Cast—cont'd

2. Tape one end of the strip to the inside of the cast.
3. Tape the other end to the outside of the cast, covering the cast edge.
4. Repeat with the other strips of tape. Overlap the edges to make a smooth surface.

Itching

Sometimes the skin under the cast will feel itchy. Do not put anything inside the cast to scratch the skin. Children are often tempted to put forks, knives, food crumbs, combs, and other objects in the cast. Notify your health professional if any object is stuck in the cast. If the skin itches, some things that may make the child more comfortable include the following:

1. Blow COOL air from a hair dryer into the cast.
2. Rub the opposite arm or leg.
3. Rub the skin around the cast edges.

BATHS

Children in body casts and full leg casts should receive sponge baths. A child with a lower leg or arm cast may be bathed, or may take a shower if the cast is well covered or kept out of the water. The cast must remain dry. It can be wrapped with a plastic covering or a waterproof cast cover. The plastic cover should be removed and stored safely after the bath or shower. If a plaster cast becomes wet, it will soften and may need to be replaced. When a fiberglass cast becomes wet, it should be thoroughly dried with a fan or hair dryer on the cool setting. If a cast liner is used, the child may get the cast wet. Your health professional will tell you if you need to keep the cast dry.

CAST CARE

The surface of fiberglass casts can be easily wiped clean with a damp cloth. However, plaster casts cannot be cleaned. If the cast will be on for a long time, cloth coverings such as a large, stretchy sock or part of an opaque stocking (tights) can be used to protect the cast. These coverings can then be washed and replaced. If a cover is used, it must be

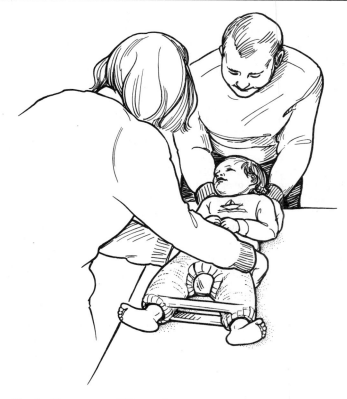

Fig. 4 Two persons lifting and moving a child in a body cast. The bar between the legs is never used for this purpose.

fabric and not plastic so that air can circulate through the cast.

SPICA CASTS (BODY CAST)

Body casts are designed to keep the child's hips and thighs from moving. Special care must be taken, because the cast covers the child's abdomen (stomach area) and the child is usually unable to move about. A "window" may be cut in the cast to allow the stomach to expand after meals. The genital area will be left open to allow the child to urinate and have bowel movements without soiling the cast. To protect the cast, duct tape or plastic wrap may be taped to the cast around this opening. This allows urine and stool to be easily wiped off. The other edges of the cast can be "petalled" to keep rough edges from harming the child's skin. Cotton padding, available from beauty supply stores, can also be used as disposable cushioning inside the edges of the cast.

The child should be lifted with support under the shoulders and hips. Two people may be needed to safely lift the older infant and child (Fig. 4). When lifting, avoid twisting the child's body. Never use the bar that keeps the legs separated to lift the child. Placing pressure on this bar can damage the cast. A new cast must be put on if the cast is badly damaged.

Since the child cannot move much, diet changes may be needed. Three problems that may occur with body casts are constipation, too much weight gain, and choking. The older infant and child should be given extra liquids and a diet high in fiber, such as fresh fruits, vegetables, beans, and whole grains such as oatmeal and whole wheat bread. If diet does not help, a mild stool softener may be used.

To prevent too much weight gain, avoid sugared drinks and candy, because they add "empty" calories and may keep

COMMUNITY AND HOME CARE INSTRUCTIONS

Caring for the Child in a Cast—cont'd

the child from eating foods needed for healing and growth.

Choking is also a concern. Do not feed the child grapes, whole or round pieces of hot dogs, or nuts. These can cause the child to choke. Tell the child to chew carefully.

While in a body cast, the young child cannot move around. You must be responsible for positioning the child and meeting all other needs. Change the child's position frequently. A bean bag chair can be used to place the child upright or to turn the child from side to side. It can also be used to help the child lie on the abdomen with arms over the side to play with toys on the floor.

If the child was able to crawl or walk before being put in a cast, a car mechanic's dolly (a flatbed wagon on wheels) can be used to help the child move around. Make sure there are no stairs or loose rugs that can cause injury.

INFANTS

Feeding the infant in a body cast requires some planning. You can support the child with your arm under the neck and head. Place the infant's hips and legs on a pillow at your side. This position can also be used for bottle- or breast-feeding. You can also hold the child's head and

shoulders in front of you with the legs behind your back. If the child is able to sit, a chair or table can be padded to help the child eat and play in a semisitting position.

For infants who are heavy wetters or for nighttime, a sanitary napkin or urine incontinence pad can be placed inside a smaller diaper for extra absorbency. Both napkin and diaper are then changed after each wetting. Ultra-absorbent sanitary pads and disposable diapers hold the most urine and keep skin the driest.

Children in body casts must be safely restrained while riding in cars. Some approved car seats can be modified, and a specially designed car restraint is available for purchase. (The Snug seat is available from Spelcast, [800] 336-7684.)

OLDER CHILDREN

Allow the child to help set the daily schedule. Within reason, the child can decide when meals, activities, schoolwork, and visits from friends take place. Since most clothing will not fit over the cast, some changes must be made. Loose-fitting shorts can be slit on the side seams and self-adhering or other simple fasteners attached so that these can be easily placed on the child.

It is too difficult for the child to use the bathroom. A bedpan or urinal should be available for the child to use.

When traveling in a car, the child should lie on the back seat; a special vest should be used with the car seat belts to restrain the child. (The E-Z On vest is available from E-Z On Products, 605 Commerce Way West, Jupiter, FL 33458; [407] 747-6920 or [800] 323-6598 [outside Florida].)

CAST REMOVAL

When the injury is healed, the cast will be removed. A cast is removed by rapid vibrations of the cast cutter. Although the machine makes a loud noise that can be scary, there is little chance that the child can be hurt by it. However, prepare the child for the cast removal. If possible, show the child how the cutter vibrates and give him a chance to get used to the noise. Tell the child there may be a tickling feeling when the cutter is used.

The skin will appear dry, pale, and scaly when the cast is removed. To soften and remove the dead skin, soak the skin in warm water and use a skin moisturizing lotion. Never scrub the skin to remove the scales. As the old skin comes off, new skin will grow.

Unit 5

COMMUNITY AND HOME CARE INSTRUCTIONS

Preventing Spread of HIV and Hepatitis B Virus Infections

The child with HIV or hepatitis B virus has an infection that other children and adults can get. To protect all people who come near the child, certain guidelines must be followed. The germ that caused the child's illness can be spread to others by contact with some of the child's body fluids. These may include blood, bloody body fluids, feces, and semen.

Your best protection against infection is good handwashing after you have taken care of the child. Always wash your hands with soap and water. Count to 10 while you are washing, then rinse with clear water and dry with a clean paper or cloth towel. If there are any cuts or other open areas on your hands, or if your health professional recommends you use them, wear gloves when touching any of the child's body fluids. Always follow any contact with the child's body fluids with good handwashing, even if gloves are worn. Always have your child wash his or her hands after touching body fluids.

Each time you care for the child, you must decide what type of safeguard to use. If the child wears diapers, the disposable, ultra-absorbent kind with leg bands should be used. If the child does not have loose, watery stools, and your hands will not come in contact with the urine or stool, then good handwashing

after changing the diaper is sufficient. However, if the child has large, loose stools, gloves should be worn to provide added protection. You must wash your hands when you are finished, even if gloves were worn. Place all diapers, gloves, wipes, tissues, and used dressings in a plastic bag and throw the bag away.

When feeding an infant, protect your clothes with a waterproof apron or cloth in case the infant has a "wet burp" or vomits.

CLEANING BODY FLUID SPILLS

If the child vomits, has a nose bleed, or has a loose stool that needs to be cleaned up, you should wear gloves. First, using paper towels, blot the spill to decrease the amount of liquid to be cleaned. Dispose of these towels in a plastic garbage bag. Pour a bleach solution (1 part household bleach mixed in 9 parts water) onto the spill area. Carefully blot with paper towels. Place these towels into a plastic bag. Wash soiled linens and clothes separately in hot water with detergent. Wash your hands with soap and water after removing gloves.

HEPATITIS B VACCINE

A vaccine is available to protect people from a type of hepatitis called hep-

atitis B. This vaccine has been added to the list of immunizations that all infants should receive. Three doses must be given. The first dose is given at birth; the child receives the second dose 1 month after the first injection, and the third dose is given 6 months after the first. It can be given at the same time as other immunizations (such as DPT, MMR, and Hib) but in different muscles. For older children who have not been immunized, especially adolescents, vaccination is now a required immunization.

SAFE SEX

Many infectious diseases can be passed to a partner during sexual activity. Once someone has a disease that can be transmitted sexually, care must be taken to stop spreading the disease. Avoid having casual sex with many partners, and tell partners if you are infected. Always use a condom during sex.

HEPATITIS A VACCINE

A vaccine is also available to protect certain people from a type of hepatitis called hepatitis A. Ask your health professional if your child should get this vaccine.

This section may be photocopied and distributed to families.

Unit 5

INSTRUCTIONS RELATED TO ADMINISTRATION OF MEDICATIONS

COMMUNITY AND HOME CARE INSTRUCTIONS

Giving Medications to Children

It is necessary for you to give the child medicine called _____ . This medicine will have

the following benefits: _____

    You will need to give the drug as follows:

        Amount _____

        How often _____

        Special instructions _____

    Your health professional has written on the chart below when the medicine should be given. Give the drug at the same time each day so that it becomes part of the daily routine for you and the child.

    For the child to have the most value from this medicine, it must be given until your health professional tells you to stop. Even though the child does not seem ill any longer, the medicine must be given for the prescribed time period.

    Some common side effects of the drug are: _____

If you have any problems that concern you, or notice any unexpected reactions from the medicine, notify your health

professional at _____

DRUG SCHEDULE

	Sunday	Monday	Tuesday	Wednesday	Thursday	Friday	Saturday
When child wakes up							
Breakfast 1 hr before							
with							
2 hr after							
Lunch 1 hr before							
with							
2 hr after							
Dinner 1 hr before							
with							
2 hr after							
Bedtime							
During night							

    Check the box for the correct day and time. If the drug is given at times that differ from the suggested ones, write in the hour where appropriate.

COMMUNITY AND HOME CARE INSTRUCTIONS

Giving Oral Medications

Your health professional has prescribed special medicine for the child that must be taken by mouth. This is a good time to teach the child about medicines as special things we take to get better. Do not tell her that the drug is candy. If the child thinks that the medicine is candy, and if the bottle is ever left in a place where she can reach it, she may take an overdose. Tell the child to take drugs ONLY from you or other special people, such as grandparents or babysitters. Store ALL drugs in a safe place such as a locked cabinet. The storage area should be cool and dry. Bathrooms are usually too warm and moist for storing tablets or capsules. ALWAYS keep drugs in the original container, with the child-proof cap tightly closed. Place drugs that need to be refrigerated on a high shelf toward the back of the refrigerator, not in the door.

TO ENCOURAGE THE CHILD

Unpleasant-tasting drugs can be mixed with a small amount of a pleasant-tasting food such as applesauce, juice, pudding, jelly, flavored ice, ice cream, or other, more flavorful foods. Allow the child to choose the food; this will encourage her to eat or drink all of the medicine. Tell the child what you have done so that she does not think the food always tastes like the drug-food combination. Do not add drugs to essential foods and liquids (milk, formula, orange juice, cereal) because the child may refuse them later. When mixing a drug with food or liquids, add it to a *small* amount (1 or 2 teaspoons) so that the child will only have to eat or drink that small amount to get all of the medicine. Offer the child a drink of water or other liquid to rinse away the taste of the drug.

If the drug tastes unpleasant, the child can suck on a small ice cube or Popsicle to decrease the taste. Also, you can cut a straw in half and have the child sip the medicine through a straw or have the child pinch her nose while taking the medicine. Not smelling the drug will lessen the unpleasant taste.

Some drugs taste better if served cold rather than at room temperature.

Give the child a gold star or sticker for taking the drug. These can be placed on the drug schedule sheet that you were given. The child can keep track of the number of times she has taken the medicine and how many doses are left. The stars or stickers also provide a record of her help.

TABLETS AND CAPSULES

Many tablets are pleasantly flavored, and the child can either swallow the tablet whole or chew the tablet. If a half-tablet is prescribed, only scored tablets (those with a visible groove on the tablet) can be broken in half. An unscored tablet may break into unequal portions. Pill cutters can be used to cut the tablet in half. They are sold in most drug stores. This does not matter if the child is taking the whole tablet. Tablets may also be cut in half if they are too large for the child to swallow whole.

If the child cannot swallow the tablet, you can crush the tablet between two spoons or a spoon and a piece of wax paper. However, before crushing any tablet, check with your health professional or pharmacist to make sure the tablet can be crushed. After the tablet is crushed, you can mix it with a nonessential food such as applesauce, jam, or fruit juice. Make sure all of the crushed tablet is added. If you have added medicine to the food, tell the child.

If the medicine is a capsule, do not open the capsule unless you have been told to do so by the pharmacist or your health professional. If it can be opened, add it to food as described above. Praise the child after she has taken the medicine.

LIQUID MEDICINES

Many medicines are liquid. You can give the liquid in a measuring spoon, dropper, syringe, calibrated spoon, nipple, or medicine cup (Fig. 1). DO NOT use household teaspoons or tablespoons. These are not standard sizes and will not measure the correct amount of medicine. Use a measuring spoon or the special measuring device sometimes supplied with the drug.

Measuring spoon	Metric equivalent
¼ teaspoon	1.25 mls
½ teaspoon	2.5 mls
¾ teaspoon	3.75 mls
1 teaspoon	5 mls
1 tablespoon	15 mls
1 ounce	30 mls

Instructions

1. Read the label to make certain you have the right drug and to check the right amount of medicine to give the child. Shake the bottle well to mix the medicine if the label says to do this.
2. Pour out the exact amount of the drug into the measuring spoon.
   OR
   Fill the syringe or dropper with the drug to the right amount. Read the amount at the bottom of the semicircular line around the top of the liquid (Fig. 2).
3. Give the medicine to the child in a quiet place so that you will not be disturbed.

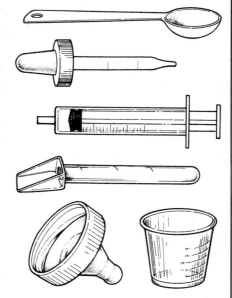

Fig. 1 Examples of items used to give liquid medications.

From Wong DL, Hess CS: *Wong and Whaley's Clinical manual of pediatric nursing*, ed 5. Copyright © 2000, Mosby, St Louis.

Unit 5

COMMUNITY AND HOME CARE INSTRUCTIONS

Giving Oral Medications—cont'd

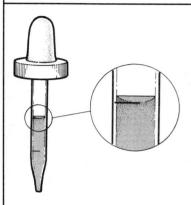

Fig. 2   Checking correct amount.

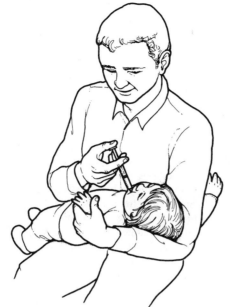

Fig. 3   Giving oral medication using a syringe. Note how the child's arms are placed.

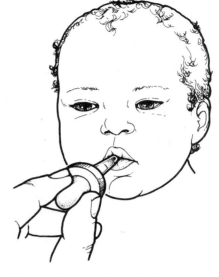

Fig. 4   Giving oral medication using a dropper.

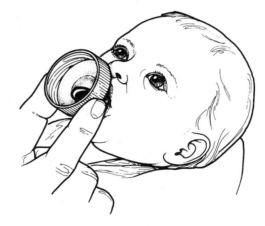

Fig. 5   Giving oral medication using a bottle nipple.

4. Tell the child what you are going to do.
5. If needed, hold the infant or young child in your lap. Place her arm closest to you behind your back. Firmly hug her other arm and hand with your arm and hand; snuggle her head between your body and your arm (Fig. 3). Sometimes you may also want to grasp her legs between yours. Your other hand remains free to give the child the drug.
6. Allow the child to sip the drug from the spoon. If it is a large amount of medicine, and the child can drink from a cup, you can measure the drug into a small cup. Make sure that the child takes all of the drug. You may have to add a small amount of water to rinse the drug from the sides of the cup.
   OR
   Gently place the dropper or syringe in the child's mouth along the inside of the cheek (Fig. 4). Allow the child to suck the liquid from the dropper or syringe. If the child does not suck, squeeze a small amount of the drug at a time. This takes longer, but the child will swallow the medicine and be less likely to spit it out or choke on it.
   OR
   Place an empty bottle nipple in the child's mouth, add the drug to the nipple, and allow the child to suck the nipple (Fig. 5).
7. Rinse the child's mouth with plain water to remove any of the sweetened drug from the gums and teeth. This can be done by wrapping a paper towel around your finger, soaking it in plain water, and then swabbing the gums, cheeks, palate, and tongue.
8. Return the drug to a safe place out of the child's reach. Place it in the refrigerator if the label says to do this.
9. Write down the time you gave the child the medicine and check for the time you need to give the next dose.
10. PRAISE THE CHILD FOR HELPING.

Unit 5

COMMUNITY AND HOME CARE INSTRUCTIONS

Giving Intramuscular (IM) Injections

Your health professional has prescribed special medicine for the child, which must be given by injection. This is a good time to teach the child about medicines as special things that we need to get better. Several things can be done to make the injection less painful:

1. Apply EMLA to the place you will give the injection 2½ hours before the medicine is due OR spray the area with the medicine ordered by your health professional right before you give the medicine.
2. Give the child something to do, such as squeezing someone's hand, humming, or counting.
3. Keep the child involved in talking, singing, or watching TV.

Equipment

Alcohol swabs
Syringe and needles
Drug stored at room temperature

Instructions

1. Gather all equipment.
2. Wash your hands with soap and water. Count to 10 while washing, then rinse with clear water and dry with a clean paper or cloth towel.
3. Open the packet containing a new syringe.
4. Clean the top of the drug bottle with alcohol.
5. Remove the cap from the syringe. Do not touch the needle.
6. Pull back the plunger and fill with the same amount of air as the drug dose (Fig. 1).
7. Put the needle into the drug bottle. Turn the bottle upside down. Push the plunger to inject the air into the drug bottle (Fig. 2).
8. With the tip of the needle in the drug, pull back the plunger to fill the syringe with the amount needed (Fig. 3).
9. Remove any air bubbles in the syringe. Hold the syringe with the needle pointing upward and firmly tap the syringe with a finger of the free hand. When all of the bubbles are at the top of the syringe, push the plunger gently to remove the bubbles.
10. Make sure the drug dosage is the right amount. Top of black rubber stopper should be on the desired amount (not bottom of stopper).
11. Remove the needle from the bottle.
12. Put the cap back on the needle loosely.
13. Use the injection spot circled in the accompanying diagram (Fig. 4).
14. Have the child lie or sit down and remove all clothing from the injection area.
15. Have someone hold the child if you think the child will not be able to lie still.
16. Using a circular motion, clean the injection spot with alcohol.
17. Let the skin dry.
18. Place your hand on the landmarks shown in Fig. 4 to locate the correct injection spot.
19. Grasp the muscle firmly between your thumb and fingers. This steadies the muscle and allows for the drug to be injected into the deepest part of the muscle.
20. Place the cap between the index and middle fingers and pull out the syringe.
21. With a quick darting motion, insert the needle into the injection spot (Fig. 5).
22. Pull back the plunger and check to see if there is any blood in the syringe.
    a. If there is blood, remove the needle, change needles, and begin again after making sure the medication dose is still right. Place the needle in an area slightly away from the first spot.
    b. If there is no blood, push the plunger slowly until the syringe is empty.

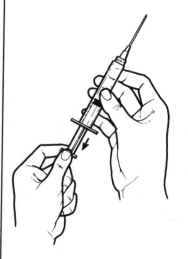

Fig. 1 Filling the syringe with air.

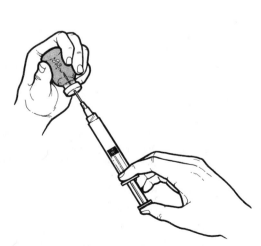

Fig. 2 Putting air into the drug bottle.

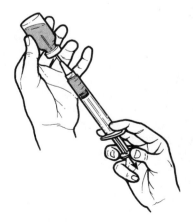

Fig. 3 Filling the syringe with the drug.

This section may be photocopied and distributed to families.

COMMUNITY AND HOME CARE INSTRUCTIONS

Giving Intramuscular (IM) Injections—cont'd

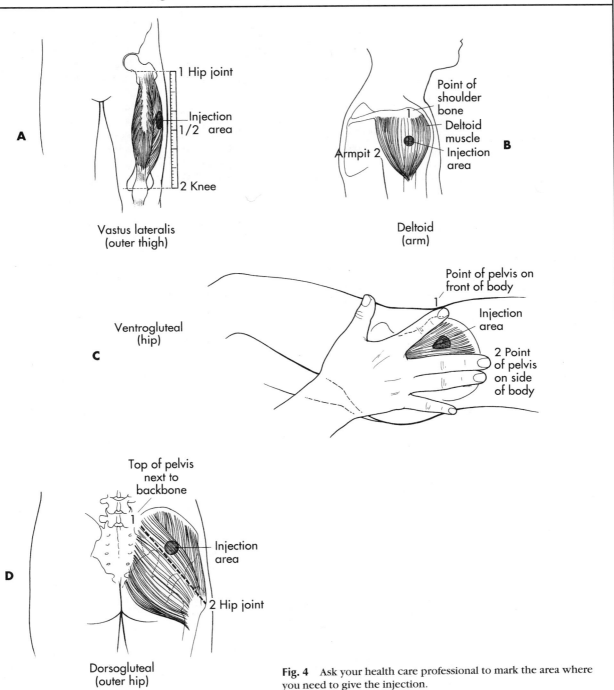

Fig. 4   Ask your health care professional to mark the area where you need to give the injection.

Continued

Unit 5

COMMUNITY AND HOME CARE INSTRUCTIONS

Giving Intramuscular (IM) Injections—cont'd

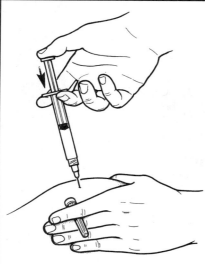

23. Remove the syringe quickly from the site, and gently rub the area with a dry sterile pad or a clean tissue.
24. Place a small bandage on the injection spot.
25. Comfort the child and make sure that he knows the drug is necessary to get better. It is important that the child does not think that the injections are punishment.
26. PRAISE THE CHILD FOR HELPING.

27. Return the drug to a safe place out of the child's reach.
28. Throw the used needle and syringe into a puncture-resistant container, such as an empty plastic milk carton. Return full carton to health professional for disposal.
29. Write down the date and time of the dose and which injection site was used. Check the time that the next dose needs to be given. Use a different area for the next injection.

Fig. 5   Injection of drug.

COMMUNITY AND HOME CARE INSTRUCTIONS

Giving Subcutaneous (Sub Q) Injections

Your health professional has prescribed special medicine for the child, which must be given by injection. This is a good time to teach the child about medicines as special things that we need to get better. Several things can be done to make the injection less painful.

1. Apply EMLA to the place you will give the injection 2½ hours before the medicine is due OR spray the area with the medicine ordered by your health professional right before you give the medicine.
2. Give the child something to do, such as squeezing someone's hand, humming, or counting.
3. Keep the child involved in talking, singing, or watching TV.

Equipment

Alcohol swabs
Syringe and needles
Medicine stored at room temperature

Instructions

1. Gather all equipment.
2. Wash your hands with soap and water. Count to 10 while washing, then rinse with clear water and dry with a clean paper or cloth towel.
3. Open the packet containing a new syringe.

4. Clean the top of the drug bottle with alcohol.
5. Remove the cap from the syringe. Do not touch the needle.
6. Pull back the plunger and fill with the same amount of air as the drug dose (Fig. 1).
7. Put the needle into the drug bottle. Turn the bottle upside down. Push the plunger to inject the air into the medication bottle (Fig. 2).
8. With the tip of the needle in the drug, pull back the plunger to fill the syringe with the amount needed (Fig. 3).
9. Remove any air bubbles in the syringe. Hold the syringe with the needle pointing up and firmly tap the syringe with a finger of the free hand. When all of the bubbles are at the top of the syringe, push the plunger gently to remove the bubbles.
10. Make sure the drug dosage is the right amount. Top of black rubber stopper should be on the desired amount (not bottom of stopper).
11. Remove the needle from the bottle.
12. Put the cap back on the needle loosely.

13. Have the child lie or sit down and remove all clothing from the injection area.
14. Have someone hold the child if you think the child will not be able to lie still.
15. Using a circular motion, clean the injection spot with alcohol.
16. Let the skin dry.
17. Grasp the skin around the injection spot firmly, raising only the skin ½ to 1 inch (Fig. 4).
18. Place the cap between the two fingers (index and middle fingers) that are grasping the skin and pull out the syringe.
19. With a quick darting motion, insert the needle bevel up (see inset) into the injection site at a 90-degree angle.*
20. Release your grasp on the child's skin.*
21. Pull back the plunger and check to see if there is any blood in the syringe.*
    a. If there is blood, remove the needle, change needles, and begin again after making sure the medication dose is still right. Place the needle in an area slightly away from the first spot.
    b. If there is no blood, push the plunger slowly until the syringe is empty.

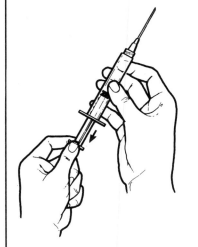

Fig. 1 Filling the syringe with air.

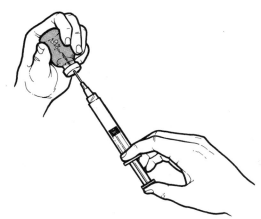

Fig. 2 Putting air into the drug bottle.

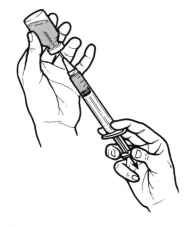

Fig. 3 Filling the syringe with the drug.

*NOTE: Your practitioner may suggest using a 45-degree angle and not pulling back on the syringe (to aspirate for blood). In either case, continue grasping the skin during the injection.

This section may be photocopied and distributed to families.

Continued

Unit 5

COMMUNITY AND HOME CARE INSTRUCTIONS

Giving Subcutaneous (Sub Q) Injections—cont'd

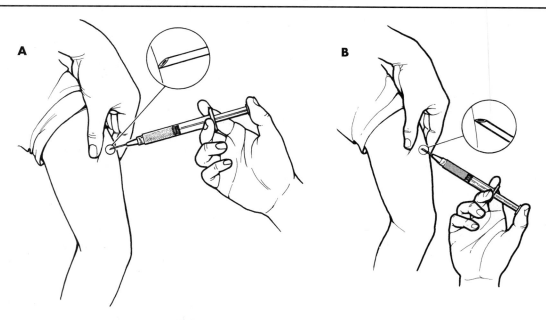

Fig. 4 Injection of drug with bevel of needle pointing up (insets). **A,** Using 90-degree angle. **B,** Using 45-degree angle.

22. Remove the syringe quickly from the site, and gently rub the area with a dry sterile pad or a clean tissue.
23. Place a small adhesive bandage on the injection spot.
24. Comfort the child and make sure that he knows the drug is necessary to get better. It is important that the child does not think that the injections are punishment.
25. PRAISE THE CHILD FOR HELPING.
26. Return the drug to a safe place out of the child's reach.
27. Throw the used needle and syringe into a puncture-resistant container, such as an empty plastic milk carton. Return full carton to health professional for disposal.
28. Write down the date and time of the dose and which injection site was used. Check the time that the next dose needs to be given. Use a different area for the next injection.

Unit 5

COMMUNITY AND HOME CARE INSTRUCTIONS

Caring for an Intermittent Infusion Device

A small tube (catheter) was placed in the child for the administration of intravenous (IV) drugs at home. This tube is known as an intermittent infusion device. Look at the spot where the tube enters the skin several times each day. Notify your health professional at _____ if you observe any of the following signs around the device:

- Redness
- Swelling/puffiness
- Leaking/drainage
- Red streak along the skin near the device
- Pain around the entry spot

A clear adhesive or tape dressing is usually placed over the device to protect it. The child may wash around the fingers, but should not get the dressing or any exposed part of the tube wet. During a bath or shower, cover the tube and dressing with plastic wrap, such as Saran Wrap, or a plastic bag to keep the area dry. The device may need to be changed by your health professional, especially if any problems develop.

These instructions describe the use of needleless devices on the syringe and medicine bottle (also called a vial). The type of the needleless devices you use may differ from the type described here, but the same basic methods are used for all of them. Be sure to ask your health professional to show you how your device works. Information for using a needle on the syringe is also given, but be very careful to avoid sticking yourself or someone else with the needle.

FLUSHING

The inside of the catheter must be rinsed (flushed) with a solution, usually heparin (a special drug called an anticoagulant), or saline (a special saltwater solution) to prevent any blood clots from forming, which can clog the tube. The small amount of solution that you are using will rinse the entire length of the tube. The tube must be flushed _____ time(s) each day and after any drug or fluid is given through the tube.

Equipment

Needleless cannula and syringe or needle and syringe
Alcohol swabs
Bottle of solution at room temperature
Needleless adapter for the bottle

Instructions

1. Gather equipment that you will need on a clean dry surface.
2. Wash your hands with soap and water. Count to 10 while washing, then rinse with clear water and dry with a clean paper or cloth towel.
3. Open the package of alcohol swabs.
4. Wipe the top of the bottle with one of the swabs for about 10

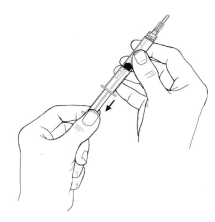

Fig. 1 Filling the syringe with air by pulling back on plunger.

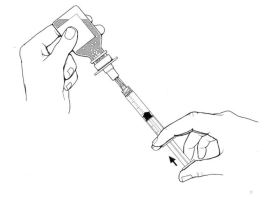

Fig. 2 Putting air into the drug bottle by pushing forward on the plunger.

seconds. Let the bottle top dry. Do not touch the bottle top after you have cleaned it.

5. Open the package of the bottle adapter and push the pointed end straight into the rubber top of the bottle. It may take some force to do this, but do not try to twist the adapter into the bottle top.
6. Open the package containing a new syringe and remove the cap from the bottom of the syringe. Do not touch the exposed part.
7. Open the package of the needle cannula by pulling apart the wrapping at the top of the package. Connect the bottom of the syringe to the opening of the cannula by twisting the two pieces together.
8. Remove the cover of the cannula. Do not touch any part of it. If you do touch it, use another new one.
9. If you are using a syringe with a needle, you do not need the bottle adapter. Just follow steps 6 through 8, substituting the needle for the cannula. Sometimes the syringe and needle are already attached.
10. Pull back the plunger and fill with the same amount of air as the dose (Fig. 1).
11. Put the cannula into the adapter or the needle into the rubber stopper of the bottle. Turn the bottle upside down. Push the plunger to inject the air into the bottle (Fig. 2).

Continued

From Wong DL, Hess CS: *Wong and Whaley's Clinical manual of pediatric nursing*, ed 5. Copyright © 2000, Mosby, St Louis.

Unit 5

COMMUNITY AND HOME CARE INSTRUCTIONS

Caring for an Intermittent Infusion Device—cont'd

12. With the tip of the cannula or needle in the solution, pull back the plunger to fill the syringe with the amount needed (Fig. 3).
13. Remove any air bubbles in the syringe. Hold the syringe with the cannula or needle pointing up and firmly tap the syringe with a finger of the free hand. When all of the bubbles are at the top of the syringe, push the plunger gently to remove the bubbles.
14. Make sure you are using the right amount of solution.
15. Remove the syringe from the bottle and place the cover back on the cannula or needle.

16. With the second alcohol swab, wipe the cap on the catheter or on the end of extra tubing that has been attached to the catheter for about 10 seconds. Let the cap dry. Do not touch it after you have cleaned it.
17. Insert the cannula or needle in the cap. If you are using the cap on the device, hold the plastic just below the rubber cap to make it easier to insert the cannula or needle (Fig. 4).
18. Slowly push the plunger of the syringe to put the solution into the tubing.

19. STOP pushing if there is pressure or pain. Call your health professional and go to step 21.
20. If there is extra tubing, hold the clamp on the tubing with your free hand. Slide the clamp to close the tubing as you push the last 0.2 cc of solution (Fig. 5).
21. Remove the syringe from the cap.
22. PRAISE THE CHILD FOR HELPING.
23. Return the solution to a safe place out of the child's reach.
24. Write down the date and time of the dose and check the time that the next dose needs to be given.
25. Follow your health professional's instructions for throwing away the used equipment. If you used needles, put them into a rigid container, like a used bleach bottle, to prevent other people, like garbage collectors, from being stuck. Make sure you do not mix the container with other materials to be recycled. You may want to label the container, "NOT FOR RECYCLING."

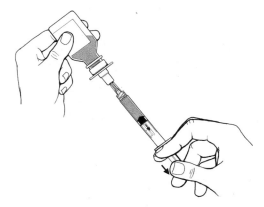

Fig. 3   Filling the syringe with solution by pulling back on the plunger.

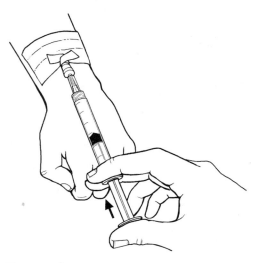

Fig. 4   Injecting solution into the intermittent infusion device by pushing slowly forward on the plunger.

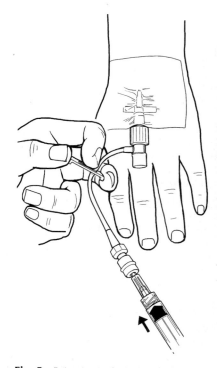

Fig. 5   Injecting solution into the tubing attached to the infusion device by pushing slowly forward on the plunger and closing the clamp as the last 0.2 cc is given.

Caring for a Central Venous Catheter

A catheter (tube) was placed in your child so that an intravenous line will be available for long-term treatment. This tube can be used to give medications, fluids, nutrients, and possibly for obtaining blood specimens. Several different types of catheters can be used, such as the Broviac or the Groshong. Both types of catheters are inserted under the skin and into a major blood vessel near the heart (Fig. 1).

SPECIAL CONSIDERATIONS

A young child, either the child with the tube or a playmate, may want to handle the tube and, as a result, may accidentally pull it out. To prevent the child from playing with the tube, keep a T-shirt on the child, use one-piece outfits such as overalls, or select outfits that open in the back. Never leave the child alone when she is undressed. Keep all sharp objects, especially scissors, out of the reach of young children in the home.

When the child is bathed, keep the skin dry where the tube enters the body. Plastic wrap can be taped over a gauze dressing, or a transparent dressing can be used to protect the site.

All people who care for the child should be taught about the catheter. At school tell both the child's teacher and the school nurse so that an adult can help the child if needed.

Your health professional should be notified if the tube becomes damaged.

The tube should be repaired as soon as possible because of the risk of infection. If the child has a Broviac catheter, clamp the tube at once. The Groshong catheter does not need to be clamped.

FLUSHING THE TUBE

The care of each catheter is slightly different. These written instructions will help you to care for the tube at home. Catheter care should always be done in a quiet place where you will not be disturbed. If the child is active, you will need a helper. The helper can keep the child still while you do the catheter care.

The inside of the Broviac must be flushed (rinsed) with a heparin (a special drug called an anticoagulant) solution. This will help prevent any blood clots from forming. If blood clots form, the tube may become plugged. The small amount of heparin that you are using will rinse the entire length of the tube. If the child has a Groshong catheter, no heparin flushes are needed, only weekly saline (special saltwater) rinses. The Broviac must be flushed _____ time(s) each day, and either tube is rinsed after giving any drug or fluid through the tube.

These instructions describe the use of needleless devices on the syringe and medicine bottle (also called a vial). The type of needleless device you use may differ from the type described here, but the same basic methods are used for all of them. Be sure to ask your health

professional to show you how your device works. Information for using a needle on the syringe is also given, but be very careful to avoid sticking yourself or someone else with the needle.

Equipment

Needleless cannula and syringe or
Needle and syringe (10 ml size)
2 antiseptic swabs/wipes
Bottle of heparin at room temperature (Broviac) or
Bottle of sterile saline at room temperature (Groshong)
Needleless adapter for the bottle

Instructions

1. Gather equipment that you will need and place on a clean, dry surface.
2. Wash your hands with soap and water. Count to 10 while washing, then rinse with clear water and dry with a clean paper or cloth towel.
3. Open the package of antiseptic swabs.
4. With one of the swabs, scrub the top of the solution bottle for about 10 seconds. Let the bottle top dry. Do not touch the bottle top after you have cleaned it.
5. Open the package of the bottle adapter and push the pointed end straight into the rubber top of the bottle. It may take some force to do this, but do not try to twist the adapter into the bottle top.
6. Open the package containing a new syringe and remove the cap from the bottom of the syringe. Do not touch the exposed part.
7. Open the package of the needle cannula by pulling apart the wrapping at the top of the package. Connect the bottom of the syringe to the opening of the cannula by twisting the two pieces together.
8. Remove the cover of the cannula. Do not touch any part of it. If you do touch it, use another new one.
9. If you are using a syringe with a needle, you do not need the bottle adapter. Just follow steps 6 through 8, substituting the needle for the cannula. Sometimes the syringe and needle are already attached.

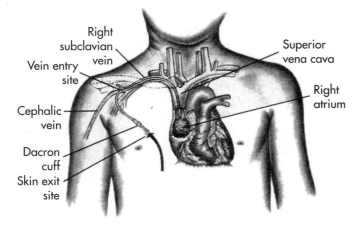

Fig. 1 Placement of central catheter.

Right subclavian vein
Vein entry site
Cephalic vein
Dacron cuff
Skin exit site
Superior vena cava
Right atrium

Continued

From Wong DL, Hess CS: *Wong and Whaley's Clinical manual of pediatric nursing,* ed 5. Copyright © 2000, Mosby, St Louis.

Unit 5

COMMUNITY AND HOME CARE INSTRUCTIONS

Caring for a Central Venous Catheter—cont'd

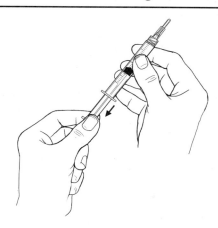

Fig. 2 Filling the syringe with air by pulling back on plunger.

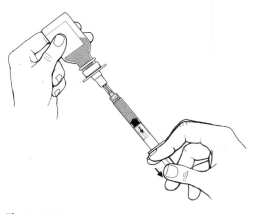

Fig. 4 Filling the syringe with solution by pulling back on the plunger.

10. Pull back the plunger and fill the syringe with the same amount of air as needed (Fig. 2).
11. Insert the cannula into the adapter or the needle into the rubber stopper of the bottle. Turn the bottle upside down. Push the plunger to inject the air into the bottle (Fig. 3).
12. With the tip of the cannula or needle in the solution, pull back the plunger to fill the syringe with the amount needed (Fig. 4).
13. Remove any air bubbles in the syringe. Hold the syringe with the cannula or needle pointing up and firmly tap the syringe with a finger of the free hand. When all the bubbles are at the top of

the syringe, push the plunger gently to remove the bubbles.
14. Make sure the heparin or saline is the right amount.
15. Remove the syringe from the bottle.
16. Place the cannula or cover over the needle and set aside.
17. With the second alcohol swab, wipe the cap on the catheter for about 10 seconds. Let the cap dry. Do not touch it after you have cleaned it.
18. Insert the cannula or needle in the cap.
19. Slowly push the plunger of the syringe to put the solution into the tubing (Fig. 5).
20. STOP pushing if there is pressure or pain. Call your health professional and go to step 22.

21. Hold the clamp on the tubing with your free hand. Slide the clamp to close the tubing as you push the last 0.2 cc of solution.
22. Remove the syringe from the cap.
23. PRAISE THE CHILD FOR HELPING.
24. Return the solution to a safe place out of the child's reach.
25. Write down the date and time of the dose and check the time that the next dose needs to be given.

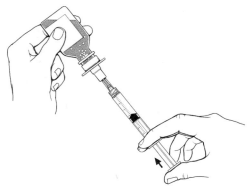

Fig. 3 Putting air into the drug bottle by pushing forward on the plunger.

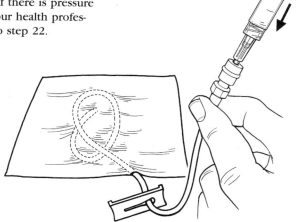

Fig. 5 Injecting solution into central venous catheter by pushing slowly forward on the plunger.

Unit 5

COMMUNITY AND HOME CARE INSTRUCTIONS

Caring for a Central Venous Catheter—cont'd

26. Follow your health professional's instructions for throwing away the used equipment. If you used needles, put them into a rigid container, like a used bleach bottle, to prevent other people, like garbage collectors, from being stuck. Make sure you do not mix the container with other materials to be recycled. you may want to label the container, "NOT FOR RECYCLING."

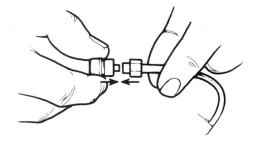

Fig. 7   Attaching new injection cap.

CHANGING THE INJECTION CAP

This should be done _____ time(s) per week. If the cap is changed at the time of rinsing, the heparin or saline is given through the new injection cap.

Equipment

Antiseptic swab
Injection cap

Procedure

1. Gather the equipment you will need.
2. Wash your hands with soap and water. Count to 10 while washing, then rinse with clear water and dry with a clean paper or cloth towel.
3. Clamp the tube midway between the skin and the end of the tube or on the reinforced clamping sleeve that is on some catheters; do not clamp a Groshong catheter.
4. With the swab, clean around the tip of the tube below the injection cap.
5. Open the new injection cap package.
6. Remove the used injection cap from the tube and attach the new injection cap (Figs. 6 and 7).
7. Remove the clamp from the catheter (not needed with Groshong).

DRESSING CHANGE

After the catheter has been in your child for a short time, a dressing may or may not be placed over the area where it enters the skin. Your health professional will tell you if a dressing is needed and how often to change it. Usually, a clear, transparent dressing is used. This lets you see the child's skin around the tube. Look at the skin around the tube each day. Call your health professional at once if you see any redness, drainage, or swelling; if the area around the tube is painful; or if the child has a temperature above 100.4° F.

Equipment

Adhesive remover pad
Transparent dressing
Antiseptic swabs
Bag for disposing of used supplies and dressing
Tape

Instructions

1. Gather the equipment on a clean, dry surface.
2. Wash your hands with soap and water. Count to 10 while washing, then rinse with clear water and dry with a clean paper or cloth towel.
3. Gently peel off the edges of the old dressing using adhesive remover, if necessary. Peel off one edge at a time.
   Another way to remove the dressing is to grasp opposite corners of the plastic film and pull them away from each other to stretch and loosen the film. After the film begins to loosen, grasp the other two corners of the film and pull. This method is easier and more comfortable than pulling the dressing up and off the skin.
4. Carefully look at the skin around the tube.
5. Using each antiseptic swab only once, clean the skin where the tube enters the body. Use a circular motion starting at the tube and moving out about 3 inches from the tube (Fig. 8).

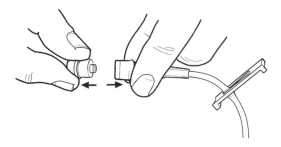

Fig. 6   Removing used cap.

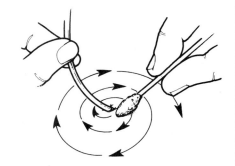

Fig. 8   Cleaning the skin in a circular motion, beginning at the catheter and moving outward.

Unit 5

Continued

COMMUNITY AND HOME CARE INSTRUCTIONS

Caring for a Central Venous Catheter—cont'd

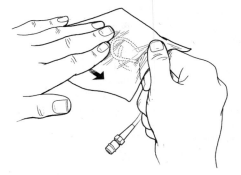

6. Loop the tube around the entry site, leaving the injection cap below the dressing.

7. Carefully place the dressing on the child's skin. Hold the dressing in both hands. When the top of the dressing is on the skin, slowly bring the dressing toward the bottom of the window frame, making sure that it attaches to the skin (Fig. 9).

8. Secure the end of the tube with tape to keep it from dangling.

9. Place all used items in a paper bag. Close the bag and throw it away.

10. PRAISE THE CHILD FOR HELPING.

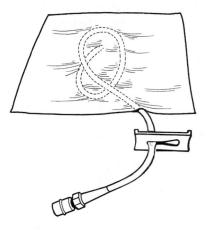

Fig. 9 Applying transparent dressing, beginning at the top and carefully bringing the dressing to the bottom.

COMMUNITY AND HOME CARE INSTRUCTIONS

Giving Rectal Medications—Suppositories

Medicines can be given rectally if the child cannot eat or drink. If you have been told to give only half of a suppository, cut the suppository in half *lengthwise.*

Equipment

Suppository
Warm water

Instructions

1. Gather equipment.
2. Wash your hands with soap and water. Count to 10 while washing, then rinse with clear water and dry with a clean paper or cloth towel.

3. Remove the wrapper from the suppository.
4. The index finger or the pinky (fifth finger) should be used to put in the suppository. Use the pinky if the child is small. Make sure the fingernail is short and smooth. As a covering, you can use plastic wrap or a plastic sandwich bag on the finger. Disposable gloves and finger cots can also be bought and used.
5. Remove the child's underpants or diaper.
6. With water, wet the finger or covering you will use to insert the suppository.

7. Wet the suppository with warm (not hot) water. Do not use Vaseline or any other kind of grease or lubricant. These may affect how the medicine works.
8. Insert the suppository, with the flat (not pointed) end first, 1 inch into the child's rectum (Fig. 1). If the child finds this uncomfortable, put pointed end first in rectum.
9. If the child is too young to help, hold the buttocks together for at least 5 minutes. This prevents the suppository from being pushed out.
10. Wash your hands as above.
11. PRAISE THE CHILD FOR HELPING.

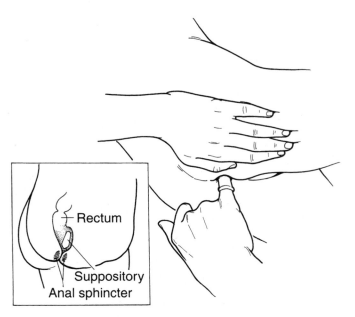

Rectum

Suppository
Anal sphincter

Fig. 1 Using smallest finger to insert rectal suppository with blunt end first.

This section may be photocopied and distributed to families.
From Wong DL, Hess CS: *Wong and Whaley's Clinical manual of pediatric nursing,* ed 5. Copyright © 2000, Mosby, St Louis.

Unit 5

COMMUNITY AND HOME CARE INSTRUCTIONS

Giving Eye Medications

Your health professional has prescribed a special drug for the child's eye(s). For this drug to have the most benefit, it is important that you closely follow these procedures.

Equipment

Dropper
Medicine at room temperature
Clean tissue, clean washcloth, warm water

Instructions for Eye Drops

1. Gather equipment.
2. Wash your hands with soap and water. Count to 10 while washing, then rinse with clear water and dry with a clean paper or cloth towel.
3. Remove any discharge from the eye with a clean tissue.
4. If the eye has crusted material around it, wet a washcloth with warm water and place this over the eye. Wait about 1 minute. Gently wipe the eye from the nose side outward with the washcloth, place it on the eye, and wait again. If you cannot remove the crusting, rewet the washcloth. Then try to gently remove the crusted drainage. Continue using the warm, moist washcloth and gently wiping until all of the crusting is removed. If both eyes need cleaning, use separate cloths for each eye. Launder the washcloth(s) before using again.
5. Have the child lie on his back on a flat surface. If the child will not lie still, you can hold the child by sitting on a flat surface such as the floor or bed. Place the child on his back with his head between your legs and his arms under your legs. If needed, you can cross your lower legs over the child's legs to keep him from moving. Place a pillow under the child's shoulders, or a rolled up towel under his neck so that his head is tilted back and to the same side as the eye to be treated (right eye, turn head to right; left eye, turn head to left). The eye drops should flow *away* from the child's nose.

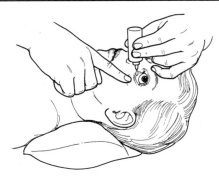

Fig. 1   Dropper and hand position for giving eye drops.

6. Open the bottle of eye drops. Do not let the dropper portion touch anything.
7. Tell the child to look up and to the other side (away from the eye into which you are putting the drops). Choose something specific for the child to look at. If the child is young, you can make a game of giving the eye drops. Tell the child to open his eyes on the count of 3. Then count to 3. When you say 3, drop the eye drops into the child's eye. Even if the child will not open the eyes on 3, keep him lying down until he decides to open the eyes. The medicine will flow in the eye.
8. Note that the wrist of the hand you will be using to give the drops is placed on the child's forehead. This will help steady your hand.
9. Gently pull down the child's lower eyelid with the other hand by placing gentle downward pressure below the eyelashes (Fig. 1).
10. Position the bottle so that the drug will fall into the lower eyelid, *not* directly onto the eyeball.
11. Squeeze the bottle for the required number of drops.
12. Tell the child to close the eye, then to blink. This helps spread the drug around the eye.
13. Remove any extra drug with a clean tissue, wiping from the nose outward. Putting gentle pressure on the inner corner of the

eye for 1 minute prevents any medicine from dripping into the back of the throat and causing an unpleasant taste.

14. If both eyes are to be given the drug, repeat with the other eye.
15. Hold and comfort the child.
16. PRAISE THE CHILD FOR HELPING.
17. Write down the time you gave the child the drug and check for the time you need to give the next dose.

Instructions for Ointments

When both drops and ointment are needed, give the drops before the ointment. If the ointment is used only once each day, apply the ointment at bedtime since it will blur the child's vision.

1. Follow steps 1 through 9 for eye drops.
2. Position the tube at the inner part of the eye near the nose (Fig. 2).
3. Squeeze a ribbon of the ointment onto the inside of lower eyelid. Begin at the side of the eye near the nose and go toward the outer edge of the eye.
4. Give the tube a half-turn. This helps "cut" the ribbon of medicine.
5. Finish with steps 12 through 17 for eye drops.

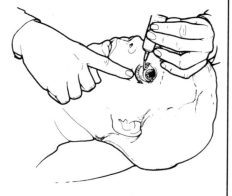

Fig. 2   Tube and hand position for applying eye ointment.

COMMUNITY AND HOME CARE INSTRUCTIONS

Giving Ear Medications

Your health professional has prescribed a special drug for the child's ear(s). For this drug to have the most benefit, it is important that you follow these instructions.

Equipment

Medicine
Container of warm water
Clean tissue or cotton-tipped applicator and cotton ball if desired

Instructions

1. Gather equipment.
2. Wash your hands with soap and water. Count to 10 while washing, then rinse with clear water and dry with a clean paper or cloth towel.
3. Place the drug bottle in warm water. Cold drops in the ear are uncomfortable.
4. Feel a drop to make sure the drug is warm, not too cold or too hot.
5. Have the child lie on the side opposite the ear into which you will be putting the drug (right ear, on left side; left ear, on right side). If the child will not lie still, you can hold the child by sitting on a flat surface, such as the floor or bed. Place the child on her back with her head between your legs and her arms under your legs. If needed, you can cross your lower legs over the child's legs to keep her from moving.
6. Check the ear to see if any drainage is present. If there is drainage, remove it with a clean tissue or cotton-tipped applicator. DO NOT clean any more than the outer ear.
7. Open the bottle of eardrops. Do not let the dropper portion touch anything.

8. The wrist of the hand you will be using is placed on the cheek or head. This will help steady your hand.
9. You will need to straighten the child's ear canal. For children who are 3 years old and under, pull the outer ear *down* and toward the *back* of the head (Fig. 1). For older children, pull the outer ear *up* and toward the *back* (Fig. 2).
10. Position the bottle so that the drops will fall against the side of the ear canal.
11. Squeeze the bottle for the right number of drops.
12. Keep the child lying on that side with the medicated ear up for 1 minute. Gently rub the skin in front of the ear (Fig. 3). This helps the drug flow to the inside of the ear.
13. If any drug has spilled on the skin, wipe the outer ear. A cotton ball can be loosely placed in the ear, but it must be changed each time drops are given.

14. If both ears need the drug, repeat with the other ear after the 1-minute wait.
15. Hold and comfort the child.
16. PRAISE THE CHILD FOR HELPING.
17. Write down the time you gave the child the drug and check for the time you need to give the next dose.

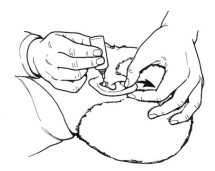

Fig. 2   Hand and dropper position for older children, with earlobe pulled up and back.

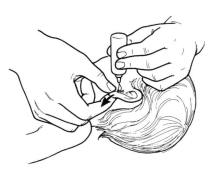

Fig. 1   Hand and dropper position for children 3 years old and younger, with earlobe pulled down and back.

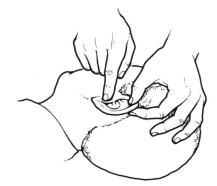

Fig. 3   Rubbing ear to help drug flow to inside of ear.

This section may be photocopied and distributed to families.

Unit 5

COMMUNITY AND HOME CARE°INSTRUCTIONS

Giving Nose Drops

Your health professional has prescribed a special drug. This drug is placed in the child's nose. If the child is having trouble breathing and eating because of a "stuffy nose," these nose drops may help the child. For this drug to have the most benefit, you should follow these instructions.

Equipment

Drug at room temperature
Clean tissues, clean washcloth, warm
  water

Instructions

1. Gather equipment.
2. Wash your hands with soap and water. Count to 10 while washing, then rinse with clear water and dry with a clean paper or cloth towel.
3. Remove any mucus from the nose with a clean tissue.

4. If the nose has crusted material around it, wet a washcloth with warm water and place this around the nose. Wait about 1 minute. Gently wipe the nose with the washcloth. If you cannot remove the crusting, rewet the washcloth and again place it around the nose. Continue using the warm, moist washcloth and gently wiping until all of the crusting is removed. Launder the washcloth before using it again.
5. Place the child on his back.
6. If the child will not lie still, have a helper hold the child. If you are alone, you can hold the child by sitting on a flat surface such as the floor or a bed. Place the child on his back with his head between your legs and his arms under your legs. If needed, you can cross your lower legs over the child's

legs to keep him from moving (Fig. 1).
7. Tilt the child's head backward by placing a pillow or rolled-up towel under the child's shoulders or letting the head hang over the side of a bed or your lap (Fig. 2).
8. Open the bottle of nose drops.
9. Place the right number of drops in each side of the nose.
10. Keep the child's head tilted back for at least 1 minute (slowly count to 60) to prevent gagging or tasting the drug.
11. Hold and comfort the child.
12. PRAISE THE CHILD FOR HELPING.
13. Return the drug to a safe place out of the child's reach.
14. Write down the time you gave the child the drug and check for the time you need to give the next dose.

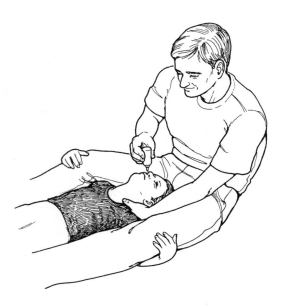

Fig. 1 Safely holding child while giving nose drops.

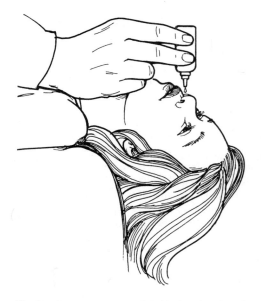

Fig. 2 Correct position of child's head and neck for giving nose drops.

This section may be photocopied and distributed to families.

From Wong DL, Hess CS: *Wong and Whaley's Clinical manual of pediatric nursing*, ed 5. Copyright © 2000, Mosby, St Louis.

Unit 5

COMMUNITY AND HOME CARE INSTRUCTIONS

Applying EMLA

Your health professional has prescribed a topical anesthetic medicine called EMLA, which stands for "Eutectic Mixture of Local Anesthetics." A topical anesthetic means a medicine that is placed on normal, healthy skin to make it numb. EMLA contains two anesthetics, lidocaine and prilocaine. Be sure to tell your health professional if your child has an allergy to either of these medicines before using EMLA. Use only the amount of EMLA that has been prescribed.

EMLA comes in two forms, a cream and an Anesthetic Disc. Both numb the skin so that the pain of a needle is greatly decreased or avoided. The choice for using either the cream or the disc depends on where it is used. The Disc is best for flat surfaces and for numbing areas that are no larger than about 1 inch. It is easier to apply than the cream because it contains the anesthetic in a peel and stick adhesive dressing. The cream must be covered with the dressing that comes with the 5-gram tube. There is also a 30-gram tube that is useful if you need to apply the cream several times. The dressing, called Tegaderm, is a clear plastic film with adhesive (sticky) edges. If you do not have this dressing, you can cover the cream with ordinary plastic film, like Saran Wrap, and seal the edges of the plastic to the skin with tape. You cannot use ordinary Band-Aids because the cream will leak out.

Equipment

EMLA Anesthetic Disc or
EMLA cream with Tegaderm dressing
Plastic film and tape (if needed)
Ball point pen or marker
Tissue or paper towel

General Instructions

1. Make sure that the area in which you apply the EMLA is clean and dry and that the skin has no open areas or sores. Do not apply the medicine near the eye, in the ear, or in the mouth.
2. If you are not sure of where to apply EMLA, ask your health professional to mark the place on the drawing in Fig. 1.

3. For a blood sample or when an IV is needed, apply to two or more areas in case your child may need more than one try to get into the vein.
4. If your child is young and afraid of needles, you can tell your child that EMLA is like a "magic cream that takes hurt away." Tap or lightly scratch area of skin to show your child that "skin is now awake." After removing the EMLA, again tap or lightly scratch the skin to show your child that "the skin is now asleep" so that it cannot feel a needle.
5. To prevent children from playing with the cream under the clear dressing, cover it with a tissue or paper towel and a little tape.
6. Leave EMLA on the skin for at least 60 minutes for a puncture, such as a vein or finger stick; and at least 2 to 2½ hours for an intramuscular (IM) injection or biopsy. EMLA may need to be kept on longer if your child has dark or thicker skin.
7. After removing the Disc or cream, see if the skin is pale or reddened. If there is no visible skin change, leave EMLA on longer, but not longer than 4 hours.
8. PRAISE THE CHILD FOR HELPING.
9. Return the drug to a safe place out of the child's reach.

Instructions for EMLA Anesthetic Disc

1. Make sure that the area to be anesthetized is clean and dry. Take hold of the aluminum flap at the corner of the Anesthetic Disc and bend it backwards (Fig. 2). Next, take hold of the corner of the beige-colored Anesthetic Disc layer.
2. Pull the two layers apart, separating the adhesive surface from the protective liner. Make sure that you do not touch the white, round disc, which contains EMLA (Fig. 3).
3. Press firmly around the edges of the Anesthetic Disc to be sure it sticks to the skin (Fig. 4). Tap lightly on the Disc to make sure that it touches the skin.
4. Mark on the edge of the Anesthetic Disc the time that you applied EMLA (Fig. 5).

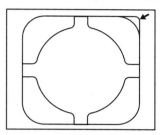

Fig. 2 Applying the Anesthetic Disc: Take hold of the aluminum flap at the corner of the Disc and bend it backwards. Next, take hold of the corner of the beige-colored Disc layer.

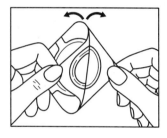

Fig. 3 Pull the two layers apart. Do not touch the white, round Disc, which contains EMLA.

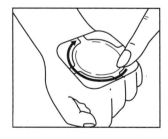

Fig. 4 Press firmly around the *edges* of the Anesthetic Disc to ensure good adhesion to the skin. Lightly tap on the Disc to make sure it touches the skin.

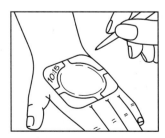

Fig. 5 Mark the time of application along the edge of the Anesthetic Disc.

Unit 5

Continued

From Wong DL, Hess CS: *Wong and Whaley's Clinical manual of pediatric nursing*, ed 5. Copyright © 2000, Mosby, St Louis.

COMMUNITY AND HOME CARE INSTRUCTIONS

Applying EMLA—cont'd

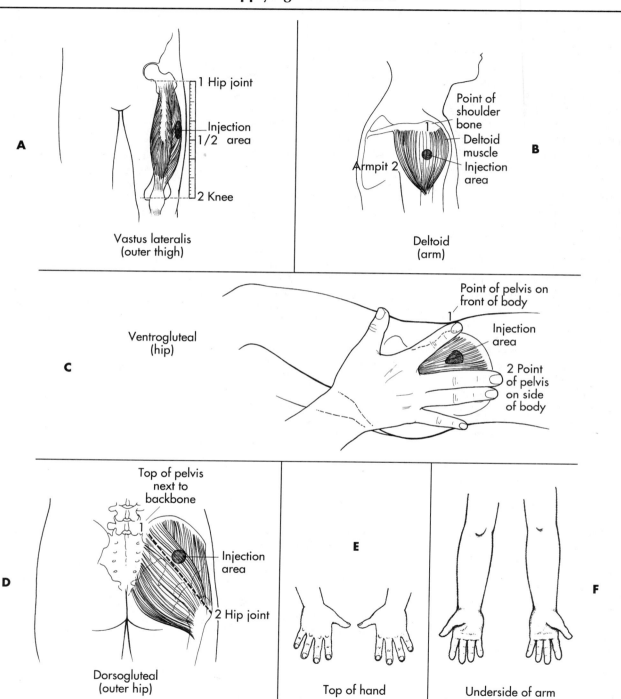

A

1 Hip joint

Injection
1/2 area

2 Knee

Vastus lateralis
(outer thigh)

B

Point of
shoulder
bone

Deltoid
muscle

Injection
area

Armpit 2

Deltoid
(arm)

Ventrogluteal
(hip)

C

Point of pelvis on
front of body

1

Injection
area

2 Point
of pelvis
on side
of body

D

Top of pelvis
next to
backbone

1

Injection
area

2 Hip joint

Dorsogluteal
(outer hip)

E

Top of hand

F

Underside of arm

Fig. 1   Ask your health care professional to mark the area where you need to apply EMLA. The numbers
on Figs. **A-D** mark the places used to find the injection areas. (Figs. **E** and **F** reproduced with permission
of Astra Pharmaceuticals, L.P., 725 Chesterbrook Blvd., Wayne, PA 19087.)

Unit 5

COMMUNITY AND HOME CARE INSTRUCTIONS

Applying EMLA—cont'd

5. Remove the Disc by gently pulling one corner of the dressing up and away from the skin. Wipe off the cream with a tissue. The numbing effect can last 1 hour or more after removing the dressing.

Instructions for EMLA Cream

1. Unscrew the cap and puncture the metal covering of the tube with the point on the top of the cap.
2. Apply half of the 5-gram tube in a thick layer to about a 2 inch by 2 inch area of skin where the procedure will be done (Fig. 6). If the puncture area is very small, such as a finger stick, you can use a third of the tube.
3. Remove the center cut-out piece of the Tegaderm (Fig. 7).
4. Peel the paper liner from the paper framed dressing (Fig. 8).
5. Cover the EMLA cream so that you get a thick layer underneath. Do not spread out the cream. Smooth down the dressing edges carefully and be sure it is secure to avoid leakage (Fig. 9).
6. Remove the paper frame (Fig. 10). Mark directly on the occlusive dressing the time you applied the cream.
7. To remove the Tegaderm dressing, grasp opposite sides of the film and pull the sides away from each other to stretch and loosen the film. After the film begins to loosen, grasp the other two sides of the film and pull. This method is easier and more comfortable than pulling the dressing up and off the skin.
8. Wipe off the EMLA cream with a tissue. The numbing effect can last 1 hour or more after removing the dressing.

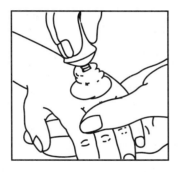

Fig. 6 Applying EMLA Cream: Apply 2.5 g of cream (half the 5-g tube) in a thick layer at the site.

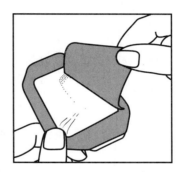

Fig. 7 Take an occlusive dressing (provided with the 5-g tubes only) and remove the center cut-out piece.

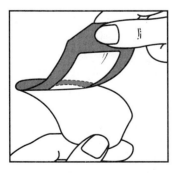

Fig. 8 Peel the paper liner from the paper framed dressing.

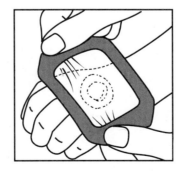

Fig. 9 Cover the EMLA Cream so that you get a thick layer underneath. Smooth the dressing edges carefully to avoid leakage.

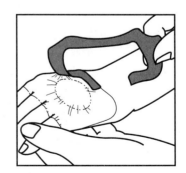

Fig. 10 Remove the paper frame. Mark the time of application directly on the occlusive dressing. (Figs. 2-10 reproduced with permission of Astra Pharmaceuticals, L.P., 725 Chesterbrook Blvd., Wayne, PA 19087.)

Unit 5

INSTRUCTIONS RELATED TO ALTERNATIVE FEEDING TECHNIQUES AND ELIMINATION

COMMUNITY AND HOME CARE INSTRUCTIONS

Giving Nasogastric Tube Feedings

For the child to obtain enough food to grow, you must feed her by tube. If the child is active, you will need someone to hold the child while you insert the tube. After the tube is securely in place, you should hold and cuddle the child during the feeding.

You should give the child _____ ounces of _____ every _____ hours.

Call your health professional at _____ if any of the following occur:

- Vomiting
- Change in color of stomach contents
- Increased amount of stomach contents before feeding
- Increased bowel movements
- You are unable to put in the tube
- The child becomes very irritable
- Two meals are missed due to too much food in the stomach

Equipment

Liquid food at room temperature and water in pour container
Feeding tube
½-inch tape
Water
Syringe
Stethoscope

Instructions

1. Gather equipment.
2. Wash your hands with soap and water. Count to 10 while washing, then rinse with clear water and dry with a clean paper or cloth towel.
3. Cut a piece of tape. You will need this to mark the right distance and to hold the tube in place during the feeding.
4. Tell the child (even if infant) what you will be doing.
5. Place the child on your lap, on her right side, or reclining in an infant seat.
6. Use a pacifier for the infant to enjoy sucking during the feeding.
7. Measure the tube for the exact distance you will have to insert it.
   a. Hold the tip of the tube on the child's stomach (midway between the belly button and the highest point of the lower rib cage).
   b. Extend the tube up to the child's earlobe, then out to the nose (Fig. 1).
   c. Mark the spot at the nose with the piece of tape.
8. Dip the tip of the tube in clear water to moisten.

9. Insert the tip of the tube into one nostril, guiding it toward the back of the child's throat.
10. If the child is able to help, have her swallow the tube to help it pass.
11. Quickly insert the tube to the tape mark on the tube. If the child begins coughing or has any other problems, remove the tube at once.
12. Tape the tube to the child's upper lip and cheek (Fig. 2). If the child wants to pull the tube, tape it down the back to keep it out of reach. Be sure the tube is not compressed or kinked.
13. Check the placement of the tube:
    a. Place 5 cc of air in the syringe. Connect the syringe to the tube.
    b. Place the stethoscope over the child's stomach area.
    c. Inject the air quickly into the tube while listening for the sound of gurgling through the stethoscope.
    d. Remove the air by gently pulling back on the plunger to the 5 cc mark.
    e. If stomach contents appear in the tube as you pull back on the plunger, the tube is in the correct place.

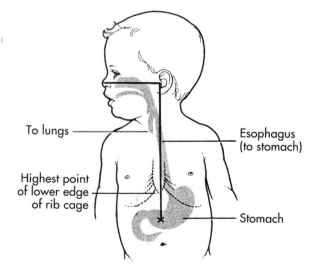

Fig. 1 Measuring length of tube to insert: from midway between belly button and highest point of lower rib cage; to earlobe; to nose.

To lungs

Esophagus (to stomach)

Highest point of lower edge of rib cage

Stomach

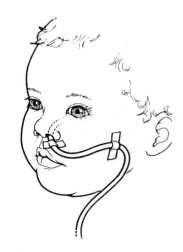

Fig. 2 Taping tube to keep from injuring child's nose.

From Wong DL, Hess CS: *Wong and Whaley's Clinical manual of pediatric nursing*, ed 5. Copyright © 2000, Mosby, St Louis.

Unit 5

COMMUNITY AND HOME CARE INSTRUCTIONS

Giving Nasogastric Tube Feedings—cont'd

f. If you are unable to see any stomach contents in the tube, place the child on the left side or advance the tube a short distance. Pull back on plunger again to check for stomach contents.

g. If more than one fourth of the last feeding is still present, return the food to the stomach and wait 30 to 60 minutes. When there is less than one fourth of the amount of food, return the stomach contents and feed the child.

14. Check the temperature of the food; it should be room temperature.
15. Disconnect the syringe from the tube and remove the plunger from the syringe.
16. Reconnect the syringe to the tube.
17. Fill the syringe with the right amount of food.

18. If necessary, push gently with the plunger to start the flow of food; then remove the plunger and allow the food to flow by itself.
19. The bottom of the syringe should never be held higher than the child's chin, or 6 inches above the level of the child's stomach (Fig. 3).
20. Continue adding food until the right amount has been fed. Do not allow the syringe to become empty.
21. When the food is at the bottom of the syringe, add 1 to 2 teaspoons (5 to 10 ml) of water to rinse the tube.
22. Place the clamp on the tube if it will be left in place between feedings.
23. Hold, cuddle, and burp the child.
24. PRAISE THE CHILD FOR HELPING.
25. Write down the time and amount of the child's feeding. Use the other nostril for the next insertion.

TO REMOVE THE TUBE

1. Loosen the tape that is holding the tube.
2. Fold the tube and pinch it tightly together.
3. Pull the tube out quickly.
4. Hold, cuddle, and burp the child.

CARE OF THE NASOGASTRIC TUBE AND SYRINGE

Wash with soap and water, and rinse the inside well with clear water. Dry the syringe, plunger, and tube. Put plunger in syringe when dry and store everything in a clean, dry container (e.g., plastic bag, margarine container).

If the tube remains in place between feedings, look at the nose before each feeding for redness. *Always* check to make sure the tube is in the right place before adding formula (step 13). Change the tube every _____ days.

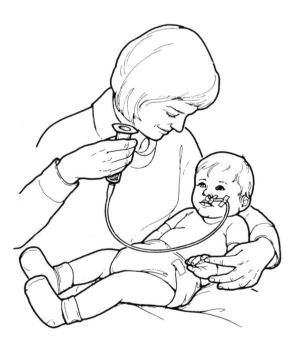

Fig. 3 Comforting child during feeding. Note the bottom of the syringe is at the level of child's shoulder.

Unit 5

COMMUNITY AND HOME CARE INSTRUCTIONS

Giving Gastrostomy Feedings

To help the child get enough food to grow, an opening was made into the child's stomach. There are several types of gastrostomy feeding devices. Your health professional chose the one that is best for your child. It is very important that the brand and size of the feeding and/or decompression tube match the device in the child. If a gastrostomy tube has been put into this opening, you can now feed the child through this. If your child has a skin level device instead of a tube, instructions for feeding are on p. 621. You should hold and cuddle the child during the feeding.

You should give the child _____ ounces of _____ every _____ hours.

Call your health professional at _____ if any of the following occur:

- Vomiting
- Change in color of stomach contents
- Increased amount of stomach contents before feeding
- Change in color of mucus
- Increased bowel movements
- The child becomes very irritable
- Increased redness around gastrostomy site
- Two meals are missed due to too much food in the stomach

GASTROSTOMY TUBE FEEDING

Equipment

Liquid food at room temperature in pour container
Water to rinse tube
Syringe

Instructions

1. Gather equipment.
2. Wash your hands with soap and water. Count to 10 while washing, then rinse with clear water and dry with a clean paper or cloth towel.
3. Tell the child (even if infant) what you will be doing.
4. Place the child on your lap or reclining in an infant seat. The older child can sit in a chair or on a bed.
5. Use a pacifier for the infant to enjoy sucking during the feeding.
6. Attach the syringe to the gastrostomy tube.
7. Unclamp the tube.
8. Pull back gently on the plunger to see the amount of food left in the child's stomach.
9. If more than one fourth of the last feeding is still present, return the food to the stomach and wait 30 to 60 minutes. When there is less than one fourth of the amount of food, feed the child.
10. Remove the plunger from the syringe. Hold syringe/tubing below stomach level when filling syringe to prevent excess air getting into stomach.
11. Fill syringe with the right amount of food.
12. A gentle push with the plunger of the syringe may be necessary to start the flow of food; then remove the plunger and allow the food to flow by itself.
13. Never hold the bottom of the syringe higher than the child's chin (Fig. 1).
14. Continue adding food to the syringe until you have finished the right amount. Do not let the syringe become empty.
15. When the food is at the bottom of the syringe add water (1 to 2 teaspoons [5 to 10 ml] or the amount specified by your health professional) to rinse the tube and keep it from clogging.
16. Clamp the tube and remove the syringe.
17. Gently pull the tube to allow the balloon to rest against the inside of the stomach at the opening.
18. Tape the tube to prevent it from advancing or allowing stomach contents to leak on the skin.
19. Hold and cuddle child after the feeding.
20. PRAISE THE CHILD FOR HELPING.

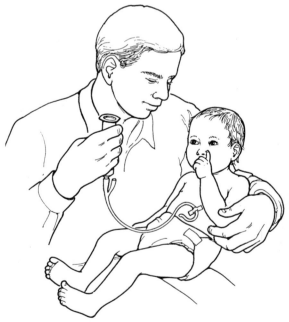

Fig. 1 Feeding the child with a gastrostomy tube. Note the bottom of the syringe is at the level of child's shoulder.

From Wong DL, Hess CS: *Wong and Whaley's Clinical manual of pediatric nursing*, ed 5. Copyright © 2000, Mosby, St Louis.

Unit 5

COMMUNITY AND HOME CARE INSTRUCTIONS

Giving Gastrostomy Feedings—cont'd

Wash the syringe in soap and warm water using a bottle brush. Rinse the inside well with clear water. Dry the syringe and plunger. Put plunger in syringe when dry and store in a clean dry container between feedings (e.g., plastic bag, margarine container).

Care of a Gastrostomy Tube

The gastrostomy tube should be changed _____ . If the tube accidentally comes out, it should be replaced as quickly as possible. A moist gauze bandage can be placed over the opening until you can get to a quiet place where you can reinsert the tube. When you are away from home and the child will need to be fed, you should carry an extra gastrostomy tube with you in case something happens to the tube that is in place.

Equipment

Gastrostomy tube
Water for lubricant
Small syringe
Water or air if needed for balloon
Tape

Removing the Tube

Remove the tube just before feeding so that there will be only a small amount of liquid in the child's stomach.
1. Gather equipment.
2. Wash your hands with soap and water. Count to 10 while washing, then rinse with clear water and dry with a clean paper or cloth towel.
3. Tell the child what you will be doing.
4. Lay the child flat to ensure a straight tract to insert tube into.
5. Attach the small syringe to the tube at point A (Fig. 2).
6. Unclamp the tube and withdraw the air/water from the balloon.
7. Reclamp the tube and quickly remove it, holding the tip up to prevent stomach contents from dripping.
8. Place it out of the child's reach while you place the new tube.

Inserting the Tube

1. Wet the tip of the clean tube with water.
2. Put the tip of the tube through the opening into the child's stomach.
3. Insert the tube beyond the balloon on the tip (Fig. 3).
4. Connect the syringe, containing ___ cc of air or water, to point A.
5. Inject the air or water into the tube.
6. Gently pull on the tube to make sure the balloon is inflated and the tube is in position.
7. Tape the tube securely to the child's abdomen.
8. Clamp the new tube until you are ready for the next feeding
    The gastrostomy tube that you have removed should be cleaned in soap and water. Rinse the inside of the tube well with clear water. Dry the tube and store in a clean, dry container (e.g., plastic bag, margarine container).

SKIN LEVEL DEVICE FEEDING
Equipment

Liquid food at room temperature in pour container
Tubing
Clamp
Water to rinse tube
Syringe
Decompression tube if needed

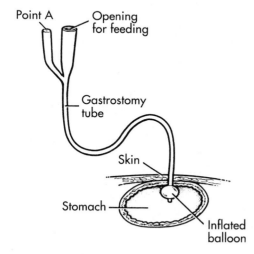

Fig. 2 Diagram of a gastrostomy tube. Point A is used to inflate the balloon. The other opening is for the feeding syringe.

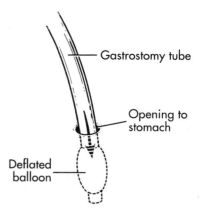

Fig. 3 Gastrostomy tube in stomach with balloon deflated.

Unit 5

This section may be photocopied and distributed to families.

Continued

COMMUNITY AND HOME CARE INSTRUCTIONS

Giving Gastrostomy Feedings—cont'd

Instructions

1. Gather equipment.
2. Wash your hands with soap and water. Count to 10 while washing, then rinse with clear water and dry with a clean paper or cloth towel.
3. Tell the child (even if infant) what you will be doing.
4. Place the child on your lap or reclining in an infant seat. The older child can sit on a chair or a bed.
5. Use a pacifier for the infant to enjoy sucking during the feeding.
6. If the stomach seems full and gassy, air can be removed by putting the decompression tube into the device. If formula comes out, wait 1 hour before feeding, and try again.
7. Feed the child if the stomach does not seem full and gassy, or if formula does not come up the tubing when the air is removed.
8. Attach syringe to the tubing.
9. Secure the clamp near the bottom of the tube.
10. Open the safety plug of the device.
11. Fill the syringe and tube with formula. This keeps too much air from going into the stomach.
12. Connect the tubing to the device.
13. Unclamp the feeding tube.
14. A gentle push with the plunger may be necessary to start the flow of food; then remove the plunger and allow the food to flow by itself.
15. Never hold the bottom of the syringe higher than the child's chin.
16. Continue adding food to the syringe until you have finished the right amount. Do not let the syringe become empty.

17. When the food is at the bottom of the syringe, add 1 to 2 teaspoons (5 to 10 ml) of water to rinse the tube.
18. Remove the tube from the device.
19. Replace the safety plug on the device.
20. Hold and cuddle the child after the feeding.
21. PRAISE THE CHILD FOR HELPING.

Rinse the tubing and syringe with water after each feeding. Each day, wash the syringe and tube in warm, soapy water. Use a bottle brush for the syringe, and pipe cleaners can be used for the tubing. Rinse the inside well with clear water. If a milky coating is on the inside of the syringe or tubing, use a solution of 1 part vinegar to 2 parts water to clean the inside before the soapy wash and rinse.

Care of the Skin Level Device

Clean around the site each day with mild soap and water. Turn the button around in a complete circle to make sure it is completely cleaned. Dry the area and leave it exposed to air for about 20 minutes so it can dry completely.

Medications can plug the device. Medicines in tablet form should be crushed well and mixed with water or food before putting them in the syringe. Thick liquids can be mixed with warm water to make them thinner. The medicine should be given before the feeding, to make sure the medicine goes into the stomach. If it is not time for a feeding, rinse the tubing with 1 to 2 teaspoons (5 to 10 ml) of water after giving the medicine.

If the device comes out, it is not an emergency. Do not throw the device away. Save it for your health professional

to look at. Place a moist gauze pad over the opening. If the device comes out during office hours, call your health professional for instructions. If it is after office hours, place a gastrostomy tube into the opening as you were taught or follow the instructions on page 621. Use the gastrostomy tube for feedings until you can contact your health professional.

SKIN CARE

Keep the skin around the gastrostomy tube or skin level device clean and dry. A bandage does not have to be put over the area, but this may be needed to keep the child from pulling on the tube. A cloth diaper can be wrapped around the child's abdomen and secured with tape. This will keep the child from playing with the tube. Other ways to keep the tube out of reach are to use one-piece outfits, tube tops, the tops of panty hose, or children's tights with the legs cut off.

Zinc ointment, Duoderm-CGF (a thin dressing that can be kept on the skin for 7 days), Pro Shield Plus, or Ilex Dermalyte Protective Barrier Ointment can be used on the skin around the tube. This will provide protection for the skin in case there is a small leakage of gastric fluid. If the area becomes red or sore, call your health professionals at _____ for further directions.

CLOTHING

Dress the child in loose-fitting clothing that does not press the gastrostomy tube against the skin. Bib-type overalls are preferable to pants. The overalls cover the tube, making it less likely that the child or other children will play with the tube. Also, wearing overalls avoids tight elastic around the child's waist.

Unit 5

COMMUNITY AND HOME CARE INSTRUCTIONS

Performing Clean Intermittent Bladder Catheterization*

The child is unable to empty the bladder of urine. A catheter (tube) can be put into the bladder to let the urine come out by itself. This will help the child to remain dry and will help prevent bladder infections. Catheterization should be done when the child wakes up in the morning, before bedtime, and every _____ hours during the day. If the child is unable to do the catheterization alone, someone at school should be taught to help the child. Stopping fluids 2 hours before bedtime may help the child stay dry through the night.

A record should be kept of all that the child drinks and the amount of urine that was obtained by catheterization. (See sample on p. 625.) A description of the urine is helpful so that you can notice changes that may be caused by an infection. Look at the urine to see if it is cloudy or clear, pale yellow or dark amber. Smell it to tell if a strange odor is present.

Call your health professional at _____ if any of these occur:

- Temperature above 101° F
- Trouble inserting the tube
- Change in the amount of urine
- Change in the way the urine looks or smells
- Pain with insertion

Equipment

Catheter and storage container
Soap and water with washcloth or unscented towelettes or baby wipes
Urine container
Water-soluble lubricant

Instructions for Boys

1. Have equipment ready; keep the tube in its container until you are ready to use it.
2. Wash your hands with soap and water. Count to 10 while washing, then rinse with clear water and dry with a clean paper or cloth towel.
3. Tell the child what you will be doing.
4. Catheterization can be done sitting, standing, or lying down.
5. Remove or arrange the child's clothing so that it will not get wet and the urine can flow.
6. Wet the first 2 inches of the tube, either by placing lubricant on your finger and spreading it on the tube, or by dipping the catheter into the lubricant on a clean tissue or paper towel.
7. Hold penis straight; if the child is uncircumcised, pull the foreskin back as far as it will go without forcing it.
8. Wipe the tip of the penis with towelette, baby wipe, or a clean washcloth with soap and water.
9. Hold the penis upright. Push the tube into the urinary opening gently (Fig. 1). Just before the bladder you may feel some resistance. Do not push the tube in and out if resistance is met. Hold the tube and continue to move it in slowly, using gentle but firm pressure until the muscle relaxes.
10. Tell the child to take a deep breath and slowly let it out. This helps the child to relax.
11. Continue to insert the catheter until urine begins to flow. Then insert the tube about another ½ inch and hold it there until urine stops flowing.
12. Push the foreskin forward if needed. Never leave it pulled back.
13. Let all of the urine flow out.
14. Tell the child to squeeze his belly as if he were having a bowel movement; blow bubbles or a pinwheel; or press on child's tummy with your hand. This helps empty all of the urine out of the bladder.
15. Slowly remove the tube; if urine begins to flow again, stop removing the tube and allow it to empty.
16. Wash your hands and the catheter with soap and water. Rinse the inside of the tube well with clear water.
17. PRAISE THE CHILD FOR HELPING.
18. Dry the catheter with a clean paper or cloth towel and store in a clean, dry container (e.g., plastic bag or margarine container).
19. Write down the time; whether the underwear/diaper was wet, damp, or dry; and the amount and the way the urine looks.
20. Never reuse a catheter that appears rough, stiff, worn, discolored, or damaged in any way.
21. Your health professional will tell you how often a new catheter should be used.

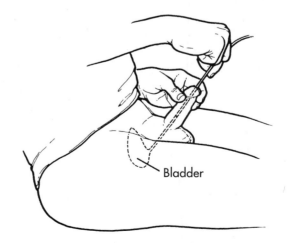

Fig. 1   A boy doing intermittent self-catheterization.

*You can use these instructions if your child does self-catheterization. But be sure your child washes his or her hands before and after the procedure.
This section may be photocopied and distributed to families.

From Wong DL, Hess CS: *Wong and Whaley's Clinical manual of pediatric nursing,* ed 5. Copyright © 2000, Mosby, St Louis.

Continued

Unit 5

COMMUNITY AND HOME CARE INSTRUCTIONS

Performing Clean Intermittent Bladder Catheterization*—cont'd

Instructions for Girls

1. Gather equipment; keep the tube in its container until you are ready to use it.
2. Wash your hands with soap and water. Count to 10 while washing, then rinse with clear water and dry with a clean paper or cloth towel.
3. Tell the child what you will be doing.
4. Remove or arrange the child's clothing so it will not get wet and urine can flow.
5. Position the girl as comfortably as possible, either lying down, with her knees bent in a "frog-like" position; or sitting, with legs spread apart for self-catheterization.
6. Separate the labia with the thumb and forefinger and locate the urinary opening (urethra) (Fig. 2). A mirror can be used to teach the child self-catheterization.

7. Wash the labia one or two times with the unscented towelette, baby wipe, or a washcloth with warm soap and water. Be sure to wash from front to back and never go back and forth across the opening.
8. Wet the first 2 inches of the tube, either by placing lubricant on your finger and spreading it on the tube, or by dipping the catheter into the lubricant on a clean tissue or paper towel.
9. Insert the tube gently into the urethra until urine begins to flow. Then move it slowly about another ½ inch (Fig. 3).
10. Allow all of the urine to flow out.
11. Tell the child to squeeze her belly as if she were having a bowel movement; blow bubbles or a pinwheel; or press on her tummy with your hand. This helps empty all of the urine out of the bladder.

12. Slowly begin to remove the tube when the urine stops. More urine will flow as you remove the tube.
13. Wash your hands and the catheter with soap and water. Rinse the inside of the tube well with clear water.
14. Dry the tube with a clean paper or cloth towel and store in a clean, dry container (e.g., plastic bag or margarine container).
15. PRAISE THE CHILD FOR HELPING.
16. Write down the time; whether the underwear/diaper was wet, damp, or dry; the amount of urine; and the way the urine looks.
17. Never reuse a catheter that appears rough, stiff, worn, discolored, or damaged in any way.
18. Your health professional will tell you how often a new catheter should be used.

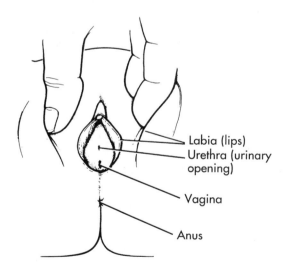

Labia (lips)
Urethra (urinary opening)
Vagina
Anus

Fig. 2 Female anatomy showing urinary opening (urethra).

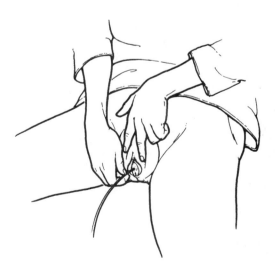

Fig. 3 A girl doing intermittent self-catheterization.

*You can use these instructions if your child does self-catheterization. But be sure your child washes his or her hands before and after the procedure.

Unit 5

COMMUNITY AND HOME CARE INSTRUCTIONS

Performing Clean Intermittent Bladder Catheterization*—cont'd

Sample Record

Day and time	Amount fluid in	Amount fluid out	Wet/damp/dry	Appearance

COMMUNITY AND HOME CARE INSTRUCTIONS

Caring for the Child with a Colostomy

The child has had surgery that has changed the way in which he has a bowel movement. An opening was made in the abdomen and the bowel was attached to the skin. This allows the bowel to empty through the opening (stoma) instead of the rectum. Therefore the area must be kept clean to prevent the skin from becoming irritated. An ostomy appliance (pouch) is placed over the stoma to collect the stool.

You will need to do the ostomy care for the infant and young child. The child can assist according to his developmental level. For example, the child can gather the equipment and hand you supplies. As the child grows, allow him to increase his responsibility in the care of the ostomy. By the age of 8 or 10 years, most children can do the care by themselves.

Ostomy care should be taught to other people who will be caring for the child. At school, tell both the child's teacher and the school nurse so that adult help is available if needed. An extra set of clothing can be kept at the school in case the ostomy appliance leaks. This will help spare the child any embarrassment.

Dress the child in loose-fitting clothing that does not press on the colostomy. Bib-type overalls or dresses are preferable to pants. The overalls or dress will cover the ostomy and avoid the elastic waistband on pants, which may irritate the ostomy.

Call your health professional at ____ if any of these occur:
- Bleeding from the stoma more than usual when cleaning stoma
- Bleeding from skin around stoma
- Change in bowel pattern
- Change in the size of the stoma
- Change in color of stoma
- Temperature above 100.4° F

OSTOMY CARE (WITH A POUCH/APPLIANCE)

The pouch will remain intact for different lengths of time. The pouch should be changed on a routine schedule or sooner, if it leaks. Each time the pouch is changed the area needs to be clean and dry and a new barrier must be applied. During the day, the stool can be removed/rinsed from the pouch, and then the pouch can be clamped. Two-piece pouches are also available.

Equipment

Washcloth
Skin barrier/wafer
Stoma paste
Pouch/appliance
Rinse bottle

Instructions

1. Gather equipment.
2. Wash your hands with soap and water. Count to 10 while washing, then rinse with clear water and dry with a clean paper or cloth towel.
3. Tell child what you are going to do. (Have him do it if old enough. Be sure he washes his hands before and after the procedure.)
4. Remove old pouch and skin barrier.
5. Wash the skin and gently pat dry.
6. Look for any redness or irritation.
7. Cut the skin barrier to size.
8. Apply the skin barrier. If using the type with an adhesive backing, remove the paper seal first.
9. Remove the covering from the adhesive backing on the pouch.
10. Center the pouch over the stoma and press gently, moving from the stoma edge out.
11. Close the end of the pouch with a clamp or rubber band.
12. PRAISE THE CHILD FOR HELPING.
13. Wash your hands as above.

Emptying the Pouch

1. When the pouch is one-third filled with stool, open the lower end of the pouch over the toilet or another container and let the stool drain out.
2. Rinse the inside of the pouch each day with a squeeze bottle of cool water to remove all the stool. Fill the pouch with a small amount of clear water and swish it around to thoroughly clean pouch. Then empty pouch over the toilet or a diaper.
3. Make a wick from toilet tissue to dry the inside lower 1 inch of the pouch. Wipe off the outside and reattach the clamp or rubber band.
4. PRAISE THE CHILD FOR HELPING.
5. Wash your hands as above.

SKIN CARE

Protection of the skin around the colostomy is a very important part of the child's care. If the skin around the colostomy becomes irritated (moist or red), it is important to help heal the area as fast as possible. A barrier should always be used to keep the stool off the skin. A barrier can be made by mixing zinc oxide ointment and karaya powder. The paste can be smoothed on the skin around the ostomy. Duoderm-CGF is a ready-made wafer-type barrier that is placed on the skin for up to 7 days.

Proshield Plus* can be used on moist skin and under an ostomy pouch. To help the pouch stay on securely, an adhesive spray must be used before the pouch is applied. Proshield Plus can also be applied over medicated creams if they are needed to treat an infection.

If a pouch is not used, petrolatum (Vaseline) is applied over the ointment to keep the diaper from sticking to the ointment. When stool is on the skin around the ostomy, clean off the stool and petrolatum, but keep the barrier ointment on to protect the healing skin. Apply more petrolatum before diapering the child.

*Available from Healthpoint Medical, San Antonio, Texas, (800) 441-8227.

This section may be photocopied and distributed to families.

Giving an Enema

An enema is needed when stool must be removed from the bowel or intestine. However, simple constipation in children should not be treated with enemas but with changes in the child's diet. Increasing the amount of liquids to at least 1 quart each day and the amount of fiber in foods (especially whole grains, bran cereals, fresh vegetables, and fruit with the skin on) should increase the size and number of the child's bowel movements.

Large amounts of milk, rice, bananas, and cheese can cause constipation. The child should eat small amounts of these items. If your child is an infant, ask your health professional before changing the feedings.

If the child has persistent constipation, a complete medical evaluation is necessary to determine the cause. If you have been told by a health professional to give an enema (usually only one or two enemas in a day) to the child, use these instructions.

Age	Amount of Lukewarm Water	Approximate Amount of Salt	Distance to Insert Tube
Infant	½-1 cup (120-240 ml)	¼-½ tsp (1.25-2.5 ml)	1 in (2.5 cm)
2-4 yr	1-1½ cups (240-360 ml)	½-¾ tsp (2.5-3.75 ml)	2 in (5.0 cm)
4-10 yr	1½-2 cups (360-480 ml)	¾-1 tsp (3.75-5.0 ml)	3 in (7.5 cm)
11 yr	2-3 cups (480-720 ml)	1-1½ tsp (5.0-7.5 ml)	4 in (10 cm)

ENEMA BAG

Equipment

Lukewarm water (water that feels
 comfortably warm)
Salt
Measuring spoon
Enema bag or kit
Lubricant such as Vaseline or KY Jelly
Potty chair or toilet

Instructions

1. Gather equipment.
2. Wash your hands with soap and water. Count to 10 while washing, then rinse with clear water and dry with a clean paper or cloth towel.
3. Refer to the above chart for the right amount of water and salt for the child's age; never use plain tap water.
4. Mix the lukewarm water and salt.
5. Measure the rectal tube for the correct distance.
6. Check to make sure the tube is clamped shut. Then fill the enema container with the solution.
7. Place the child in one of the following positions:
   a. Lying face down on belly with the knees and hips bent toward the chest (Fig. 1).
   b. Lying on the left side with the left leg straight and the right leg bent at the hip and knee and placed comfortably on top of the left leg (Fig. 2).
   c. Sitting on the potty chair or toilet (Fig. 3).

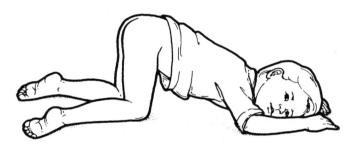

Fig. 1 "Knee-chest" position for receiving an enema.

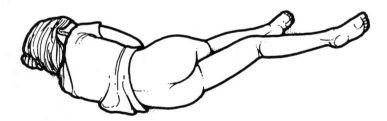

Fig. 2 Side-lying position for receiving an enema.

8. Unclamp tube to allow the liquid to flow through and remove air that is present. Clamp the tube.
9. Place a small amount of lubricant on your finger or on a tissue and spread the lubricant around the tip of the tube, being careful not to plug the holes with lubricant (Fig. 4).
10. Gently put the tube into the child's rectum to the marked distance (Fig. 5).
11. Holding the bottom of the container no more than 4 inches above the child, open the clamp and allow the liquid to flow. You may have to hold the tube in place.
12. When the container is empty, remove the tube.
13. Have the child keep the liquid inside for 3 to 5 minutes. If the child is too young to follow instructions, then hold the buttocks together to keep the liquid inside.
14. Help the child to the toilet or potty chair, or allow the child to release the liquid into a diaper.
15. PRAISE THE CHILD FOR HELPING.
16. Write down the appearance of the results of the enema.
17. Wash your hands as above.

Continued

From Wong DL, Hess CS: *Wong and Whaley's Clinical manual of pediatric nursing*, ed 5. Copyright © 2000, Mosby, St Louis.

COMMUNITY AND HOME CARE INSTRUCTIONS

Giving an Enema—cont'd

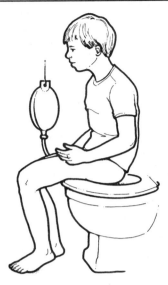

Fig. 3   Position for receiving an enema on toilet.

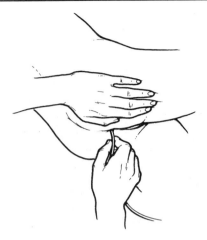

Fig. 5   Gently placing the tube in the child's rectum. Make sure the tube is not put in farther than the marked distance.

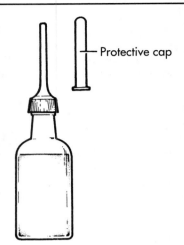

— Protective cap

Fig. 6   Pre-packaged enema with the protective cap removed.

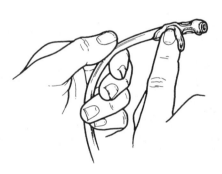

Fig. 4   Putting lubricant on the tip of the enema tube.

PREPACKAGED ENEMA

Ready-to-use enemas are available in varying amounts and solutions for infants, children, and adults. Use the amount and type of solution recommended by your health care professional.

Equipment

Basin of warm water
Prepackaged enema
Potty chair or toilet

Instructions

1. Warm the liquid in a basin of warm water.

2. Wash your hands with soap and water. Count to 10 while washing, then rinse with clear water and dry with a clean paper or cloth towel.
3. Place the child in one of the following positions:
   a. Lying face down on belly with the knees and hips bent toward the chest (Fig. 1).
   b. Lying on the left side with the left leg straight and the right leg bent at the hip and knee and placed comfortably on top of the left leg (Fig. 2).
   c. Sitting on the potty chair or toilet (Fig. 3).
4. Remove the cap (Fig. 6). Put the tip, which is already lubricated, into the child's rectum the right distance (Fig. 7).
5. Gently squeeze the enema container to empty. A small amount will remain in the container after squeezing.
6. Remove the tip.
7. Have the child keep the liquid inside for 3 to 5 minutes. If the child is too young to follow instructions, then hold the buttocks together to keep the liquid inside.

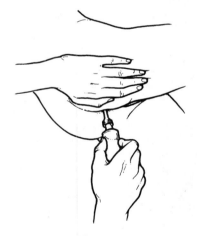

Fig. 7   Gently placing tip of prepackaged enema in the child's rectum.

8. Help the child to the toilet or potty chair, or allow the child to release the solution into a diaper.
9. PRAISE THE CHILD FOR HELPING.
10. Write down the appearance of the results of the enema.
11. Wash your hands as in step 2.

INSTRUCTIONS RELATED TO MAINTAINING RESPIRATORY FUNCTION

Suctioning the Nose and Mouth

The child needs help to keep the mouth and nose clear of mucus. Suctioning equipment, a humidifier, and other supplies will be needed. While the child is in the hospital, you should practice using the same suction machine that you will be using at home. This allows you a chance to become familiar with the equipment. You will also need a mucus trap or nasal aspirator that can be used to remove mucus when you and the child are away from home. Practice with these items while the child is in the hospital.

Certain guidelines are helpful for the child who has problems clearing mucus from the back of the nose and mouth (pharynx). To keep the mucus liquid so that it is easy to remove by both suctioning and coughing, added moisture is needed. Encourage the child to drink at least 1 quart (four 8-ounce cups) of liquid a day and place a cool mist humidifier in the room where the child sleeps. Change the water in the humidifier each day and clean the humidifier regularly, according to the manufacturer's instructions.

All of the people who provide care for the child must know how to suction the child so that they can assist you. On each telephone in the house, tape emergency phone numbers such as 911 (if available in your area), the local hospital, your health professional, and any other numbers that are necessary. Notify your health professional at _____ if any of the following occur:

- Temperature above 100.4° F
- Presence of yellow or green mucus
- Change in the smell of the mucus
- Increased amount of mucus
- The child is very irritable
- The child is having difficulty breathing

SUCTIONING

Suctioning keeps the airway (nose and mouth, Fig. 1) clear of mucus to help the child breathe more easily. Suctioning is not done routinely, but only when needed. Suction when the following occur:

- The child is having trouble breathing
- The child appears very restless

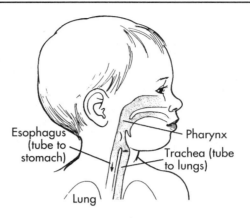

Fig. 1 Child's airway. Suctioning should clear the pharynx of mucus.

- The child has difficulty eating or sucking
- The child's color becomes paler
- The child's nostrils flare (spread out)
- You hear the sound of air bubbling through the mucus

When the child has a cold, more mucus is produced, so you will probably need to suction more often. The child may cough or gag when you insert or remove the suction catheter. Gently tell the child when you are almost finished. If the child is old enough, teach him how to help you by holding the supplies.

Preparing the Supplies

Clean jars and containers:
Wash plastic containers and glass jars with lids in a dishwasher or in hot, soapy water and rinse well. Use a clean towel to dry or allow to air dry. Keep a supply of containers washed and dried.

Salt solution (saline):
Boil water for 5 minutes. Add ¾ teaspoon of salt to each 2 cups of water when you are heating the water. Let cool, then pour into a clean glass jar and cover. Store the sterile saline in the refrigerator.

Equipment

Suction machine with tubing
Suction catheters
Saline or water (cool)
White vinegar
Clean container for rinsing catheter

Instructions

1. Gather all the equipment you will need.
2. Wash your hands with soap and water. Count to 10 while washing, then rinse with clear water and dry with a clean paper or cloth towel.
3. Open the suction catheter package and connect the catheter to the suction machine.
4. Make sure the suction machine is plugged in and working.
5. Measure the tube for the distance you will have to insert it. Place the tip of the catheter at the child's ear lobe and mark the distance to the tip of the child's nose. Hold the catheter at this mark (Fig. 2).

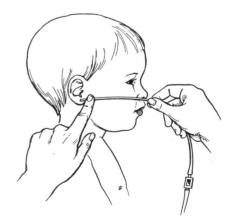

Fig. 2 Measuring length to insert suction catheter.

From Wong DL, Hess CS: *Wong and Whaley's Clinical manual of pediatric nursing,* ed 5. Copyright © 2000, Mosby, St Louis.

Continued

Unit 5

COMMUNITY AND HOME CARE INSTRUCTIONS

Suctioning the Nose and Mouth—cont'd

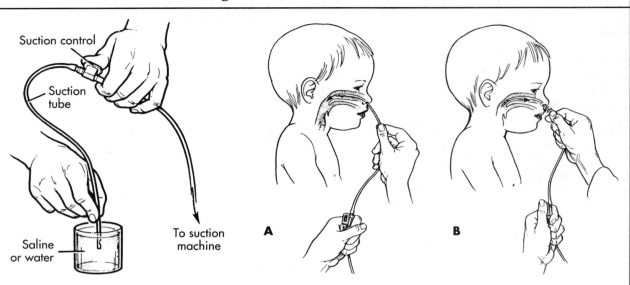

Fig. 3   Rinsing and lubricating catheter with thumb on suction control.

Fig. 4   **A,** Inserting catheter with thumb off suction control. **B,** Removing catheter with thumb on suction control.

6. Place the tip of the catheter in the sterile saline and place your thumb over the opening to obtain suction. The saline wets the catheter (Fig. 3).
7. Tell the child to take a deep breath.
8. With your thumb off the opening (no suction), insert the suction catheter in one nostril up to the measured distance (Fig. 4, *A*).
9. Place your thumb on the suction port to obtain suction.
10. Rotate or twist the catheter as you remove it with a slow steady motion (Fig. 4, *B*). Both inserting the catheter and suctioning should take no longer than 5 seconds. Remember, the child may not breathe while you are suctioning. Try holding your breath whenever your thumb is on the suction port. This will be a reminder to you for timing.
11. Look at the mucus. Check the color, smell, and consistency for any change.
12. Rinse the suction catheter in the sterile saline or water with your thumb on the suction port.

13. Allow the child to take a few deep breaths.
14. Repeat steps 7 through 13 up to two times if needed (for large amounts of mucus), then repeat for the other nostril.
15. After suctioning the nose, you can use the same catheter to clear the child's mouth.
16. Place the tip of the catheter in the saline and place your thumb over the opening to obtain suction.
17. Tell the child to take a deep breath.
18. With your thumb off the opening (no suction), insert the suction catheter in the child's mouth along one side of the mouth until it reaches the back of the throat.
19. Place your thumb on the suction port to obtain suction.
20. Rotate or twist the catheter as you remove it with a slow steady motion. Both inserting the catheter and suctioning should take no longer than 5 seconds. Remember, the child may not breathe while you are suctioning. Try holding your breath whenever your thumb is on the

suction port. This will be a reminder to you for timing.
21. Look at the mucus. Check the color, smell, and consistency for any change.
22. Rinse the suction catheter in the saline or water with your thumb on the suction port.
23. Allow the child a chance to take a few deep breaths.
24. Repeat steps 17 through 23 up to three times.
25. Hold and comfort the child.
26. PRAISE THE CHILD FOR HELPING.
27. After each use, throw away the saline or water and clean the container. The suction machine should be clean and ready for the next time that you will have to use it.
28. Your health professional will instruct you on the care of the suction catheters, or use the method described below.
29. Wash your hands as in step 2.

COMMUNITY AND HOME CARE INSTRUCTIONS

Suctioning the Nose and Mouth—cont'd

INSTRUCTIONS FOR CLEANING THE SUCTION CATHETERS

1. Rinse the suction catheters in cool tap water. Do not use hot water because it "cooks" the mucus, which makes it more difficult to remove.
2. Place the catheters in a clean jar filled with hot, soapy water.
3. Rinse both the inside and outside of the tube under hot, running water. Hold the tube with kitchen tongs so that you don't burn yourself.
4. Shake off the excess water.
5. Mix 1 part white vinegar and 3 parts water in a clean container.
6. Place the clean catheters in this solution for 30 minutes.
7. Remove the catheters from the liquid and rinse thoroughly with clean water.
8. Shake off the excess water.
9. Place on a clean paper towel to dry. When the tube is completely dry, place it in a clean plastic bag.
10. Close the bag and store until the next time you suction the child.
11. If you notice any moisture in the bag, repeat the entire cleaning procedure.

INSTRUCTIONS FOR USING A NASAL ASPIRATOR

When the child's nose is plugged with loose, runny mucus, the nasal aspirator is very helpful in removing it. The aspirator can also be used when the nose is plugged with dry, crusted mucus. Nose drops must first be used to moisten the mucus before it can be removed. Saline nose drops are the safest product to use. These can be purchased or made at home. To make the nose drops at home, mix ¾ teaspoon (4 ml) salt with 1 pint (2 cups or 500 ml) tap water or the mixture prescribed by your health professional. The solution can be stored in any clean, covered container, but should be mixed fresh each day. Use a clean eye dropper to put the solution into the

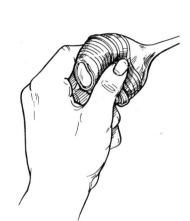

Fig. 5 Squeezing nasal aspirator to remove air.

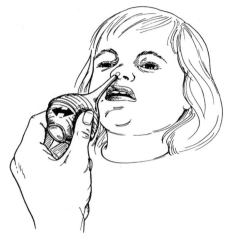

Fig. 6 Releasing grasp to suck mucus from nose.

child's nose, or wet a cotton ball and let the saline drip into the nose. Once the dried mucus is softened, then the nasal aspirator can be used.

Instructions

1. Squeeze the rounded end of the bulb to remove air (Fig. 5).
2. Place the tip of the bulb snugly into one side of the nose (nostril).
3. Let go of the bulb slowly; the bulb will suck the mucus out of the nose (Fig. 6).
4. When the bulb is reinflated, remove it from the nose (Fig. 7).
5. Squeeze the bulb into a tissue to get rid of the mucus.
6. Repeat steps 1 through 5 for the other side of the nose.
7. Hold and comfort the child.
8. Repeat this process as often as needed to keep the nose clear.

Cleaning the Nasal Aspirator

Clean the nasal aspirator by filling it with tap water. Then squeeze the bulb to remove the water and the mucus. Refill the bulb with water and boil for 10 minutes. Let the bulb cool and squeeze out the water before using it again.

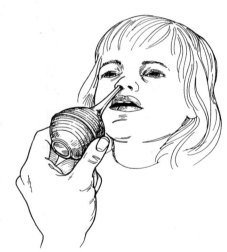

Fig. 7 Removing aspirator from nose when bulb is reinflated.

Unit 5

Performing Postural Drainage

Mucus is a protective covering of the inside of the lungs and airways. Mucus traps dust and dirt in the air that we breathe and helps prevent these from irritating the lung. When an infection or other irritation is present, the body produces more thick mucus to help the lungs get rid of the infection. Some illnesses, such as cystic fibrosis, also cause too much thick mucus. When this thick mucus blocks the airways, breathing becomes more difficult. To help the body get rid of the extra mucus, postural drainage is done. This series of activities helps move thick mucus from the lungs into the trachea (windpipe) where it can be coughed out. The airways can be compared to a freshly opened catsup bottle. Even when the bottle is held upside down, it takes several sharp blows to the bottom of the bottle to make the catsup start flowing.

The postural drainage needs to be carried out _____ times per day. This should be done when the child wakes up; before bedtime; and about 1½ hours before lunch and the evening meal. It should not be done after meals since the exercises and coughing may cause the child to vomit. The exercises should be finished 30 to 45 minutes before the meal, so that the child has a chance to rest and feel like eating.

The child must be placed in several different positions for the postural drainage. You must adapt the procedure for the child's age and strength. Each session should usually last 20 to 30 minutes and involve four to six positions. The remaining positions are then used at the other postural drainage times throughout the day.

TECHNIQUES YOU WILL NEED

Cupping (Percussion)

Position your hand as if you were holding a liquid or powder, then turn it upside down (Fig. 1). When the child is in the drainage position, rapidly strike the child's chest with your hand. The entire oval of your hand should make contact with the child's chest. If your child is very small, you may be given a special device to use instead of your hand. The drawings that follow have a shaded area to show where to place your hand for each position. Cupping is carried out for about 1 minute in each position. Have the child wear a shirt so that your hand does not touch the child's bare skin during cupping. Remember, cupping is not the same as hitting. When done right,

cupping does not hurt the child or cause the skin to become red, which occurs when the skin is slapped.

Vibration

Learning to vibrate may take a little practice. First, place one of your hands on top of the other; then rapidly tighten and loosen the muscles of your lower arm (Fig. 2). This creates a vibration that, when applied to the skin, is passed through to the lungs to loosen mucus. Now, have the child take a deep breath and while she is breathing out, place your hands over the lung segment to be drained and vibrated. An electric vibrator (massager) or a padded electric toothbrush (for infants) can be used as well as your hands for vibration.

POSITIONING AIDS

Infants and small children can be positioned in your lap. For older children, a padded slant board can be used. If a slant board is not available, a bed or couch at a comfortable height can be used. Pillows are helpful to position the child comfortably.

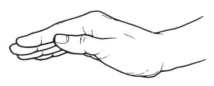

Fig. 1   Correct hand position for cupping.

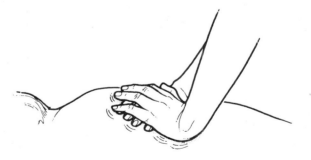

Fig. 2   Correct position of hands for vibrating.

This section may be photocopied and distributed to families.

Unit 5

COMMUNITY AND HOME CARE INSTRUCTIONS

Performing Postural Drainage—cont'd

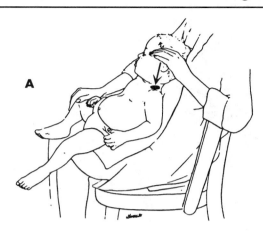

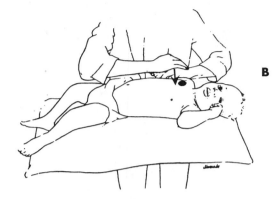

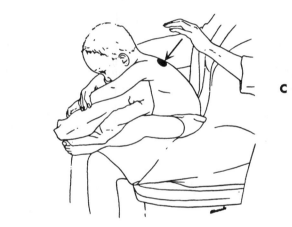

Instructions

1. Place the child in the position in Fig. 3, *A.*
2. Tell the child to take several deep breaths. The child can also use special blow bottles, try to blow up a balloon, or blow bubbles. These help the child to take deep breaths and may cause the child to cough.
3. Cup the area shaded in the picture for about 1 minute.
4. After cupping have the child take a deep breath and vibrate the area as she breathes out. Repeat this for three breaths. If the child is too young to understand how to breathe deeply and slowly, just vibrate during a few breaths.
5. Tell the child to cough. Since she may not be able to cough when lying down, help her to a sitting position to produce a good, deep cough.
6. Repeat steps 1 through 5 for each of the other positions (Fig. 3, *B* through *I*).
7. Only one side is shown above, but remember that the procedure must be repeated for both left and right sides.
   REMEMBER: Spend about 20 to 30 minutes at each session. Watch the child carefully for signs of tiredness. The postural drainage should be stopped before she becomes tired. It can be continued after the child has had an opportunity to rest.

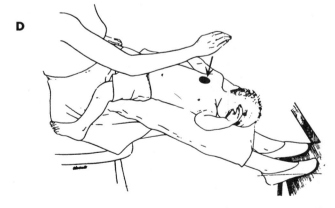

Fig. 3 Positions for postural drainage. (Modified from Cystic Fibrosis Foundation: *Infant segmental bronchial drainage,* Rockville, MD, The Foundation. Reprinted with permission.)

Unit 5

Continued

COMMUNITY AND HOME CARE INSTRUCTIONS

Performing Postural Drainage—cont'd

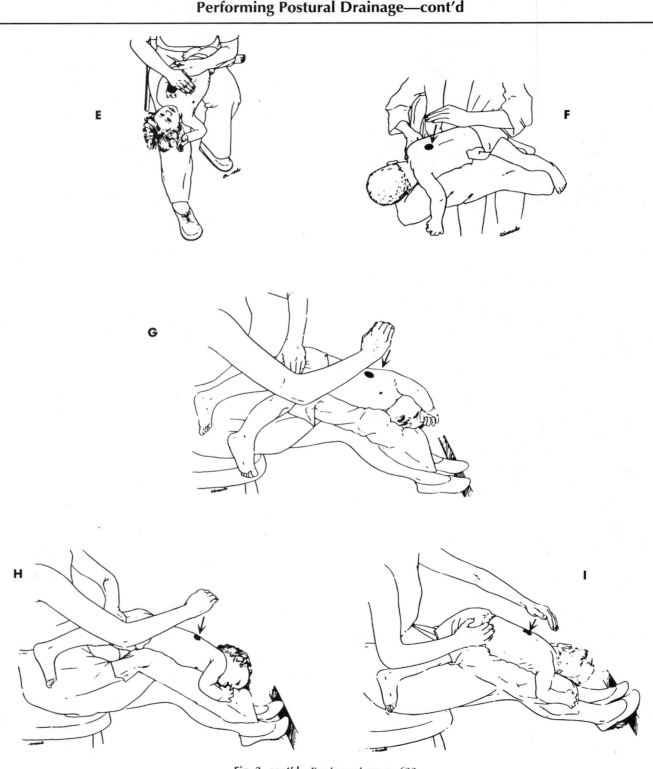

Fig. 3, cont'd   For legend see p. 633.

For legend see p. 633.

COMMUNITY AND HOME CARE INSTRUCTIONS

Caring for the Child with a Tracheostomy

A small opening (stoma) was made in the child's windpipe (or trachea, Fig. 1) to help her breathe easier. The tracheostomy ("trach") will require special care while you are at home. Suctioning equipment, a humidifier, and other supplies will be needed. While the child is in the hospital, you should practice using the same suction machine (and monitor) that you will be using at home. This helps you to become familiar with the equipment.

Supplies that you will need when you are outside the house are the following: a mucus trap that can be used when the suction machine is not available, sterile saline, water-soluble lubricant, trach tube with ties attached, scissors, and emergency phone numbers. These items should be kept in a "to-go bag" that is ready at all times. Practice with these items while the child is in the hospital.

SPECIAL CONSIDERATIONS

Certain precautions are needed for the child with a trach. Since the air that the child breathes no longer passes through the nose and mouth, it is no longer warmed, moistened, and filtered before it enters the lungs. To keep the mucus liquid, so that it is easy to remove by both suctioning and coughing, added moisture is needed. Your health professional will advise you on the amount of liquid that should be given to the child to drink throughout the day.

When the child is out in hot, dry, or cold weather, or on very windy days, wrap a handkerchief or scarf around the child's neck. This will help warm and filter the air the child breathes. Humidifying/filtering devices can also be bought. To keep food and liquids from falling into the trach, use a cloth bib with short ties when the child is eating.

Communication

The trach makes it harder for the child to make her needs known. Nursery monitors or intercoms can be used to listen for changes in the child's breathing. This may signal that the child needs you.

Older children can use bells to call you, or "talking" boards, where they can point to different words. If the child is old enough to write, the child may choose to communicate in this way. Some children are able to talk by placing their finger over the trach for short periods of time.

Skin Care

The moist secretions from the trach can irritate the skin. It is important to keep the area around the tracheostomy clean and dry to prevent skin irritation and infection. Wash the skin with soap and water and dry well. Change the trach ties each day or if they become wet or dirty. Tie the knot in a new place each time to keep from irritating the skin. Do not apply any ointments or other medications on the skin unless you are told to do so by your health professional.

Safety

Careful adult supervision is needed when the child is near water. Tub baths can be given, but be careful not to allow water into the trach. Swimming and boating must be avoided; however, the child can use a wading pool with supervision.

Any smoke, aerosol sprays, powder, or dust can irritate the lining of the child's trachea. Therefore the child should not be in the same room with anyone who is smoking or where aerosol sprays (such as hairspray and antiperspirants) are being used. Strong cleaning liquids such as ammonia are also irritating. Hair from animals that shed can clog the child's trachea. Avoid stuffed animals and toys with small parts that can be removed and put into the trach by a curious child.

All of the people who provide care for the child must be aware of how to suction the trach so that they can help you. Anyone caring for the child alone must also know cardiopulmonary resuscitation (CPR). Tape a list of emergency phone numbers to each telephone in the house. Include 911 (if available in your area), the local hospital, your health professional, and any others that are needed.

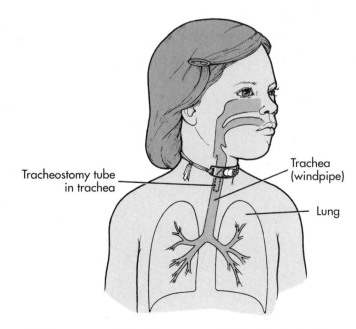

Tracheostomy tube in trachea

Trachea (windpipe)

Lung

Fig. 1   Diagram of breathing system with "trach" tube in place.

NOTE: For some children, additional instructions on stoma care and/or use of monitor may be needed. Home Care Instructions are available for CPR and postural drainage.

This section may be photocopied and distributed to families.

From Wong DL, Hess CS: *Wong and Whaley's Clinical manual of pediatric nursing,* ed 5. Copyright © 2000, Mosby, St Louis.

Continued

COMMUNITY AND HOME CARE INSTRUCTIONS

Caring for the Child with a Tracheostomy—cont'd

Call your health professional at _____
_____ if any of the following occur for 12 to 24 hours:

- The child is very irritable
- The child is having trouble breathing
- Temperature above 100.4°F
- Yellow or green mucus from trach or stoma
- Bright red blood from the trach
- Change in the smell of the mucus
- Increased amount of mucus
- Tracheostomy comes out and you are unable to replace it

SUCTIONING

You will need to suction the child's trach to keep the airway clear of mucus. Suctioning helps the child to breathe more easily. Suctioning should be done when the child wakes up and before sleep. Suction the child when any of the following occur:

- She is having trouble breathing
- She appears very restless
- She has trouble eating or sucking
- Her color becomes paler
- Her nostrils flare (spread out)
- You hear either the sound of air bubbling through the mucus or stridor (whistling)

When the child has a cold, more mucus is produced so you will need to suction more often. But suction only when needed; suctioning too often can cause the body to make more mucus.

Preparing the Supplies

Clean jars and containers:
Wash plastic containers or glass jars with lids in a dishwasher or hot soapy water and rinse well. Use a clean towel to dry or allow to air dry. Keep a supply of them washed and dried.

Sterile saline:
Boil water for 5 minutes. Add ¾ teaspoon of noniodized salt (check the ingredients on the box) to each 16 oz (2 cups) of water when you are heating the water. Let cool, then pour into a clean glass jar and cover. Store the sterile saline in the refrigerator.

Tracheostomy ties:
Use ½-inch seam binding, which is available in the sewing department of many stores. Self-sticking (Velcro) ties are also available, but are safe only if the child cannot pull them apart.

Equipment

Suction machine with tubing
Cardiorespiratory monitor (if ordered)
Suction catheters
Clean plastic container for rinsing catheter
NOTE: Ask your health professional if you should wear gloves.

Instructions

1. Gather all the equipment you will need.
2. Wash your hands with soap and water. Count to 10 while washing, then rinse with clear water and dry with a clean paper or cloth towel.
3. Open the suction catheter package and connect the catheter to the suction machine.
4. Make sure the suction machine is plugged in and working. Check that the suction pressure is not above 80 mm Hg for infants or 120 mm Hg for older children.
5. Before suctioning, you must measure the right distance to insert the tube. Holding the extra trach in one hand, place the suction catheter next to the trach tube. Slowly push the catheter until it is ¼ inch longer than the trach tube. Hold this spot with your fingers. Now measure the

distance from the tip of the catheter to the spot you are holding. Write it down _____ . This is how far you should place the catheter each time you suction.

6. Place the tip of the catheter in the sterile saline or water and place your thumb over the opening to get suction. The sterile saline lubricates the catheter (Fig. 2).
7. With your thumb off the opening (no suction), insert the suction catheter to a distance ¼ inch longer than the tube (about 2 to 3 inches in an infant or small child, Fig. 3).
8. Place your thumb on the suction port to obtain suction. Rotate or twist the catheter as you remove it with a slow, steady motion (Fig. 4). Both inserting the catheter and suctioning should take no longer than 3 or 4 seconds. Remember, the child cannot breathe during suctioning. As a reminder, count 1-one thousand, 2-one thousand, and so on.
9. Look at the mucus. Check the color, smell, and thickness for any change.
10. Rinse the suction catheter in the sterile saline or water with your thumb on the suction port.

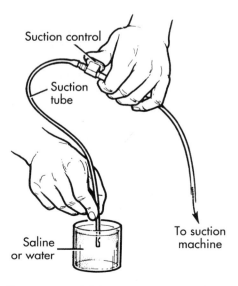

Fig. 2   Rinsing and lubricating suction catheter with thumb on suction control.

Suction control
Suction tube
Saline or water
To suction machine

COMMUNITY AND HOME CARE INSTRUCTIONS

Caring for the Child with a Tracheostomy—cont'd

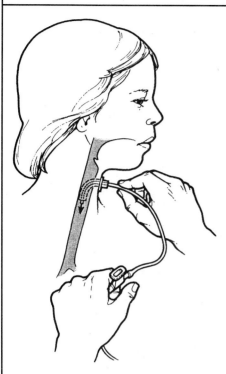

Fig. 3   Putting the suction catheter in trach tube with thumb off suction control. Catheter is inserted no more than ¼ inch longer than tube.

11. Allow about 30 seconds before suctioning again.
12. Repeat steps 5 through 11 up to three times.
13. Hold and comfort the child.
14. PRAISE THE CHILD FOR HELPING.
15. After each use, discard the saline and clean the container. Clean the suction machine to have it ready for the next time.
16. Use the following instructions, or ask your health professional to discuss the care of the suction catheters.
17. Wash your hands with soap and water. Count to 10 while washing, then rinse with clear water and dry with a clean paper or cloth towel.

CHANGING THE TRACHEOSTOMY TUBE

A plastic or metal tracheostomy tube may be used. Your health professional will provide you with any specific instructions needed.

The tracheostomy tube is changed routinely to allow for a thorough cleaning of the tube. The change should be done 2 to 3 hours after meals to avoid any chance of the child vomiting. When you change the tube, check the skin around the trach for any redness, swelling, cuts, or bruises.

Change the trach tube in a quiet place where you will not be disturbed. If the child is active, you will need someone to hold the child.

Equipment

Clean trach tube with trach ties attached (Fig. 5) and obturator, if needed
Suction machine with catheters
Sterile saline in clean container
Pipe cleaners
Hot, soapy water
White vinegar

Instructions for Changing the Tube

1. Gather all the equipment you will need.
2. Wash your hands with soap and water. Count to 10 while washing, then rinse with clear water and dry with a clean paper or cloth towel.
3. Place the child in an infant seat or sitting upright.
4. If the child is unable to help, have your helper hold the child's arms while the tube is being changed.
5. Suction the trach until it is clear. (See instructions for suctioning.)
6. Untie or carefully cut the old trach ties. Use scissors with rounded tips.
7. Remove the trach tube (Fig. 6).
8. Quickly check the skin.

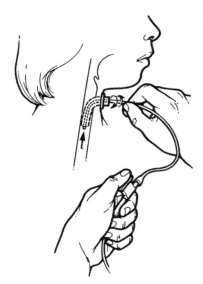

Fig. 4   Twisting catheter while removing it from trach tube with thumb on suction control.

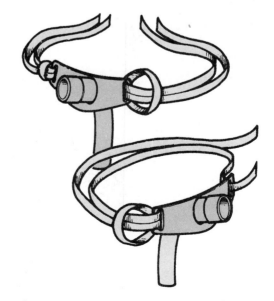

Fig. 5   Trach tube with ties. Knot will be tied either in back *(top example)* or on side *(bottom example).*

Caring for the Child with a Tracheostomy—cont'd

9. Quickly dip the clean trach tube in the sterile saline and shake to remove excess water.

10. Insert the clean tracheostomy tube (with or without an obturator) into the opening (stoma).

11. Remove obturator, if used.

12. Secure the tracheostomy ties, either at the side or back of the neck. Change the position of the knot each time the tube or ties are changed. Make sure that the ties are snug enough to let you put only one finger under them (Fig. 7).

13. If you are unable to put the new tube in, reposition the child's neck, dip the tube into the saline, and try again. If you still cannot get the tube in, check if the child is in distress. If the child is not in distress call your health professional. If the child is having trouble breathing, call the emergency numbers and begin rescue breathing, if necessary.

14. Hold and comfort the child.

15. PRAISE THE CHILD FOR HELPING.

16. Wash your hands with soap and water. Count to 10 while washing, then rinse with clear water and dry with a clean paper or cloth towel.

NOTE: The child may cough or gag during the insertion or removal of the tracheostomy tube. Gently tell the child when you are almost finished. If the child is old enough, teach her how to help you by handing you the supplies.

Your health professional will instruct you on the care of the suction catheters, or use the method described below.

INSTRUCTIONS FOR CLEANING THE SUCTION CATHETERS

1. Rinse the suction catheters in cool tap water. Do not use hot water because it "cooks" the mucus and makes it more difficult to remove.

2. Place the catheters in a clean jar filled with hot, soapy water.

3. Rinse both the inside and outside of the tube under hot, running water. Hold the tube with kitchen tongs so that you don't burn yourself.

4. Rinse the inside and outside with sterile saline.

5. Shake off the excess water.

6. Mix 1 part white vinegar and 3 parts water in a clean container.

7. Place the clean catheters in this solution for 30 minutes.

8. Remove the catheters from the liquid and rinse thoroughly with clean water.

9. Shake off the excess water.

10. Place on a clean paper towel to dry. When the tubes are completely dry, place them in a clean plastic bag.

11. Close the bag and store until the next time you suction the child.

12. If you notice any moisture in the bag, repeat the entire cleaning procedure.

INSTRUCTIONS FOR CLEANING THE TRACHEOSTOMY TUBE

1. Rinse the trach tube in cool tap water. Hot water "cooks" the mucus, which makes it harder to remove.

2. Place the trach tube in a clean jar filled with hot, soapy water.

3. Scrub the tube with pipe cleaners while it is in the jar.

4. While holding it by the area where the ties are attached, rinse both the inside and outside of the tube under hot, running water. You can hold it with kitchen tongs so that you do not burn yourself.

5. Rinse the inside and outside of the tube with sterile saline.

6. Shake off the excess water.

7. Mix 1 part white vinegar and 3 parts water in a clean container.

8. Place the clean tube in this solution for 30 minutes.

9. Remove the tube from the liquid and rinse thoroughly with clean water.

10. Shake off the excess water.

11. Place inside a clean paper towel to dry. Keep the trach tube in a safe place so that it can dry undisturbed.

12. When the tube is completely dry, place it in a clean plastic bag.

13. Close the bag and store until the next tube change.

14. If you notice any moisture in the bag, repeat the entire cleaning procedure.

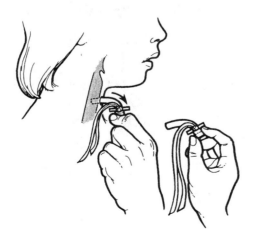

Fig. 6 Removing trach tube with left hand. Right hand has clean trach tube ready to insert.

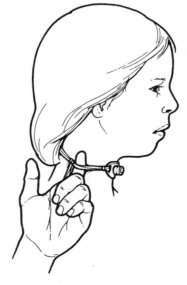

Fig. 7 Trach ties are tight enough if only one finger fits under them.

Unit 5

Home Apnea Monitoring

Prolonged apnea is defined as a lack of breathing for 20 seconds or more, or a shorter time period if the child develops a bluish or pale color, or the heart rate drops, or both. Many infants will not breathe for approximately 15 seconds. This is considered normal when the child does not have any color change or a significant drop in heart rate and begins breathing without stimulation.

When the child has apnea, it is necessary for his breathing and heart rate to be monitored at home using special equipment called an apnea monitor. You also need to keep a record and write down a description of each apneic episode. This description includes the date, time, and the child's condition. This record will help your health professional to evaluate the need for continued home monitoring.

Equipment

Apnea monitor (respiratory and heart rate)
Electrodes/belt
Clock or watch with second hand in the room where the baby sleeps
Apnea recording sheet and pencil or pen near monitor
Emergency numbers attached to all telephones in the house

Follow the manufacturer's instructions for applying the electrodes or belt to the child and setting up the monitor. The monitor requires electricity to operate. Most monitors are equipped with battery packs that allow you to take short trips with the child. Carefully read the manufacturer's instructions for the care of the batteries. All adults in the home should be familiar with the monitor, CPR, and the following information. You will be taught about the care and use of your specific monitor.

The monitor can be used anywhere in the home and is easily moved. Place the monitor on a sturdy, flat surface in the room, out of the reach of any other children. The monitor will sound an alarm if breathing stops for more than 20 seconds. When an alarm sounds, you must determine if the infant has stopped breathing; if the child is able to begin breathing without stimulation; and if the machine is working properly.

Placement of Electrodes/Belt

Correct placement of the electrodes is important for the monitor to be useful.

Place your index and middle fingers just below the child's nipple (use only one finger for small infants). Slide the fingers over to the side edge of the child's chest. Place one electrode here. Do the same for the other side and place the second electrode (Fig. 1). If your monitor has a belt, the electrodes are attached to the belt and then the belt is placed on the child's chest. Put the belt on the child, making sure the electrodes are placed as described above.

Care of Skin Electrodes

If skin electrodes are used, they should be changed every 2 to 3 days or when they become loose. To change the electrodes, carefully peel them off the child's chest. Wash the skin with soap and water to remove all of the adhesive, and dry thoroughly. Attach the monitor leads to the new electrodes before you apply them to the skin. Peel the backing of one of the electrodes and apply it to the skin. Attach the other electrode in the same manner. Notify your health professional if there are signs of redness at the site of the electrodes.

Procedure for Alarms Sounding

1. Calmly check the time.
2. Do not touch the child. Observe the child for another 10 seconds. If the child is not awake:
   a. Look at the child's color to see if it is the usual color.
   b. Place your ear by the child's nose and mouth and listen for air moving.
   c. Look to see if the child's chest is moving.

3. If the child's color is good and the child is breathing without difficulty, wait 10 seconds, then check the monitor to make sure the connections are intact and reset the alarms. Write down the event on the record sheet.
4. If there is a change in the skin color or the child has not resumed breathing, rub the child's back or chest. Wait 10 seconds and look to see if the infant begins breathing. If he does, observe him for another 10 seconds. If the color and breathing have returned to normal, check the monitor to make sure the connections are intact and reset the alarms. Write down the event on the record sheet.
5. If the child has not resumed breathing, gently slap the bottom of his feet. Never vigorously shake the child. Wait 10 seconds and look to see if he begins breathing. If he does, observe for another 10 seconds. If the color and breathing have returned to normal, check the monitor to make sure the connections are intact and reset the alarms. Write down the event on the record sheet.
6. If the child has not responded to measures such as slapping the feet, begin CPR.

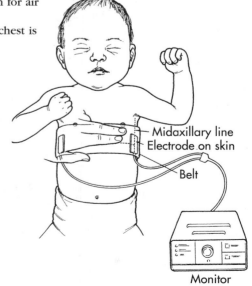

Fig. 1 Placement of electrodes or belt for apnea monitoring.

From Wong DL, Hess CS: *Wong and Whaley's Clinical manual of pediatric nursing,* ed 5. Copyright © 2000, Mosby, St Louis.

Unit 5

Infant Cardiopulmonary Resuscitation (CPR)*

Cardiopulmonary resuscitation (CPR) is a way to do some of the work of the heart and lungs for a short time. The heart pumps the blood around the body to provide oxygen and nutrients to the different body systems. The lungs are a transfer spot: as the blood flows through the lungs, oxygen is picked up by the blood and carbon dioxide is released. When the infant breathes, oxygen is brought into the body and carbon dioxide is breathed out.

Before beginning CPR, you must assess the infant to determine if both breathing and the heart have stopped. CPR is done when the infant's heart and breathing have stopped. You can breathe for the infant by blowing air into the lungs. Between breaths, the chest falls and air flows out of the lungs. You can do the work of the heart by doing a chest compression. The heart can be squeezed between the breastbone and the backbone to force blood out of the heart and into the arteries that carry it to the rest of the body. When you remove the pressure, the heart fills with blood so that the next squeeze (compression) will force additional blood out to the body.

All of the infant's caregivers must be able to perform CPR so that you can have relief and help if needed. Prepare for an emergency before it happens. Tape emergency information and telephone numbers to each phone in the house. Include 911 (if available in your area), the phone number that you are calling from, the address, and directions to the house. When calling in an emergency, be sure to give all of this information in addition to a description of what happened, who is involved, and the condition of the infant. Do not hang up the phone until the emergency operator tells you to do so.

Equipment
Emergency telephone numbers
Bulb syringe

ASSESSMENT
1. If trauma is suspected, do not move infant's head or neck. Avoid moving him unless he is in danger of further injury. If you need to turn the infant over, roll the head and torso as a unit, supporting head and neck to prevent movement that could cause further injury.
2. Try to wake the infant. Tap the infant, say his name loudly, clap your hands, or flick the bottom of his feet and look for a response or movement. Do not shake the infant.
3. Shout for help.
4. If infant is still unresponsive, begin CPR at once by opening the infant's airway (see below).
5. If there is someone else with you, have that person call the emergency telephone number (911) for help. If you are alone, do not stop to call, but begin CPR immediately. Do CPR for 1 minute, then call the emergency number as quickly as possible.

AIRWAY
1. Place the infant on his back on a *firm surface.*
2. Properly position the head and open the airway by placing your hand on the forehead and placing the fingers (not thumb) of your other hand under the bony part of the lower jaw near the middle of the chin. Be careful not to push the forehead too far back or to put too much pressure on the skin under the jaw. Make sure the infant's lips are open. Then lift and slightly tilt the head backward to a sniffing or nose pointing to the ceiling position. Proper positioning is essential to allow air to enter the windpipe to the lungs (Fig. 1).
3. If vomit is present, you must clear the infant's mouth before you breathe for the infant.
4. Quickly remove any mucus or vomit with your fingers or a bulb syringe after turning the infant's head to the side. If using a bulb syringe, squeeze it before placing it in the mouth, then release the pressure in the bulb to remove the material.

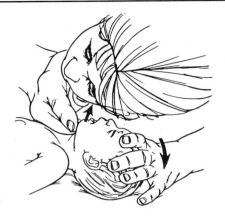

Fig. 1 Proper positioning to open the infant's airway.

a. If you see an object, vomit, or mucus, insert a finger of your other hand inside the mouth.
b. Move your finger toward you across the back of the throat. This sweeping action will help remove foreign objects.

BREATHING
5. Once the mouth is clear, reposition the head and observe the chest to determine if the infant has begun breathing. Place your ear close to the infant's mouth and look, listen, and feel for breathing for 3 to 5 seconds.
6. If breathing has not begun, you must breathe for the infant:
a. Open your mouth wide. Cover the infant's nose and mouth with your mouth (Fig. 2).

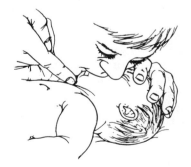

Fig. 2 Covering the nose and mouth for breathing.

Figures are reproduced with permission from Chandra NC, Hazinski MF: *Textbook of basic life support for healthcare providers,* Dallas, 1994, American Heart Association.

*These guidelines should not be used as substitutes for basic life support (BLS) training. It is important that you participate in an infant/child CPR class in your community.

This section may be photocopied and distributed to families.

From Wong DL, Hess CS: *Wong and Whaley's Clinical manual of pediatric nursing,* ed 5. Copyright © 2000, Mosby, St Louis.

Infant Cardiopulmonary Resuscitation (CPR)*—cont'd

b. Give two slow breaths about 1 to 1½ seconds in length, pausing to inhale between them. Each breath should be just enough to make the chest rise.

7. If you do not see the chest rise, reposition the head and try again. After repositioning the head, if you still cannot see the chest rise, then follow the instructions for caring for the choking infant (p. 645).

8. If the infant vomits, turn his head to the side and clean out the mouth with your finger or the bulb syringe.

CIRCULATION

9. After giving two breaths and seeing the chest rise, if the infant does not start breathing on his own, check his pulse.

10. Lightly place your index and middle fingers on the inside of the infant's elbow on the side closest to his body (Fig. 3). Feel for a pulse for 5 seconds. Practice this before an emergency arises to become used to finding the pulse.

11. When there is a pulse but no breathing, continue rescue breathing until the infant starts breathing. For an infant, the rate should be one breath every 3 seconds, or 20 per minute. Rescue breathing may be all that is needed to restart the infant's breathing. If breathing resumes, see step 18.

12. Begin cardiac compressions if there is no pulse.

13. Locate the correct position for chest compressions. Use one hand to hold the infant's head in the correct position. (See Fig. 1). Using the other hand, draw an imaginary line connecting the infant's nipples and place two fingers at a spot one finger's width below the imaginary line on the breastbone (Fig. 4).

14. Using your middle and ring fingers, press straight down on the breast bone for a distance of ½ to 1 inch. Repeat this 5 times. After each 5 compressions, stop and give the infant one breath of air (Fig. 5).

15. Compress the chest at least 100 times per minute. To keep from going too fast, count 1, 2, 3, 4, 5 in your head.

16. After about 1 minute, stop and check the infant to see if he has begun breathing or has a pulse. Call the emergency number (911) if you are alone. If you need to move the infant to get help or to get out of danger, try not to stop CPR for more than 5 seconds.

17. CPR may be stopped only if one of the following occurs:
    a. The infant begins breathing and the heart rate returns to normal.
    b. You are relieved by someone who can do CPR.
    c. You reach medical assistance and other action is begun.
    d. You are exhausted.

18. *Recovery position*—If the infant begins breathing on his own and there is no suspected injury, place infant on his side with the head resting on his arm and with the top leg slightly bent at the knee and resting on the firm surface. (See recovery position, Fig. 6.) Write down a description of what occurred and immediately call the emergency phone number (911).

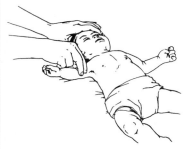

Fig. 3 Checking the arm (brachial) pulse.

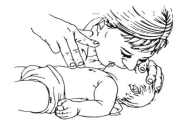

Fig. 5 Combining breathing with chest compressions.

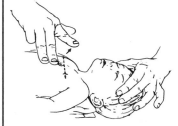

Fig. 4 Finding the proper location for chest compressions.

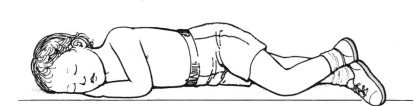

Fig. 6 Recovery position.

COMMUNITY AND HOME CARE INSTRUCTIONS

Child Cardiopulmonary Resuscitation (CPR)*†

Cardiopulmonary resuscitation (CPR) is a way to do some of the work of the heart and lungs for a short time. The heart pumps the blood around the body to provide oxygen and nutrients to the different body systems. The lungs are a transfer spot: as the blood flows through the lungs, oxygen is picked up by the blood and carbon dioxide is released. When the child breathes, oxygen is brought into the body and carbon dioxide is breathed out.

Before beginning CPR, you must assess the child to determine if both breathing and the heart have stopped. CPR is done when the child's heart and breathing have stopped. You can breathe for the child by blowing air into the lungs. Between breaths, the chest falls and air flows out of the lungs. You can do the work of the heart by doing a chest compression. The heart can be squeezed between the breastbone and the backbone to force blood out of the heart and into the arteries that carry it to the rest of the body. When you remove the pressure, the heart fills with blood so that the next squeeze (compression) will force additional blood out to the body.

All of the child's caregivers must be able to perform CPR so that you can have relief and help if needed. Prepare for an emergency before it happens. Tape emergency information and telephone numbers to each phone in the house. Include 911 (if available in your area), the phone number that you are calling from, the address, and directions to the house. When calling in an emergency, be sure to give all of this information in addition to a description of what happened, who is involved, and the condition of the child. Do not hang up the phone until the emergency operator tells you to do so.

Equipment

Emergency telephone numbers

ASSESSMENT

1. If trauma is suspected, do not move the child's head or neck. Avoid moving child unless she is in danger of further injury. If you need to turn the child over, roll the head and torso as a unit, supporting head and neck to prevent movement that could cause further injury.
2. Try to wake the child. Tap the child, say her name loudly, clap your hands, or shake gently to look for a response or movement.
3. Shout for help.
4. If child is still unresponsive, begin CPR at once by opening the child's airway (see below).
5. If there is someone else with you, have them call the emergency telephone number (911) for help. If you are alone, do not stop to call, but begin CPR immediately. Do CPR for 1 minute, then call the emergency numbers as quickly as possible. *If the child is 8 years old or older, call the emergency telephone number (911) for help before beginning CPR. ***

AIRWAY

1. Place the child on her back on a *firm* surface.
2. Properly position the head and open the airway by placing your hand on the forehead and placing the fingers (not thumb) of your other hand under the bony part of the lower jaw near the middle of the chin. Then lift and slightly tilt the head backward to a sniffing or nose pointing to the ceiling position. Be careful not to push the forehead too far back or to put too much pressure on the skin under the jaw. Make sure the child's lips are open. Proper positioning is essential to allow air to enter the windpipe to the lungs (Fig. 1).

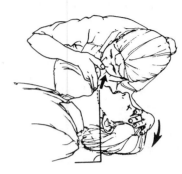

Fig. 1 Proper positioning to open the child's airway.

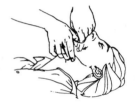

Fig. 2 Finger sweep to remove object from mouth.

3. If vomit is present, you must clear the child's mouth before you breathe for the child.
4. Quickly remove any mucus or vomit with your fingers after turning the child's head to the side.
   a. If you see an object, vomit, or mucus, insert a finger of your other hand inside the mouth (Fig. 2).
   b. Move your finger toward you across the back of the throat. This sweeping action will help remove foreign objects.

Figures reproduced with permission from Chandra NC, Hazinski MF: *Basic life support for healthcare providers,* Dallas, 1994, American Heart Association.

*Instructions are for children between 1 and 8 years old. The sections in italics are for children older than 8 years.

†These guidelines should not be used as substitutes for basic life support (BLS) training. It is important that you participate in an infant/child CPR class in your community.

This section may be photocopied and distributed to families.

Unit 5

COMMUNITY AND HOME CARE INSTRUCTIONS

Child Cardiopulmonary Resuscitation (CPR)—cont'd

BREATHING

5. Once the mouth is clear, reposition the child's head and observe the chest to determine if breathing has begun. Place your ear close to the child's mouth and look, listen, and feel for breathing for 3 to 5 seconds.

6. If breathing has not begun, you must breathe for the child:
   a. Open your mouth and cover the child's mouth with your mouth (Fig. 3). For a larger child, pinch the nose closed with the thumb and forefinger of the hand you have on the forehead.
   b. Give two slow breaths about 1 to 1½ seconds in length, pausing to inhale between them. Each breath should be just enough to make the chest rise.

7. If you do not see the chest rise, reposition the head and try again. After repositioning the head, if you still cannot see the chest rise, then follow the instructions for caring for the choking child. (See p. 648.)

8. If the child vomits, turn her head to the side and clean out the mouth with your finger.

CIRCULATION

9. After giving two breaths and seeing the chest rise, if the child does not start breathing on her own, check her pulse.

10. Lightly place your index and middle fingers on the child's windpipe. Slide your fingers into the groove between the windpipe and the neck muscles (Fig. 4). Feel for a pulse for 5 to 10 seconds. Practice this before an emergency arises to become used to finding the pulse.

11. When there is a pulse but no breathing, rescue breathing should be started and continued until the child resumes breathing. For a child 1 to 8 years old, the rate should be one breath every 3 seconds, or 20 per minute.
    For children 8 years and older, the rate should be one breath

every 5 seconds, or 12 per minute. Rescue breathing may be all that is needed to restart the child's breathing. If breathing resumes, see step 18.

12. Begin cardiac compressions if there is no pulse.

13. Locate the correct position for chest compressions. Use one hand to maintain the child's head position. Using two fingers of your other hand, find the place on the child's lower chest where the ribs meet the breast bone. Feel the notch: you must avoid pressing at this spot. Place the heel of your hand on the breast bone between the nipple line (an imaginary line connecting the nipples) and the notch. The fingers of the hand on the chest should be pointing away from you, across the child's chest (Fig. 5).
    For children 8 years and older, place the hand closest to the child's head on the breastbone next to the index finger on the chest. Then place the hand that you used to mark the place on the child's chest on top of your other hand. Your fingers can be

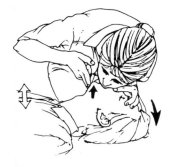

Fig. 3 Covering the mouth and pinching the nose for breathing.

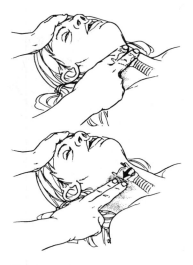

Fig. 4 Finding proper location of neck pulse.

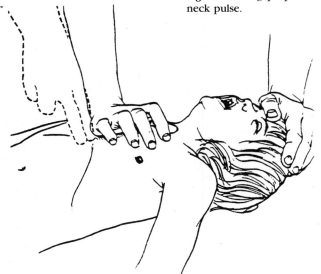

Fig. 5 Locating position for chest compression in the child.

Unit 5

Child Cardiopulmonary Resuscitation (CPR)—cont'd

interlaced or straight; your arms must be straight and your shoulders above your hands (Figs. 6 and 7).

14. Using one hand, press straight down on the breastbone for a distance of 1 to 1½ inches. Repeat this 5 times. After each 5 compressions, stop and give the child one breath of air. Keep your other hand on the head to maintain the head in the right position. *For children 8 years and older, using both hands, press*

straight down on the breastbone for a distance of 1½ to 2 inches. Repeat this 15 times. After each 15 compressions, give the child two breaths of air. Remember to correctly reposition the head when you breathe for the child. (See step 2 and Fig. 8.)

15. Compress the chest 100 times per minute. To keep from going too fast, count 1, 2, 3, 4, 5 in your head.

16. After about 1 minute, stop and check the child to see if he has begun breathing. Then check the pulse for 5 seconds. *For children 8 years and older, after 4 cycles of 15 compressions and two breaths, stop and check pulse.* Call the emergency number (911) as quickly as possible if you are alone. If you need to move the child to get help or to get out of danger, try not to stop CPR for more than 5 seconds.

17. CPR may be stopped only if one of the following occurs:
    a. The child begins breathing and the heart rate returns to normal.
    b. You are relieved by someone who can do CPR.
    c. You reach medical assistance and other action is begun.
    d. You are exhausted.

18. *Recovery position*—If breathing resumes and there is no suspected injury, roll the child onto his side moving the head, shoulders, and trunk at the same time without twisting. Place the child's head resting on his hand and slightly bend the top leg at the knee, resting it on the floor or surface (see Fig. 9). If the child begins breathing on his own, write down a description of what occurred and immediately call the emergency phone number (911).

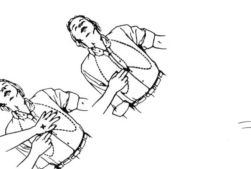

Fig. 6 Locating chest compression position in the child over 8 years of age.

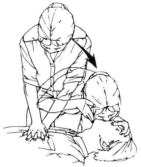

Fig. 8 Performing chest compressions and breathing for the child over 8 years of age.

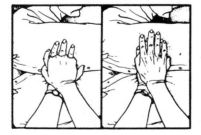

Fig. 7 Chest compression in the child over 8 years of age.

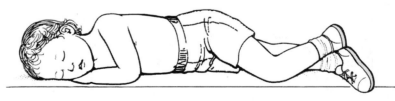

Fig. 9 Recovery position.

COMMUNITY AND HOME CARE INSTRUCTIONS

Caring for the Choking Infant*

Choking is a very serious, life-threatening event. If the infant begins to choke or is having difficulty breathing, immediate action is needed. When the airway is blocked, the infant cannot cry or make sounds. If the infant is coughing, his color is pink, and he can make sounds, no action may be needed.

AWAKE AND ALERT (CONSCIOUS) INFANT

1. Look at the infant to see if he is having difficulty breathing.
2. If the infant is not making sounds, appears to be choking, has a dusky color, and difficulty breathing, take action immediately:
   a. Position the infant face down on your forearm. Hold the head and neck firmly with one hand. If the infant is large, it may be necessary to support his weight on your thigh.
   b. Give up to five quick blows between the shoulder blades with the heel of your hand (Fig. 1).
3. If this does not remove the object, give up to five chest thrusts.
   a. Draw an imaginary line connecting the child's nipples.
   b. Place your fingers on the breastbone, one finger's width below the imaginary line (Fig. 2).
   c. Using your middle and ring fingers, thrust straight down on the breastbone a distance of ½ to 1 inch (Fig. 3).

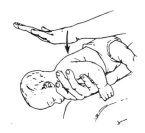

Fig. 1 Back blows in the infant.

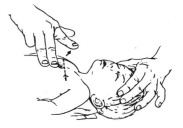

Fig. 2 Location of position for chest thrusts in the infant.

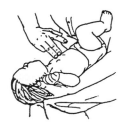

Fig. 3 Performing chest thrusts in the infant.

4. Repeat steps 2 and 3 until the airway is clear and the infant begins breathing or until the infant becomes unconscious. If the infant becomes unconscious, call the emergency number (911) at once.

INFANT BECOMES UNCONSCIOUS

1. If the infant becomes unconscious, place him on a *firm,* flat surface and call for help.
2. Check the inside of the infant's mouth to see if there is a foreign object.
3. Open the infant's mouth, using your thumb and fingers to grasp both the tongue and lower jaw and lift up gently (Fig. 4).
4. If you see an object, insert a finger of your other hand inside the infant's mouth and move your finger toward you across the back of the infant's throat (Fig. 5). This

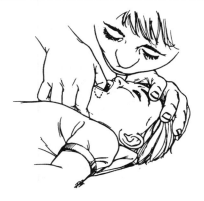

Fig. 4 Opening the mouth to look for an object.

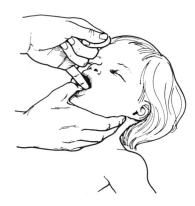

Fig. 5 Removing foreign object with finger.

sweeping action will help remove the foreign object. Be careful not to push it farther into the throat. If no object is seen, do not sweep out the mouth.

5. If the infant does not begin breathing, properly position the head and open the airway by placing your hand on the forehead and place the fingers (not thumb) of your other hand under the bony part of the lower jaw near the middle of the chin. Then lift and slightly tilt the head backward to a sniffing or nose

Unit 5

Figures reproduced with permission from Chandra NC, Hazinski MF: *Textbook of basic life support for healthcare providers,* Dallas, 1994, American Heart Association.

*These guidelines should not be used as substitutes for basic life support (BLS) training. It is important that you participate in an infant/child CPR class in your community.

This section may be photocopied and distributed to families.

Continued

COMMUNITY AND HOME CARE INSTRUCTIONS

Caring for the Choking Infant—cont'd

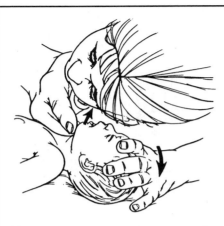

Fig. 6   Proper position for opening the airway.

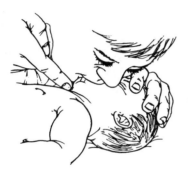

Fig. 7   Covering the nose and mouth for breathing.

pointing to ceiling position. Proper positioning is essential to allow the air to enter the windpipe to the lungs (Fig. 6).

6. If vomit is present, you must clear the infant's mouth before you give the breath.

7. Cover the infant's mouth and nose with your mouth. Give one breath and watch to see if the chest rises (Fig. 7). If the chest does not rise with the breath, place the infant on your forearm with his face down. Give him up to five quick blows between the shoulder blades with the heel of your hand. (See Fig. 1.)

8. Quickly turn the infant onto his back and give up to five chest thrusts.
    a. Draw an imaginary line connecting the child's nipples.
    b. Place your finger on the breastbone, one finger's width below the imaginary line. (See Fig. 2.)
    c. Using your index and middle fingers, thrust straight down on the breastbone a distance of ½ to 1 inch. (See Fig. 3.)

9. Quickly place the infant on a firm, flat surface and check the infant's mouth again. If an object is seen, attempt to remove it with a finger sweep. (See steps 3 and 4.)

10. Properly position the head (See step 5.) and give a breath. Watch to see if the chest rises (Fig. 7).

11. Keep repeating steps 2 through 10 until the infant's airway is cleared and you can see his chest rise with your breath. Give a second breath.

12. When the obstruction is removed, check the brachial pulse for 5 to 10 seconds by placing your fingers on the inside of the upper arm (Fig. 8).

13. If the pulse is present but breathing is absent, breathe for the infant once every 3 seconds or 20 times each minute. (See Fig. 7.)

14. If the pulse is absent, start cycles of chest compressions and breaths (Fig. 9). Continue your actions until the infant begins breathing and the pulse returns, or until emergency help arrives.

INFANT FOUND UNCONSCIOUS

1. Try to wake the infant. Tap the infant, say his name loudly, clap your hands, or flick the bottom of his feet to look for a response or movement. Do not shake the infant.

2. Shout for help.

3. Begin CPR at once if infant is still unresponsive.

4. If there is someone else with you, have that person call the emer-

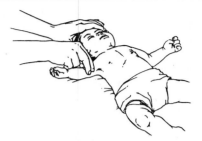

Fig. 8   Checking the arm (brachial) pulse.

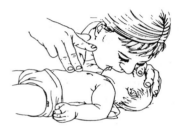

Fig. 9   Performing chest compressions and breathing for the infant.

gency telephone number (911) for help. If you are alone, do not stop to call, but begin CPR immediately. Do CPR for 1 minute, then call the emergency number as quickly as possible.

5. Place the infant on his back on a *firm* surface.

6. Properly position the head and open the airway by placing your hand on the forehead. Place the fingers (not thumb) of your other hand under the bony part of the lower jaw near the middle of the chin. Be careful not to push the forehead too far back or to put too much pressure on the skin under the jaw. Make sure the infant's lips are open. Then lift and slightly tilt the head backward to a sniffing or nose pointing to the ceiling position. Proper positioning is essential to allow air to enter the windpipe to the lungs (Fig. 6).

Unit 5

Caring for the Choking Infant—cont'd

7. If vomit is present, you must clear the infant's mouth before you breathe for the infant.

8. Quickly remove any mucus or vomit with your fingers or a bulb syringe after turning the infant's head to the side. If using a bulb syringe, squeeze it before placing it in the mouth, then release the pressure on the bulb to remove the material.
   a. If you see an object, vomit, or mucus, insert a finger of your other hand inside the mouth.
   b. Move your finger toward you across the back of the throat. This sweeping action will help remove foreign objects.

9. Once the mouth is clear, reposition the head and observe the chest to determine if the infant has begun breathing. Place your ear close to the infant's mouth and look, listen, and feel for breathing for 3 to 5 seconds.

10. If the infant does not begin breathing, give him a breath. Watch to see if the chest rises. (See Fig. 7.)

11. If the chest does not rise, reposition the infant's head and try to breathe again.

12. If the chest still does not rise, place the infant on your forearm with his face down. Give him up to five quick blows between the shoulder blades with the heel of your hand. (See Fig. 1.)

13. Quickly turn the infant onto his back and give up to five chest thrusts.
    a. Draw an imaginary line connecting the child's nipples.
    b. Place your finger on the breastbone, one finger's width below the imaginary line. (See Fig. 2.)
    c. Using your index and middle fingers, thrust straight down on the breastbone a distance of ½ to 1 inch. (See Fig. 3.)

14. Check the infant's mouth again. If an object is seen, attempt to remove it with a finger:
    a. Open the infant's mouth by grasping the tongue and lower jaw between your thumb and fingers. (See Fig. 4.)
    b. If you see an object, insert the index finger of your other hand inside the mouth on the side farthest from you and move your finger toward you across the back of the infant's throat. This sweeping motion will help remove the foreign object. Be careful not to push it farther into the throat. (See Fig. 5.)

15. Properly position the head and give a breath. Watch to see if the chest rises. (See Fig. 7.)

16. Keep repeating steps 8 through 15 until the infant's airway is cleared and you can see that his chest rises with your breath. Give a second breath.

17. Check the brachial pulse for 5 seconds by placing your fingers on the inside of the upper arm. (See Fig. 8.)

18. If the pulse is present but breathing is absent, breathe for the infant once every 3 seconds or 20 times each minute. (See Fig. 7.)

19. If the pulse is absent, start compressions. (See Fig. 9.) Continue your actions until the infant begins breathing and the pulse returns, or until emergency help arrives.

20. If the infant resumes breathing on his own, place him on his side with head resting on hand or arm and top leg slightly bent at the knee resting on the surface (Fig. 10). If the infant begins breathing on his own, write down a description of what occurred and immediately call the emergency phone number (911).

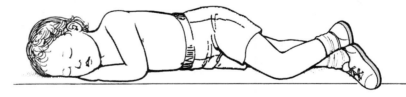

Fig. 10 Recovery position.

Unit 5

COMMUNITY AND HOME CARE INSTRUCTIONS

Caring for the Choking Child*

Choking is a very serious, life-threatening event. If a child begins to choke, or is having difficulty breathing, immediate action is needed. When the airway is blocked, the child cannot talk or make noises. If the child is coughing forcefully and can make sounds, no action is needed. If the child is not awake and alert, begin immediately with the directions for the unconscious child.

AWAKE AND ALERT (CONSCIOUS) CHILD—SITTING OR STANDING

1. Ask the child if he is choking. Check if he can talk or make noise. See if child is showing the universal sign of choking by clutching neck. If the child cannot make any sounds, then begin emergency treatment.
2. Stand or kneel behind the child (Fig. 1).
3. Wrap your arms around the child's waist. Make one hand into a fist.
4. Put your fist, with the thumb side against the child's skin, on the abdomen just above the belly button. Make sure you are well below the breastbone.
5. Grab the fist with your other hand. Press into the child's abdomen with upward thrusts until the object comes out or until the child loses consciousness.

6. Each thrust should be a separate movement. This allows enough force to help the child expel the object.
7. If the child still cannot breathe, continue the thrusting while calling for help.
8. Continue your actions until the object is removed, help arrives, or the child becomes unconscious. If the child becomes unconscious, call the emergency telephone number (911) at once.

AWAKE AND ALERT (CONSCIOUS) CHILD—LYING DOWN

1. If the child is on the floor, ask if the child is OK. If she cannot breathe or talk, place the child flat on her back.
2. Kneel on the floor at the child's feet. On a larger child you can straddle the legs.
3. Put the heel of one hand on the child's abdomen just above the belly button. Make sure you are well below the breastbone.
4. Put your other hand on top of the first hand and press into the child's abdomen with a quick upward thrust (Fig. 2).
5. Repeat the thrusts until the object comes out or until the child becomes unconscious. Each thrust should be a separate movement. This allows enough force to help the child expel the object.

6. Repeat steps 3, 4, and 5 until the object is removed, help arrives, or the child becomes unconscious. If the child becomes unconscious, call the emergency number (911) at once.

CHILD BECOMES UNCONSCIOUS

1. If the child is not already on the floor, place the child on a *firm,* flat surface such as the floor.
2. Kneel on the floor next to the child.
3. Open the child's mouth. Use your thumb and fingers to grasp both the tongue and lower jaw and lift (Fig. 3).
4. If you can see an object, insert a finger of your other hand inside the child's mouth. Move your finger toward you across the back of the throat and remove the object (Fig. 4). This sweeping

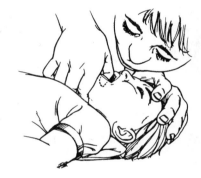

Fig. 3   Opening the mouth to look for an object.

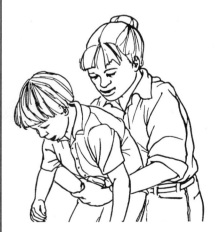

Fig. 1   Proper hand placement for abdominal thrusts.

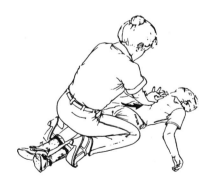

Fig. 2   Hand placement for abdominal thrusts with the child lying down.

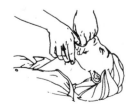

Fig. 4   Removing foreign object with finger.

Figures are reproduced with permission from Chandra NC, Hazinski MF: *Textbook of basic life support for healthcare providers,* Dallas, 1994, American Heart Association.

*These guidelines should not be used as substitutes for basic life support (BLS) training. It is important that you participate in an infant/child CPR class in your community.

This section may be photocopied and distributed to families.

Unit 5

COMMUNITY AND HOME CARE INSTRUCTIONS

Caring for the Choking Child—cont'd

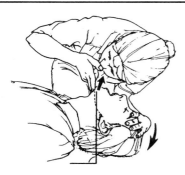

Fig. 5 Opening the airway and checking for breathing.

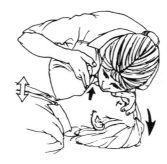

Fig. 6 Covering the mouth and pinching the nose for breathing.

action will help remove the foreign object. Be careful not to push it further into the throat. If no object is seen, do not sweep out the mouth.

5. If the child does not begin breathing, open the airway and try to breathe for the child.
   a. To open the airway, gently lift the chin with the fingers of one hand on the lower jaw near the middle of the chin, while pushing down on the forehead with your other hand. Tilt the child's head into a sniffing or nose pointing to the ceiling position.
   b. Lift the chin so that the teeth are almost together while listening for breathing (Fig. 5).
   c. If the child does not begin breathing at once, pinch the child's nostrils with your thumb and forefinger while keeping the child's head in the right position.
   d. Open your mouth wide, take a deep breath, make a tight seal over the child's mouth, and try to breathe for child (Fig. 6).
   e. Watch to see if the child's chest rises with your breath.
   f. If the child's chest still does not rise, get ready to do abdominal thrusts.
6. Kneel on the floor at the child's feet. On a larger child you can straddle the child's legs. (See Fig. 2.)

7. Put the heel of one hand on the child's abdomen just above the belly button. Make sure you are well below the breastbone.
8. Put your other hand on top of the first hand and press into the child's abdomen with a quick upward thrust.
9. Repeat up to five abdominal thrusts if needed. Each thrust should be a separate movement. This allows enough force to help the child expel the object.
10. Repeat steps 3 through 9 until the object is removed and the child is breathing, or until emergency help arrives. As soon as the obstruction is removed, give the child one breath. If the chest rises, give another breath, then check for a pulse.

    If a pulse is present and the child is not breathing, give one rescue breath every 3 seconds for a child 1 to 8 years old or one rescue breath every 5 seconds for a child 8 years or older until the child resumes breathing. If the pulse is absent, begin chest compressions as described in Child Cardiopulmonary Resuscitation. (See p. 643.) Continue CPR until emergency help arrives or until the child begins breathing and the pulse returns.

CHILD FOUND UNCONSCIOUS

1. Try to wake the child. Tap the child, say his name loudly, clap your hands, or shake gently to look for a response or movement.
2. Call for help. If someone comes to help, tell them to call the emergency telephone number (911).
3. If the child is not already on the floor, place the child on a *firm,* flat surface such as the floor.
4. Kneel on the floor next to the child.
5. If the child is not breathing, open the airway and try to breathe for the child:
   a. To open the airway, gently lift the chin with one hand while pushing down on the forehead with your other hand. Tilt the child's head into a sniffing or nose to the ceiling position.
   b. Lift the chin so the teeth are almost together while listening for breathing (Fig. 5).
   c. If the child does not breathe after 5 seconds, pinch the child's nostrils with your thumb and forefinger while keeping the child's head in the right position.
   d. Open your mouth wide, take a deep breath, make a tight seal over the child's mouth, and attempt to breathe for the child. (See Fig. 6.)
   e. Watch to see if the child's chest rises with your breath.
   f. If the child's chest does not rise, reposition the head and try to give a second breath. If the chest still does not rise, get ready to do abdominal thrusts.
   g. If you are alone, call the emergency telephone number (911).
6. Kneel on the floor at the child's feet. On a larger child you can straddle the child's legs. (See Fig. 2.)
7. Put the heel of one hand on the child's abdomen just above the belly button. Make sure you are well below the breastbone.
8. Put your other hand on top of the first hand and press into the child's abdomen with a quick upward thrust. (See Fig. 2.)

Unit 5

Continued

COMMUNITY AND HOME CARE INSTRUCTIONS

Caring for the Choking Child—cont'd

9. Repeat up to five abdominal thrusts if needed. Each thrust should be a separate movement. This allows enough force to help the child expel the object.

10. Open the child's mouth and check for a foreign object. Use your thumb and fingers to grasp both the tongue and lower jaw and lift. (See Fig. 3.)

11. If you can see an object, put a finger of your other hand inside the child's mouth. Move your finger toward you across the back of the throat and remove the object. (See Fig. 4.)

12. Repeat steps 5 through 11 until the object is removed and the child is breathing, or until emergency help arrives. As soon as the obstruction is removed, give the child one breath. If the chest rises, give another breath, then feel for a pulse (Fig. 7).

    If a pulse is present and the child is not breathing, give one rescue breath every 3 seconds until the child resumes breathing. If the pulse is absent, begin

chest compressions as described in Child Cardiopulmonary Resuscitation. (See p. 643.) Continue CPR until emergency help arrives or until the child begins breathing and the pulse returns.

13. If the child resumes breathing on his own, place him on his side by rolling the head, shoulders, and trunk together without twisting. Place the child's head resting on his head and slightly bend the top leg at the knee, resting it on the floor or surface (Fig. 8). If the child begins breathing on his own, write a description of what occurred and immediately call the emergency number (911).

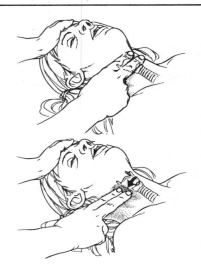

Fig. 7 Finding location of neck pulse.

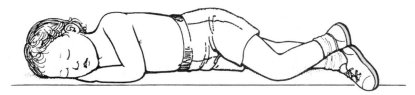

Fig. 8 Recovery position.

Reference Data

ABBREVIATIONS USED IN LABORATORY TESTS

Abbreviation	Term
cap	capillary
CHF	congestive heart failure
conc.	concentration
CSF	cerebrospinal fluid
d	day; diem
EDTA	ethylenediaminetetraacetic acid
g	gram
m	meter
hr	hour
L, l	liter
mEq	milliequivalent
min	minute
mm	millimeter
mm^3	cubic millimeter
mo	month
mol	mole
mmol	millimole
mosmol	milliosmole
s	second
SI	International System of Units
Therap.	therapeutic
U	International Unit of enzyme activity
vol	volume
wk	week
yr	year
>	greater than
≥	greater than or equal to
<	less than
≤	less than or equal to
±	plus/minus
≈	approximately equal to

PREFIXES DENOTING DECIMAL FACTORS

Prefix	Symbol	Amount
deci	d	one tenth (10^{-1})
centi	c	one hundredth (10^{-2})
milli	m	one thousandth (10^{-3})
micro	μ	one millionth (10^{-6})
nano	n	one billionth (10^{-9})
pico	p	one trillionth (10^{-12})
femto	f	one quadrillionth (10^{-15})

COMMON LABORATORY TESTS*

Test/Specimen	Age/Sex/Reference	Conventional Units		International Units (SI)	
		Normal Ranges			
Acetaminophen					
Serum or plasma	Therap. conc.	10-30 µg/ml		66-200 µmol/L	
	Toxic conc.	>200 µg/ml		>1300 µmol/L	
Ammonia nitrogen					
Plasma or serum	Newborn	90-150 µg/dl		64-107 µmol/L	
	0-2 wk	79-129 µg/dl		56-92 µmol/L	
	>1 mo	29-70 µg/dl		21-50 µmol/L	
	Thereafter	15-45 µg/dl		11-32 µmol/L	
Urine, 24 hr		500-1200 mg/d		36-86 mmol/d	
Antistreptolysin O titer (ASO)					
Serum	2-4 yr	<160 Todd units			
	School-age children	170-330 Todd units			
Base excess					
Whole blood	Newborn	(−10)-(−2) mmol/L		(−10)-(−2) mmol/L	
	Infant	(−7)-(−1) mmol/L		(−7)-(−1) mmol/L	
	Child	(−4)-(+2) mmol/L		(−4)-(+2) mmol/L	
	Thereafter	(−3)-(+3) mmol/L		(−3)-(+3) mmol/L	
Bicarbonate (HCO_3)					
Serum	Arterial	21-28 mmol/L		21-28 mmol/L	
	Venous	22-29 mmol/L		22-29 mmol/L	
		Premature (mg/dl)	**Full term (mg/dl)**	**Premature (µmol/L)**	**Full term (µmol/L)**
Bilirubin, total					
Serum	Cord	<2.0	<2.0	<34	<34
	0.1 d	8.0	<6.0	<137	<103
	1-2 d	12.0	<8.0	<205	<137
	2-5 d	16.0	<12.0	<274	<205
	Thereafter	2.0	0.2-1.0	<34	3.4-17.1
Bilirubin, direct (conjugated)					
Serum		0-0.2 mg/dl		0-3.4 µmol/L	
Bleeding time					
Blood from skin puncture					
Ivy	Normal	2-7 min		2-7 min	
	Borderline	7-11 min		7-11 min	
Simplate (G-D)		2.75-8 min		2.75-8 min	
Blood volume					
Whole blood	Male	52-83 ml/kg		0.052-0.083 L/kg	
	Female	50-75 ml/kg		0.050-0.075 L/kg	
C-reactive protein (CRP)					
Serum	Cord	52-1330 ng/ml		52-1330 µg/L	
	2-12 yr	67-1800 ng/ml		67-1800 µg/L	
Calcium, ionized					
Serum, plasma, or whole blood	Cord	5.0-6.0 mg/dl		1.25-1.50 mmol/L	
	Newborn, 3-24 hr	4.3-5.1 mg/dl		1.07-1.27 mmol/L	
	24-48 hr	4.0-4.7 mg/dl		1.00-1.17 mmol/L	
	Thereafter	4.8-4.92 mg/dl		1.12-1.23 mmol/L	

Modified from Behrman RE and others, editors: *Nelson textbook of pediatrics*, ed 15, Philadelphia, 1996, WB Saunders.
*For a description of abbreviations see p. 652.

Continued

Unit 6

		Conventional Units	International Units (SI)
Test/Specimen	**Age/Sex/Reference**	**Normal Ranges**	
Calcium, total			
Serum	Cord	9.0-11.5 mg/dl	2.25-2.88 mmol/L
	Newborn, 3-24 hr	9.0-10.6 mg/dl	2.3-2.65 mmol/L
	24-48 hr	7.0-12.0 mg/dl	1.75-3.0 mmol/L
	4-7 d	9.0-10.9 mg/dl	2.25-2.73 mmol/L
	Child	8.8-10.8 mg/dl	2.2-2.70 mmol/L
	Thereafter	8.4-10.2 mg/dl	2.1-2.55 mmol/L
Carbon dioxide, partial pressure (P_{CO_2})			
Whole blood, arterial	Newborn	27-40 mm Hg	3.6-5.3 kPa
	Infant	27-41 mm Hg	3.6-5.5 kPa
	Thereafter: Male	35-48 mm Hg	4.7-6.4 kPa
	Female	32-45 mm Hg	4.3-6.0 kPa
Carbon dioxide, total (tCO_2)			
Serum or plasma	Cord	14-22 mEq/L	14-22 mmol/L
	Premature (1 wk)	14-27 mEq/L	14-27 mmol/L
	Newborn	13-22 mEq/L	13-22 mmol/L
	Infant, child	20-28 mEq/L	20-28 mmol/L
	Thereafter	23-30 mEq/L	23-30 mmol/L
Cerebrospinal fluid (CSF)			
Pressure		70-180 mm water	70-180 mm water
Volume	Child	60-100 ml	0.06-0.10 L
	Adult	100-160 ml	0.10-0.16 L
Chloride			
Serum or plasma	Cord	96-104 mmol/L	96-104 mmol/L
	Newborn	97-110 mmol/L	97-110 mmol/L
	Thereafter	98-106 mmol/L	98-106 mmol/L
Sweat	Normal (homozygote)	<40 mmol/L	<40 mmol/L
	Marginal (e.g., asthma, Addison disease, malnutrition)	45-60 mmol/L	45-60 mmol/L
	Cystic fibrosis	>60 mmol/L	>60 mmol/L
Cholesterol, total	1-3 yr	45-182 mg/dl	1.15-4.70 mmol/L
	4-6 yr	109-189 mg/dl	2.80-4.80 mmol/L

		Percentiles			*Percentiles*		
		5	**75**	**95**	**5**	**75**	**95**
	Male:						
	6-9 yr	126	172	191 mg/dL	3.26	4.45	4.94 mmol/L
	10-14 yr	130	179	204 mg/dL	3.36	4.63	5.28 mmol/L
	15-19 yr	114	167	198 mg/dL	2.95	4.32	5.12 mmol/L

		Percentiles			*Percentiles*		
		5	**75**	**95**	**5**	**75**	**95**
	Female:						
	6-9 yr	122	173	209 mg/dL	3.16	4.47	5.41 mmol/L
	10-14 yr	124	174	217 mg/dL	3.21	4.50	5.61 mmol/L
	15-19 yr	125	175	212 mg/dL	3.23	4.53	5.48 mmol/L

		Conventional Units	International Units (SI)
Clotting time (Lee-White)			
Whole blood		5-8 min (glass tubes)	5-8 min
		5-15 min (room temp)	5-15 min
		30 min (silicone tube)	30 min

Test/Specimen	Age/Sex/Reference	Conventional Units	International Units (SI)
		Normal Ranges	
Creatine kinase (CK, CPK)			
Serum	Cord blood	70-380 U/L	70-380 U/L
	5-8 hr	214-1175 U/L	214-1175 U/L
	24-33 hr	130-1200 U/L	130-1200 U/L
	72-100 hr	87-725 U/L	87-725 U/L
	Adult	5-130 U/L	5-130 U/L
Creatinine			
Serum	Cord	0.6-1.2 mg/dl	53-106 µmol/L
	Newborn	0.3-1.0 mg/dl	27-88 µmol/L
	Infant	0.2-0.4 mg/dl	18-35 µmol/L
	Child	0.3-0.7 mg/dl	27-62 µmol/L
	Adolescent	0.5-1.0 mg/dl	44-88 µmol/L
	Adult: Male	0.6-1.2 mg/dl	53-106 µmol/L
	Female	0.5-1.1 mg/dl	44-97 µmol/L
Urine, 24 hr	Premature	8.1-15.0 mg/kg/24 hr	72-133 µmol/kg/24 hr
	Full term	10.4-19.7 mg/kg/24 hr	92-174 µmol/kg/24 hr
	1.5-7 yr	10-15 mg/kg/24 hr	88-133 µmol/kg/24 hr
	7-15 yr	5.2-41 mg/kg/24 hr	46-362 µmol/kg/24 hr
Creatinine clearance (endogenous)			
Serum or plasma and urine	Newborn	40-65 ml/min/1.73 m^2	
	<40 yr: Male	97-137 ml/min/1.73 m^2	
	Female	88-128 ml/min/1.73 m^2	
Digoxin			
Serum, plasma; collect at least 12 hr after dose	Therap. conc.		
	CHF	0.8-1.5 ng/ml	1.0-1.9 nmol/L
	Arrhythmias	1.5-2.0 ng/ml	1.9-2.6 nmol/L
	Toxic conc.		
	Child	>2.5 ng/ml	>3.2 nmol/L
	Adult	>3.0 ng/ml	>3.8 nmol/L
Eosinophil count			
Whole blood, capillary blood		50-350 cells/mm^3 (µl)	50-350 × 10^6 cells/L
Erythrocyte (RBC) count			
Whole blood	Cord	3.9-5.5 million/mm^3	3.9-5.5 × 10^{12} cells/L
	1-3 d	4.0-6.6 million/mm^3	4.0-6.6 × 10^{12} cells/L
	1 wk	3.9-6.3 million/mm^3	3.9-6.3 × 10^{12} cells/L
	2 wk	3.6-6.2 million/mm^3	3.6-6.2 × 10^{12} cells/L
	1 mo	3.0-5.4 million/mm^3	3.0-5.4 × 10^{12} cells/L
	2 mo	2.7-4.9 million/mm^3	2.7-4.9 × 10^{12} cells/L
	3-6 mo	3.1-4.5 million/mm^3	3.1-4.5 × 10^{12} cells/L
	0.5-2 yr	3.7-5.3 million/mm^3	3.7-5.3 × 10^{12} cells/L
	2-6 yr	3.9-5.3 million/mm^3	3.9-5.3 × 10^{12} cells/L
	6-12 yr	4.0-5.2 million/mm^3	4.0-5.2 × 10^{12} cells/L
	12-18 yr: Male	4.5-5.3 million/mm^3	4.5-5.3 × 10^{12} cells/L
	Female	4.1-5.1 million/mm^3	4.1-5.1 × 10^{12} cells/L
Erythrocyte sedimentation rate (ESR)			
Whole blood			
Westergren (modified)	Child	0-10 mm/hr	0-10 mm/hr
	<50 yr: Male	0-15 mm/hr	0-15 mm/hr
	Female	0-20 mm/hr	0-20 mm/hr
Wintrobe	Child	0-13 mm/hr	0-13 mm/hr
	Adult: Male	0-9 mm/hr	0-9 mm/hr
	Female	0-20 mm/hr	0-20 mm/hr

Continued

Unit 6

		Conventional Units		International Units (SI)	
Test/Specimen	**Age/Sex/Reference**	**Normal Ranges**			
Fibrinogen					
Plasma	Newborn	125-300 mg/dl		1.25-3.00 g/L	
	Thereafter	200-400 mg/dl		2.00-4.00 g/L	
Galactose					
Serum	Newborn	0-20 mg/dl		0-1.11 mmol/L	
Urine	Newborn	≤60 mg/dl		≤3.33 mmol/L	
	Thereafter	<14 mg/24 hr		<0.08 mmol/24 hr	
Glucose					
Serum	Cord	45-96 mg/dl		2.5-5.3 mmol/L	
	Newborn, 1 d	40-60 mg/dl		2.2-3.3 mmol/L	
	Newborn, >1 d	50-90 mg/dl		2.8-5.0 mmol/L	
	Child	60-100 mg/dl		3.3-5.5 mmol/L	
	Thereafter	70-105 mg/dl		3.9-5.8 mmol/L	
Whole blood	Adult	65-95 mg/dl		3.6-5.3 mmol/L	
CSF	Adult	40-70 mg/dl		2.2-3.9 mmol/L	
Urine (quantitative)		<0.5 g/d		<2.8 mmol/d	
(Qualitative)		Negative		Negative	
Glucose tolerance test (GTT), oral Serum					

		Normal	**Diabetic**	**Normal**	**Diabetic**
Dosages					
Adult: 75 g	Fasting	70-105 mg/dl	>115 mg/dl	3.9-5.8 mmol/L	>6.4 mmol/L
Child: 1.75 g/kg of ideal	60 min	120-170 mg/dl	≥200 mg/dl	6.7-9.4 mmol/L	≥11 mmol/L
weight up to maximum	90 min	100-140 mg/dl	≥200 mg/dl	5.6-7.8 mmol/L	≥11 mmol/L
of 75 g	120 min	70-120 mg/dl	≥140 mg/dl	3.9-6.7 mmol/L	≥7.8 mmol/L

		Conventional Units		International Units (SI)	
Growth hormone (hGH, somatotropin)					
Plasma	Cord	10-50 ng/ml		10-50 µg/L	
Fasting, at rest	Newborn	10-40 ng/ml		10-40 µg/L	
	Child	<5 ng/ml		<5 µg/L	
	Adult: Male	<5 ng/ml		<5 µg/L	
	Female	<8 ng/ml		<8 µg/L	
Hematocrit (HCT, Hct)					
Whole blood	I d (cap)	48%-69%		0.48-0.69 vol. fraction	
	2 d	48%-75%		0.48-0.75 vol. fraction	
	3 d	44%-72%		0.44-0.72 vol. fraction	
	2 mo	28%-42%		0.28-0.42 vol. fraction	
	6-12 yr	35%-45%		0.35-0.45 vol. fraction	
	12-18 yr: Male	37%-49%		0.37-0.49 vol. fraction	
	Female	36%-46%		0.36-0.46 vol. fraction	
Hemoglobin (Hb)					
Whole blood	1-3 d (cap)	14.5-22.5 g/dl		2.25-3.49 mmol/L	
	2 mo	9.0-14.0 g/dl		1.40-2.17 mmol/L	
	6-12 yr	11.5-15.5 g/dl		1.78-2.40 mmol/L	
	12-18 yr: Male	13.0-16.0 g/dl		2.02-2.48 mmol/L	
	Female	12.0-16.0 g/dl		1.86-2.48 mmol/L	
Hemoglobin A (HbA)					
Whole blood		>95% of total		0.95 fraction of Hb	

Test/Specimen	Age/Sex/Reference	Conventional Units	International Units (SI)
		Normal Ranges	
Hemoglobin F (HbF)			
Whole blood	1 d	63%-92% HbF	0.63-0.92 mass fraction HbF
	5 d	65%-88% HbF	0.65-0.88 mass fraction HbF
	3 wk	55%-85% HbF	0.55-0.85 mass fraction HbF
	6-9 wk	31%-75% HbF	0.31-0.75 mass fraction HbF
	3-4 mo	<2%-59% HbF	<0.02-0.59 mass fraction HbF
	6 mo	<2%-9% HbF	<0.02-0.09 mass fraction HbF
	Adult	<2.0% HbF	<0.02 mass fraction HbF
Immunoglobulin A (IgA)			
Serum	Cord blood	1.4-3.6 mg/dl	14-36 mg/L
	1-3 mo	1.3-53 mg/dl	13-530 mg/L
	4-6 mo	4.4-84 mg/dl	44-840 mg/L
	7 mo-1 yr	11-106 mg/dl	110-1060 mg/L
	2-5 yr	14-159 mg/dl	140-1590 mg/L
	6-10 yr	33-236 mg/dl	330-2360 mg/L
	Adult	70-312 mg/dl	700-3120 mg/L
Immunoglobulin D (IgD)			
Serum	Newborn	None detected	None detected
	Thereafter	0-8 mg/dl	0-80 mg/L
Immunoglobulin E (IgE)			
Serum	Male	0-230 IU/ml	0-230 kIU/L
	Female	0-170 IU/ml	0-170 kIU/L
Immunoglobulin G (IgG)			
Serum	Cord blood	636-1606 mg/dl	6.36-16.06 g/L
	1 mo	251-906 mg/dl	2.51-9.06 g/L
	2-4 mo	176-601 mg/dl	1.76-6.01 g/L
	5-12 mo	172-1069 mg/dl	1.72-10.69 g/L
	1-5 yr	345-1236 mg/dl	3.45-12.36 g/L
	6-10 yr	608-1572 mg/dl	6.08-15.72 g/L
	Adult	639-1349 mg/dl	6.39-13.49 g/L
Immunoglobulin M (IgM)			
Serum	Cord blood	6.3-25 mg/dl	63-250 mg/L
	1 mo-4 mo	17-105 mg/dl	170-1050 mg/L
	5 mo-9 mo	33-126 mg/dl	330-1260 mg/L
	10 mo-1 yr	41-173 mg/dl	410-1730 mg/L
	2-8 yr	43-207 mg/dl	430-2070 mg/L
	9-10 yr	52-242 mg/dl	520-2420 mg/L
	Adult	56-352 mg/dl	560-3520 mg/L
Iron			
Serum	Newborn	100-250 µg/dl	17.90-44.75 µmol/L
	Infant	40-100 µg/dl	7.16-17.90 µmol/L
	Child	50-120 µg/dl	8.95-21.48 µmol/L
	Thereafter: Male	50-160 µg/dl	8.95-28.64 µmol/L
	Female	40-150 µg/dl	7.16-26.85 µmol/L
	Intoxicated child	280-2550 µg/dl	50.12-456.5 µmol/L
	Fatally poisoned child	>1800 µg/dl	>322.2 µmol/L
Iron-binding capacity, total (TIBC)			
Serum	Infant	100-400 µg/dl	17.90-71.60 µmol/L
	Thereafter	250-400 µg/dl	44.75-71.60 µmol/L
Lead			
Whole blood	Child	<10 µg/dl	<0.48 µmol/L
Urine, 24 hr		<80 µg/L	<0.39 µmol/L

Continued

Unit 6

Test/Specimen	Age/Sex/Reference	Conventional Units		International Units (SI)
		Normal Ranges		
Leukocyte count (WBC count) (Whole blood)		×1000 cells/mm³ (µl)		×10⁹ cells/L
	Birth	9.0-30.0		9.0-30.0
	24 hr	9.4-34.0		9.4-34.0
	1 mo	5.0-19.5		5.0-19.5
	1-3 yr	6.0-17.5		6.0-17.5
	4-7 yr	5.5-15.5		5.5-15.5
	8-13 yr	4.5-13.5		4.5-13.5
	Adult	4.5-11.0		4.5-11.0
		×1000 cells/mm³ (µl)		×10⁹ cells/L
CSF	Premature	0-25 mononuclear		0-25
		0-100 polymorphonuclear		1-100
		0-1000 RBC		0-1000
	Newborn	0-20 mononuclear		0-20
		0-70 polymorphonuclear		0-70
		0-800 RBC		0-800
	Neonate	0-5 mononuclear		0-5
		0-25 polymorphonuclear		0-25
		0-50 RBC		0-50
	Thereafter	0-5 mononuclear		0-5
Leukocyte differential count Whole blood				
	Myelocytes	0%	0 cells/mm³ (µl)	Number fraction 0
	Neutrophils—"bands"	3%-5%	150-400 cells/mm³ (µl)	Number fraction 0.03-0.05
	Neutrophils—"segs"	54%-62%	3000-5800 cells/mm³ (µl)	Number fraction 0.54-0.62
	Lymphocytes	25%-33%	1500-3000 cells/mm³ (µl)	Number fraction 0.25-0.33
	Monocytes	3%-7%	285-500 cells/mm³ (µl)	Number fraction 0.03-0.07
	Eosinophils	1%-3%	50-250 cells/mm³ (µl)	Number fraction 0.01-0.03
	Basophils	0%-0.75%	15-50 cells/mm³ (µl)	Number fraction 0-0.0075
Mean corpuscular hemoglobin (MCH) Whole blood				
	Birth	31-37 pg/cell		0.48-0.57 fmol/L
	1-3 d (cap)	31-37 pg/cell		0.48-0.57 fmol/L
	1 wk-1 mo	28-40 pg/cell		0.43-0.62 fmol/L
	2 mo	26-34 pg/cell		0.40-0.53 fmol/L
	3-6 mo	25-35 pg/cell		0.39-0.54 fmol/L
	0.5-2 yr	23-31 pg/cell		0.36-0.48 fmol/L
	2-6 yr	24-30 pg/cell		0.37-0.47 fmol/L
	6-12 yr	25-33 pg/cell		0.39-0.51 fmol/L
	12-18 yr	25-35 pg/cell		0.39-0.54 fmol/L
	18-49 yr	26-34 pg/cell		0.40-0.53 fmol/L

Unit 6

Test/Specimen	Age/Sex/Reference	Conventional Units	International Units (SI)
		Normal Ranges	
Mean corpuscular hemoglobin concentration (MCHC)			
Whole blood	Birth	30%-36% Hb/cell or g Hb/dl RBC	4.65-5.58 mmol or Hb/L RBC
	1-3 d (cap)	29%-37% Hb/cell or g Hb/dl RBC	4.50-5.74 mmol or Hb/L RBC
	1-2 wk	28%-38% Hb/cell or g Hb/dl RBC	4.34-5.89 mmol or Hb/L RBC
	1-2 mo	29%-37% Hb/cell or g Hb/dl RBC	4.50-5.74 mmol or Hb/L RBC
	3 mo-2 yr	30%-36% Hb/cell or g Hb/dl RBC	4.65-5.58 mmol or Hb/L RBC
	2-18 yr	31%-37% Hb/cell or g Hb/dl RBC	4.81-5.74 mmol or Hb/L RBC
	>18 yr	31%-37% Hb/cell or g Hb/dl RBC	4.81-5.74 mmol or Hb/L RBC
Mean corpuscular volume (MCV)			
Whole blood	1-3 d (cap)	95-121 μm^3	95-121 fl
	0.5-2 yr	70-86 μm^3	70-86 fl
	6-12 yr	77-95 μm^3	77-95 fl
	12-18 yr: Male	78-98 μm^3	78-98 fl
	Female	78-102 μm^3	78-102 fl
Osmolality			
Serum	Child, adult:	275-295 mOsmol/kg H_2O	
Urine, random		50-1400 mOsmol/kg H_2O, depending on fluid intake; after 12 hr fluid restriction: >850 mOsmol/kg H_2O	
Urine, 24 hr		$\approx$300-900 mOsmol/kg H_2O	
Oxygen, partial pressure (Po_2)			
Whole blood, arterial	Birth	8-24 mm Hg	1.1-3.2 kPa
	5-10 min	33-75 mm Hg	4.4-10.0 kPa
	30 min	31-85 mm Hg	4.1-11.3 kPa
	>1 hr	55-80 mm Hg	7.3-10.6 kPa
	1 d	54-95 mm Hg	7.2-12.6 kPa
	Thereafter (decreases with age)	83-108 mm Hg	11-14.4 kPa
Oxygen saturation (Sao_2)			
Whole blood, arterial	Newborn	85%-90%	Fraction saturated 0.85-0.90
	Thereafter	95%-99%	Fraction saturated 0.95-0.99
Partial thromboplastin time (PTT)			
Whole blood (Na citrate)			
Nonactivated		60-85 s (Platelin)	60-85 s
Activated		25-35 s (differs with method)	25-35 s
pH			**H+ concentration**
Whole blood, arterial	Premature (48 hr)	7.35-7.50	31-44 nmol/L
	Birth, full term	7.11-7.36	43-77 nmol/L
	5-10 min	7.09-7.30	50-81 nmol/L
	30 min	7.21-7.38	41-61 nmol/L
	>1 hr	7.26-7.49	32-54 nmol/L
	1 d	7.29-7.45	35-51 nmol/L
	Thereafter	7.35-7.45	35-44 nmol/L
	Must be corrected for body temperature		

Continued

Unit 6

Test/Specimen	Age/Sex/Reference	Conventional Units	International Units (SI)
		Normal Ranges	
pH—cont'd			
Urine, random	Newborn/neonate	5-7	0.1-10 μmol/L
	Thereafter	4.5-8 (average ≈6)	0.01-32 μmol/L (average ~1.0 μmol/L)
Stool		7.0-7.5	31-100 nmol/L
Phenylalanine			
Serum	Premature	2.0-7.5 mg/dl	120-450 μmol/L
	Newborn	1.2-3.4 mg/dl	70-210 μmol/L
	Thereafter	0.8-1.8 mg/dl	50-110 μmol/L
Urine, 24 hr	10 d-2 wk	1-2 mg/d	6-12 μmol/d
	3-12 yr	4-18 mg/d	24-110 μmol/d
	Thereafter	trace-17 mg/d	trace-103 μmol/d
Plasma volume			
Plasma	Male	25-43 ml/kg	0.025-0.043 L/kg
	Female	28-45 ml/kg	0.028-0.045 L/kg
Platelet count (thrombocyte count)			
Whole blood (EDTA)	Newborn (After 1 wk, same as adult)	$84\text{-}478 \times 10^3/mm^3$ (μl)	$84\text{-}478 \times 10^9/L$
	Adult	$150\text{-}400 \times 10^3/mm^3$ (μl)	$150\text{-}400 \times 10^9/L$
Potassium			
Serum	Newborn	3.0-6.0 mmol/L	3.0-6.0 mmol/L
	Thereafter	3.5-5.0 mmol/L	3.5-5.0 mmol/L
Plasma (heparin)		3.4-4.5 mmol/L	3.4-4.5 mmol/L
Urine, 24 hr		2.5-125 mmol/L (varies with diet)	2.5-125 mmol/L
Protein			
Serum, total	Premature	4.3-7.6 g/dl	43-76 g/L
	Newborn	4.6-7.4 g/dl	46-74 g/L
	1-7 yr	6.1-7.9 g/dl	61-79 g/L
	8-12 yr	6.4-8.1 g/dl	64-81 g/L
	13-19 yr	6.6-8.2 g/dl	66-82 g/L
Total			
Urine, 24 hr		1-14 mg/dl	10-140 mg/L
		50-80 mg/d (at rest)	50-80 mg/d
		<250 mg/d (after intense exercise)	<250 mg/d after exercise
Total			
CSF		Lumbar: 8-32 mg/dl	80-320 mg/L
Prothrombin time (PT)			
One-stage (Quick)			
Whole blood (Na citrate)	In general	11-15 s (varies with type of thromboplastin)	11-15 sec
	Newborn	Prolonged by 2-3 sec	Prolonged by 2-3 sec
Two-stage modified (Ware and Seegers)			
Whole blood (Na citrate)		18-22 sec	18-22 sec
RBC count (See erythrocyte count)			
Red blood cell volume			
Whole blood	Male	20-36 ml/kg	0.020-0.036 L/kg
	Female	19-31 ml/kg	0.019-0.031 L/kg

Test/Specimen	Age/Sex/Reference	Conventional Units	International Units (SI)
		Normal Ranges	
Reticulocyte count			
Whole blood	Adults	0.5%-1.5% of erythrocytes or 25,000-75,000/mm³ (µl)	0.005-0.015 (number fraction)
			25,000-75,000 × 10⁶/L
Capillary	1 d	0.4%-6.0%	0.004-0.060 (number fraction)
	7 d	<0.1%-1.3%	<0.001-0.013 (number fraction)
	1-4 wk	<0.1%-1.2%	<0.001-0.012 (number fraction)
	5-6 wk	<0.1%-2.4%	<0.001-0.024 (number fraction)
	7-8 wk	0.1%-2.9%	0.001-0.029 (number fraction)
	9-10 wk	<0.1%-2.6%	<0.001-0.026 (number fraction)
	11-12 wk	0.1%-1.3%	0.001-0.013 (number fraction)
Salicylates			
Serum, plasma	Therap. conc.	15-30 mg/dl	1.1-2.2 mmol/L
	Toxic conc.	>30 mg/dl	>2.2 mmol/L
Sedimentation rate (See erythrocyte sedimentation rate)			
Sodium			
Serum or plasma	Newborn	134-146 mmol/L	134-146 mmol/L
	Infant	139-146 mmol/L	139-146 mmol/L
	Child	138-145 mmol/L	138-145 mmol/L
	Thereafter	136-146 mmol/L	136-146 mmol/L
Urine, 24 hr		40-220 mmol/L (diet dependent)	40-220 mmol/L
Sweat	Normal	<40 mmol/L	<40 mmol/L
	Indeterminate	45-60 mmol/L	45-60 mmol/L
	Cystic fibrosis	>60 mmol/L	>60 mmol/L
Specific, gravity			
Urine, random	Adult	1.002-1.030	1.002-1.030
	After 12 hr fluid restriction	>1.025	>1.025
Urine, 24 hr		1.015-1.025	
Theophylline			
Serum, plasma	Therap. conc.		
	Bronchodilator	10-20 µg/ml	56-110 µmol/L
	Premature apnea	6-10 µg/ml	28-56 µmol/L
	Toxic conc.	>20 µg/mL	>166 µmol/L
Thrombin time			
Whole blood (Na citrate)		Control time ±2 sec when control is 9-13 sec	Control time ±2 sec when control is 9-13 sec
Thyroxine, total			
Serum	Full-term infants:		
	1-3 d	8.2-19.9 µg/dL	106-256 nmol/L
	1 wk	6.0-15.9 µg/dL	77-205 nmol/L
	1-12 mo	6.1-14.9 µg/dL	79-192 nmol/L
	Prepubertal children:		
	1-3 yr	6.8-13.5 µg/dL	88-174 nmol/L
	3-10 yr	5.5-12.8 µg/dL	71-165 nmol/L
	Pubertal children and adults	4.2-13.0 µg/dL	54-167 nmol/L

Continued

Test/Specimen	Age/Sex/Reference	Conventional Units		International Units (SI)	
		Normal Ranges			
Tourniquet test (capillary fragility)		<5-10 petechiae in 2.5 cm circle on forearm (halfway between systolic and diastolic); pressure maintained for 5 min; 0-8 petechiae in 6 cm circle (50 torr for 15 min); 10-20 petechiae in 5 cm circle (80 mm Hg)		<5-10 petechiae in 2.5 cm circle on forearm (halfway between systolic and diastolic); pressure maintained for 5 min; 0-8 petechiae in 6 cm circle (50 torr for 15 min); 10-20 petechiae in 5 cm circle (80 mm Hg)	
Triglycerides (TG) Serum, after ≥12 hr fast		**mg/dl**		**g/L**	
		M	F	M	F
	Cord blood	10-98	10-98	0.10-0.98	0.10-0.98
	0-5 yr	30-86	32-99	0.30-0.86	0.32-0.99
	6-11 yr	31-108	35-114	0.31-1.08	0.35-1.14
	12-15 yr	36-138	41-138	0.36-1.38	0.41-1.38
	16-19 yr	40-163	40-128	0.40-1.63	0.40-1.28
	20-29 yr	44-185	40-128	0.44-1.85	0.40-1.28
Triiodothyronine, free Serum	Cord	20-240 pg/dl		0.3-3.7 pmol/L	
	1-3 d	200-610 pg/dl		3.1-9.4 pmol/L	
	6 wk	240-560 pg/dl		3.7-8.6 pmol/L	
	Adults (20-50 yr)	230-660 pg/dl		3.5-10.0 pmol/L	
Triiiodothyronine, total (T_3RIA) Serum	Cord	30-70 ng/dl		0.46-1.08 nmol/L	
	Newborn	72-260 ng/dl		1.16-4.00 nmol/L	
	1-5 yr	100-260 ng/dl		1.54-4.00 nmol/L	
	5-10 yr	90-240 ng/dl		1.39-3.70 nmol/L	
	10-15 yr	80-210 ng/dl		1.23-3.23 nmol/L	
	Thereafter	115-190 ng/dl		1.77-2.93 nmol/L	
Urea nitrogen Serum or plasma	Cord	21-40 mg/dl		7.5-14.3 mmol urea/L	
	Premature (1 wk)	3-25 mg/dl		1.1-9 mmol urea/L	
	Newborn	3-12 mg/dl		1.1-4.3 mmol urea/L	
	Infant/child	5-18 mg/dl		1.8-6.4 mmol urea/L	
	Thereafter	7-18 mg/dl		2.5-6.4 mmol urea/L	
Urine volume Urine, 24 hr	Newborn	50-300 ml/d		0.050-0.300 L/d	
	Infant	350-550 ml/d		0.350-0.550 L/d	
	Child	500-1000 ml/d		0.500-1.000 L/d	
	Adolescent	700-1400 ml/d		0.700-1.400 L/d	
	Thereafter: Male	800-1800 ml/d		0.800-1.800 L/d	
	Female	600-1600 ml/d (varies with intake and other factors)		0.600-1.600 L/d	
WBC (See leukocyte)					

SELECTED RESOURCES ON PEDIATRIC PAIN

FEDERAL GUIDELINES ON PAIN

Acute pain management: operative or medical procedures and trauma

Quick reference guide for clinicians: acute pain management in adults: operative procedures

Quick reference guide for clinicians: acute pain management in infants, children and adolescents: operative and medical procedures

Pain control after surgery: a patient's guide

Management of cancer pain

Quick reference guide for clinicians: management of cancer pain: adults

Managing cancer pain: patient guide

Management of cancer pain: infants, children, and adolescents. (Not published; for excerpts, see *Journal of Pharmaceutical Care in Pain and Symptom Control* 2(1): 75-103, 1994.)

Resources contain federal medical practice guidelines written by a panel of experts. Available at no charge from the **Agency for Health Care Policy and Research (AHCPR)** Publications, PO Box 8527, Silver Spring, MD 20907; (800) 358-9295; www.ahcpr.gov

PROFESSIONAL ORGANIZATIONS

AHCPR Guidelines on Pain: Nursing Implications. Booklet and two audiotapes describing the development and clinical applications of the guidelines; from **APS** (see below)

Principles of Analgesic Use in the Treatment of Acute Pain and Cancer Pain, ed 4, 1999. Booklet describing consensus guidelines for treating pain; available from American Pain Society **(APS)**, 4700 W. Lake Dr., Glenview, IL 60025-1485; (847) 375-4715; fax (847) 375-6315; e-mail: info@ampainsoc.org; www.ampainsoc.org/; or from Purdue Frederick Company, 100 Connecticut Ave., Norwalk, CT 06850-3950; (800) 733-1333 or (203) 853-0123, ext. 7378 or 7314; www.partnersagainstpain.com

Management of Acute Pain: a Practical Guide. A book describing effective pain management strategies; available from the **International Association for the Study of Pain (IASP)**, 909 NE 43rd St., Suite 306, Seattle, WA 98105-6020; (206) 547-6409; e-mail: IASP@locke.hs.washington.edu; www.halcyon.com/iasp

Cancer Pain Relief and Palliative Care in Children (in English; French and Spanish in preparation). World Health Organization in conjunction with IASP. 1998, ISBN 92-4-154512-7, 76 pp. Sw.fr.18-. Order from: WHO Distribution and Sales, 1211 Geneva 27, Switzerland. Price in developing countries: Sw.fr.12.60. In the US: $16.20 + $5 shipping and handling; Order no. 1150459, WHO Publications Center USA, 49 Sheridan Ave., Albany, NY 12210, USA; (518) 436-9686; fax (518) 436-7433; e-mail: QCORP@compuserve.com

Joint Commission on Accreditation of Healthcare Organizations (JCAHO) has established pain assessment and management standards and a toll-free hot line at (800) 994-6610 to encourage patients, their families, caregivers and others to share concerns regarding quality of care issues at accredited health care organizations. Complaints (may be anonymous) may be sent by e-mail to *complaint@jcaho.org;* by fax to the Office of Quality Monitoring at (630) 792-5636; or by mail to the Office of Quality Monitoring, Joint Commission, One Renaissance Blvd, Oakbrook Terrace, IL,

60181. The pain standards are available from: www.jcaho.org/standard/pm_hap.html

The Use of Opioids for the Treatment of Chronic Pain. A consensus statement from the American Academy of Pain Medicine and the American Pain Society **(APS)**; from *Clinical Journal of Pain* 13(1):6-8, 1997; see also **Opioids and chronic pain** (editorial), Wilson, PR, *Clinical Journal of Pain* 13(1):1-2, 1997

LEGAL IMPLICATIONS

Pain management on trial. Cushing M, *American Journal of Nursing* 92(2):21-22, 1992.

Must we make the courts our last resort? Lipman AG, (editorial), *Journal of Pharmaceutical Care in Pain and Symptom Control* 5(1):1-3, 1997

Pain management: legal risks and ethical responsibilities. Rich BA, *Journal of Pharmaceutical Care in Pain and Symptom Control* 5(1):5-20, 1997

OTHER SELECTED RESOURCES

A Child in Pain: How to Help, What to Do. By Leora Kuttner, 1996; a book written for consumers that focuses on the effects, assessment, and treatment of pain in children; available from Hartley & Marks, PO Box 147, Pt. Roberts, WA 98281; (800) 277-5887

Adolescent Pediatric Pain Tool (APPT). Assessment includes use of human figure drawing, Word-Graphic Rating Scale, and choice of descriptive words; available from Pediatric Pain Study, University of California School of Nursing, Dept. of Family Health Care Nursing, San Francisco, CA 04143-0606; (415) 476-4040

Building an Institutional Commitment to Pain Management: The Mayday Resource Manual for Improvement. An excellent compilation of resource material to promote institutional support of pain management; all of the sample resource tools are available on a disc; available from Wisconsin Cancer Pain Initiative, 3675 Medical Sciences Center, University of Wisconsin Medical School, 1300 University Avenue, Madison, WI 53706; (608) 262-0978, fax (608) 265-4014; e-mail: wcpi@facstass.wisc.edu

Children's Cancer Pain Can Be Relieved: a Guide for Parents and Families; and **Jeff Asks About Cancer Pain.** Booklets that provide parents and older children with facts about pain and its management in pediatric cancer. **Handbook of Cancer Pain Management.** A booklet describing types of cancer pain, assessment, and treatment, with a section on children's pain; available from Wisconsin Cancer Pain Initiative, 3675 Medical Sciences Center, University of Wisconsin Medical School, 1300 University Avenue, Madison, WI 53706; (608) 262-0978, fax (608) 265-4014; e-mail: wcpi@facstass.wisc.edu

Circumcision: Information for Parents. Pamphlet describes the benefits and risks of the procedure and the importance of providing analgesia for the infant. Available from the American Academy of Pediatrics, Division of Pediatrics, 141 Northwest Point Blvd., PO Box 747, Elk Grove Village, IL 60009-0747; (800) 433-9016; fax (847) 228-1281; www.aap.org

Clinical Reference Guide For Health Care Providers; Sickle Cell Related Pain: Assessment and Management Conference Proceedings; Sickle Cell Related Pain: As-

sessment and Management—A Guide for Patients and Parents. An excellent compilation of resource material to promote pain management in people with SCD; available from the New England Regional Genetics Groups (NERGG), PO Box 670, Mt. Desert, ME 04660; (207) 288-2704; fax (207) 288-2705; or Mary Aten (617) 243-3033; e-mail: maryaten@mediaone.net

Compounding Specialist. For information about specially compounded medications, such as Tetracaine 1% Sucker (80 mg), contact Deril J. Lees, R.Ph., **The Apothecary Shoppe,** 3707 East 51st St, Tulsa, OK 74135; (800) 610-2003 in U.S. or (918) 665-2003; fax (918) 665-8283. (See also **Professional Compounding Centers of America (PCCA),** (800) 331-2498; fax (800) 874-5760; www.thecompounders.com)

Epidural analgesia for acute pain management: a self-directed learning program and pre- and post-test answers and explanations. By Chris Pasero, MS, RN; the objectives for the program are to identify the nurse's role in assessing and managing acute pain of adult patients and to identify how to care for adult patients who are receiving epidural analgesia; available from the American Society of Pain Management Nurses (ASPMN), 7794 Grow Drive, Pensacola, FL 32514-7072; (888) 34ASPMN; fax (850) 484-8762; e-mail ASPMN@aol.com

Guidelines for Standard of Care of Acute Painful Episodes in Patients with Sickle Cell Disease. By Ballis SK, Carlos TM, Dampier C, and Guidelines Committee: Harrisburg, PA, 1996, Commonwealth of Pennsylvania Department of Health; available from Samir K, Ballas, MD, Cardeza Foundation, 1015 Walnut St., Philadelphia, PA 19107

Guidelines for Treatment of Cancer Pain: The Pocket Edition of the Final Report of the Texas Cancer Council's Workgroup on Pain Control in Cancer Patients. By C. Stratton Hill, Jr., MD, (1997); available free from the Texas Cancer Council, PO Box 12097, Austin, TX 78711; (512) 463-3190; fax (512) 475-2563

Managing Pain Before it Manages You. By Margaret A. Caudill, MD, PhD., 1995; available from The Guilford Press, A Division of Guilford Publications, Inc., 72 Spring Street, New York, NY 10012

McCaffery: Contemporary Issues in Pain Management. Four videotapes focus on pain management in the elderly; improving the quality of pain management; epidural analgesia for chronic pain; and preventing and managing opioid-induced respiratory depression. **McCaffery on Pain: Nursing Assessment and Pharmacological Intervention in Adults.** Four videotapes focus on nursing assessment of the patient with pain; the three analgesic groups: practical considerations; use of opioid analgesic; and undertreatment of pain. A resource manual also accompanies the videotapes; available for purchase from Williams & Wilkins Electronic Media, 428 E. Preston St., Baltimore, MD 21202; (800) 527-5597

No More Crying: Reducing Distress During Venipuncture. Videotape describes distraction, limit-setting, and positive reinforcement to reduce the distress associated with procedures; available for rental or purchase from Carle Medical Communications, 611 W. Park St., Urbana, IL 61801; (217) 384-4838; fax (217) 384-8280; www.baxleymedia.com

No Fears, No Tears: Children with Cancer Coping with Pain. Videotape demonstrates the use of distraction and imagery to reduce distress from various procedures; available from Canadian Cancer Society, (604) 872-4400; fax (604) 879-4533; for information on **No Fears, No Tears—13 Years Later,** contact Leora Kuttner, PhD, (604) 736-8801; fax (604) 294-9986; e-mail: leora_kuttner@sfu.ca or order directly from www.burnessc.com/nofears

Oucher pain scales. Available from the Association for the Care of Children's Health (ACCH), PO Box 25707, Alexandria, VA 22313; (703) 684-6179 or (800) 808-ACCH (2224); fax (703) 684-1589; www.acch.org

Pain in Infants: Confronting the Challenges. By Bonnie J. Stevens, PhD, RN; videotape describes assessment strategies and analgesic intervention for neonates and infants; available for purchase from Williams & Wilkins Electronic Media, 428 E. Preston St., Baltimore, MD 21202; (800) 527-5597

Pain, Pain, Go Away: Helping Children with Pain. By Patrick J. McGrath, G. Allen Finley, and Judith Ritchie, booklet teaches parents about pain in children and helps parents request better pain care. Available from the Association for the Care of Children's Health, PO Box 25707, Alexandria, VA 22313; (703) 684-6179 or (800) 808-ACCH (2224); fax (703) 684-1589; www.acch.org

Pain Relief: How to Say No to Acute, Chronic, and Cancer Pain! By Jane Cowles, 1993; a book written for consumers that focuses on the prevention, assessment, and individualized treatment of pain in children and adults; available from MasterMedia Limited, 17 East 89th St., New York, NY 10128; (800) 334-8232

Pain Resource Center. Serves as a clearinghouse to disseminate information and resources to improve the quality of pain management; from City of Hope National Medical Center, Pain Resource Center, 1500 East Duarte Road, Duarte, CA 91010; (626) 359-8111, ext. 3829; fax (626) 301-8941; e-mail: mayday_pain@smtplink.coh.org; http://mayday.coh.org

Perioperative Analgesia Approaching the 21st Century. Study guide and audiocassette reviews current and emerging approaches, such as preemptive analgesia, for surgery; available from the American Pain Society **(APS),** 4700 W. Lake Dr., Glenview, IL 60025; (847) 375-4715; fax (847) 375-6315; e-mail: info@ampainsoc.org; www.ampainsoc.org/

Pediatric Pain Awareness Initiative (PPAI). A multidisciplinary group of health care professionals whose purpose is to raise the awareness of parents and professionals about managing pain in children; information packets are available for consumers and professionals by calling (888) 569-5555

Pediatric Pain Letter. By Patrick J. McGrath, PhD, and G. Allen Finley, MD; a quarterly review of the literature on pain in infants, children and adolescents that presents a series of structured abstracts accompanied by critical commentaries; questions and subscriptions may be addressed to Julie Goodman, Managing Editor, Pediatric Pain Letter, Psychology Department, Dalhousie University, Halifax, Nova Scotia, B3H 4J1; e-mail: jgoodman@is2.dal.ca

Pediatric Pain: Taming the Hurt. By Marian E. Broome, PhD, RN; videotape reviews principles of pain assessment and both pharmacologic and cognitive-behavioral pain management strategies; available for purchase from Williams & Wilkins Electronic Media, 428 E. Preston St., Baltimore, MD 21202; (800) 527-5597

Quality of Mercy: a Case for Better Pain Management. Videotape highlights problems in infant pain control and cancer and burn pain; available for rental or purchase from Filmakers Library, 124 East 40th St., New York, NY 10016; (212) 808-4980; fax (212) 808-4983; e-mail: info@filmakers.com; www.filmakers.com

Questions parents and concerned professionals might ask of their local health care institutions. A one-page sheet that addresses questions to effectively raise awareness about infant pain control; in Butler, NB: How to raise professional awareness of the need for adequate pain relief for infants, *Birth* 12(1):38-41, 1988

Report of the Consensus Conference on the Management of Pain in Childhood Cancer. A collection of articles addressing pain assessment and management; in *Pediatrics*

86(5):supplement, 1990; available from American Academy of Pediatrics, PO Box 927, Elk Grove Village, IL 60009-0927; (800) 433-9016; (847) 228-1281; www.aap.org

Therapeutic Electro Membrane (TEM). A high-technology electron reservoir membrane that, upon contact with the human body, releases the electrons in the form of micro-current impulses; the reservoir is in a soft dressing that is applied over the painful area for 48 hours; TEM relieves acute or chronic musculoskeletal pain, including soft tissue injuries, sports injuries, arthritis, back pain, fibromyalgia, neurogenic pain, and myofacial pain; available from Helio Medical Supplies, Inc., 2080A Walsh Ave., Santa Clara, CA 95050; (888) PAINTEM; e-mail: eileen@heliomed.com

Whaley and Wong's Pediatric Pain Assessment and Management. By Donna Wong, PhD, RN; videotape focuses on process of QUESTT for pain assessment and Six Rights for pharmacologic pain relief; available from Mosby, 11830 Westline Industrial Drive, St. Louis, MO 63146; (800) 426-4545; fax (800) 535-9935; www.mosby.com

When Children Have to Die . . . Pediatric Palliative Care. A special thematic issue from *Journal of Palliative Care* 12(3), Autumn 1996; editorial inquiries may be sent to the Editor-in-Chief, Journal of Palliative Care, Center for Bioethics, Clinical Research Institute of Montreal, 110 Pine Avenue West, Montreal, QC, Canada H2W 1R7; e-mail: stamous@ircm.umontreal.ca

Wong-Baker FACES Pain Rating Scale Reference Manual. Describes development and research of the scale; available from the **Pain Resource Center,** City of Hope National Medical Center, 1500 East Duarte Road, Duarte, CA 91010;

(626) 359-8111, ext. 3829; fax (626) 301-8941; e-mail: mayday_pain@smtplink.coh.org; to obtain permission to use the scale, contact: Julie Lawley, WB Saunders, The Curtis Center, Independence Square West, Philadelphia, PA 19106; (800) 523-1649, ext. 8302; fax (215) 238-8483; or *www. mosby.com/WOW/.* A compilation of many pain scales, including the FACES, is available free from Purdue Frederick Company, 100 Connecticut Ave., Norwalk, CT 06850-3950; (800) 733-1333 or (203) 853-0123, ext. 7378 or 7314; www.partnersagainstpain.com

Wong-Baker FACES Pain Rating Scale Pins. The cost for 1 to 99 pins is $5 U.S. each. U.S. postage and handling for up to 50 pins is $5; postage for 51 to 99 pins is $8. The cost for orders of 100 or more is $4 each. Postage and handling is $10 for 100 pins, and for each additional set of 50 pins is $5. Pins may be purchased in gold, red, or blue and with coding of 0-5 for all colors and 0-10 for red only. Please specify color and coding or one will be chosen. Orders can be sent to Linda Toth, PO Box 2984, Sanford, NC 27331; (919) 498-1158; fax (919) 498-3993. Make check payable to *Linda Toth.*

Wong on Web. Internet access to numerous documents and other resource data compiled by Donna Wong, *www.mosby.com/WOW/.*

OTHER EXCELLENT AND PRACTICAL TEXTS

McCaffery M, Pasero C: *Pain: clinical manual,* ed 2, St Louis, 1999, Mosby.

Yaster M and others: *Pediatric pain management and sedation handbook,* St Louis, 1997, Mosby.

ABBREVIATIONS AND ACRONYMS
General Abbreviations

A substantial number of words and phrases are abbreviated in nursing practice for convenience in communication. Although most of the abbreviations are familiar to health professionals, many are not. In addition, students unfamiliar with the vocabulary used by health professionals are at a particular disadvantage when interpreting communications. This extensive list is compiled to facilitate this process. Because many of the abbreviations can represent several different words or phrases, the user is advised to use caution in their interpretation. For example, *per os* can be interpreted as *by mouth* or *in left eye; D/C* can mean *discharge* or *discontinue.* The meaning of unfamiliar abbreviations should be confirmed with the people who wrote them. If the author of a particular abbreviation is unavailable, check the abbreviation in a dictionary of medical abbreviations, or use a list of hospital-approved abbreviations to verify its meaning. (See also p. 675 for selected abbreviations for drugs.)

AA	Automobile accident; Alcoholics Anonymous
AAMD	American Association on Mental Deficiency
Ab	Antibody
ABG	Arterial blood gases
ABR	Auditory brainstem response
ac	*Ante cibum* (before meals)
ACCH	Association for the Care of Children's Health
ACLS	Advanced cardiac life support
ACT	Activated clotting time
ACTH	Adrenocorticotropic hormone

AD	Autosomal dominant; atopic dermatitis; *auris dextra* (right ear)
ADA	Adenosine deaminase (deficiency disease)
ADC	Aid to Dependent Children
ADD	Attention deficit disorder
ADDH	Attention deficit disorder, hyperactivity
ADH	Antidiuretic hormone
ADHD	Attention deficit-hyperactivity disorder
ADI	Acceptable daily intake
ADL	Activities of daily living
ad lib	*Ad libitum* (as desired)
ADP	Adenosine diphosphate
ADR	Adverse drug reaction
ADS	Attention deficit syndrome; antidiuretic substance
AEP	Auditory evoked potential
AF	Atrial fibrillation
AFB	Acid-fast bacillus
AFDC	Aid to families with dependent children
AFP	Alpha-fetoprotein
Ag	Antigen, *argentum* (silver)
AGA	Appropriate for gestational age
AGC	Absolute granulocyte count
AGN	Acute glomerulonephritis
AHC	Acute hemorrhagic conjunctivitis
AHD	Autoimmune hemolytic disease
AHF	Antihemophilic factor; antihemolytic factor
AHG	Antihemophilic globulin; antihuman globulin

AI	Aortic insufficiency		BEAM	Brain electrical activity map
AID	Artificial insemination by donor		BEI	Butanol-extractable iodine
AIDS	Acquired immune deficiency syndrome		BFP	Biologic false positive
AIH	Artificial insemination by husband		BG	Blood glucose
AJ	Ankle jerk		BHI	Biosynthetic human insulin
ALG	Antilymphocytic globulin		bid	*Bis in die* (twice a day)
ALL	Acute lymphoid leukemia		BJ	Biceps jerk
ALS	Advanced life support		BM	Bowel movement; bone marrow
ALT	Alanine aminotransferase		BMD	Bone marrow depression
AMA	Against medical advice; American Medical Association		BMR	Basal metabolic rate
			BNBAS	Brazelton Neonatal Behavioral Assessment Scale
AMEND	Aiding Mothers Experiencing Neonatal Death		BOA	Behavioral observation audiometry; born out of asepsis
AMI	Acute myocardial infarction			
AML	Acute myelogenous leukemia		BPD	Bronchopulmonary dysplasia
amp	Ampule		BRAT	Bananas, rice cereal, applesauce, toast
AMP	Adenosine monophosphate		BRP	Bathroom privileges
ANA	Antinuclear antibody; American Nurses Association		BS	Blood sugar; bowel sounds; breath sounds
			BSA	Body surface area; bovine serum albumin
ANLL	Acute nonlymphocytic leukemia		BSE	Breast self-examination
ANS	Autonomic nervous system; anterior nasal spine		BSER	Brainstem-evoked response
			BSI	Biologic substance(s) isolation; body substance isolation
AODM	Adult onset diabetes mellitus			
AOM	Acute otitis media		BSID	Bayley Scales of Infant Development
AP	Anteroposterior; antepartum; atrioperitoneal		BT	Bleeding time
APON	Association of Pediatric Oncology Nurses		BTPS	Body temperature and pressure, saturated (with water)
aq	*Aqua* (water)			
AR	Autosomal recessive		BUN	Blood urea nitrogen
ARC	AIDS-related complex		BW	Birth weight
ARD	Acute respiratory disease		BWF	Basic waking frequency
ARDS	Adult respiratory distress syndrome		BWS	Battered woman syndrome
ARF	Acute renal failure; acute respiratory failure		Bx	Biopsy
ARV	AIDS-associated retrovirus		c	*cum* (with)
AS	Aortic stenosis; aortic sound; aqueous solution; aqueous suspension; astigmatism; ankylosing spondylitis; *auris sinistra* (left ear)		CA (Ca)	Cancer; chronologic age; calcium
			CAH	Congenital adrenal hyperplasia; chronic active hepatitis
			CAL	Chronic airflow limitation
ASAP	As soon as possible		cAMP	Cyclic adenosine monophosphate
ASD	Atrial septal defect		cap	Capsule
ASDH	Acute subdural hematoma		CAPD	Continuous ambulatory peritoneal dialysis
ASH	Asymmetric septal hypertrophy		CAT	Computed axial tomography
ASK	Antistreptokinase		CAV	Congenital absence of vagina; croup-associated virus
ASO	Antistreptolysin O			
ATC	Certified athletic trainer; around the clock		CAVH	Continuous arteriovenous hemofiltration
ATG	Antithymocyte globulin		CB	Chronic bronchitis
ATN	Acute tubular necrosis		CBA	Congenital biliary atresia
ATO	Alimentary tract obstruction		CBC	Complete blood count
ATP	Autoimmune thrombocytopenia (purpura); adenosine triphosphate		CBD	Closed bladder drainage
			CBF	Cerebral blood flow
ATPS	Ambient temperature and pressure, saturated (with water)		CBPU	Care by parent unit
			CBV	Cerebral blood volume; cerebral blood (flow) velocity
ATV	All-terrain vehicle			
AU	*Auris uterque* (each ear)		CC	Chief complaint; caucasian child; common cold; critical condition; color and circulation; creatinine clearance
Av	Average; avoirdupois			
AV (A-V)	Atrioventricular			
AVM	Arteriovenous malformation		CCMS	Clean-catch midstream specimen
AWD	Abdominal wall defect		Ccr	Creatinine clearance
BA	Bronchial asthma; bone age		CCS	Crippled Children's Services
BAEP	Brainstem auditory evoked potential		CD	Communicable disease; celiac disease; cutdown
BAER	Brainstem auditory evoked response			
BAT	Brown adipose tissue		CDC	Centers for Disease Control and Prevention
BBB	Blood-brain barrier		CDGA	Constitutional delay of growth and adolescence
BBT	Basal body temperature			
BC	Blood culture		CDH	Congenital dislocated hip; congenital diaphragmatic hernia
BCG	Bacille Calmette-Guérin (tuberculin vaccine)			
BCS	Battered child syndrome		CDP	Continuous distending pressure
BD	Bronchial drainage; birthday; birth defect		C-E	Croup-epiglottitis syndrome
BE	Barium enema			

CF	Cystic fibrosis; cardiac failure; complement fixation
CFF	Cystic Fibrosis Foundation
CFU	Colony-forming units
CHAP	Child Health Assessment Program
CHB	Complete heart block
CHC	Child health conference; community health center
CHD	Congenital heart disease; childhood disease; coronary heart disease
CHF	Congestive heart failure
CHL	Crown-heel length
CI	Cardiac index; cardiac insufficiency; cerebral infarction
CID	Cytomegalic inclusion disease; combined immune deficiency
CIE	Countercurrent immunoelectrophoresis
CINAHL	Cumulative Index to Nursing and Allied Health Literature
CK	Creatine kinase
CL	Cleft lip
CLBBB	Complete left bundle branch block
CLD	Chronic lung disease; chronic liver disease
CL (P)	Cleft lip with or without cleft palate
CLP	Cleft lip and cleft palate
cm	Centimeter
CMA	Cow's milk allergy
CMI	Cell-mediated immunity
CML	Chronic myelocytic leukemia
CMPI	Cow's milk protein intolerance
CMR	Cerebral metabolic rate
CMV	Cytomegalovirus
CN	Clinical Nurse
CNA	Canadian Nurses Association
CNM	Certified Nurse Midwife
CNS	Central nervous system; Clinical Nurse Specialist
CNSD	Chronic nonspecific diarrhea
CO	Cardiac output; carbon monoxide
COA	Children of alcoholics
Cocci	Coccidioidomycosis
COHb	Carboxyhemoglobin
COLD	Chronic obstructive lung disease
COPD	Chronic obstructive pulmonary disease
COR	Conditioned orientation reflex
CP	Cleft palate; cerebral palsy; capillary pressure; cor pulmonale; Certified Prosthetist; constant pressure; child psychiatrist; closing pressure (spinal tap); chronic pyelonephritis
CPAP	Continuous positive airway pressure
CPAV	Continuous positive airway ventilation
CPD	Cephalopelvic disproportion; childhood polycystic disease
CPK	Creatine phosphokinase
CPM	Continuous passive motion
CPN	Certified Pediatric Nurse
CPP	Cerebral perfusion pressure
CPPV	Continuous positive pressure ventilation
CPR	Cardiopulmonary resuscitation
CPS	Cycles per second; Child Protective Services
CPSC	Consumer Product Safety Commission
CPT	Chest physiotherapy
CRBBB	Complete right bundle branch block
CRD	Child restraint devices
CRF	Corticotropin-releasing factor
CRP	C-reactive protein

CRS	Congenital rubella syndrome
CS	Clinical Specialist; cesarean section
C&S	Culture and sensitivity
CSA	Colony-stimulating activity
CSD	Cat scratch disease
CSF	Cerebral spinal fluid; cerebrospinal fluid
CSII	Continuous subcutaneous insulin infusion
CSN	Certified School Nurse
CSOM	Chronic serous otitis media
CT	Computed tomography; circulation time; clotting time; coated tablet; compressed tablet; corneal transplant; Coombs test
CTT	Computerized transaxial tomography
CUG	Cystourethrogram
CV	Closing volume
CVA	Cerebrovascular accident; costal vertebral angle
CVI	Common variable immunodeficiency
CVO_2	Mixed venous oxygen content
CVP	Central venous pressure
CVR	Cerebral vascular resistance
CVS	Clean voided specimen; chorionic villi sampling
CW	Crutch walking
C/W	Consistent with
CXR	Chest x-ray
DA	Developmental age
DASE	Denver Articulation Screening Examination
DAW	Dispense as written
db	Decibel
DC D/C	Discontinue; discharge; dichorionic
D & C	Dilatation and curettage
DCT	Direct Coombs test
DD	Dry dressing; differential diagnosis; discharge diagnosis; discharge by death; diaper dermatitis
DDH	Developmental dysplasia of the hip
DDST	Denver Developmental Screening Test
DDST-R	Denver Developmental Screening Test, revised
DFA	Diet for age
DH	Diaphragmatic hernia
DHHS	Department of Health and Human Services
DI	Diabetes insipidus
D/I	Direct/indirect ratio (bilirubin)
DIC	Disseminated intravascular coagulation
DIP	Desquamated interstitial pneumonitis
DKA	Diabetic ketoacidosis
dl	Deciliter
DLIS	Digoxin-like immunoreactive substance
DM	Diabetes mellitus; diastolic murmur
DMD	Duchenne muscular dystrophy
DNHW	Department of National Health and Welfare (Canada)
DNR	Do not resuscitate
DOA	Date of admission; dead on arrival
DOB	Date of birth
DOD	Date of discharge; date of death
DOE	Dyspnea on exertion
DP	Dorsalis pedis (artery)
DPNB	Dorsal penile nerve block
DPT	Diphtheria-pertussis-tetanus (vaccine)
DQ	Developmental quotient
DRG	Diagnosis-related group(s)
DS	Down syndrome
DSA	Digital subtraction angiography
DSD	Dry sterile dressing

Unit 6

DSDB	Direct self-destructive behavior
DSM	Diagnostic and Statistical Manual of Mental Disorders
DT	Delirium tremens
DTR	Deep tendon reflex
DU	Diagnosis undetermined
DV	Dilute volume
D&V	Diarrhea and vomiting
DW	Distilled water
D5W	Dextrose 5% in water
Dx	Diagnosis
DZ	Dizygotic
EA	Esophageal atresia
EAM	External acoustic meatus
EBL	Estimated blood loss
EBM	Expressed breast milk
EBV	Epstein-Barr virus
ECC	Emergency cardiac care; extracorporeal circulation
ECD	Endocardial cushion defect
ECF	Extracellular fluid; extended care facility
ECG	Electrocardiogram
ECM	Erythema chronicum migrans
ECMO	Extracorporeal membrane oxygenation
ED	Emergency department
EDC	Estimated date of confinement
EDD	Estimated date of delivery
EEE	Eastern equine encephalitis
EEG	Electroencephalogram
EENT	Eye, ear, nose, throat
EF	Extended field (irradiation)
EFA	Essential fatty acid
EFE	Endocardial fibroelastosis
EFM	Electronic fetal monitoring
EGS	Electric galvanic stimulator
EHBA	Extrahepatic biliary atresia
E-IPV	Enhanced (potency)-IPV
ELBW	Extremely low birth weight
ELISA	Enzyme-linked immunosorbent assay
elix	Elixir
EMG	Electromyogram
EMI	Electromagnetic interference
EMM	Expressed mother's milk
EMR	Educable mentally retarded
EMS	Emergency medical services
EMT	Emergency medical technician
ENA	Extractable nuclear antigens
EOA	Examination, opinion, and advice
EOM	Extraocular movement; extraocular muscle
EP	Extraperitoneal, evoked potential; erythrocyte protoporphyrin
EPA	Erect posteroanterior
EPCA	Epidural patient controlled analgesia
EPI	Echo-planar imaging
EPSDT	Early and Periodic Screening, Diagnosis, and Treatment
ER	Emergency room; external rotation; expiratory reserve; equivalent roentgen (unit)
ERA	Electric response audiometry
ERG	Electroretinography
ERPF	Effective renal plasma flow
ERV	Expiratory reserve volume
ESI	Early Screening Inventory
ESR	Erythrocyte sedimentation rate
ESRD	End-stage renal disease
ET	Endotracheal; esotropia; eustachian tube

ETA	Estimated time of arrival
E$_T$CO$_2$	End-tidal carbon dioxide concentration
ETOH	Ethyl alcohol
ETT	Endotracheal tube
EV	Enterovirus
FAAN	Fellow in American Academy of Nursing
FAB	French-American-British
FAE	Fetal alcohol effect
FAS	Fetal alcohol syndrome
FB	Foreign body
FBA	Foreign body aspiration
FBS	Fasting blood sugar
FDA	Food and Drug Administration
FEP	Free erythrocyte porphyrins
FET	Forced expiratory technique
FEV$_1$	Forced expiratory volume, 1 second
FEV$_5$	Forced expiratory volume, 5 seconds
FEVC	Forced expiratory volume capacity
FFA	Free fatty acids
FFP	Fresh-frozen plasma
FH, FHx	Family history
FHS	Fetal hydantoin syndrome
Fio$_2$, FIO$_2$	Forced inspiratory oxygen; fraction of inspired oxygen
FISH	Fluorescent in-situ hybridization
FLK	Funny-looking kid
FLM	Fetal lung maturity
FMD	Fibromuscular dysplasia
FMH	Family medical history
FMS	Fat-mobilizing substance
FNP	Family Nurse Practitioner
FRC	Functional residual capacity
FS	Full strength
FSH	Follicle-stimulating hormone
FSP	Fibrin split products
FSS	Family short stature
FTA-ABS	Fluorescent treponemal antibody absorption (test)
FTSG	Full-thickness skin graft
FTT	Failure to thrive
F/U	Follow-up
FUE	Fever of unknown etiology
FUO	Fever of unknown origin
FVC	Forced vital capacity
FWB	Full weight bearing
Fx	Fracture
FYI	For your information
GA	General anesthesia; gestational age
GABHS	Group A β-hemolytic streptococci
GAS	Group A streptococci
GBBS	Group B β-streptococci
GBM	Glomerular basement membrane
GC	Gonococci (gonorrhea); general condition; general circulation
GCS	Glasgow Coma Scale
G&D	Growth and development
GDM	Gestational diabetes mellitus
GER	Gastroesophageal reflux
GFR	Glomerular filtration rate
GGT	Gamma-glutamyl transpeptidase
GGTP	Gamma-glutamyl transpeptidase
GH	Growth hormone
GHB, GHb	Glycosylated hemoglobin
GHD	Growth hormone deficiency
GHRF	Growth hormone releasing factor
GH-RH	Growth hormone releasing hormone
GI	Gastrointestinal

GOT	Glutamic-oxaloacetic transaminase
G6PD	Glucose-6-phosphate dehydrogenase
GSE	Gluten-sensitive enteropathy
GSW	Gunshot wound
gtt	*Guttal (drops)*
GTT	Glucose tolerance test
GU	Genitourinary
GVH	Graft-vs-host
GVHD	Graft-vs-host disease
GVHR	Graft-vs-host reaction
h	*Hora (hour)*
HA	Headache
H-A	Hartmannella-Acanthamoeba
HAV	Hepatitis A virus
Hb	Hemoglobin
HB	Heart block
HBGM	Home blood glucose monitoring
HBIG	Hepatitis B immune globulin
HBO	Hyperbaric oxygen
HbOC	Haemophilus b conjugate vaccine (diphtheria CRM_{19}– protein conjugate)
HBsAg	Hepatitis B surface antigen
HBV	Hepatitis B virus; honey bee venom
HC	Hyperosmolar coma
hCG	Human chorionic gonadotropin
HCI	Home care instructions
HCM	Health care management
Hct	Hematocrit
HD	Heart disease
HDCV	Human diploid cell virus
HDL	High-density lipoprotein
HDN	Hemorrhagic disease of the newborn
HEENT	Head, eye, ear, nose, and throat
HELLP	Hemolysis elevated liver low platelets
HFJV	High-frequency jet ventilation
HFO	High-frequency oscillation
HFOV	High-frequency oscillatory ventilation
HFPPV	High-frequency positive pressure ventilation
HFV	High-frequency ventilation
Hgb	Hemoglobin
HGH (hGH)	Human growth hormone
HHHO	Hypothyroidism, hypoxia, hypogonadism, obesity
HHNC	Hyperosmolar, hyperglycemic, nonketogenic coma
HHNK	Hyperosmolar, hyperglycemic, nonketotic dehydration
H/I	Hypoxia-ischemia
Hib (HIB)	*Haemophilus influenzae* type B
HIE	Hypoxic-ischemic encephalopathy
HISG	Human immune serum globulin
HIV	Human immunodeficiency virus
HL	Hearing level
HLA	Human leukocytic antigen; histocompatibility locus antigen
HMD	Hyaline membrane disease
HMO	Health maintenance organization
HO	House officer
HOB	Head of bed
HOME	Home Observation for Measurement of the Environment
HOPI	History of previous (prior) illness
HPA	Hypothalamic-pituitary-adrenal (axis)
HPB	Health Protection Branch (of Canada)
HPC	Healed primary complex
HPLC	High-power liquid chromatography
HPN	Hypertension

HPV	Human parvovirus; human papillomavirus
HR	Heart rate
HRA	Health risk appraisal
HRF	Health-related facility
HRIG	Human rabies immune globulin
hs	*Hora somni* (hour of sleep; bedtime)
HS	Heart sounds; herpes simplex; house surgeon
HSA	Health systems agency; human serum albumin
HSBG	Heel stick blood gases
HSE	Herpes simplex encephalitis
HSN	Herpes simplex neonatorum
HSP	Henoch-Schönlein purpura
HSV	Herpes simplex virus
HTLV-III	Human T-lymphotropic virus type III
HTN	Hypertensive; hypertension
HTPN	Home total parenteral nutrition
HTSI	Human thyroid stimulator immunoglobulin
HUS	Hemolytic uremic syndrome
Hx	History
IA	Imperforate anus; internal auditory; intraarterial; intraarticular; infantile apnea
IAA	Insulin autoantibodies
IABP	Intraaortic balloon pump
IAFI	Infantile amaurotic familial idiocy
IAR	Interagency referral
IBC	Iron-binding capacity
IBD	Inflammatory bowel disease
IBO	In behalf of
IBS	Irritable bowel syndrome
IBW	Ideal body weight
IC	Intracutaneous
ICA	Islet cell antibodies
ICC	Intermittent clean catheterization
ICD	International Classification of Diseases
ICF	Intracellular fluid
ICN	Intensive care nursery
ICP	Intermittent catheterization program; intracranial pressure
ICS	Intercostal space
ICSH	Interstitial cell-stimulating hormone
ICU	Intensive care unit
ID	Identification; intradermal; initial dose; infective dose; ineffective dose; inside diameter
IDD	Insulin-dependent diabetes
IDDM	Insulin-dependent diabetes mellitus
IDM	Infant of diabetic mother
IDP	Infant development program
I/E ratio	Inspiratory-expiratory ratio
IEP	Individualized education program; immunoelectrophoresis
IF	Involved field (irradiation); immunofluorescence
IFA	Indirect fluorescent antibody
IFSP	Individualized family service plan
Ig (IG)	Immune globulin
IGIV	Immune globulin intravenous
IgS	Immunoglobulin system
IGT	Impaired glucose tolerance
IH	Infectious hepatitis
IHA	Indirect hemagglutination
IHSS	Idiopathic hypertrophic subaortic stenosis
IIA	Interrupted infantile apnea
IM	Intramuscular; internal medicine; infectious mononucleosis; intramedullary
IMV	Intermittent mandatory ventilation
IND	Investigational New Drug

Unit 6

INV	Influenza vaccine
IOL	Intraocular lens
IPH	Intraparenchymal hemorrhage
IPPB	Intermittent positive pressure breathing
IPPD	Intermedial purified protein derivative (tuberculin test)
IPV	Inactivated polio virus (vaccine)
IQ	Intelligence quotient
IRB	Institutional Review Board
IRV	Inspiratory reserve volume
ISADH	Inappropriate secretion of ADH
ISC	Intermittent self-catheterization; intermittent servo control
ISDB	Indirect self-destructive behavior
ISF	Interstitial fluid
ISG	Immune serum globulin
ISP	Infant stimulation program
IT	Intrathecal
ITP	Idiopathic thrombocytopenia; idiopathic thrombocytopenic purpura
ITQ	Infant Temperament Questionnaire
IU	Immunizing unit; international unit
IUCD	Intrauterine contraceptive device
IUD	Intrauterine device
IUFD	Intrauterine fetal death
IUGR	Intrauterine growth retardation
IV	Intravenous
IVC	Inferior vena cava
IVCD	Intraventricular conduction defect
IVDU	Intravenous drug use
IVGG	Intravenous gamma-globulin
IVH	Intraventricular hemorrhage
IVP	Intravenous pyelogram
IVT	Intravenous transfusion
IWL	Insensible water loss
JA	Juvenile arthritis
JAS	Juvenile ankylosing spondylitis
JCAHO	Joint Commission on Accreditation of Healthcare Organizations
JCP	Juvenile chronic polyarthritis
JND	Just noticeable difference
JOD	Juvenile-onset diabetes
JODM	Juvenile-onset diabetes mellitus
JRA	Juvenile rheumatoid arthritis
KD	Kawasaki disease
17-KGS	17-Ketogenic steroid
KIDS	Kansas Infant Development Screen
17-KS	17-Ketosteroids
KUB	Kidney, ureter, and bladder
KVO	Keep vein open
LA	Left atrium
LAE	Left atrial enlargement
LAP	Left arterial pressure
LATS	Long-acting thyroid stimulator
LAV	Lymphadenopathy-associated virus
LBCD	Left border of cardiac dullness (sternal border)
LBM	Lean body mass
LBW	Low birth weight; lean body weight
LCM	Left costal margin
LD	Lethal dose; light difference (perception); left deltoid
L&D	Labor and delivery
LDH	Lactic dehydrogenase
LDL	Low-density lipoprotein
LE	Lupus erythematosus; left eye; LE prep; lower extremity
LES	Lower esophageal sphincter; Life Expectancy Survey
LFD	Light for dates
LG	Left gluteal
LGA	Large for gestational age
LH	Luteinizing hormone
LH-RH	Luteinizing hormone releasing hormone
LIP	Lymphoid interstitial pneumonitis
LJM	Limited joint movement
LKS	Liver, kidneys, spleen
LLBCD	Left lower border of cardiac dullness
LLE	Left lower extremity
LLL	Left lower lobe
LLQ	Left lower quadrant
LLT	Left lateral thigh
LMC	Left midclavicular line
LMD	Local medical doctor
LMN	Lower motor neuron
LMP	Last menstrual period
LNMP	Last normal menstrual period
LOC	Level of consciousness; loss of consciousness; locus of control; laxative of choice
LOM	Left otitis media; loss of movement; limitation of motion
LOS	Length of stay
LP	Lumbar puncture
LPN	Licensed Practical Nurse
LQ	Lower quadrant
LRE	Least restrictive environment
LRI	Lower respiratory infection
LS	Lecithin; sphingomyelin
LSB	Left sternal border; left scapular border
LTB	Laryngotracheobronchitis
LTH	Luteotropic hormone
LUE	Left upper extremity
LUL	Left upper lobe
LUOQ	Left upper outer quadrant
LUQ	Left upper quadrant
LV	Left ventricle
LVG	Left ventrogluteal
LVH	Left ventricular hypertrophy
LVN	Licensed vocational nurse
LVO	Left ventricular output
M	Molar; mean; muscle; male
M²	Meters squared (square meters)
MA	Mental age; menstrual age
MABP	Mean arterial blood pressure
MAC	Maximum allowable concentration
MAMC	Midarm muscle circumference
MAP	Mean arterial pressure; mean airway pressure; most appropriate placement
MAS	Meconium aspiration syndrome
MAWP	Mean arterial wedge pressure
MBC	Minimum bactericidal concentration
MBP	Mean blood pressure
MC	Mucocutaneous lymph node syndrome; maternal child; monochorionic
MCDI	Minnesota Child Development Inventory
mcg	Microgram
MCH	Mean corpuscular (cell) hemoglobin; maternal and child health
MCHC	Mean corpuscular (cell) hemoglobin concentration
MCL	Midclavicular line
MCNS	Minimal change nephrotic syndrome
MCSA	McCarthy Scales of Children's Abilities

MCT	Medium-chain triglyceride; mean circulatory time
MCV	Mean corpuscular (cell) volume; mean clinical value
MD	Muscular dystrophy; medical doctor; manic depression; myocardial disease
MDA	Minimal daily allowance
MDI	Medium dose inhalants; metered dose inhaler
MDR	Minimal daily requirement
MDRP	Multidrug-resistant pathogens
MEBM	Maternally expressed breast milk
MED	Minimal effective dose; minimal erythema dose
mEQ	Milliequivalents
MFD	Minimal fatal dose
mg	Milligram
MGN	Membranous glomerulonephritis
MH	Melanocytic hormone
MHC	Major histocompatibility complex
MI	Mitral insufficiency; myocardial infarction; myocardial ischemia; mental illness
MIC	Minimum inhibitory concentration
mics	Micrograms
MID	Minimum infective dose
MIF	Migration-inhibiting factor
MLC	Mixed lymphocyte culture
MLD	Minimum lethal dose; median lethal dose
MLNS	Minimal lesion nephrotic syndrome
MM	Mucous membrane; multiple melanoma; myocardial infarction; myocardial ischemia; mitral insufficiency
MMEF	Maximal midexpiratory flow
MMPI	Minnesota Multiphasic Personality Inventory
MMR	Morbidity and Mortality Report
MNP	Mononuclear phagocyte
MO	Medical officer
MOD	March of Dimes
MODM	Mature-onset diabetes mellitus
MOF	Multiple organ failure
MOSF	Multiple organ system failure
MPAP	Mean pulmonary artery pressure
MPD	Maximum permissible dose
MPI	Minnesota Preschool Inventory
MPS	Mucopolysaccharidosis
MR	Mental retardation; may repeat; measles, rubella; mitral regurgitation; magnetic resonance
MRD	Minimum reacting dose
MRI	Magnetic resonance imaging
MRSA	Methicillin-resistant *Staph aureans*
MS	Mitral stenosis; multiple sclerosis; mitral sounds; musculoskeletal
MS-1	Hepatitis A
MS-2	Hepatitis B
MSAF	Meconium stained amniotic fluid
MSAFP	Maternal serum alpha-fetoprotein
MSL	Midsternal line
MSP	Münchausen syndrome by proxy
MST	McCarthy Screening Tests
MTT	Mean transit time
MVA	Motor vehicle accident
MVP	Moisture vapor permeable (dressing)
MVV	Maximum voluntary ventilation
MZ	Monozygotic
N	Normal
n	Number

NA	Nutritional assessment; not applicable
NAD	No abnormalities noted; no appreciable disease
NAI	Nonaccidental injury
NANB	Non-A, non-B (hepatitis)
NAPNAP	National Association of Pediatric Nurse Associates and Practitioners
NASN	National Association of School Nurses
NB	Newborn
NBAS	Newborn Behavioral Assessment Scale
NBN	Newborn nursery
NCDB	National Center Drugs and Biologics
NCDC	National Center for Disease Control
NCHS	National Center for Health Statistics
NCVS	Nerve conduction velocity studies
ND	Not done
NEC	Necrotizing enterocolitis
NFT	Nonorganic failure to thrive
NG	Nasogastric
NGU	Nongonorrheal urethritis
NH	Neonatal hepatitis
NHL	Non-Hodgkin lymphoma
NICU	Neonatal intensive care unit
NIDDM	Non–insulin-dependent diabetes mellitus
NIH	National Institutes of Health
NIMH	National Institute of Mental Health
NKA	No known allergies
nl	Normal (value)
NLN	National League for Nursing
NLTR	Non–life-threatening reaction
NM	Neonatal mortality
NMR	Nuclear magnetic resonance; neonatal mortality rates
NND	New and Nonofficial Drugs
NNS	Nonnutritive sucking
NO	Nitric oxide
NOFT	Nonorganic failure to thrive
NOP	Not otherwise provided for
NOS	Not otherwise specified
NP	Nasopharynx; new patient; not palpable; nerve palsy; Nurse Practitioner
NPN	Nonprotein nitrogen
NR	Normal range; nonreactive; no report; no respirations; not remarkable; no resuscitation; not refillable; normal reaction
NREM	Nonrapid eye movement
NS	Normal saline; not significant
NSAID	Nonsteroidal antiinflammatory drug
NSFTD	Normal spontaneous full-term delivery
NSR	Normal sinus rhythm
NSU	Nonspecific urethritis
NT	Nasotracheal
NTB	Necrotizing tracheobronchitis
NTD	Neural tube defect
NTM	Nontuberculous mycobacterium
NTP	Normal temperature and pressure
NUG	Necrotizing ulcerative gingivitis
NVSS	Normal variant short stature
NWB	Non–weight-bearing
NYD	Not yet diagnosed
OASDL	Ordinary activities and skills of daily living
OBS	Organic brain syndrome
OC	Oral contraceptive; oculocephalic (doll's eye reflex)
OCD	Over-the-counter drug; obsessive-compulsive disorder

Unit 6

OCP	Ova, cysts, and parasites
OD	*Oculus dexter* (right eye); once daily; overdose; outside diameter; optical density
OFC	Occipitofrontal circumference
OG	Orogastric
OHS	Orally administered hydration solution(s)
OI	Opportunistic infection; osteogenesis imperfecta
OJ	Orange juice
OM	Otitis media; opportunistic mycoses
OME	Otitis media with effusion
OOB	Out of bed
O&P	Ova and parasites
OPC	Outpatient clinic
OPD	Outpatient department
OR	Operating room
ORIF	Open reduction internal fixation
OS	*Oculus sinister* (left eye)
OSA	Obstructive sleep apnea
OSB	Open spina bifida
OT	Ocupational therapy; orotracheal; old tuberculin; old term
OTC	Over the counter
OU	*Oculi unitas* (both eyes)
OV	Oculovestibular (cold water caloric test)
P	Probability
PA	Posteroanterior; pernicious anemia; primary amenorrhea; pulmonary artery; prolonged action; physician's assistant
PAC	Premature atrial contraction
Paco$_2$	Carbon dioxide pressure (tension), arterial
PACU	Postanesthesia care unit
PAIDS	Pediatric AIDS
PALS	Pediatric advanced life support
PANESS	Physical and neurologic examination for soft signs
Pao$_2$	Oxygen pressure (tension), arterial
PAP	Primary atypical pneumonia; Papanicolaou smear; passive-aggressive personality; pulmonary artery pressure
PAPVR	Partial anomalous pulmonary venous return
PAR	Post anesthesia room
PAT	Paroxysmal atrial tachycardia
PAW	Mean airway pressure
PAWP	Pulmonary artery wedge pressure
PB	Peripheral blood
PBA	Percutaneous bladder aspiration
PBB	Polybrominated biphenyls
PBGT	Personal blood glucose testing
PBI	Protein-bound iodine
PBS	Phosphate-buffered saline
pc	*Post cibos* (after meals)
PC	Purulent conjunctivitis; present complaint
PCA	Patient controlled analgesia
PCB	Polychlorinated biphenyls
PCC	Poison Control Center
PCM	Protein-calorie malnutrition
Pco$_2$	Partial pressure (tension), carbon dioxide
PCP	Patient care plan, *Pneumocystis carinii* pneumonia
PCR	Polymerase chain reaction
PCT	Prothrombin consumption test
PCV	Packed cell volume
PCWP	Pulmonary capillary wedge pressure
PD	Pupillary distance
PDA	Patent ductus arteriosus
PDC	Private diagnostic clinic

PDI	Preschool Development Inventory
PDNB	Penile dorsal nerve block
PDQ	Prescreening Developmental Questionnaire
PDR	Physicians' Desk Reference
PE	Physical examination; pressure equalizing; probable error; pulmonary embolism; port of entry; point of entry; physical education; pelvic examination
PEEP	Positive end-expiratory pressure
PEEX	Pediatric Early Elementary Examination
PEFR	Peak expiratory flow rate
PEG	Percutaneous endoscopic gastrostomy; pneumoencephalogram
PEN	Parenteral/enteral nutrition
PERL	Pupils equal and react to light
per os	By mouth
PERRLA	Pupils equal, round, react to light and accommodation
PET	Positron emission tomography
PETT	Positron emission transaxial tomography
PF	Pulmonary flow
PFC	Persistent fetal circulation
PFNB	Percutaneous fine needle biopsy
PFT	Pulmonary function test
PG	Prostaglandin; phosphatidylglycerol
PH	Past history; previous history; public health
pH	Power of hydrogen
PHA	Phytohemagglutinin
PHN	Public Health Nurse
PHV	Peak height velocity
PI	Pulmonary insufficiency; present illness
PICC	Percutaneously inserted central catheter
PICU	Pediatric intensive care unit
PID	Pelvic inflammatory disease
PIE	Pulmonary interstitial emphysema
PIH	Pregnancy-induced hypertension
PIP	Peak inspiratory pressure; proximal interphalangeal
PIPP	Peak inspiratory plateau pressure
PKD	Polycystic kidney disease
PKU	Phenylketonuria
PLH	Pulmonary lymphoid hyperplasia
PM	Postmortem
PMC	Pseudomembranous colitis
PMD	Private medical doctor; past (previous) medical doctor
PMH	Past medical history
PMI	Point of maximum impulse (intensity)
PMN	Polymorphonuclear neutrophil
PMR	Psychomotor retardation; perinatal mortality rate; physical medicine and rehabilitation
PNA	Pediatric Nurse Associate
PND	Paroxysmal nocturnal dyspnea; postnasal drip
PNM	Postnatal mortality
PNP	Pediatric Nurse Practitioner
PNPR	Positive-negative pressure respiration
p.o.	*Per os* (by mouth)
PO	Postoperative; phone order
Po$_2$	Partial pressure (tension), oxygen
POA	Primary optic atrophy
POMR	Problem-oriented medical record
POR	Problem-oriented record
PP	Partial pressure; patient profile; peripheral pulses; postpartum; postprandial; presenting problem
PPC	Progressive patient care
PPD	Purified protein derivative

PPHN	Persistent pulmonary hypertension of the newborn	**RATG**	Rabbit anti-thymocytic globulin
PPLO	Pleuropneumonia-like organism	**RBC**	Red blood cell
PPPA	Poison Prevention Packaging Act	**RBD**	Right border dullness
PPS	Peripheral pulmonic stenosis	**RBE**	Relative biologic effectiveness
PPT	Partial prothrombin time	**RBF**	Renal blood flow
PPV	Positive pressure ventilation	**RBS**	Random blood sugar
PR	Perfusion rate; peripheral resistance; progress report; pulse rate; public relations	**RC**	Rice cereal; red cell
		RCC	Red cell concentrate
PRA	Plasma renin activity	**RCM**	Right costal margin
PRBC	Packed red blood cells	**RD**	Retinal detachment; respiratory disease; right deltoid
PRESS	Preschool Readiness Experimental Screening Scale	**RDA**	Recommended dietary allowance
PRN, prn	*Pro re nata* (as necessary); as circumstance may require	**RDS**	Respiratory distress syndrome
		RDSI	Revised Developmental Screening Inventory
PROM	Passive range of motion; premature rupture of membranes	**RE**	Regional enteritis; rear end (accident); right eye; rectal examination
PRP	Persistent recurrent pneumonia	**REE**	Resting energy expenditure
PRP-D	Polysaccharide of *Haemophilus influenzae* type b conjugated to diphtheria toxoid	**REM**	Rapid eye movement
		RF	Rheumatic fever; rheumatoid factor
PS	Pulmonic stenosis; pyloric stenosis	**RG**	Right gluteal
P/SH	Personal social history	**RHD**	Rheumatic heart disease; relative hepatic dullness
PSMA	Progressive spinal muscular atrophy	**RIA**	Radioimmunoassay; radioactive immunoassay
PSP	Phenolsulfonphthalein test	**RICE**	Rest, ice, compression, elevation
PSR	Psychological Stimulus Response	**RICM**	Right intercostal margin
PSRO	Professional Standards Review Organization	**RLE**	Right lower extremity
PSSD	Psychosocial dwarfism	**RLF**	Retrolental fibroplasia
PT	Physical therapy (therapist); prothrombin time	**RLQ**	Right lower quadrant
PTA	Prior to admission; plasma thromboplastin antecedent; percutaneous transluminal angioplasty	**RLT**	Right lateral thigh
		RMA	Rhythmic motor activities
		RML	Right mediolateral; right middle lobe
PTC	Plasma thromboplastin component; phenylthiocarbamide	**RMR**	Resting metabolic rate
		RMSF	Rocky Mountain spotted fever
PTH	Parathyroid hormone; pseudohyperparathyroidism	**RN**	Registered Nurse
		RN, C	Registered Nurse, Certified
PTT	Partial thromboplastin time	**RN, CS**	Registered Nurse, Certified Specialist
PUD	Peptic ulcer disease	**RO**	Rule out; routine order
PUO	Pyrexia of undetermined (unknown) origin	**ROM**	Range of motion; right otitis media
PV	Parainfluenza virus	**ROP**	Retinopathy of prematurity
PVC	Premature ventricular contraction; polyvinyl chloride	**ROS**	Review of systems
		R-PDQ	Revised Prescreening Developmental Questionnaire
PVD	Percussion, vibration, and drainage	**RPF**	Renal plasma flow
PVH	Periventricular hemorrhage	**RPR**	Rapid plasma reagin
PVP	Pulmonary venous pressure	**RR**	Respiratory rate; recovery room; radiation response; rust ring
PVR	Peripheral vascular resistance; pulmonary vascular resistance		
PVS	Percussion, vibration, and suction	**RS**	Review of symptoms; Reye syndrome; Reiter syndrome
PWB	Partial weight-bearing	**RSB**	Right sternal border
PWM	Pokeweed mitogen	**RSV**	Respiratory syncytial virus
PWP	Pulmonary wedge pressure	**RT**	Respiratory therapy (therapist); room temperature
PWS	Port-wine stain; Prader-Willi syndrome		
Px	Pneumothorax; prognosis	**RTA**	Renal tubular acidosis
q	*Quaque* (every)	**RTI**	Respiratory tract infection
qd	*Quaque die* (every day)	**RTUS**	Real-time ultrasound
qh	*Quaque hora* (every hour)	**RUE**	Right upper extremity
q2h	Every 2 hours	**RUL**	Right upper lobe
qid	*Quater in die* (four times a day)	**RUOQ**	Right upper outer quadrant
qn	Every night	**RUQ**	Right upper quadrant
qns	Quantity not sufficient	**RV**	Residual volume; right ventricle
qod	Every other day	**Rv**	Rotavirus
QPIT	Quantitative pilocarpine iontophoresis test	**RVG**	Right ventrogluteal
qs	Quantity sufficient	**RVH**	Right ventricular hypertrophy
RA	Rheumatoid arthritis; return appointment; renal artery; right arm; right atrium; rectal atresia; repeat action; room air	**RVV**	Rubella vaccine virus
		Rx	Prescription; *recipe* (take)
		s	*Sine* (without)
RAE	Right atrial enlargement	**SAC**	Short arm cast
RAST	Radioallergosorbent test		

SAD	Sugar and acetone determination
SAH	Subarachnoid hemorrhage
SAM	Surface active material; Society for Adolescent Medicine
Sao_2	Saturated arterial oxygen
sb	Strabismus
SBE	Subacute bacterial endocarditis
SC	Subcutaneous; servo control
SCB	Strictly confined to bed
SCD	Sudden cardiac death; sickle cell disease
SCFE	Slipped capital femoral epiphysis
SCID	Severe combined immune deficiency disease
SCM	Sternocleidomastoid muscle
SCU	Special care unit
SCV	Smooth, capsulated, virulent
SD	Standard deviation; septal defect; spontaneous delivery; sudden death; shoulder disarticulation
SEA	Seronegative enthesopathy and arthropathy (syndrome)
SES	Socioeconomic status
SFD	Small for dates
SG	Specific gravity; Swan-Ganz
SGA	Small for gestational age
SGOT	Serum glutamic-oxaloacetic transaminase
SGPT	Serum glutamic-pyruvic transaminase
SH	Social history; self help; serum hepatitis; shoulder
SI	*Système International a' Unités*
SIADH	Syndrome of inappropriate ADH
SIDS	Sudden infant death syndrome
SIG	Serum immune globulin
SIMV	Synchronized intermittent mandatory ventilation
SKL	Serum killing levels
SKSD	Streptokinase/streptodornase (control test)
SLC	Short leg cast
SLD	Specific learning disability
SLE	Systemic lupus erythematosus; St. Louis encephalitis
SLUD	Salivation, lacrimation, urination, defecation
SLWC	Short leg walking cast
SMA	Smooth muscle antibodies; sequential multiple analyzer
SMBG	Self-monitoring blood glucose
SM-C	Somatomedin-C
SNF	Skilled nursing facility
SNP	School Nurse Practitioner
SNS	Sympathetic nervous system
SOB	Short of breath; see order book
SOM	Serous otitis media
S/P	Status post
SPA	Suprapubic aspiration; salt poor albumin
SPF	Sun protection factor
SPL	Sound pressure levels
SPT	Sweat patch test
SQ	Subcutaneous
SR	System review; sinus rhythm; sedimentation rate; stretch reflex; schizophrenic reaction; stimulus response
S-R	Stimulus-response
SRI	Systemic reaction index
SRSA	Slow reacting substance of anaphylaxis
ss	*Semis* (one half)
S/S	Signs and symptoms
SSE	Soapsuds enema; soap solution enema
SSEP	Somatosensory evoked potential

SSI	Segmental spinal instrumentation
SSSS	Staphylococcal scalded skin syndrome
stat	*Statim* (immediately)
STC	Serum theophylline concentration
STD	Sexually transmitted disease; skin test dose; standard test dose
STS	Serologic test for syphilis
STSG	Split-thickness skin graft
STU	Skin test unit
SubQ	Subcutaneous
supp	Suppository
susp	Suspension
SV	Stroke volume
SVC	Superior vena cava
SVD	Spontaneous vaginal delivery
SVR	Systemic vascular resistance
SVT	Sinus ventricular tachycardia; supraventricular tachycardia
Sx	Symptoms
SxH	Sexual history
T_3	Triiodothyronine
T_4	Thyroxine
TA	Toxin-antitoxin; tricuspid atresia; truncus arteriosus
T&A	Tonsillectomy and adenoidectomy
tab	Tablet
TAPVR	Total anomalous pulmonary venous return
TB	Tuberculosis
TBG	Thyroxine-binding globulin
TBI	Traumatic brain injury; total body irradiation
TBLC	Term birth, living child
TBM	Total body mass
Tbn	Tuberculin
TBSA	Total body surface area
TBT	Tracheobronchial tree
TBW	Total body water
TcB	Transcutaneous bilirubinometer
TCDB	Turn, cough, deep breathe
$tcPaco_2$	Transcutaneous carbon dioxide pressure (tension)
$tcPao_2$	Transcutaneous oxygen pressure (tension)
TCU	Transitional care unit
Td	Adult tetanus and diphtheria
TD	Typhoid dysentery
TDM	Therapeutic drug monitoring
T_E	Expiratory time
TEF	Tracheoesophageal fistula
TEN	Toxic epidermal necrolysis
TENS	Transcutaneous electrical nerve stimulation
TEV	Talipes equinovarus
TEWL	Transevaporative water loss
Tg	Thyroglobulin
TG	Triglyceride(s)
TGA	Transposition of great arteries
TGE	Theoretical growth evaluation
TGV	Transposition of great vessels
TI	Tricuspid insufficiency
TIA	Transient ischemic attack
tid	*Ter in die* (three times a day)
TIPP	The Injury Prevention Program
TKO	To keep open
TLC	Tender loving care; total lung capacity; total lymphocyte count; thin layer chromatography
TM	Tympanic membrane; temperature by mouth; tender midline; transmetatarsal; temporomandibular

TMR	Trainable mentally retarded
TNI	Total nodal irradiation
TNR	Tonic neck reflex
TO	Target organ; telephone order
TOF	Tetralogy of Fallot
TORCH	Toxoplasmosis, (other), rubella, cytomegalovirus, herpes simplex
TORCHES	Toxoplasmosis, rubella, cytomegalovirus, herpes simplex, syphilis
Torr	Millimeters of mercury
TPN	Total parenteral nutrition
TPR	Temperature, pulse, respiration; total perfusion resistance
TRH	Thyrotropin releasing hormone
TS	Terminal sensation; test solution; tricuspid stenosis; Tourette syndrome
TSF	Triceps skinfold
TSB	Total serum bilirubin
TSE	Testicular self-examination
TSH	Thyroid stimulating hormone
TSS	Toxic shock syndrome
TT	Transit time; tuberculin tested
TU	Tuberculin units; toxic unit; transmission unit
TV	Total volume; tidal volume
Tx	Treatment; therapy
UA	Urinalysis
UAC	Umbilical artery catheters
UCHD	Usual childhood diseases
UD	Urethral discharge
UDT	Undescended testicle
UGI	Upper gastrointestinal
U/L	Upper/lower body ratio
ULC	Unique-looking child
UMN	Upper motor neuron
UNO	United Network for Organ Sharing
UP	Universal precautions
UPC	Unplanned pregnancy counseling
UQ	Upper quadrant
UrA	Uric acid
URI	Upper respiratory infection
US	Ultrasound
USA	Ultrasonic aerosol (nebulization)
USPHS	United States Public Health Service
UTI	Urinary tract infection
UV	Ultraviolet
UVA	Ultraviolet A
UVB	Ultraviolet B
VA	Visual acuity
VAD	Venous access devices
VAR	Visual-aural range
VC	Vital capacity

VCA	Viral capsid antigen
VCG	Vectorcardiography
VCT	Venous clotting time
VCUG	Voiding cystourethrogram
VD	Venereal disease
VDG	Venereal disease, gonorrhea
VDRL	Venereal Disease Research Laboratory
VDRR	Vitamin D-resistant rickets
VDS	Venereal disease, syphilis
VDT	Video display terminal
VE	Vesicular exanthema
VEP	Visual evoked potential
VF	Visual fields
VG	Ventricular gallop
VIG	Vaccinia immune globulin
VLBW	Very low birth weight
VLDL	Very low-density lipoprotein
VM	Vasomotor; vestibular membrane
VNA	Visiting Nurses Association
VO	Verbal order
VP	Venous pressure
VPC	Ventricular premature complex
VRA	Visual reinforced audiometry
VS	Vital signs
VSD	Ventricular septal defect
VSGA	Very small for gestational age
VSS	Vital signs stable
V_r	Tidal volume
VUR	Vesicoureteral reflux
VZIG	Varicella zoster immune globulin
VZV	Varicella zoster virus
WAIS	Wechsler Adult Intelligence Scale
WB	Whole blood
WBC	White blood cell count
WEE	Western equine encephalitis
WHM	Women's health movement
WHO	World Health Organization
WIPI	Word intelligibility by picture identification
WISC-R	Wechsler Intelligence Scale for Children—Revised
WNL	Within normal limits
WPPSI	Wechsler Preschool and Primary Scale of Intelligence
WPW	Wolff-Parkinson-White syndrome
WRAT	Wide Range Achievement Test
XLMR	X-linked mental retardation
XLR	X-linked recessive
XTB	X-ray treated blood
ZIG	Zoster immune globulin
ZIP	Zoster immune plasma

Drugs

Using acronyms or abbreviations to designate drugs is an unsafe practice; because many abbreviations are similar to others and are not universally known to users. Any drug order, written or transcribed, should be written out clearly and legibly. Some notable exceptions are BAL, EDTA, and NPH.

ACh	Acetylcholine
ARA-A	Vidarabine
ARA-C	Cytarabine
ASA	Acetylsalicylic acid (aspirin)
BAL	British Antilewisite (dimercaprol)
CaEDTA	Calcium disodium edetate

CBZ	Carbamazepine
CPZ	Chlorpromazine
DDAVP	Desmopressin acetate
DES	Diethylstilbestrol
DF, DFO	Deferoxamine
DIG	Digoxin
DPT	Demerol-phenergan-thorazine
DTaP	Diphtheria, tetanus, acellular pertussis vaccine
DTP	Diphtheria, tetanus, pertussis
EDTA	Edetate disodium; ethylenediaminetetraacetic acid

EES	Erythromycin ethylsuccinate	**Pb**	Phenobarbital
EMLA	Eutectic mixture of local anesthetics	**PCN**	Penicillin
Epi	Epinephrine	**PCP**	Phencyclidine
HbCV	Haemophilus b conjugate vaccine	**PRP-D**	Diphtheria toxoid Hib conjugate (ProHIBit)
HBIG	Hepatitis B immune globulin	**PRP-HbOC**	Diphtheria CRM 197 protein Hib conjugate (Hib-TITER)
HBV	Hepatitis B virus vaccine (Recombivax HB and Energix-B)	**PRP-OMP**	Meningococcal protein Hib conjugate (Pedvax HIB)
HCT	Hydrocortisone; hydrochlorothiazide	**PTU**	Propylthiouracil
HCTZ	Hydrochlorothiazide	**PVP**	Povidone-iodine solution
Hib	Haemophilus influenza type B	**PZ**	Protamine zinc
INH	Isoniazid	**RIG**	Rabies immune globulin
IPV	Inactivated poliovirus vaccine	**SRT**	Sustained-release theophylline
KCl	Potassium chloride	**SSKI**	Saturated solution of potassium iodide
LSD	Lysergic acid diethylamide	**TAO**	Troleandomycin
MMR	Measles, mumps, rubella	**TAT**	Tetanus antitoxin
MOM	Milk of magnesia	**Td**	Tetanus, diphtheria (reduced dose) vaccine
MS	Morphine sulfate	**TD**	Tetanus, diphtheria (full dose) vaccine
MTX	Methotrexate	**THAM**	Tromethamine
MTZ	Tapazole	**TIG**	Tetanus immune globulin
MVI	Multivitamins (without fat-soluble vitamins)	**TOPV**	Trivalent oral poliovirus
NPH	Neutral-protamine-Hagedorn; isophane	**TRIS**	Tris (hydroxymethyl) aminomethane
NTG	Nitroglycerine	**VMA**	Vanillylmandelic acid
OPV	Oral poliovirus vaccine	**VZV**	Varicella zoster virus
PABA	Para-aminobenzoic acid		
PAS	Para-aminosalicylic acid		

Index

A